Patient **Education** and **Wellness**

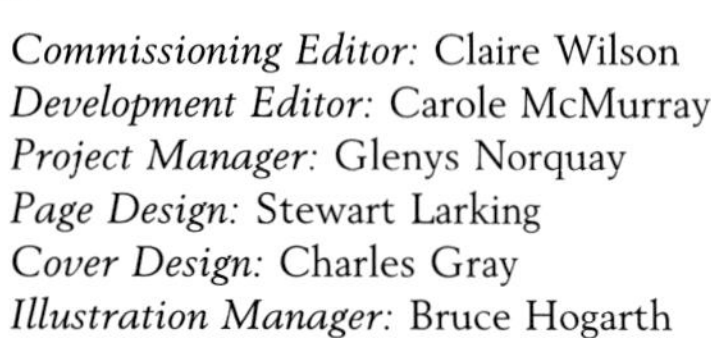

Commissioning Editor: Claire Wilson
Development Editor: Carole McMurray
Project Manager: Glenys Norquay
Page Design: Stewart Larking
Cover Design: Charles Gray
Illustration Manager: Bruce Hogarth

Patient **Education** and **Wellness**

A handbook for manual therapists

Jennifer Jamison MBBCh PhD EdD FICC(Hon) EdD FACNEM
Formerly Professor of Primary Care, Division of Health Sciences, Murdoch University, Perth, Western Australia, Australia

Chapter 3 contributed by

Cheryl Hawk DC PhD
Professor and Dean of Research, Southern California University of Health Sciences, California, USA

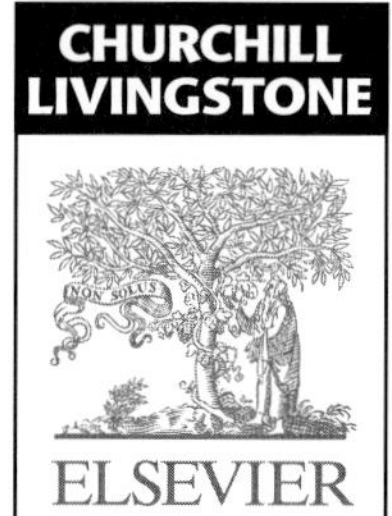

CHURCHILL LIVINGSTONE

ELSEVIER

Edinburgh London New York Oxford Philadelphia St Louis Sydney Toronto 2010

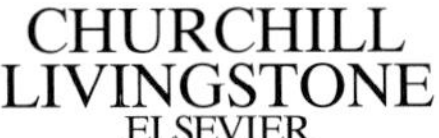

© 2010 Elsevier Ltd. All rights reserved.

No part of this publication may be reproduced or transmitted in any form or by any means, electronic or mechanical, including photocopying, recording, or any information storage and retrieval system, without permission in writing from the publisher. Details on how to seek permission, further information about the Publisher's permissions policies and our arrangements with organizations such as the Copyright Clearance Center and the Copyright Licensing Agency, can be found at our website: www.elsevier.com/permissions.

This book and the individual contributions contained in it are protected under copyright by the Publisher (other than as may be noted herein).

ISBN 978 0 7020 4041 2

British Library Cataloguing in Publication Data
A catalogue record for this book is available from the British Library

Library of Congress Cataloging in Publication Data
A catalog record for this book is available from the Library of Congress

Notices
Knowledge and best practice in this field are constantly changing. As new research and experience broaden our understanding, changes in research methods, professional practices, or medical treatment may become necessary.

Practitioners and researchers must always rely on their own experience and knowledge in evaluating and using any information, methods, compounds, or experiments described herein. In using such information or methods they should be mindful of their own safety and the safety of others, including parties for whom they have a professional responsibility.

With respect to any drug or pharmaceutical products identified, readers are advised to check the most current information provided (i) on procedures featured or (ii) by the manufacturer of each product to be administered, to verify the recommended dose or formula, the method and duration of administration, and contraindications. It is the responsibility of practitioners, relying on their own experience and knowledge of their patients, to make diagnoses, to determine dosages and the best treatment for each individual patient, and to take all appropriate safety precautions.

To the fullest extent of the law, neither the Publisher nor the authors, contributors, or editors, assume any liability for any injury and/or damage to persons or property as a matter of products liability, negligence or otherwise, or from any use or operation of any methods, products, instructions, or ideas contained in the material herein.

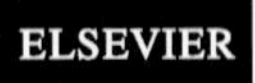

your source for books, journals and multimedia in the health sciences

www.elsevierhealth.com

Working together to grow libraries in developing countries

www.elsevier.com | www.bookaid.org | www.sabre.org

ELSEVIER   BOOK AID International   Sabre Foundation

The Publisher's policy is to use **paper manufactured from sustainable forests**

Printed in China

Contents

Points to ponder!

- *Self-care represents a sea change in healthcare.*
- *Wellness requires responsible self-care.*

The 2008 report of the World Health Organization draws attention to the growing need for an increased emphasis on primary health care.[1] The report discusses how the early approaches of improving hygiene, water, sanitation and health education in primary health care have now been replaced by a need to promote healthier lifestyles and mitigate the health effects of social and environmental hazards. It debunks the belief that primary health care is a cheap alternative requiring a modest investment. It recognizes that although primary health care requires considerable investment, it delivers better value for money than the alternatives.

Primary care is a hub from which patients are guided through the health system. A major feature of primary care in the 21st century is its person-centredness. Successful primary care is perceived to put 'people at the centre of health care, harmonizing mind and body, people and systems'. People-centred primary care provides a regular point of entry into the health system and offers comprehensive and integrated care catering for a wide range of health problems. It supplies continuity of care, making it possible to build an enduring relationship of trust between people and their health care providers. Successful person-centred primary care is achieved in ongoing relationships between patients and health professionals within which patients participate in decision making about their health and health care.

Primary care affords opportunities for disease prevention and health promotion as well as early detection of disease – not merely treating common ailments. It is provided by health professionals with diverse backgrounds, all of whom have specific and sophisticated biomedical and social skills. Primary practitioners are educators and motivators. Person-centred primary health care providers enable lay persons to use evidence-based information to make health-promoting lifestyle choices, avoid hazardous alternatives and recognize early evidence of dysfunction. Primary health care providers introduce consumers to, and facilitate them to undertake, self-care.

Self-care promises to transform both the tired health care system of the 20th century and those who practise it. Given the shift from acute infectious conditions to chronic non-communicable disorders, an ageing population and financially strained health care, self-care is rapidly being transformed from an option to a necessity. Successful self-care requires a change in the role of both health consumer and health professional; it shifts the emphasis from treatment to prevention, from dependent patient to active consumer. Self-care, by focusing on the individual rather than the condition, moves the emphasis from the passive recipient to interactive self-reliant client. It is only when individuals take personal responsibility for their wellbeing that the necessary population shift from high to low risk can be achieved. This text provides primary practitioners and patients with resources to aid them achieve the health shift fundamental to a sustainable health care system.

This book provides a blueprint for implementing self-care. It hypothesizes that a change in biomedical thinking is a prerequisite for addressing global health problems. Drawing on constructs used in complementary and alternative medicine and supported by scientific research in psychoneuroimmunology, a solution based on the infomedical model is proposed. This solution changes the clinical focus from disease care to health promotion and requires that the patient take personal responsibility for promoting their wellbeing. The impetus for self-care arises from a cognitive shift, its potency lies in the behavioural changes it effects.

Part 1 of the text alerts the primary practitioner to the evolving role of the health professional and the changing needs of the consumer in primary health care. It outlines strategies to enable patients to embrace self-care. The practitioner is made aware of the challenges facing health care in the 21st century and is provided with guidelines on how to assume the role of a facilitator who motivates and acts as a resource for evidence-based information.

Parts 2 to 4 of the text provide health professionals with resources they can use to inform and motivate patients. Part 2 identifies healthy lifestyle choices and considers how each contributes to wellness. It explores lifestyle choices and identifies green flags signalling healthy options. It considers how diet, spinal care, physical activity, sleep, mental fitness and sexual prudence all contribute to wellness. Part 3 examines how risky lifestyle choices jeopardize well-being. It identifies orange flags that signal hazardous options. It discusses how substance abuse, tobacco, alcohol, stress and environmental hazards can compromise health and reduce longevity. Part 4 focuses on detecting dysfunction. It identifies risk markers which suggest that the organism is being stressed and homeostasis is compromised. The more technologically advanced the diagnostic tool, the greater the potential to interrupt the progression of the disease process. Part 4 identifies the red flags of impending disease and suggests, at best, how homeostasis may be restored, or, at worst, how disease progression may be limited. Risk markers for inflammation, obesity, diabetes, hypertension, ischaemic heart disease and osteoporosis are identified and their health implications discussed.

Resources for patient education and motivation are provided on a CD. It provides health professionals with handouts to alert, inform, motivate and guide patients to pursue a long, healthy life. The CD constitutes a handy toolbox to enable health professionals to provide more cost-effective person-centred primary care. The Pathway to Wellness template provides an overview of resources available on the CD.

Reference

1. World Health Organization. The World Health Report 2008 – Primary health care (now more than ever). <http://www.who.int/whr/2008/en/index.html> Accessed 12.02.08.

List of Posters

PART 1

Sketching a path to wellness

Points to Ponder !

- The health care system is struggling to cope with the needs of an ageing population.
- The situation is likely to worsen as government coffers increasingly rely on a shrinking workforce.
- A sustainable health care system requires not only that the emphasis changes from treatment to prevention but also that individuals actively strive for wellness.

Part 1 delineates problems threatening health care and identifies some strategies individuals can employ to meet the challenges ahead. It provides the theoretical background upon which the practical information in the remainder of the text is based. Chapter 1 considers how changes in demography and disease prevalence coupled with technological and therapeutic advances in medicine have paradoxically resulted in an ailing health care system. Chapter 2 considers how a paradigm shift may provide the basis for developing a sustainable health care system. It explores how an integrated approach which draws from conventional health care and complementary and alternative medicine (CAM) therapies may provide an answer and identifies a new role for 'patients'. Chapter 3 focuses on chiropractic and describes how this vitalistic profession draws from the biomedical model to offer health care straddling discrepant paradigms. Chapter 4 identifies the mindset required for achieving a sustainable health care system with respect to both the cognitive framework in which care is offered by clinicians and the personal responsibility assumed by patients. It explores the changed relationship between patient and practitioner, the individual and their health status. Chapter 5 looks at the clinical encounter and considers how the practitioner can use communication to create a therapeutic environment conducive to a wellness lifestyle. Chapter 6 identifies the dimensions of wellness, explores the dynamic nature of wellbeing, and identifies the necessity for patients to adopt a self-care ethos. Chapter 7 considers how individuals may take increased responsibility for their wellbeing and outlines guidelines for undertaking safe self-care. Chapter 8 looks at strategies used to empower individuals to undertake self-care and identifies the vital role for health professionals in promulgating a sustainable health care system.

A health care system in crisis

Advances in medicine have revolutionized health care. Technology has made it possible to detect early pathological changes before signs or symptoms are discernible. While advances in diagnostic medicine have made it possible to detect potentially pathological changes while they are reversible, improvements in therapy have made remission of some previously fatal diseases feasible. Early diagnosis, drugs, radiotherapy and surgery prolong the lives of cancer patients. Patients, who in another health care era would have died, survive with any number of transplanted organs. The sophisticated system of health care developed in the 20th century does, however, come at a cost. Conventional health care systems disproportionately focus on disease rather than health, on the hospital rather than the community clinic. Instead of comprehensive service provided by a generalist, health care tends to be fragmented and specialized. Health is perceived as a commodity and health services are becoming increasingly commercialized.

Health: a costly government expenditure item

Health expenditure per capita in 2004 in the US was US$6102; in Canada, US$3165; in Germany, US$3005; in Australia, US$2876; in the UK, US$2546; and in New Zealand, US$2083.[1] As shown in Tables 1.1 and 1.2 the health care budget is an important item in gross domestic product (GDP) expenditure of both well and less developed countries. Health care expenditure is an important indicator of the capacity of a health care system to service a population's needs. Yet, despite the US spending a greater proportion of its GDP on health care than do many other countries, the US lacks a satisfactory health care system.[2] Michael Moore's film on health care in the US lays bare the sad state of America's health care system. He describes how Americans slip across the border to Canada for health care they cannot afford in their own country and how prisoners in Guantanamo Bay received better health care than American citizens. In spite of having the most costly health care system in the world, health care provided in the US is considered inferior to that available in Canada, Australia and the UK. The US rated lowest with respect to quality, access, efficiency, equity, and healthy lives.[1] Access to health services is a major problem in this country. The US, unlike the UK and Canada, does not offer universal health coverage insurance. While insured Americans enjoy rapid access to specialized health care services, lower-income earners have difficulty gaining access to affordable health care. On the other hand, government-subsidized health

Table 1.1 The cost of health care in well-developed countries*

	Canada	USA	UK	Australia
Gross national income per capita (ppp internat $)	36,280	44,070	33,650	33,940
Government expenditure on health as % of total expenditure on health	70.4	45.8	87.4	67.2
Total expenditure on health as % GDP	10	15.3	8.4	8.7
Hospital beds/10,000 population	34	32	39	40

*2006 Figures derived from http://www.who.int/whosis/data/

Table 1.2 The cost of health care in less-developed countries*

	USA (for comparison)	South Africa	Zimbabwe	China
Gross national income per capita (ppp internat $)	44,070	8900	?	4460
Government expenditure on health as % of total expenditure on health	45.8	41.9	52.6	42
Total expenditure on health as % GDP	15.3	8.6	8.4	4.5
Hospital beds /10,000 population	32	28	30	22

*2006 Figures derived from http://www.who.int/whosis/data/

care, although ensuring access for all, does not necessarily provide timely care for non-acute cases. While patients in the UK, Canada and Australia have little to no financial burden, they experience long wait times for specialized services. So problematic are hospital waiting lists that rather than making use of the government-funded Medicare system, many Australians choose to take out and bear the cost of private health insurance.

It is not only hospital care draining the health care budget. In Australia in the 2003–04 financial year, although hospital services accounted for more than one-third, pharmaceuticals consumed over one-tenth of the recurrent health budget.[3] The Australian government provides a subsidized universal system of pharmaceutical provision, the Pharmaceutical Benefits Scheme (PBS).[4] Despite incorporating patient copayments, with differentials for the general population compared with concessional beneficiaries, the PBS devours around 14% of total government health care. It has been estimated that pharmaceutical prescriptions are up by 41% over the latest decade. An untoward consequence of

successful medical intervention has been creation of a population group whose ability to function depends on regular medication. Prescription drug use is escalating and its impact on the health care dollar is cause for concern. The disproportionate distribution of the health care dollar to secondary and tertiary levels of health care leaves little for primary health care services. In contrast to the vast amounts spent on hospitals and pharmaceuticals, the Australian government allocated a mere 1.7% of recurrent health expenditure in 2003–04 to disease prevention and health promotion.[3] The disproportionate expenditure on disease care versus health promotion is also apparent in the US.

Davis has identified a disjunction between what Americans pay for health care services and the contribution those services make to longer and healthier lives, relief of pain and anxiety, and quality of life.[5] Compared with other industrialized nations, the US spends twice as much per capita but ranks 19th on mortality amenable to medical care. It was proposed that greater health gains would be possible if all Americans had access to modern medicine and had a source of primary care that ensured they received all appropriate care. The lack of national health insurance was deemed, in addition to denying lower-income families access to hospital services, to undermine access to preventive care and better health outcomes. Americans without health insurance are less likely than those with coverage to receive preventive care services at appropriate ages.[6]

Modern medicine has been extremely successful at managing disease and prolonging the lives of sick people. The downside to this success is the evolution of a health care system which focuses on disease rather than health care. The disease care system has started to unravel. Medical advances, whether they be diagnostic or therapeutic, are costly. The overall growth of health expenditure per Australian grew by an average 3.8% each year between the 1997–98 and 2002–03 financial years.[3] At that time, although over two-thirds of health care costs were shouldered by the Australian government, dissatisfaction with the ability of the current health care system to care for the nation's health was growing. The ability of any government to satisfactorily fund a population's demand for contemporary medical care is currently questionable. The situation is predicted to steadily worsen given demographic trends.

Changing demography: straining government resources

In the 15 years from 1990 to 2005, population growth rates decreased in both highly and less developed nations (see Tables 1.3 and 1.4). During this period, the growth rate in Australia dropped from 1.5% to 1.1%; in Canada, from 1.3% to 1.0%; in the US, from 0.3% to 0.5%; in China, from 1.4% to 0.6%; in South Africa, from 2.3% to 0.8%; and in Zimbabwe, from 3.0% to 0.7%.[7] The UK proved the exception, where the growth rate rose from 0.3% to 0.5%. Growth rates dropped despite people living for longer. In 2000, average life expectancy at birth was highest for Australians (80 years), followed by Canadians (79 years) and those living in the UK (78 years). In these countries the infant mortality rates also dropped during this period. In fact, the infant mortality rate in Canada dropped from 8 per 1000 live births in 1990 to 5 per 1000 in 2000, where it remained in 2006. Australia reported similarly low infant mortality statistics over the same period (8, 5 and 5), as did the USA (10, 7 and 7) and the UK.[8,6,5] In 2000 in these four countries the probability of dying before the age of 5 years was low, around 6 per 1000 live births. The apparent paradox of decreased population growth in nations with reduced mortality among the young and increased longevity is explained by reduced fertility rates, helped somewhat by active contraception, e.g. in the UK the prevalence of contraceptive use was reported to be 82%. These altered statistics are best visualized in the changing demographic pattern. The pyramid shape used to describe population distribution no longer provides a satisfactory fit for developed countries. The previously dominant demographic population pyramid, with its large base of young people and relatively small peak of elderly people, is now assuming a form more reminiscent of a skyscraper. The change is most dramatic in countries with relatively low birth rates that have a large baby boomer cohort. An inevitable outcome of this changing demographic is an increased dependency ratio.

Table 1.3 Population statistics for well-developed countries*

	Canada	USA	UK	Australia
Population annual growth	0.9	1.0	0.4	1.1
Population median age	39	36	39	37
% population >60 yrs of age	18	17	22	18
% population <15 yrs of age	17	21	18	19

*2006 Figures derived from http://www.who.int/whosis/data/

Table 1.4 Population statistics for less-developed countries*

	USA (for comparison)	South Africa	Zimbabwe	China
Population annual growth	1.0	0.7	0.8	0.6
Population median age	36	24	19	33
% population >60 yrs of age	17	7	5	11
% population <15 yrs of age	21	32	39	21

*2006 Figures derived from http://www.who.int/whosis/data/

The relative numbers of children, working-age and older persons are changing. The percentage of older people is becoming disproportionately large. In 2000 there were approximately 605 million people over the age of 60; by 2050 this number is predicted to increase to almost 2 billion.[8] Currently, the elderly constitute around 10% of the global population, with this figure being doubled in developed countries and halved in underdeveloped countries. By 2050, people 60 years of age and older are projected to make up 22% of the world's population, with one-third of the population falling into this age group in developed countries. Not only will there be a larger number of elderly people in the future, people will be living longer. There will be more older-aged elderly persons.[8] Two-thirds of seniors who have ever lived are alive today![9] Babies born today in Australia can expect to live for over 80 years on average.[3] For females, life expectancy at birth in 2002–2004 was 83 years, and for males it was 78 years. At age 65, Australian men in 2002–2004 could expect to reach the age of 82.5 years on average and women to reach 86.1 years – respectively about 6 and 8 years more than their counterparts in the early 20th century. It is predicted that 9 out of every 100 persons will reach 80 years of age in developed regions in the next four decades.[8] By 2050, the number of the oldest old is projected to be five times as large as at present and to constitute 4% of the total population.

Based on a determination of the number of people presumed too old or too young to work, the dependency ratio provides governments with an estimate of the likely demand for future government subsidies. The youth-dependency ratio (the number of children per 100 persons of labour-force age) and the elderly-dependency ratio (the number aged 65 years or older per 100 persons of labour-force age) provide insight into the escalating burden being placed on a shrinking taxpayer base.[8] By definition, labour-force age is considered 15–64 years. The baby boomers that fired the industrialized powerhouses of developed nations are entering retirement and global demography is being transformed. Baby boomer-rich countries are particularly vulnerable to a rapid ageing transition. The dramatic increase from 14% to 21% of the population in the 65 years and older age group in Canada and the US reflects the baby boomers' progression into retirement.[8] Alarmingly, there is mounting evidence that health care systems are failing to meet their populations' health needs even before the baby boomer wave enters retirement. The inadequacy of the health care dollar to meet current health care costs is going to escalate as the taxpayer base shrinks. The shortfall in the provision of health services is predicted to soar as governments vainly attempt to provide health care for an expanding elderly population. As people age, they require more health care. On average the health care expenditure required for persons over 75 years of age is almost sixfold that of persons in the 25–45 age group.[1] The health care system of the 20th century lacks the financial wherewithal to meet the needs of the ageing population of the 21st century.

The success of disease-oriented care available in developed countries has enabled sickly adults to live for longer and sickly babies to survive. In 2006 there were 5 infant deaths for every 1000 live births in Canada, Australia and the UK; in the US this rose to 7. A low infant mortality rate is a measure of the success of a health care system. Less developed nations have a higher infant mortality rate. In South Africa the infant mortality rate increased from 45 per 1000 live births in 1990 to 50 in 2000, and to 56 in 2006. In Zimbabwe the figures are

52, 58 and 55 respectively. Populations lacking ready access to modern medical resources also have lower life expectancy (see Tables 1.3 and 1.4). In 2000, life expectancy at birth in South Africa was 58 years, in Zimbabwe it was 45 years.

Disease-oriented care has achieved remarkable success at both extremes of life. Medicine's success is ironically largely responsible for its current predicament. By saving lives that would have been lost, medical intervention has fostered the growth of a population which requires ongoing, often costly, health care. For governments to continue to provide such benefits and make care accessible to all requires a transformation in the current approach to health care provision. The escalating crisis in health care needs resolution. Old approaches are unlikely to solve the problem, new strategies are needed. More effective and efficient use of the health care dollar needs to be made. Health care costs need to be capped.

The changing face of disease

The prevalence of disease shifts from communicable to non-communicable disease as countries develop. Table 1.5 demonstrates how there are relatively few years of lives lost due to infectious diseases in Australia, Canada, the UK and the US. In contrast, Table 1.6 shows that inhabitants of South Africa and Zimbabwe are at considerable risk of dying from communicable diseases. Disability adjusted life years (DALY) are often used to measure the health status of populations. One DALY represents the loss of the equivalent of 1 year of full health. In low-income countries the top five causes of DALYs are: lower respiratory disorders, diarrhoea, HIV/AIDS, malaria, and prematurity and low birth weight. In higher-income countries these are: unipolar disorders, ischaemic heart disease, cerebrovascular disease, Alzheimer's and other dementias, and alcohol-related disorders.[10] Table 1.6 shows that tuberculosis and HIV/AIDS are rampant in South Africa and Zimbabwe. In contrast, China boasts a remarkably low number of deaths attributable to HIV/AIDS. China's success in handling the global AIDS epidemic demonstrates the potency of government policy in health care. China's one child policy not only appears to have restricted its birth rate but also may have limited AIDS transmission if the condom was the contraceptive measure. The prevalence of contraception in China is 90.2%, while in South Africa and Zimbabwe it is 60.3% and 60% respectively. Government measures to control tuberculosis in China, while fairly successful, pale compared with that achieved in controlling AIDS. AIDS is spread by unsafe sex or exposure to infected blood products; tuberculosis is spread by droplets. AIDS cannot be cured; many strains of tuberculosis are amenable to drug therapy. Closer examination of this apparent absurdity draws attention to the possibility that

Table 1.5 Condition-related mortality rates in well-developed countries*

	USA	UK	Canada	Australia
Years of life lost (%) due to non-communicable diseases	75	82	80	77
Years of life lost (%) due to communicable diseases	9	10	6	5
Prevalence of tuberculosis per 100,000 population	3	12	4	7
Age-standardized mortality rate for HIV/AIDS (per 100,000 population)	5	<10	<10	<10
Age-standardized mortality rate due to non-communicable diseases (per 100,000 population)	460	434	388	362
Age-standardized mortality rate for cancer (per 100,000 population)	134	143	138	127
Age-standardized mortality rate for cardiovascular disease (per 100,000 population)	188	182	141	140
Age-standardized mortality rate for injuries (per 100,000 population)	47	26	34	35

*2002 Figures derived from http://www.who.int/whosis/data/

Table 1.6 Condition-related mortality rates in less-developed countries*

	USA (for comparison)	South Africa	Zimbabwe	China
Years of life lost (%) due to non-communicable diseases	75	15	7	56
Years of life lost (%) due to communicable diseases	9	77	90	23
Prevalence of tuberculosis per 100,000 population	3	998	597	210
Age-standardized mortality rate for HIV/AIDS (per 100,000 population)	5	675	1384	2
Age-standardized mortality rate due to non-communicable diseases (per 100,000 population)	460	808	585	665
Age standardized mortality rate for cancer (per 100,000 population)	134	154	122	148
Age-standardized mortality rate for cardiovascular disease (per 100,000 population)	188	410	347	291
Age-standardized mortality rate for injuries (per 100,000 population)	47	120	103	79

*2002 Figures derived from http://www.who.int/whosis/data/

making prudent behavioural choices may have a greater health impact than medical interventions. Preventing rather than attempting to cure can make a substantial contribution to enhanced health.

Success in management of communicable diseases is attributable to environmental and personal hygiene, immunization and antimicrobial drugs. With the exception of Zimbabwe, the countries listed have high rates of immunization; it is only the well-developed countries that have sustainable access to good sanitation. In China 35% of the population, in South Africa 41% and in Zimbabwe 54% of the population lack satisfactory access to good sanitation. Well-developed nations offer all their citizens access to a sustainable improved water supply. A safe water supply and good sanitation would go a long way to controlling the diarrhoea encountered in underdeveloped areas. Improved environmental engineering is one reason for the reduction in infant deaths in China. The 37 infant deaths per 1000 live births in 1990, dropped to 30 by 2000 and decreased to 20 in 2006. In 2000 the probability of dying before the age of 5 years in China was 37 per 1000 live births. Communicable diseases take a high toll on young lives. Non-communicable diseases are more prone to increase morbidity and mortality in older age groups. While environmental

engineering may resolve some problems in less-developed countries, different solutions need to be canvassed for managing the problem of non-communicable disease in developed nations.

Whereas well-developed countries seem to have achieved marked success in the control of infectious diseases, they are floundering when it comes to controlling non-communicable disorders. Unlike the outcome of infectious diseases, which tend to result in either cure or death, the end result of non-communicable disorders is often a chronic condition whose persistence relentlessly drains the health care purse. The demand on a health care system for management of chronic conditions differs both in cost and in nature from that required to control acute conditions. Surgery may often resolve problems created by injuries, antimicrobials will halt many infections. Acute disorders are more often than not quickly resolved. The natural history of treated chronic conditions is exacerbations and remissions with gradually increasingly disability. Acute and chronic diseases differ substantially in the impact they have on the health care system due to their discrepant natural history and prognosis (see Table 1.7).

While the availability of dollars is a necessary prerequisite to solving the problem, money alone

Table 1.7 Acute versus chronic disease*

	Acute disease	Chronic illness
Onset	Abrupt	Usually gradual
Cause	Single	Multiple
Duration	Limited	Lengthy, indefinite
Prognosis	Usually accurate	Often uncertain
Intervention	Short term, often curative	Long term, palliative
Outcome	Cure	Ongoing care
Knowledge	Professional authority	Shared
Patient role	Passive, dependent	Active participant

*Adapted with permission from Holman H, Lorig K. Patients as partners in managing chronic disease. Partnership is a prerequisite for effective and efficient health care. British Medical Journal 2000;320(7234):526–527.

does not predict clinical outcome. In 1998, despite the US spending more health care dollars, the death rate due to conditions amenable to medical care was between 25% and 50% higher than in Canada and Australia.[1] As expenditure is clearly not the sole determinant of good health care, an American study attempted to quantify factors that contributed to premature death.[11] The authors suggested that behavioural patterns contributed 40%, genetic predisposition 30%, social circumstance 15%, health care 10% and environmental exposure 5%. They concluded that 'the single greatest opportunity to improve health and reduce premature deaths lies in personal behavior'.[11] The US Department of Health and Human Services publication *Healthy People 2010* seemed to concur. This publication identified the leading health indicators as physical activity, overweight and obesity, tobacco use, substance abuse, responsible sexual behaviour, mental health, injury and violence, environmental quality, immunization and access to health care.[12] A number of these indicators can be modified by personal choices. Key lifestyle choices impacting on life expectancy have been identified as smoke-/tobacco-free living; 30 minutes physical activity a day; and a diet that emphasizes fruits and vegetables, lean meats, and low-fat dairy products.[13] Lifestyle choices influence health.[14]

Health: a personal choice but a community imperative

Individuals can reduce their risk of developing disease by selecting healthy, and avoiding risky, lifestyle options. The cost of caring for young people at high risk is 2.39 times that for those at low risk. The costs of caring for the elderly at high risk is almost threefold that of caring for those at low risk. Demand on the health care budget could be reduced by lowering the overall population risk. Many risks can be modified. Analysis of a 2004–2005 national health survey in Australia found that 86% of adults ate too little vegetables, 46% devoured too few fruits, 54% were overweight or obese, 34% had very low levels of physical activity, 13% consumed alcohol at risky levels and 23% were smokers. Almost 97% of the adult population surveyed had at least one of these modifiable risk factors.[15] Although the proportion of the population at risk may vary by country, these risk factors are encountered worldwide. Globally, 60% of all deaths are due to chronic disease and these risk factors are important contributors to the pathogenesis of chronic diseases. Chronic diseases such as heart disease, strokes, cancer, chronic respiratory disease and diabetes took 35 million lives in 2005 and half of these occurred in persons under 70 years of age.[16] Although the more lavish and sedentary lifestyles of affluent societies are conducive to developing many non-communicable diseases, as seen in Table 1.6, chronic disease is not the prerogative of well-developed nations. Somewhat surprisingly, 80% of chronic disease deaths occur in low- and middle-income countries. The WHO reports that physical inactivity causes 2 million deaths each year, that tobacco use is the single largest cause of cancer and that there is a causal relationship between alcohol and more than 60 types of disease and injury. It is not only Australians that make risky life choices (see Table 1.8).

Compared to a young person with few or no risks, the cost of providing health care to persons 65 years and older is 6.82 fold higher for those at 'high risk' compared to 2.22 times higher for those with few or no risks. Health care for high-risk elderly persons is particularly costly. While many health risks can be modified, population ageing cannot be halted. Around 12.5% of the Australian population is now over the age of 65; by 2047 the proportion of the Australian population aged

Table 1.8 Modifiable risk by country*

	Year	Canada	UK	Zimbabwe	China
Annual per capita (age >15 yrs) alcohol consumption (litres pure alcohol)	2003/6	7.8	11.75	4.41	5.2
Prevalence male obesity >15 yrs of age	2002/5	15.9	22.3	3.9	2.4
Prevalence female obesity >15 yrs of age	2002/5	13.9	23	19.4	3.4

*Figures derived from http://www.who.int/whosis/data/

65 and over is projected to increase to 25%.[17] A similar scenario could be painted for the US, Canada, UK and other well-developed countries. Self-insured US corporations provide worksite health promotion programmes to maintain and/or to improve their employees' health status. This business strategy is justified on the basis that individuals with more high-risk behaviours incur higher costs than those with low-risk behaviours.[18,19] An Australian health fund calculated care of members with medium- or high-risk lifestyle behaviours increased that fund's total expenditure by 13.5%.[20] They concluded that health risk reduction and low-risk maintenance constituted an important strategy for improving/maintaining the health and wellbeing of their membership and for potential savings in health care costs. The Australian figure is somewhat lower than that calculated by US funds. Excess health care costs associated with higher health risks in US studies varied between 21% and 31%, with a mean close to 25%.[21,22] There is good evidence that individuals who change lifestyle behaviours improve their health status and reduce their health care costs.[23,24]

Davis urges the US to invest in healthy children and a healthy workforce as this would pay dividends with respect to both healthier lives and greater economic productivity.[5] Diverting a greater proportion of the health care dollar to health promotion and disease prevention is a step towards achieving this. A sustainable health care system would seem to be based upon a low-risk population.

The path towards a low-risk population

Two fundamental changes need to be canvassed in order to achieve a low-risk population. Firstly, the disease care orientation of the 'health' care system needs to be revisited; secondly, the role of the individual in health care needs to be reappraised. The goal of health care, instead of aiming to provide satisfactory disease care, should be to increase the quality of life years. Efforts to increase longevity, instead of aiming to achieve a long life, should seek to add years of healthy life. Ideas to achieve this may come from innovations within conventional medicine or be drawn from CAM. The White House Commission on Complementary and Alternative Medicine Policy considered it necessary to, among other things, 'evaluate the possible role of CAM approaches in supporting health and wellness'.[25] Specific recommendations included the idea that 'the Healthy People Consortium should form a working group to evaluate the potential impact of safe and effective CAM practices and products on the nation's leading health indicators…' and that 'research on the role of CAM in wellness and health promotion, the application of CAM principles and practices, and the role of CAM practitioners in the management of chronic disease should be expanded'.

While recognition of CAM practitioners in conventional health care may boost the number of registered health professionals, expand the range of diagnostic procedures and therapeutic techniques available, and enhance a health promotion orientation, this alone is unlikely to solve the problems confronting the health care system. A more fundamental change is needed if countries are to shift their populations towards the low-risk pole of the health disease spectrum. It is in the national interest for authorities to encourage individuals to take personal responsibility for their wellbeing.

Recognizing that the contradiction between acute care practices and chronic disease problems can no longer be ignored, one approach proposed to reduce demand on the UK health care service is creation of a 'fully-engaged' population that makes responsible health choices to manage their own health and health care. A wide range of policies in the NHS in England are directed towards facilitating creation of a fully engaged scenario. To reach a stage of full engagement a population is postulated to need to pass through the phases of health literacy, health promotion, self-care, chronic disease self-management, patient and finally citizen involvement.[26] Health literacy is the ability to understand one's own health and to make sound decisions. Knowledge is not necessarily transformed to action and therefore community-based trainers to help individuals change unhealthy habits are proposed. Other initiatives projected are making health information integral to health care encounters, involving community organizations, and building health communication partnerships such as the Expert Patient Programme in which trained volunteers provide self-care management for chronic conditions such as diabetes or arthritis. The aim is a sustainable health care system which uses government and community organizations to support patients engaged with their own care. The desired outcome is increased life expectancy, more efficient use of resources and high level of public commitment to making healthy lifestyle choices.

In the UK, enhancing patient understanding is seen as the first step to achieving a low-risk population. Instead of being disease-focused, a patient-centred approach is needed. Taking the patient's views into account has been demonstrated to result in higher satisfaction, better compliance, and greater continuity of care.[27] Programmes that enhance the ability of patients with chronic disease to participate in their health care have been developed and shown to be worthwhile.[28] One successful self-management education programme addressed topics ranging from continuous use of medication, pain control and learning to interpret changes in the disease and its consequences, through use of medical and community resources, to various behavioural changes, including those required to adapt to social and workplace dislocations and cope with emotional reactions. Participants in this programme experienced fewer symptoms, improved their physical activity and required significantly less medical attention.[28] Self-care groups in which patients set the agenda for recurrent meetings with their principal doctor have increased the quality of life and reduced use of medical services. Remote medical

management via the telephone or electronic communication has been shown to reduce cost and improve the health status of participants compared with patients receiving usual care. In each instance the patient takes the central role and assumes increased personal responsibility. Similarly, to marshal a low-risk population, individuals will need to assume a central role in their health management.

There is convincing evidence that those making healthy lifestyle choices can reduce their risk of disease. A nutritious diet, prudent use of alcohol, avoidance of tobacco and drug misuse, adequate physical activity, maintaining an appropriate body weight and practising safe sex are all matters of personal choice. Healthy lifestyle choices are a well-recognized therapeutic measure advocated by health professionals. Nonetheless, patients receiving Western health care largely perceive it to be their physician's responsibility for getting them well. The dependent patient role is well established in Western medicine. The 'taking a tablet' solution is far less demanding than changing an unhealthy habit. For individuals to take primary responsibility for their health requires a substantial change in thinking. While advice on healthy living is readily available,[29–31] as demonstrated in Table 1.8, persuading 'healthy' people to implement this advice is more problematic. It has been estimated that between 20% and 80% of patients do not adhere to their medical regimens and that economic costs due to this phenomenon range from US$ 25 to 100 billion a year in, amongst others, lost productivity, additional treatment and hospital admission costs.[27] As patients who feel ill are tardy when asked to comply with their medical treatment, getting individuals who feel well to change their habits poses a daunting task.

While much works needs to be done in persuading individuals to voluntarily adopt healthy habits, much success has been achieved in motivating consumers in well-developed countries to submit to screening programmes to ensure that early pathology is detected. Early detection and intervention to control hypertension, diabetes and cancer can dramatically change the natural history of these conditions. National screening programmes are available for certain conditions. Table 1.9 shows how Western women are electing to enter screening programmes in an effort to reduce their risk of dying from breast or cervical cancer through early diagnosis and timely treatment of covert disease. The UK offers national public health screening programmes for early detection of conditions

Table 1.9 Female preventive care by country*

	Year	CAN	UK	AUST	SA	ZIM	CHINA
% Women who have had mammography	2006	71	75	57	6	2	16
% Women who have had Pap smear	2002/3	74	70	61	17	19	21

CAN – Canada; AUST – Australia; SA – South Africa; ZIM – Zimbabwe.
*Figures derived from http://www.who.int/whosis/data/

ranging from bowel cancer to diabetic retinopathy, from Down syndrome to fetal anomalies.[32] Analysis of 22 randomized controlled studies suggested that alerting individuals to their personal risk was most likely to increase uptake of screening tests in individuals at high risk.[33] Personalized risk is based on the individual's own risk factors for a condition and may be calculated using epidemiological data. It can be presented as an absolute or relative risk, a risk score, or categorized into high-, medium- and low-risk groups.

The way ahead

It would seem that clinical care in a 21st century health care system will place increased emphasis on health literacy and personal responsibility. It would seem that the goal of health care will be to enhance wellness and shift a population's health norm to one of low risk. The health care system cannot indefinitely service a high-risk population. With a growth rate of 6–7%, global pharmaceutical sales were expected to reach US$ 735–745 billion in 2008.[34] In 2006, the US, the European Union and Japan spent US$ 287, US$ 250 and US$ 273 per capita, respectively, on medical equipment.[34] This expenditure will continue as long as health care services a high-risk population. Demographic changes demand reform of both the health care system and individuals' lifestyle choices. Health care expenditure needs to be redistributed from high-cost, technologically advanced medical care to lower-cost community intervention; individuals need to select health-promoting options. To achieve a wellness transformation an effective health care system needs to be staffed by health professionals who are skilled health educators and compelling motivators. Behaviour change of health professionals and consumers holds the key to converting an ailing into a sustainable health care system.

References

1. Davis K, Schoen C, Schoenbaum S, et al. *Mirror, Mirror on the Wall: An International Update on the Comparative Performance of American Health Care.* New York: Commonwealth Fund; 2007.

2. See http://www.michaelmoore.com/sicko/health-care-proposal/; Accessed 15.11.2008.

3. *Australian Institute of Health and Welfare. Australia's Health 2006. The Tenth Biennial Health Report of the Australian Institute of Health and Welfare.* Canberra: AIHW; 2006. Canberra. AIHW cat. no. AUS 73 http://www.aihw.gov.au/publications/aus/ah06/ah06-c00.rtf Accessed 15.11.2008.

4. Duckett SJ. Drug policy down under: Australia's pharmaceutical benefits scheme. *Health Care Financ Rev.* 2004;25(3):55–67.

5. Davis K. Health and Wealth: Measuring Health System Performance, Invited Testimony, Senate Committee on Commerce, Science, and Transportation, Subcommittee on Interstate Commerce, Trade, and Tourism, Hearing on "Rethinking the Gross Domestic Product as a Measurement of National Strength" http://www.cmwf.org/Content/Publications/Testimonies/2008/Mar/Testimony–Health-and-Wealth–Measuring-Health-System-Performance.aspx; 2008 March 12 Accessed 30.03.2009.

6. *Commonwealth Fund. Insurance coverage and receipt of preventive care.* http://www.commonwealthfund.org/snapshotscharts/snapshotscharts_show Accessed 15.11.2008.

7. *WHO, WHO Statistical Information System (WHOSIS).* http://www.who.int/whosis/data Accessed 16.11.2008.

8. Mirkin B, Weinberger MB. The demography of population ageinghttp://www.un.org/esa/population/publications/bulletin42_43weinbergermirkin.pdf Accessed 17.11.2008.

9. *AgeWorks University of Southern California.* http://www.ageworks.com/course_demo/200/module2/module2b.htm Accessed 03.11.2008.

10. WHO, *The global burden of disease 2004 update.* http://www.who.int/healthinfo/global_burden_disease/2004_report_update/en/index.html Accessed 10.11.2008.

11. Schroeder SA. Shattuck Lecture. We can do better—improving the health of the American people. *N Engl J Med.* 2007;357 (12):1221–1228.

12. *Healthy People 2010.* http://www.healthypeople.gov/LHI/lhiwhat.htm Accessed 15.11.2008.

13. *Cardiovision 2020.* http://www.cardiovision2020.org Accessed 15.11.2008.

14. Rudd K, Roxon N. *Fresh Ideas, Future Economy: Preventive Health Care for our Families and Our Future Economy.* Canberra: ALP; 2007. *http://www.alp.org.au Accessed 01.11.2008.*

15. *AIHW, Chronic diseases and associated risk factors in Australia.* http://www.aihw.gov.au/publications/index.cfm/title/10319 Accessed 13.11.2008.

16. WHO, *Chronic disease and health promotion.* http://www.who.int/chp/en/ Accessed 15.11.2008.

17. *The Intergenerational Report 2007.* http://www.treasury.gov.au/igr/IGR2007.asp Accessed 13.11.2008.

18. Yen LT, Edington DW, Witting P. Associations between health risk appraisal scores and employee medical claims costs in a manufacturing company. *Am J Health Promot.* 1991;6:46–54.

19. Goetzel RZ, Anderson DR, Witmer RW, Ozminkowski RJ, Dunn J, Wasserman J. and HERO Research Committee. The relationship between modifiable health risks and health care expenditures. *J Occup Environ Med.* 1998;40:843–854.

20. Musich S, Hook D, Barnett T, Edington D. The association between health risk status and health care costs among the membership of an Australian health plan. *Health Promot Int.* 2003;18:57–65.

21. Anderson DR, Whitmer RW, Goetzel RZ, Ozminkowski RJ, Wasserman J, Serxner S. and the HERO Research Committee. The relationship between modifiable health risks and group-level health care expenditures. *Am J Health Promot.* 2000;15:45–52.

22. Edington DW. Emerging research: a view from one research center. *Am J Health Promot.* 2001;15:341–349.

23. Musich SA, Adams L, Edington DW. Effectiveness of health promotion programs in moderating medical costs in the USA. *Health Promot Int.* 2000;15:5–15.

24. Pronk NP, Goodman MJ, O'Connor PJ, Martinson BC. Relationship between modifiable health risks and short-term health care changes. *JAMA.* 1999;282:2235–2239.

25. White House Commission on Complementary and Alternative Medicine Policy. *Final Report.* Washington, DC: White House Commission on Complementary and Alternative Medicine Policy; 2002.

26. Cayton H. The flat-pack patient? Creating health together. *Patient Educ Couns.* 2006;62 (3):288–290.

27. Fuertes JN, Mislowack A, Bennett J, Paul L, et al. The physician-patient working alliance. *Patient Educ Couns.* 2007;66(1):29–36.

28. Holman H, Lorig K. Patients as partners in managing chronic disease. Partnership is a prerequisite for effective and efficient health care. *BMJ.* 2000;320 (7234):526–527.

29. *UK Department of Health.* http://www.dh.gov.uk/en/Publicationsandstatistics/Publications/PublicationsPolicyAndGuidance/DH_089737 Accessed 03.11.2008.

30. *Medline plus.* http://www.nlm.nih.gov/medlineplus/healthscreening.html Accessed 15.11.2008.

31. *American Cancer Society, Guide to quitting smoking.* http://www.cancer.org/docroot/ped/content/ped_10_13x_guide_for_quitting_smoking.asp Accessed 15.11.2008.

32. *National Library of Health.* http://www.library.nhs.uk/screening Accessed 15.11.2008.

33. Edwards AG, Evans R, Dundon J, Haigh S, Hood K, Elwyn GJ. Personalised risk communication for informed decision making about taking screening tests. *Cochrane Database Syst Rev.* 2006;(4) CD001865.

34. WHO. *The World Health Report 2008: Primary Health Care Now More Than Ever.* Geneva: WHO; 2008. *http://www.who.int/whr/2008/whr08_en.pdf Accessed 02.12.2008.*

Canvassing solutions

2

Underdeveloped countries are challenged to reduce infant mortality and infectious diseases; in industrialized countries the health care system is confounded by an ageing population plagued by a plethora of chronic diseases. While underdeveloped countries may benefit from greater access to Western medicine, in advanced countries technologically advanced health care is failing to meet the population's health needs. In Australia it has been suggested there is 'an urgent need for major workforce reform'.[1] The US has already taken action. By the early 1970s, the US had attempted to address their growing health care problems by expanding the scope of practice of non-physician health professionals and by encouraging the growth of corporate health care entities.

American workforce reform is shaped by managed care organizations and the employment of nurse practitioners and physician assistants.[2] By preparing health professionals in these roles, the US health care system seeks to provide the community with access to more-affordable good-quality care.

The tasks performed by these mid-level professionals typically includes history-taking, physical examination, ordering laboratory and radiological investigations, prescribing medication, and counselling.[3,4] Nurse practitioners and physician assistants diagnose and treat disease working within the framework of a medical model of health care. Working mainly at the level of primary care, it is anticipated that nurse practitioners and physician assistants can manage 50% to 75% of all primary care visits.[5] It is hoped that further savings will be made in future by training these professionals in various medical specialties.[6] Even though reliance on these health professionals has doubled over the last two decades to reach approximately 100,000 nurse practitioners and 60,000 physician assistants, health care in the US remains in dire straits. Despite patients being satisfied with the care provided by mid-level practitioners,[7] this innovation within a biomedical framework has failed to address the underlying problem.

State support of a more corporatized health care system is another US initiative. By switching allegiance from physicians to corporations, the state has supported commercialization of health care. Managed health care corporations have sprung up and capitated payments have replaced fee-for-service remuneration. While the stated aim of managed health organizations for promoting the use of capitated payments is to improve service efficiency and curb costs, the effect has been to curtail the professional autonomy of physicians. Until relatively recently, the US federal and state governments had given physicians professional autonomy, subsidized and expanded physician training, required that licensed physicians supervise non-physician clinicians, and helped the profession maintain its revenue through sponsored established fee-for-service federal insurance programme payments for the elderly and poor. While the state no longer supports physicians' privileged position, it has retained principles implicit in the biomedical model of health care. The heath care reforms in the US have maintained a mechanistic perspective and the body continues to be viewed as a composite of interrelated and upgradeable or replaceable parts. Reforms based on an industrial model in which health care is perceived as a production process with patients as customers is doomed to fail, as the predominant health need is care for persons with chronic disease and disability. The idea that health care is a commodity and patients are consumers is unlikely to resolve the dilemmas confronting health care. The solution may need to be sought outside of the framework of conventional health care. It may be necessary to canvass the potential of complementary and alternative medicine (CAM) to provide the answer.

CAM: the way ahead?

CAM is not state supported yet its popularity in Western society is growing.[8] Consumers of health care are increasingly choosing to consult CAM practitioners in conjunction with, or as an alternative to, conventional health professionals.[9] Population trends would seem to suggest that CAM practitioners may serve as a desirable resource to met the perceived need in conventional health care as a 'range of new health practitioners who can deliver patient-friendly care'.[10] Integration of CAM into conventional health care does, however, mount a major challenge to the sacred tenets of the biomedical model upon which Western medicine is based.

The biomedical model adheres to the principles of reductionism, determinism, dualism and materialism. Reductionists believe complex phenomena are ultimately derived from a single primary principle and that analysing matter into its component parts leads to understanding. The practical implications of this perspective are that all disease manifestations can be conceptualized in terms of physical and chemical principles. The clinical focus becomes biological/biochemical relationships. Materialists perceive physical matter as the only reality and

hence only objective information is valid. The result is a positivist scientific paradigm in which explanations are couched in biological terms and based upon measurable changes. Determinism portrays causation as being exclusively characterized by a linear mechanistic link. This implies the existence of unilinear cause–effect relationships which lead to predictable outcomes. This view is bolstered by dualism, derived from the Cartesian view that mind and body are detached. Care of the mind is relegated to the specialties of psychiatry and psychology. The division between body and spirit is even starker, with spiritual care being relegated to the clergy. The result has been a dehumanized form of care in which disease, rather than the patient, is central to the clinical encounter. Conventional medicine, with its focus on the physical self, functions in a cognitive framework not designed to meet the emotional and spiritual needs of patients trying to cope with chronic disorders.

In sharp contrast to conventional medicine, CAM practitioners embrace the notion of vitalism. Vitalism is a doctrine which maintains that the processes of life cannot be explained by the laws of physics and chemistry alone, and that life is in some part self-determining. CAM adherents reject the notion of dualism and conceptualize the patient as a dynamic interaction of physical, chemical and spiritual forces. Monism decries separation of mind and body. The result at the clinical level is a shift in focus from disease-centred to patient-centred care. Holism takes this creed a step further and views the individual and his environment as inseparable parts of a greater whole. Health and disease are seen to result not only from aberrant physiology and dysfunctional psychology but also from the totality of man's physical, chemical and emotional interaction with social, natural/environmental and spiritual forces. Man is viewed as part of a local and global self-organizing system capable of self-renewal and self-transcendence. In this system, unilinear cause–effect relationships are rejected and replaced by the construct of interactionism, leading to the notion of mutual causality. Change and continuity are equally real and each component is an indivisible portion of the whole. Determinism is traded for indeterminism; clinical certainty is supplanted by ambiguity. Such beliefs are consistent with postmodernism which suggests the world cannot be understood in terms of a single framework but that understanding comes from accepting a disjointed plurality of values and beliefs.

Acknowledgement that multiple and diverse interacting health/disease triggers influence well-being has far-reaching implications for health care. Patient management is elevated to a new level of complexity. At one level, rigorous evaluation of patients' lifestyle choices and behaviours is required; on another, laboratory investigations may be expanded to include more esoteric evaluations of energy fluctuations and/or electromagnetic changes. CAM therapies go beyond chemical interactions. CAM allows for, indeed embraces, energy-based medicine, whether this be implemented by changing the physical structure of homeopathic remedies through succussion or by balancing chi through acupuncture needling. Indeed, at a therapeutic level, interventions to restore homeostasis may range from the use of pharmaceuticals, neutraceuticals and herbs, through massage, chiropractic, osteopathy and therapeutic touch, to counselling.

At the clinical level, an immediate benefit of a CAM system of health care would be to shift the focus from the disease to the individual and rejuvenate the healing power of the clinical consultation. The power of the physician alone to make a patient feel better, irrespective of medication, is one of the most important factors in the consultation; nonetheless, it is largely overlooked as a therapeutic tool in conventional health care.[11] In conventional health care circles, awareness is growing that information processing within the nervous system does not discriminate between symbols and physical structures. Realization that brain neurobiology can be altered by mental imagery has opened a whole new avenue of research in orthodox medicine. As evidence of an orderly relationship between autonomic, neuro-endocrinologic and immunologic responses to acute psychological stressors accumulates,[12–14] recognition that the previously denigrated placebo effect of a consultation may be explained by working through mental rather than bodily mechanisms is being bolstered.

Post-modern thinking has enhanced the credibility of CAM practices. By introducing the notion of multifactorial interacting causes rather than unilinear cause–effect relationships, the certainty consistent with a positivist approach has been undermined. By shifting the focus away from the disease onto the patient, recognition that subjective, and not only objective data, provides valid information has transformed research paradigms considered acceptable in health care. While the double-blind placebo-controlled clinical trial remains the gold standard in biomedicine, the results provided by case series have assumed the mantel of respectability. Clinical observations previously regarded as irrelevant at best, or suspect at worst, are increasingly acquiring respectability. Chiropractic is one profession benefiting from these changes.

Chiropractic: a foot in both camps

Chiropractic straddles the conventional and CAM health care systems. Chiropractic differs from most CAM professions in that it is regulated by statute in a number of jurisdictions, including the USA, UK and Australia. Furthermore, while chiropractic science is compatible with a positivist biomechanical paradigm, chiropractic philosophy is based on vitalistic principles and conforms more readily to a CAM approach to health care. While the notion of the human body being self-regulating and having the ability to heal itself is not foreign to conventional health care, the construct of innate intelligence is. Insofar as chiropractic offers conservative manual therapy for spinal problems, it has increasingly achieved recognition within conventional health care circles as a scientifically sound therapeutic option. On the other hand, its viability as a therapeutic option for the management of non-musculoskeletal conditions remains questionable. Nonetheless, with some marked exceptions,[15] many regard chiropractic as a clinically effective discipline that offers particularly effective management of pain attributable to mechanical problems of the spine, particularly the low back and neck.

Musculoskeletal diseases represent a major health problem throughout the world – indeed, it has been suggested that no other group of disorders affects more people, leads to a higher prevalence of disability, or places a higher financial burden on health systems.[16] It is therefore lamentable that the evidence for or against the efficacy of spinal manipulation for low back and neck pain remains indecisive. Controversy persists despite many published randomized clinical trials, a substantial number of reviews and several national clinical guideline publications.[17] Nonetheless, as chiropractic care is increasingly being investigated, evidence of its cost-effectiveness is accumulating. A retrospective, outcome-based analysis over a 1-year period found spinal manipulation an effective treatment for mechanical neck and low back pain patients attending a private chiropractic clinic.[18] Unfortunately, the study design did not account for the natural history of low back or neck pain-related disability. Nevertheless, a pragmatic, randomized, controlled trial concurred, concluding that ongoing chiropractic care in an NHS setting may effectively reduce disability and perceived pain for a subpopulation of patients with chronic low back pain.[19] Acute patients were reported to demonstrate greater pain relief at all time points. A second study, which included both acute and chronic chiropractic patients, concurred.[20] This study reported on pain and disability outcomes for chiropractic and medical patients with low back pain for up to 48 months. Most improvement occurred by 3 months and was sustained for 12 months. Exacerbations were reported thereafter. Another review recommended spinal manipulation and mobilization as a viable option for the treatment of both low back and neck pain.[17] However, another review, published in the same year, offered a contradictory perspective. Assendelft et al's review of spinal manipulation and mobilization for mechanical neck problems led them to believe 'the evidence did not favour manipulation and/or mobilization done alone or in combination with various other physical medicine agents'.[21]

Chiropractic's care for biomechanical problems remains contentious in conservative medical circles. Furthermore, the balance of evidence justifying chiropractic's claim to offer effective care for visceral conditions is even less convincing when viewed within a biomedical framework. Despite satisfied patients reporting subjective relief, quantitative research has largely failed to produce any objective evidence of improvement. One review concluded there was insufficient evidence to support the use of manual therapies for patients with asthma.[22] Another suggested that overall there is no evidence to suggest that spinal manipulation is effective in the treatment of primary and secondary dysmenorrhoea.[23] Similarly, chiropractic wellness care provides fertile grounds for disagreement. Explanations used by chiropractors to justify their claims to enhance wellness and provide care of visceral conditions are drawn from chiropractic philosophy. Clinical practices framed by chiropractic philosophy are rejected by conventional health care. Chiropractic philosophy, governed by the doctrine of vitalism, has been primarily responsible for chiropractic being designated a CAM system of health care.

Wellness the chiropractic way

The nervous system and spinal care are viewed as fundamental to health. Traditionally, chiropractic wellness care is offered primarily in the form of maintenance care.[24] One American study reported that US chiropractors agreed that the purpose of maintenance care is to optimize health, prevent conditions from developing, provide palliative care, and minimize recurrences or exacerbations.[25] The problem associated with chiropractic wellness care is not its intent; it lies in its implementation. While there is strong agreement that the therapeutic composition of maintenance care should place virtually equal weight on exercise and adjustments/manipulation, identification of any other elements offered in a chiropractic wellness care package are ill defined. Some chiropractors offer, to the exclusion of all else, regular assessment to detect and correct subluxations, with or without spinal exercises. Others provide information on musculoskeletal risk reduction, exercise, diet, stress reduction, and injury prevention.[26] Although chiropractic has long regarded itself as a wellness profession, it has yet to clearly define what constitutes chiropractic wellness care.

According to Nelson et al.[27] 'While nearly all factions of the profession make the claim that chiropractic represents a "wellness" approach to health, some factions use this term to mean, "We will prevent disease by eliminating subluxations." Others use the term to mean, "We will prevent back pain and related disorders by providing comprehensive spine care." And still others use the term to mean, "We will prevent a variety of degenerative diseases (cardiovascular, neoplastic, etc.) by advising patients on how to live a more healthy life."' Furthermore, Nelson et al felt that chiropractic did not fare well when compared with other primary practitioners when primary care was defined as 'the provision of integrated, accessible, health care services by clinicians who are accountable for addressing a large majority of personal health care needs, developing a sustained partnership with patients, and practicing in the context of the family and the community.' In fact, they went so far as to suggest, 'Until we can demonstrate that we are effective where others are not, the proposition of chiropractic as the "wellness profession" is not defensible.'[27] The notion of wellness being achieved by regular visits to chiropractic physicians is also questionable. In a personal communication, George B McClelland, DC, Chairman ACA Board of Governors suggested that 'philosophically the idea of regular spinal manipulative therapy opposes the concept of wellness'.

The necessity for review and clarification of chiropractic as a wellness profession was further highlighted by the publication of the Institute of Alternative Futures, which in its *Future of Chiropractic Revisited: 2005 to 2010* publication identified four possible future scenarios for this profession. The most advantageous options seemed to be development of chiropractors either as musculoskeletal experts with a narrow scope of practice or as primary practitioners assuming the mantel of 'healthy life doctors' or 'wellness consultants'. Chiropractors supporting the former option fit snugly into conventional health care; those who support the latter stumble into the sphere of CAM health care. Chiropractors specializing in musculoskeletal health care strongly support evaluation of their craft using quantitative research methods. These chiropractors are unashamedly reductionist in their clinical approach. Amongst this group, there are even those who question the very existence of the chiropractic subluxation. In contrast, those who advocate the healthy life doctor approach include chiropractors who perceive subluxations as a primary cause of dysfunction and a subluxation-free existence as a fundamental prerequisite to wellness. While the practice of these chiropractors is all too often reductionist in the sense that their practice is to almost exclusively detect and adjust subluxations, their rhetoric is holistic. Indeed, within a vitalistic framework, correction of subluxations restores homeostasis and enables the body to self-heal. By restoring biomechanical balance, the chiropractic adjustment is believed to enhance total, not merely spinal, wellbeing.

Regardless of their conventional or CAM leaning, chiropractors by and large do value their primary contact status. In view of this imperative, it would seem logical for the chiropractic profession to move in the general direction of wellness rather than that of specialist musculoskeletal health care. In 2001, the American Chiropractic Association embarked on a Wellness Campaign and has actively pursued adopting an evidence-based wellness ethos ever since. By 2006, the Chiropractors Association of Australia was actively exploring how local chiropractors could express their wellness orientation. An Australian Delphi study found that respondents, when asked 'What definition of wellness do you feel best describes current chiropractic practice in Australia?', agreed that 'Historically chiropractic wellness has been seen as the optimal expression of an individual's vital capacity or the body's natural recuperative powers. Some chiropractors have traditionally seen limitations to the expression of wellness in terms of symptoms mediated by vertebral subluxation. Such limitations can be removed by chiropractic adjustment. This version of chiropractic wellness was and is delivered within the context of a chiropractic maintenance care programme. In contrast, a more contemporary chiropractic approach defines wellness in terms of biopsychosocial and holistic wellbeing. In this model, manual therapy, counselling, exercise and/or dietary advice are frequently part of the encounter.'[28] When asked 'What definition of wellness do you believe would best serve Australia's chiropractic profession in the future?', respondents indicated that wellness should be defined as 'a process whereby chiropractors assist their patients to actively participate in assuming personal responsibility for attaining and maintaining multidimensional optimal function at the level of both their general (biopsychosocial) and spinal health.'[28]

While any conventionally acceptable definition of chiropractic wellness care would need to include mainstream medical approaches to primary care, to exclude traditional chiropractic wellness constructs would alienate large sections of the chiropractic community. The challenge faced by the leaders in the chiropractic profession is therefore to achieve a united profession by formulating a practice template that respects chiropractic philosophy while submitting to the scientific rigors demanded by conventional health care. The task is to redefine chiropractic wellness care in terms that are acceptable to all – or, more realistically, most – chiropractors. A number of issues therefore need to be addressed with respect to the role that detecting and correcting subluxations plays in wellness care. The health impact of correcting asymptomatic subluxations remains unknown. Although chiropractors believe the outcome is enhanced wellness, this belief lacks scientific validation. Until the natural history of a subluxation is clarified and its role in the pathogenesis of recognized clinical conditions identified, conventional health care will regard subluxation-based wellness care with scepticism. Indeed, the underlying problem may well be linked to the possibility that a subluxation represents a disease marker rather than having a causative role in the condition.

The chiropractic profession has long believed that by removing subluxations it eliminates impediments to health. In contrast to medical care, which chiropractors perceive as largely focusing on symptoms, chiropractic claims it manages the cause of the condition. Whereas the possibility that subluxations cause disease cannot be discounted, it is probable that detection of subluxations represents the biomechanical consequence of some other pathophysiological process. Such esoteric discourse may, however, become irrelevant if the chiropractic profession accepts a definition of chiropractic wellness care that routinely incorporates a lifestyle wellness approach into subluxation-based maintenance care.

When subluxation-based maintenance care is expanded to routinely include lifestyle counselling and health risk monitoring, patients are the recipients of better health care. In the case of hypertension, it can for example be argued that subluxation-based maintenance care rather than being curative offers palliative care. While there is some evidence that chiropractic adjustments do reduce raised blood pressure in certain individuals, such benefit is short lived. Although studies ranging from case studies to randomized clinical trials confirm that adjustments reduce blood pressure and may decrease the dose required for effective antihypertensive drug therapy, the duration of any such benefit is lost once a course of chiropractic care is terminated or active chiropractic adjustments cease.[29,30] Although chiropractic adjustments may well have the capacity to achieve temporary modification of autonomic nervous system function, the problem requires a more permanent solution. If lifestyle modification is coupled with biomechanical care of the spine, the result is an improved clinical outcome. Lifestyle modifications such as exercising regularly for 61–90 minutes each week, maintaining an ideal body weight, restricting salt intake to 1 teaspoon daily and moderating alcohol consumption have all been shown to provide a long-term benefit. Indeed these lifestyle measures are the first stage in medical blood pressure management.[31] By routinely combining chiropractic adjustment with lifestyle modifications in maintenance care programmes, a number of conventional medicine's concerns are simultaneously addressed. Disquiet about whether chiropractic adjustment corrects a cause or provides evidence of dysfunction become irrelevant to patient care. An integrated approach addresses both some proven causes as well as other possible contributing factors. From the perspective of chiropractors with a philosophical orientation, it provides some justification to chiropractic's claim that it has a role in the care of certain visceral problems. From the perspective of consumers achieving meaningful long-term wellness, it changes the dynamic from practitioner dependence to increased personal responsibility. Chiropractic maintenance care that includes lifestyle change indisputably provides wellness care.

While some chiropractors whose thinking is influenced by norms of conventional health care may find the above argument persuasive, those with a strong vitalistic leaning may require further urging. A more convincing argument for these chiropractic physicians may be to reason that improved lifestyle choices increase the efficacy of chiropractic adjustments. Maintenance care restricted to correction of subluxations and postural exercises can be likened to limiting car maintenance to cleaning the spark plugs and tuning the engine. Maintenance care that includes a nutritious diet, leisure time exercise and a healthy outlook can be equated to best-practice car maintenance that also selects the correct octane fuel, has regular oil change and maintains appropriate tyre pressure. Chiropractors who choose to become a wellness consultant or healthy life doctor, by offering a more comprehensive form of wellness care, are transformed into the sort of 'new health practitioner' required by a failing health care system. This wellness chiropractor offers primary prevention by screening patients for lifestyle hazards and intervenes by informing and motivating patients to make healthy choices. Care goes beyond biomechanical wellness. It includes consideration of possible excesses and deficiencies in diet and/or physical activity; it analyses and seeks to eliminate, or limit, toxin exposure. The objective is to create a macro- and micro-environment conducive to homeostasis. By addressing risky choices and encouraging healthy lifestyle options, an internal environment is created which is conducive to the optimal expression of innate intelligence. In this scenario, secondary prevention goes beyond screening for subluxations and includes actively searching for other risk markers such as abdominal obesity, hypertension, hypercholesterolaemia, stress and depression. The aim is to detect individuals experiencing adaptive stress and to intervene to restore homeostasis before pathophysiological changes become irreversible. In contrast to subluxation-limited wellness care, the health benefits provided by the healthy life chiropractor are longer lasting and

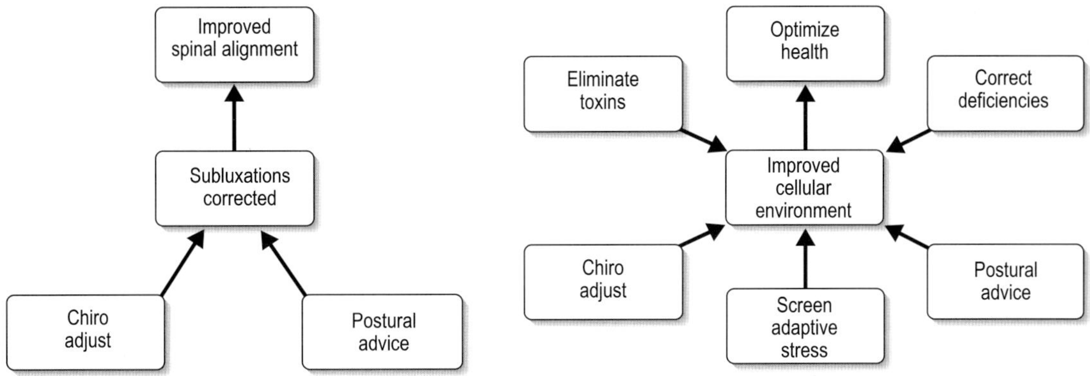

Figure 2.1 • Maintenance care: old and new.

more pervasive. By assessing and correcting poor lifestyle choices, the chiropractic physician is using multiple interventions to enhance the cellular environment (see Figure 2.1). Healthy life chiropractors rather than limiting their capacity to enhance homeostasis by restricting their intervention to spinal adjustments adopt a more holistic approach. These practitioners by implementing a more holistic approach are adhering to the principles of chiropractic philosophy while implementing their craft in a form both acceptable to and practised by enlightened medical practitioners.

While healthy life chiropractic practices may somewhat ease the burden of an ailing health care system, it is chiropractic patients who will be the main beneficiaries. A patient who presents with tension headaches and receives maintenance care confined to adjustments and relaxation advice limited to neck stretches and shoulder rolls is likely to experience more frequent and more severe headaches than the patient who, in addition to the above, is provided with stress management counselling covering both physical relaxation and mental and emotional management strategies. Patients who combine their chiropractic care with regular aerobic exercise and better time management are more likely to have fewer and less severe headaches than those who rely on chiropractic adjustments to rectify their problem. Persons who actively participate in their wellness programme cope better. Patients taking increased personal responsibility for their wellbeing experience a sense of mastery. Not only do they feel more in control, they also experience the coincidental benefits of reduced stress levels such as better sleep patterns, more energy and a reduced health risk of ischaemic heart disease.[32]

Health care: the emerging role for biophysics

By straddling conventional medicine with its reductionist and positivist approach to the management of back and neck pain and complementary and alternative medicine with its vitalistic approach to visceral conditions and wellness, the chiropractic profession shows the way for new age health care. While conventional medicine's focus is essentially restricted to care of the physical self, CAM views the body as a physical expression of an inner energetic state. Changes in the inner energetic state are reflected in the physical body and vice versa. Disease is seen to result from a disturbance of this inner energetic state. Acceptance of this construct would represent a major shift in conventional thinking. Incorporation of this construct into an integrated health care system could bring about a review of desirable clinical outcomes. Instead of the end point of medical treatment being elimination of the physical manifestations of disease or dysfunction, incorporation of CAM would seek to restore homeostasis. Instead of intervention being terminated once a biomedical 'cure' has improved inner energies, management would be continued to optimize energy flows. In an integrated health care system, treating signs and symptoms would be deemed to improve health but not restore wellness.

Conventional medicine perceives patients as physical structures governed by biochemical reactions; CAM perceives individuals as energetic beings. Molecular biochemistry is the basic unit of conventional medicine; physics is at the core of CAM. Nonetheless, conventional medicine readily acknowledges that individuals generate electrical fields; it also routinely measures electromagnetic energy using electroencephalograms (EEG) and electrocardiograms (ECG). While conventional medicine monitors electric activity in the diagnosis of heart attacks and various brain pathologies, Chinese medicine customarily uses pulse diagnosis to determine energy flow. The meridians with their acupuncture points provide Chinese medicine with an energy-based anatomical system. Acupuncturists offer an energy-based system of clinical intervention by needling acupuncture points in an effort to balance yin and yang. Stimulation of any one of many acupuncture points changes circulation at anatomically remote and apparently unrelated areas. Western medicine finds explanations used by traditional Chinese medicine as mystifying; nonetheless, intracellular signalling is believed to result from electromagnetic signalling transmitted by micro-currents generated in cells of the nervous system that surround neurons. The brain generates a DC magnetic field; AC fields are generated by ion flows in nerves and muscles. The body is electrically polarized; its centre is relatively positive with respect to its more negative periphery. Any movement and/or thought is accompanied by current flows in the nervous system. It has even been speculated that thinking about exercising certain muscles could send electrical impulses to that muscle group with resultant strengthening. Any suggestion to replace traditional physical exercise with such mental activity is, however, premature!

In additional to being energy based, CAM health care is holistic. Individuals are viewed as physical, mental and spiritual entities interacting with each other and nature. Only treating the entire person in their overall environment can restore inner balance. The individual and nature are connected and impact one upon the other. Any electrical current automatically generates a magnetic field. Not only do individuals generate weak electromagnetic fields as current flows through the body, human beings are also subject to the earth's electromagnetic field, solar and lunar electromagnetic cycles, and ionizing radiation from the sun, stars and radioactive material in rocks. In contrast to our ancestors, modern man is exposed to radiowaves, microwaves, high voltage power lines, and a myriad of AC and DC fields generated by televisions, computers and various electrical and battery-powered home appliances. All biological systems are influenced by electromagnetic fields.[33] Some are beneficial; others are not. Public concern on the potential health risks

from power-frequency fields (extremely low frequency electromagnetic fields) and from radiofrequency/microwave radiation emissions from wireless communications has been growing. Unsubstantiated, but possible, health endpoints reported to be associated with low frequency electromagnetic and/or radiofrequency fields include childhood leukaemia, brain tumours, genotoxic effects, neurological effects and neurodegenerative diseases, immune system deregulation, allergic and inflammatory responses, breast cancer, miscarriage and some cardiovascular effects.[34] The widespread use of wireless telecommunications devices, especially mobile phones, has resulted in a particularly worrisome increase in human exposure to radiofrequency fields. Mobile phones have been shown to induce changes in electrochemistry, blood–brain barrier permeability and EEG activity.[33] Despite numerous authoritative reviews, there remains no clear evidence of adverse health effects associated with radiofrequency fields and mobile phones.[35] Nonetheless, as long as some meta-analysis studies find a consistent pattern of association between mobile phone use and ipsilateral gliomas and acoustic neuromas after 10 or more years of mobile phone usage,[36] the possibility of an enhanced cancer risk cannot be excluded. The 2008 guidelines for the US and European microwave exposure from mobile phones, for the brain, of 1.6 W/kg and 2 W/kg, respectively, may well warrant review.

In contrast to the risks of excessive exposure, the benefits of appropriate levels of exposure offer new avenues of therapy. It appears that an electrical field of 0.25 volts per centimetre pulsing at 10 Hz restores normal patterns to most biological measurements.[33] Micro-pulsations of 7.83 Hz in the earth's field is the crucial timer of biocycles. Specific frequencies has been linked to various biological phenomena: a brain frequency of 8–10 Hz is associated with relaxation and meditation, a 2 Hz frequency has been linked to nerve regeneration, 10 Hz enhances ligament healing, while 15, 20 and 72 Hz stimulate capillary and fibroblast formation.[37] A double-blind trial showed that pulsed electromagnetic fields significantly enhanced healing of tibial fractures with delayed union.[38] It has been postulated that the initial transduction of electromagnetic signals occurs at the cell membrane. Clearer understanding of the mechanisms underlying the transduction of chemical energy into mechanical, electric or osmotic work is needed. Investigation of how electromagnetic signals initiate the intracellular cascade of chemical reactions that control cellular homeostasis and function may be the next frontier breached in health care. Wellness in an energy-based CAM system conceptualizes a form of health that extends beyond the individual recognizing the interrelatedness of man and the planet.

Towards a new age in health care

A health care system that meets future demands is likely to need to be characterized by preparedness to modify currently reified paradigms and willingness to be open to alternative explanations while continuing to demand scientific rigor. For conventional medicine to meet the challenges of the 21st century, it will need to grow beyond the biomedical model. Molecular biochemistry has provided a solid keystone for biology but the era may now be dawning when biophysics replaces biochemistry as the foundation of health care. With further technological advances, improved diagnostic techniques may make it possible to measure currently undetectable energy fluctuation. A scientifically sound system of energy-based care may, in time, replace the current biochemical model. Rather than seeking to balance cellular biochemistry, the task of health professionals may be to harmonize energy fields. Cellular communication may come to be understood in terms of the efficacy of energy transfer generated by chemical interaction. The well-accepted free radical theory of ageing already postulates generation of destructive reactive particles during inefficient energy extraction from food in mitochondria. New age health care, instead of measuring chemical oxidative stress markers, may measure distortions of mitochondrial energy flow. Technological advances may make measurement of energy flow a reality, but successful advancement of new age health care would require that health professions remodel cherished paradigms.

Willingness to review currently accepted explanatory systems could enhance respect for the views of others and enable productive professional interaction. Accurate verifiable observations are a pillar of safe effective care; explanations used for various phenomena can, however, be erroneous. Interventions that are currently rejected as fallacious may well achieve acceptance if interpreted within a framework different to that of biomedicine. When homeopathy is considered to be an intervention based upon chemistry, it fails the test of logic. However, if dilution and succussion of substances results in changes in the physical structure of a remedy and it is acknowledged that water is a potential carrier of electromagnetic effects, then homeopathic intervention becomes more credible and the explanation starts to justify the popularity of this system amongst satisfied patients.

Scientific rigor remains an essential prerequisite for any successful health care system. The type of research methodology regarded as appropriate for gathering information and drawing scientifically acceptable conclusion is, however, open to debate. It would seem that both positivist and naturalist approaches could contribute. While the positivist approach derived from the agricultural-botany paradigm does not accommodate subjective variables, the naturalistic approach originating from the social-anthropological paradigm recognizes and measures both subjective and objective outcomes. It is within this type of research paradigm that the contribution of CAM therapies to patient wellbeing can best be evaluated. A common research paradigm may well provide the glue that binds conventional and CAM systems of health care and produces the symbiotic relationship required for a sustainable health care system. A potential candidate for such a role is the infomedical model.[39]

The best of both worlds

The infomedical model draws from the preferred paradigms of both conventional and complementary and alternative medicine. It is characterized by interactionism, indeterminism, monism, holism and self-organization. Interactionism replaces the notion of single with multiple interacting causes of both health and disease. By considering multiple interactions, this approach makes an invaluable contribution to promoting wellness and the management of chronic diseases. Indeterminism recognizes the difficulty of accurately predicting the outcome of clinical interventions in any one patient. Acceptance of uncertainty in clinical care becomes more tolerable when processed in the context of a system that is subject to multiple rather than unilinear cause–effect relationships. Monism, which sees mind and body as inseparable, is increasingly being validated by research in the area of psychoneuroimmunology. By rejecting dualism, the infomedical model furthermore obliterates the dehumanizing effect of the biomedical model.

Holism views individuals as greater than their component parts. It serves as a reminder to health professionals that clinical outcomes are optimized by multiple rather than single health-promoting interventions. Holism may hold the key to the inexplicable 'cures' occasionally encountered in disease care. Self-organization draws from vitalism. It goes beyond the notion of homeostasis and self-renewal and entertains the possibility of self-transcendence – both for the patient and the practitioner. The infomedical model regards the patient–practitioner encounter as an emancipatory experience for both parties.

By drawing on principles from both CAM and biomedicine, the infomedical model transforms the clinical encounter. The patient is expected to be an active participant rather than a passive recipient of health care. Instead of nurturing dependency, personal responsibility is encouraged. The practitioner is also transformed in this model. The detached scientist is replaced by the participatory carer. Reliance on technology is reduced and the use of interpersonal skills increased. Clinical success is no longer measured as an objective change in a pathological unit, but a functional change judged on both objective and subjective measures. The placebo-controlled double-blind study remains the gold standard against which various clinical interventions can be judged when selecting the best treatment option for particular diseases. In addition, results from case series are used to identify treatments that patients find helpful. Instead of requiring statistical significance, management that improves function and achieves substantive significance is justified within this model. As the aim of research is no longer 'universal' truth but clinical usefulness, case series assume renewed importance by providing the framework for context-sensitive inquiry. While continuing to appreciate the invaluable contribution of quantitative research, acceptance of information derived from qualitative research adds an important dimension to health care. The infomedical model, while complying with the need for scientific rigor, accommodates the multiple health and disease triggers to which individuals are exposed. It centres the individual, rather than the disease, as the focus of the clinical encounter.

A symbiotic relationship between conventional and CAM health care is not wishful thinking. At the level of a symbiotic integrated health care system, the structure that may evolve out of an integration of these schools of thought may well be three tiered. The lowest tier would be consumer based with self-help groups aided by lower-level health professionals. The second tier would comprise community-based clinics staffed by mid-level health professionals strongly influenced by the underlying philosophies contributed by CAM. Some medically qualified practitioners are already advocating and implementing this approach in the form of integrative medicine clinics.[40] The integrative medicine clinic is staffed by a team of health professionals representing different disciplines. The medical practitioner generally acts as the primary contact gatekeeper referring patients, as required, to other team members within the clinic. The success of such a clinic depends on employing a medical practitioner with a clear appreciation of the contribution that can be made by CAM practitioners. The third tier of this postulated assimilated health care system would be hospital based. Managed by highly specialized health professionals, the third tier would be dominated by the principles derived from the biomedical model. Although care at this level may closely resemble that of the current hospital system, intervention options could be expanded to include evidence-based CAM procedures. Another difference would be that patients requiring third tier care would be accustomed to taking increased personal responsibility. Furthermore, patients who are discharged after being successfully treated would return to a health care system more capable of managing their chronic underlying condition.

A sustainable new age health care system would need to initially focus on wellness through individuals taking personal responsibility for making prudent lifestyle choices. At the primary level, the aim is wellness, defined in the positive terms of total physical, psychological, spiritual, social, economic and ecological wellbeing. The first tier of health care with its focus on personal growth would empower individuals to achieve enhanced self-healing through health-promoting lifestyle choices. The second tier could focus on the early detection of disequilibrium or adaptive stress, on screening for disease markers at a stage when pathophysiological changes are reversible. Health at this level would include, but not be confined to, 'the absence of disease'. The third tier, focused on disease care, would largely replace the current health/disease care system. Individuals requiring care at this level would suffer the consequences of irreversible pathology; care would be aimed to relieve symptoms and limit complications. While the biomedical model is likely to remain the mainstay of third tier care, it would be transformed. Diagnosis and treatment based on biochemistry could be enhanced by new energy-based technologies. By changing the focus from disease to patient, the biomedical model would be humanized by a patient-centred approach. The connectedness of individuals to each other and their environment will assume importance in diagnosis and management even at this tier of health care.

The overall impact of such a health care system would be to shift the population norm to enhanced wellness. First tier care would encourage generation of a low-risk, rather than high-risk, ageing population. Second tier care would reduce the burden of disease by correcting aberrant physiology and reversing early pathology. Third tier care would seek to limit disability in a population whose cognitive framework is one of taking increased responsibility for personal wellbeing. A sustainable health care system is one in which mutual causality is matched by reciprocal participatory interaction. A sustainable health care system is one in which the financial burden of health care is minimized by each individual actively striving to maximize their wellness potential.

In perspective

Wellness requires the status of a lifelong endeavour. Health needs to become a valued goal if the challenge of caring for an ageing population on the tax money provided by a shrinking workforce is to be met. This text seeks to provide health professionals with some of the tools required to assist patients meet the challenges of realizing their potential for wellness.

References

1. Van Der Weyden MB. Debating health workforce innovation. *Med J Aust.* 2006;184(3):100–101.
2. Atwater A, Bednar S, Hassman D, Khouri J. Nurse practitioners and physician assistants in primary care. *Dis Mon.* 2008;54(11):728–744.
3. American Academy of Physician Assistants. *Issue brief: physician assistant scope of practice.* <http://www.aapa.org>; Accessed 02.11.08.
4. American College of Nurse Practitioners. *Frequently asked questions.* <http://www.aanp.org>; Accessed 03.11.08.
5. Roblin DW, Howard D, Becker E, et al. Use of midlevel practitioners to achieve labor cost savings in the primary care practice of an MCO. *Health Serv Res.* 2004;39(3):1–15.
6. Cooper R. New directions for nurse practitioners and physician assistants in the era of physician shortages. *Acad Med.* 2007;82(9):827–828.
7. Roblin DW, Becker ER, Adams EK, et al. Patient satisfaction with primary care. Does type of practitioner matter? *Med Care.* 2004;42(6):579–590.
8. Eisenberg DM, Davis RB, Ettner SL, et al. Trends in alternative medicine use in the United States, 1990–1997: results of a follow-up national survey. *JAMA.* 1998;280:1569–1575.
9. Esch BM, Marian F, Busato A, Heusser P. Patient satisfaction with primary care: an observational study comparing anthroposophic and conventional care. *Health Qual Life Outcomes.* 2008;6:74.
10. Brooks PM, Ellis N. Health Workforce Innovation Conference. *Med J Aust.* 2006;184(3):105–106.
11. Thomas K. The placebo in general practice. *Lancet.* 1994;344:1067.
12. Shepard M. The placebo: from specificity to the non-specific and back. *Psychol Med.* 1993;23:569–578.
13. De Deyn PP, D'Hooge R. Placebos in clinical practice and research. *J Med Ethics.* 1996;22:140–146.
14. Cacioppo JT. Social neuroscience: autonomic, neuroendocrine, and immune response to stress. *Psychophysiology.* 1994;31:113–128.
15. Ernst E. The value of chiropractic. *Focus Altern Complement Ther.* 2005;10:87–88.
16. Smolen J. Combating the burden of musculoskeletal conditions. *Ann Rheum Dis.* 2004;63:329.
17. Bronfort G, Haas M, Evans RL, Bouter LM. Efficacy of spinal manipulation and mobilization for low back pain and neck pain: a systematic review and best evidence synthesis. *Spine J.* 2004;4(3):335–356.
18. McMorland G, Suter E. Chiropractic management of mechanical neck and low-back pain: a retrospective, outcome-based analysis. *J Manipulative Physiol Ther.* 2000;23(5):307–311.
19. Wilkey A, Gregory M, Byfield D, McCarthy PW. A comparison between chiropractic management and pain clinic management for chronic low-back pain in a national health service outpatient clinic. *J Altern Complement Med.* 2008;14(5):465–473.
20. Haas M, Goldberg B, Aickin M, Ganger M, Attwood M. A practice-based study of patients with acute and chronic low back pain attending primary care and chiropractic physicians: two-week to 48-month follow-up. *J Manipulative Physiol Ther.* 2004;27(3):160–169.
21. Assendelft WJJ, Morton SC, Yu EI, et al. Spinal manipulative therapy for low back pain. *Cochrane Database Syst Rev.* 2004;(1) CD00047.
22. Hondras MA, Linde K, Jones AP. Manual therapy for asthma. *Cochrane Database Syst Rev.* 2005;(2) CD001002.

23. Proctor ML, Hing W, Johnson TC, Murphy PA. Spinal manipulation for primary and secondary dysmenorrhoea. *Cochrane Database Syst Rev.* 2006;(3) CD002119.

24. Jamison JR, Rupert R. Maintenance care: towards a global description. *J Can Chiropr Assoc.* 2001;25:100–105.

25. Rupert RL. A survey of practice patterns and the health promotion and prevention attitudes of US chiropractors. Maintenance care: part I. *J Manipulative Physiol Ther.* 2000;23:1–9.

26. Hawk C, Long CR, Perillo M, Boulanger KT. A survey of US chiropractors on clinical preventive services. *J Manipulative Physiol Ther.* 2004;27:287–298.

27. Nelson CF, Lawrence DJ, Triano JJ, et al. Chiropractic as spine care: a model for the profession. *Chiropr Osteopat.* 2005;3:9.

28. Jamison JR. Wellness: defining the way ahead for chiropractic in Australia? *Chiropractic J Australia.* 2007;37:2–6.

29. Yates RG, Lamping DL, Abram NL, Wright C. Effects of chiropractic treatment on blood pressure and anxiety: a randomized, controlled trial. *J Manipulative Physiol Ther.* 1988;11(6):484–488.

30. Plaugher G, Bachman TR. Chiropractic management of a hypertensive patient. *J Manipulative Physiol Ther.* 1993;16(8):544–549.

31. Bhatt SP, Luqman-Arafath TK, Guleria R. Non-pharmacological management of hypertension. *Indian J Med Sci.* 2007;61(11):616–624.

32. Alboni P, Alboni M. [Psychosocial factors as predictors of atherosclerosis and cardiovascular events: contribution from animal models]. *G Ital Cardiol (Rome).* 2006;7(11):747–753.

33. Cosford R. Electromagnetic fields: is there any evidence for biological effects and therapeutic applications. In: Cohen M, ed. *Holistic Health Care in Practice.* Clayton: Australian Integrative Medicine Association; 2003:74–83.

34. Hardell L, Sage C. Biological effects from electromagnetic field exposure and public exposure standards. *Biomed Pharmacother.* 2008;62(2):104–109.

35. Krewski D, Glickman BW, Habash RW, et al. Recent advances in research on radiofrequency fields and health: 2001–2003. *J Toxicol Environ Health B Crit Rev.* 2007;10(4):287–318.

36. Hardell L, Carlberg M, Söderqvist K, Hansson Mild K. Meta-analysis of long-term mobile phone use and the association with brain tumours. *Int J Oncol.* 2008;32(5):1097–1103.

37. Ho MW, Stone TA, Jerman I, et al. Brief exposures to weak static magnetic field during early embryogenesis cause cuticular pattern abnormalities in Drosophila larvae. *Phys Med Biol.* 1992;37(5):1171–1179.

38. Sharrard WJ. A double-blind trial of pulsed electromagnetic fields for delayed union of tibial fractures. *J Bone Joint Surg Br.* 1990;72(3):347–355.

39. Foss L, Rothenberg K. *The Second Medical Revolution.* Boston: New Science Library; 1988.

40. Hunter J. Establishing an integrative practice. *J Comp Med.* 2008;7:22–26 67.

Integration of wellness principles into chiropractic practice in the United States

3

Cheryl Hawk, DC, PhD

Background: health care issues in the United States

In the US, health care expenditures rose to \$2.4 trillion in 2007, comprising 17% of the gross domestic product (GDP). This runaway train of expense is the disastrous result of a century or more of the operation of a disease care model. Technological and pharmaceutical solutions have been sought for everything that ails humanity, from terminal cancer to obesity. Health care quality has been for too long equated with how 'high' the technology is and how many dollars it costs. Health care professionals have been paid to deliver procedures and drugs rather than to prevent illness or help patients become responsible for improving their own health and wellbeing. Alarming sequelae of this emphasis are the 38,396 US deaths in 2006 due to drugs – including drug dependence on or poisoning from both legal and illegal drugs[1] – and the 1999 estimate of 98,000 annual deaths from medical errors, which would make medical errors the sixth leading cause of death (see Figure 3.1).[2]

Counteracting this situation is a growing movement toward disease prevention and health promotion. The national 'blueprint' for health in the US, the Healthy People initiative, provides a detailed set of measurable goals and objectives to improve the health of Americans, emphasizing prevention and health promotion rather than disease care.[3] The initiative is organized and maintained by the Office of Disease Prevention and Health Promotion of the US Department of Health and Human Services (DHHS). A broad-based coalition of more than 400 organizations, including both public and private agencies, has partnered for this initiative. All recommendations are based on the most current available scientific evidence and are arrived at through a consensus of experts and public stakeholders.

The Healthy People initiative, currently in its *Healthy People 2010* iteration, began in 1979 with the report, *Healthy People*, from the Surgeon General of the US.[3] In an ongoing process, it gathers and analyses health data to revise the nation's goals and objectives every 10 years, beginning in 1980. Public meetings were held in 2008–2009 to begin the next iteration, *Healthy People 2020*. All government agencies, including state and local public health departments, plan programmes around Healthy People objectives, and are required to document their progress toward meeting them.

Under the broad goals of increasing quality and years of healthy life and eliminating health disparities, *Healthy People 2010* delineates 28 focus areas with 467 specific, measurable objectives to direct the nation's preventive and health promotion efforts. Box 3.1 shows these focus areas. The Partners in Information Access for the Public Health Workforce, a collaboration of government agencies, public health agencies and health sciences libraries, have developed a website which links the reader to a wealth of resources for each of these focus areas (http://phpartners.org/hp/).

Such national initiatives are driven by data such as the leading causes of death and disability, as well as the underlying factors which, in effect, 'cause the causes'.

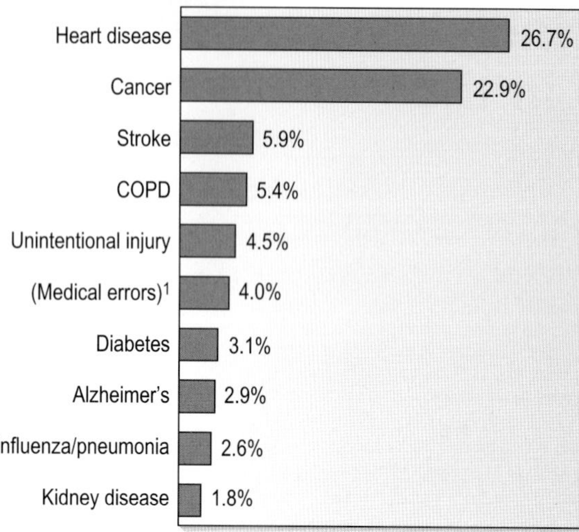

Figure 3.1 • Ten leading causes of death in the United States, 2004–5. Source: National Center for Health Statistics. *Health, United States, 2008 with Chartbook*. Hyattsville, MD: National Center for Health Statistics; 2009.[4] [1] Medical error data are 1999 estimates; source: Kohn KT, Corrigan JM, Donaldson MS. *To Err is Human: Building a Safer Health System*. Washington, DC: National Academy Press; 1999.[2]

As shown in Figure 3.1, the leading causes of death in the US are largely attributable to lifestyle factors.[4] This is demonstrated by the distribution of the determinants of health, which are behaviour, social and physical aspects of the environment, biology, policies, and interventions. Of these five determinants, behaviour and environment are responsible for over 70% of premature deaths in the US.[3] In fact, scientists at the US Centers for Disease Control and Prevention (CDC) conducted a study published in 2004 determining the 'actual' causes of death – the external factors to which the major causes of death can be attributed.[5] As summarized in Figure 3.2, over one-third of deaths are caused by tobacco use, poor diet and physical inactivity. Addressing any of these factors does not require high-tech strategies – it requires empowering individuals to make changes in their health behaviour.

Equally important to consider are the leading causes of disability, which in US adults are arthritis and back- and spine-related conditions (see Figure 3.3). In fact, the burden of musculoskeletal conditions is tremendous, accounting for more than 50% of chronic conditions skin people aged 50 and older in developed countries. In terms of lost wages and health care costs, musculoskeletal conditions account for nearly 8% of the GDP in the US.[6]

Focus areas for *Healthy People 2010*

1. Access to quality health services
2. Arthritis, osteoporosis, and chronic back conditions
3. Cancer
4. Chronic kidney disease
5. Diabetes
6. Disability and secondary conditions
7. Educational and community-based programmes
8. Environmental health
9. Family planning
10. Food safety
11. Health communication
12. Heart disease and stroke
13. HIV
14. Immunization and infectious diseases
15. Injury and violence prevention
16. Maternal, infant, and child health
17. Medical product safety
18. Mental health and mental disorders
19. Nutrition and overweight
20. Occupational safety and health
21. Oral health
22. Physical activity and fitness
23. Public health infrastructure
24. Respiratory diseases
25. Sexually transmitted diseases
26. Substance abuse
27. Tobacco use
28. Vision and hearing

Similarly to the leading causes of death, the most common causes of disability are associated with behavioural risk factors. Obesity is strongly associated with severity of symptoms and poorer outcomes in people with osteoarthritis.[7] Tobacco use, obesity, alcohol use and physical inactivity have all been suggested as contributing factors to poor outcomes in people with low back pain.[8]

Clearly, modification of behavioural risk factors is essential to improve the health of Americans as well as decrease health care costs. As evidenced by initiatives like Healthy People, US government agencies such as the DHHS and the CDC fully support an agenda which emphasizes changes in not only personal health behaviour but also policies that support such behaviour. This is consistent with the World Health Organization (WHO) advocating a paradigm shift toward integrated, preventive health

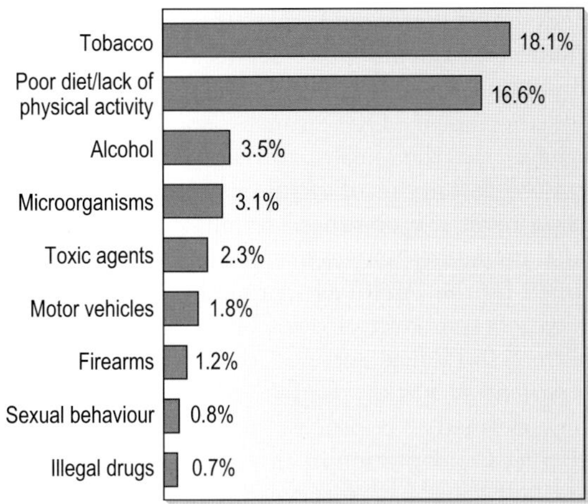

Figure 3.2 • Actual causes of death in the United States, 2000. Source: Mokdad AH, Marks JS, Stroup DR, Gerberding JL. Actual causes of death in the United States, 2000. *JAMA* 2004;291 (10):1238-1245.[5]

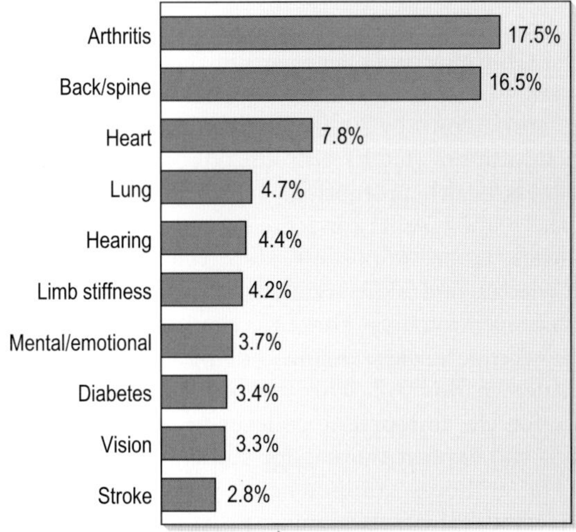

Figure 3.3 • Leading causes of disability, US adults. Source: National Center for Health Statistics, National Health Interview Survey, 2005.

care.[9] This paradigm shift is based on the worldwide increase in lifestyle-related chronic disease.

WHO recommends the following actions in order to integrate prevention into the health care system:[9]

- support a paradigm shift toward integrated, preventive health care
- implement policies that support preventive and health promotion services
- provide patients with the necessary knowledge, skills and motivation to gain self-efficacy in improving their health behaviour and health status
- include prevention in every health care encounter.

In the US, much discussion is taking place in both governmental and health care 'think tanks' and organizations about the best ways to implement the integration of prevention and health promotion into the system. The Center for American Progress, a nonpartisan research and educational organization, recommends that policies 'must focus on how best to engage individuals in their own health care'.[10] A professor at the Harvard Business School, advocating for a value-based system of health care reform, states that 'We need to radically reexamine how to organize the delivery of prevention, wellness, screening and routine health maintenance services ... We need structures for the delivery of specified prevention and wellness service bundles to defined patients population with unified reimbursement.'[11] He continues, saying that new delivery venues for prevention and health promotion services are needed, citing the success of worksite health clinics.[11] The Samueli Institute, an integrative medicine 'think tank," has developed a 'Wellness Initiative for the Nation' which makes well-thought-out and specific recommendations for shifting to a prevention and wellness paradigm that thoroughly integrates complementary and alternative medicine into the health care mainstream.[12]

Why adopt a wellness model?

Considering the exceedingly high costs of preventable death and of disability in terms of human suffering and financial resources, all health care providers need to take responsibility for contributing to the worldwide shift toward prevention. The leading actual causes of death – tobacco use, poor diet and physical inactivity – must be addressed not only at the policy level but also by direct provider–patient interactions. Since these issues affect general health and a myriad of conditions, all types of providers share this responsibility. Providers who treat patients with musculoskeletal conditions, the leading cause of disability, have a particular responsibility in this area. Doctors of Chiropractic (DCs) are perhaps uniquely qualified to address this issue, since such a high proportion of their patient population presents with musculoskeletal conditions, and there is substantial evidence that chiropractic is effective in treating them, especially those related to the spine and extremities.[13–15]

If the recommended shift toward integrated preventive health care does occur in the US, it would provide the chiropractic profession with unparalleled opportunities for integration.[16] Chiropractic in the US has traditionally operated as the 'Lone Ranger' of health care. Joining with the health care mainstream in prevention-oriented practice and community initiatives such as *Healthy People 2010* and *2020* is an opportunity for integration into the new prevention paradigm, at the ground floor.

The shift toward prevention for all providers could help the chiropractic profession integrate internally as well. Whether DCs consider themselves spine specialists, family practitioners or wellness practitioners, addressing the chief causes of death and disability is relevant to their practice. For example, tobacco use and obesity both negatively affect spine symptoms, and musculoskeletal conditions negatively affect patients' ability to be active and improve their general quality of life.

Requirements for adopting a wellness model

In order to responsibly deliver prevention and health promotion services, it is essential that chiropractors make ethical use of wellness concepts to promote patient self-efficacy rather than physician dependence. A certain segment of the profession has an idiosyncratic interpretation of 'wellness', in which the term is equated with a course of frequent and very prolonged office visits for correction of subluxations. Until there is a stronger evidence base for making claims that long-term chiropractic care does, in fact, contribute to disease prevention and health promotion, it will not help the credibility of the profession to set up such treatment plans. This does not mean that patients do not benefit from follow-up care, or that regular chiropractic care does not promote health and improved function. There is currently insufficient evidence either for or against such benefits.[17] It means that chiropractors must not overstate or misrepresent the evidence (or lack thereof) and should make rational, patient-centred decisions on the value of extended

schedules of care, and that they should always include well-documented services such as health promotion counselling as part of their care.

Furthermore, DCs must 'speak the same language' as the health care mainstream, using accepted definitions of terms. In particular, the profession must use common definitions of the terms *health promotion* and *wellness*. *Health promotion* is defined by the WHO as a process of enabling people to increase control over, and to improve, their health.[18] In clinical settings, this means *counselling the patient on healthy behaviours*. *Wellness* is commonly defined as a process of optimal functioning and creative adaptation in all aspects of life, emphasizing self-care.[19] It is important to emphasize that this is an active process in which the patient works toward health, not a passive state of receiving care from a doctor.

Chiropractors must become competent in the use of the vast and rapidly growing evidence base related to health promotion and disease prevention. Historically, like other health professions, chiropractic education has focused on symptomatic and episodic care. Chiropractic colleges are in the early stages of formally integrating this body of knowledge into the DC curriculum. In 2006, the Council on Chiropractic Education (CCE) introduced competencies in wellness/health promotion.[20] This historic addition to the requirements for accreditation of chiropractic colleges is an important step toward integrated knowledge and skills related to health promotion and prevention into the DC curricula in the US. The competencies delineated by the CCE are detailed in Box 3.2. This document creates a mandate for US chiropractic colleges to include standardized and explicit training for students in wellness.[21]

The wellness competencies were the result of concerted efforts beginning in 1999 from within the profession, specifically the Chiropractic Health Care Section of the American Public Health Association, of which the first milestone was the development from 2000–2002 of a 'Model Curriculum in Public Health' emphasizing disease prevention and health promotion. This project was supported by a cooperative agreement from the US Health Resources and Services Administration through the Association of Schools of Public Health.[22,23]

The result of the dissemination of the Model Curriculum to all US and Canadian chiropractic colleges was its adoption at several, which in turn stimulated further refinements and enhancements.[24–27] The National Board of Chiropractic Examiners also

Box 3.2

Competencies in wellness/health promotion for Doctor of Chiropractic programs in the United States required by the Council on Chiropractic Education*

Attitudes

The student must demonstrate an ability to:
- appreciate how lifestyle, health status, behavior, and psychological factors interplay in the overall health and wellness of the patient
- appreciate a multidimensional character of patient wellness, including the physical, intellectual, emotional, and spiritual dimensions
- appreciate and accept active patient participation as an essential component of health care
- effectively explain and appropriately emphasize the significant benefits that health promotion measures can have on response to treatment
- appreciate community-level health care issues and the doctor of chiropractic's role in community health care
- recognize and appreciate the significant impact that environmental influences may have on a patient's overall well being
- appreciate the broad social determinants of health.

Knowledge

The student must demonstrate an ability to:
- discuss the basic principles and perspectives of health promotion and wellness
- describe the concepts of health promotion in the context of chiropractic health care
- describe the essential components of health promotion appropriate for the needs of the patient and the public
- describe the role of the doctor of chiropractic in health promotion

- relate the specific needs of patients and the public to the lifestyle changes necessary for their health promotion
- identify the resources materials available to help educate patients and the public about health promotion and wellness
- identify the minimum screening activities for health promotion
- describe principal trends evolving in the implementation of, and health impact and affected population for each of the leading health indicators: physical activity, overweight and obesity, tobacco use, substance abuse, responsible sexual behavior, mental health, injury and violence, environmental quality, immunization, and access to health care
- describe the goals, issues, trends and disparities in the focus areas of increased quality and years of healthy life, and elimination of health disparities.

Skills

The student must demonstrate an ability to:
- communicate effectively with patients about aspects of their health including biological, psychological, social, and spiritual as part of comprehensive history taking
- use appropriate techniques to encourage patient participation in a shared responsibility for the patient's health
- implement recommended preventive screening activities
- perform common screening procedures and wellness assessments in different age groups
- provide patient counseling for health promotion and assess the outcomes of this counseling.

Source: The Council on Chiropractic Education. Standards for Doctor of Chiropractic Programs and Requirements for Institutional Status. Scottsdate, AZ: Council on Chiropractic Education, 2007.[20]

---

agreed to begin including more material on health promotion and disease prevention in the chiropractic licensing examinations, and to include questions on these topics in their *Job Analysis of Chiropractic* survey, the chief source of information on the content of chiropractic practice.[28]

The wellness competencies are being incorporated into the college curricula in various ways; they may be included in public health courses, diagnosis and assessment courses, courses on special populations such as paediatrics, geriatrics or gender health, or as part of clinical training protocols.[21,25,29] Some colleges have developed stand-alone wellness courses.[30]

For course content, all of these courses rely heavily on government resources such as those from Healthy People 2010, the United States Preventive Services Task Force, and the Centers for Disease Control and Prevention. This is necessary in order to ensure that chiropractic students can integrate with mainstream health promotion efforts as well as avail themselves of the vast extant literature on these topics. However, it is also useful for them to access resources that are specifically tailored to a chiropractic application yet are still highly evidence-based, such as *Maintaining Health in Primary Care*,[31] *Chiropractic, Health Promotion and Wellness*[32] and 'The wellness hypothesis' chapter in *The Chiropractic Theories* texbook.[33] In addition, a new public health textbook has been written from a chiropractic perspective, *Introduction to Public Health in Chiropractic*, with most of the chapter authors being DCs with dual degrees in public health and health promotion related fields.[34]

A model for chiropractic wellness, prevention and health promotion

In order to promote optimal integration into the movement toward prevention, it would be helpful for the chiropractic profession to have a model built around the concepts of prevention and health promotion. To be useful and utilizable, the model should be simple and intuitively obvious, and it must be:

- congruent with chiropractic principles and practice
- congruent with generally accepted practices and definitions
- relevant to patients' major health needs.

The US Preventive Services Task Force describes a simple model for the medical profession for clinical preventive services, which includes the components of: 1) screening for early disease and/or risk factors; 2) health behaviour counselling; and 3) immunizations and chemoprophylaxis.[35] Analogously, a model for *chiropractic* clinical preventive services would include the following components (Figure 3.4):

1. Manual procedures to promote homeostasis and optimal function.
2. Screening for early disease and risk factors.
3. Health behaviour counselling.

Underlying all three components is the concept of 'walking the walk' – the DC should model healthy behaviours while working in partnership with each patient to help him/her set wellness goals.

This is a streamlined version of a previously proposed wellness model for chiropractic proposed in 2003 in *The Chiropractic Theories*.[33] The underpinnings of this model are grounded in the principles common to complementary and alternative medicine (CAM) in general: vitalism, holism, humanism, therapeutic conservatism and naturalism.[33,36–38] Table 3.1 summarizes these grounding principles of the chiropractic wellness model.

Chiropractic Wellness Model

- Manual procedures to optimize function and promote homeostasis

- Screening for risk factors for poor health or injury

- Counselling to promote healthy behaviour and lifestyle

The doctor

- Models healthy behaviour – 'walks the walk'
- Partners with the patient to set wellness goals

Figure 3.4 • Components of a wellness model for chiropractic.

Table 3.1 Grounding principles of a chiropractic wellness model

Principle	Implications for chiropractic practice
Vitalism	• Assisting each patient's body to return to/achieve homeostasis is a necessary part of the wellness process • The purpose of chiropractic adjustments is to assist in restoring homeostasis
Holism	• Wellness is a multidimensional process • Health effects, both positive and negative, have multidimensional causes
Humanism (patient-centred care)	• The patient's needs are foremost • The patient and doctor are partners in the clinical encounter
Therapeutic conservatism	• Prevention is preferable to curative care, when possible • Anticipatory care should accompany curative care
Naturalism	• A natural lifestyle, including whole foods and avoiding drugs when possible, supports the patient's wellness process

Such a model provides a framework that is congruent with chiropractic principles yet congruent with mainstream health care, and lends itself to the development of research and educational programmes.[33,38–41]

The model should be congruent with chiropractic principles and practice

As stated above, the CCE recently adopted competencies in wellness for chiropractic education. However, even before 2006, the standards for DC programmes stated that 'the doctor of chiropractic's responsibilities as a primary care physician include wellness promotion (and) health assessment...' and 'the clinical training program must ... integrate health assessment, health maintenance and health promotion as elements of patient care.'[20] Furthermore, the Institute for Alternative Futures has stated that among the necessary conditions for the future growth of the profession are the accumulation of more evidence for the value of wellness and maintenance care, and an enhanced role in chiropractic for 'health coaching'.[42] The Association of Chiropractic Colleges, an organization to which all accredited US and Canadian chiropractic colleges belong, states that 'the purpose of chiropractic is to optimize health' and that this includes health promotion, preservation and restoration.[43] Thus. the wellness model proposed is congruent with traditional and current chiropractic principles.

It is also congruent with current chiropractic practice. The centrepiece of chiropractic care has always been manual therapy, specifically spinal adjustments to correct dysfunctional joint movement. The majority of US chiropractors also provide information and advice to patients about health behaviour, especially physical activity, diet and lifestyle.[44,45] Figures 3.5 and 3.6 further define this emphasis. Over 80% of US DCs responding to a 2004 national survey believed that all chiropractors should obtain information from patients on exercise, stress, diet, overweight/obesity and medication use. There were fewer topics the majority (over 80%) of respondents believed DCs should provide patients with information on; these topics were exercise, diet and stress.[46] For almost all topics, a higher proportion of respondents believed they should obtain or provide information than

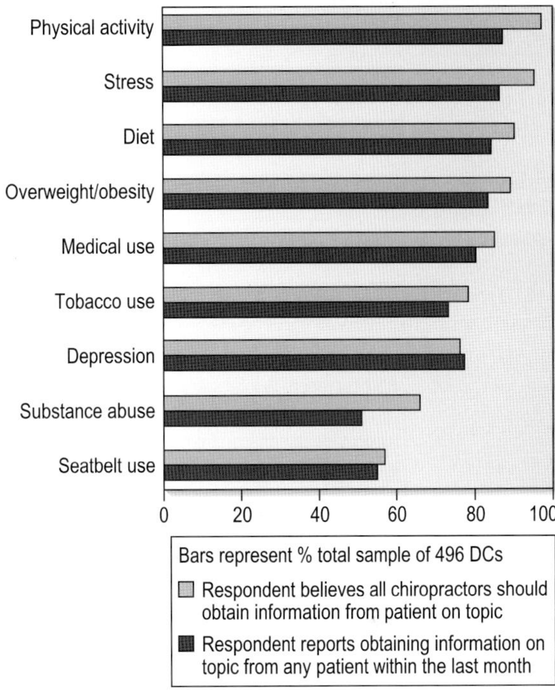

Figure 3.5 • Chiropractors' attitudes and reported behaviour related to health promotion services: proportion of respondents who agreed that chiropractors should **obtain** information from all patients in the appropriate risk category, by topic. Source: Hawk C, Long CR, Perillo M, Boulanger KT. A survey of US chiropractors on clinical prevention services. *J Manipulative Physiol Ther.* 2004;27(5):287-298.[46]

actually reported performing these services. This may indicate that they do not do health promotion counselling with all patients at every visit; however, they definitely believe that such services are within the purview of chiropractic practice.

The model should be congruent with generally accepted practices and definitions

As discussed briefly above, it is essential that chiropractors 'speak the same language' as others in the field of health promotion, disease prevention and wellness. The trend in chiropractic coursework and training to incorporate authoritative resources from such agencies as Healthy People 2010, USPSTF and the CDC is already addressing this need.[25,30] Table 3.2 provides a list of some of the most relevant resources available from the US government.

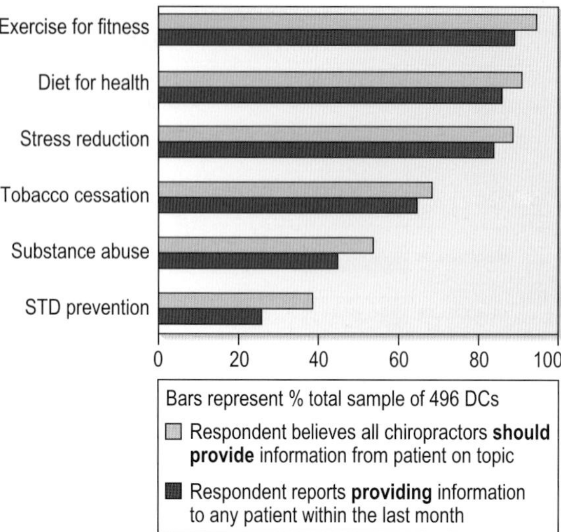

Figure 3.6 • Chiropractors' attitudes and reported behaviour related to health promotion services: proportion of respondents who agreed that chiropractors should **provide** information to all patients in the appropriate risk category, by topic. Source: Hawk C, Long CR, Perillo M, Boulanger KT. A survey of US chiropractors on clinical prevention services. *J Manipulative Physiol Ther.* 2004;27(5):287-298.[46]

Most materials are either downloadable or available either without cost or at minimal cost. Table 3.3 provides definitions for selected key terms related to wellness.[18,47,48] Figure 3.7 illustrates the relationship of the phases of prevention on the continuum of health.

Using accepted terminology and conceptual frameworks should not, however, be construed that chiropractors may not use manual procedures to promote wellness. Although there is very little evidence for such an effect at this time, there is no evidence against it.[17] What has not been adequately done is to make the connection between improved ability to function related to decreased pain, demonstrated in the many clinical studies of chiropractic care,[13–15] and an individual's quality of life and capacity to pursue their wellness goals. It is, however, important that DCs use appropriate terminology to discuss the theoretical effects of manual therapy on health. Subluxation, or joint dysfunction, is most appropriately viewed as a possible risk factor for negative health outcomes, rather than as a disease or outcome in and of itself – and one that needs to be explored in future research.[49]

Table 3.2 Resources available through US governmental agencies related to wellness, health promotion and disease prevention

Topic and Agency	Website
General prevention and health promotion	
Centers for Disease Control and Prevention	http://www.cdc.gov
Healthy People 2010	http://www.healthypeople.gov
National Cancer Institute	http://www.cancer.gov
National Center for Chronic Disease Prevention and Health Promotion	http://www.cdc.gov/nccdphp
US Preventive Services Task Force	http://www.ahrq.gov/clinic/uspstfix.htm
Overweight/obesity and physical activity	
BMI calculator	http://www.cdc.gov/nccdphp/dnpa/bmi/index.htm
BMI chart	http://www.consumer.gov/weightloss/bmi.htm
USPSTF. *Behavioral Counseling in Primary Care to Promote Physical Activity*	http://www.ahrq.gov/clinic/3rduspstf/physactivity/physactrr.htm
CDC fact sheets on physical activity	http://www.cdc.gov/nccdphp/sgr/fact.htm
CDC information on physical activity	http://www.cdc.gov/nccdphp/dnpa/physical/index.htm

Continued

Table 3.2 Resources available through US governmental agencies related to wellness, health promotion and disease prevention—cont'd

Topic and Agency	Website
Nutrition	
CDC 'Fruit and Veggies—More Matters' programme	http://www.fruitsandveggiesmatter.gov/
National Cancer Institute 5-a-day and other nutrition information	https://cissecure.nci.nih.gov/ncipubs/searchResults.asp?subject2=Nutrition
Injury prevention and control	
NCIPC fact sheets on injury topics	http://www.cdc.gov/ncipc/cmprfact.htm
Child safety brochures	http:www.cpsc.gov/cpscpub/pubs/chld_sfy.html
Child safety brochures	http:www.cpsc.gov/cpscpub/pubs/chld_sfy.html
CDC fall prevention	http://www.cdc.gov/ncipc/falls/FallPrev4.pdf
Substance abuse	
Fact sheets and posters on alcohol abuse	http://www.niaaa.nih.gov/Publications/PamphletsBrochuresPosters/English/
Tobacco cessation	
Free cessation counselling, by state	http://www.quitline.com
National Cancer Institute publications order form	https://cissecure.nci.nih.gov/ncipubs/searchResults.asp?subject2=Tobacco%2FSmoking
Surgeon General—tobacco information	http://www.surgeongeneral.gov/tobacco

Table 3.3 Definition of key terms

Term	Definition	Source
Health promotion	A process of enabling people to increase control over, and to improve, their health	WHO[a]
Phases of prevention		Woolf[b]
Primary	Preventing a negative health event from occurring	
Secondary	Screening (detecting early disease); reducing or removing risk factors	
Tertiary	Reducing sequelae of a disease, condition or injury; synonymous with 'rehabilitation'	
Risk factor	Characteristics, physiological parameters, symptoms or preclinical disease states that increase the likelihood of a particular health-related event.	Woolf[b]
Wellness	An active process through which people become aware of, and make choices toward, a more successful existence. Wellness is a process rather than a goal	National Wellness Institute[c]

[a]World Health Organization. *Ottawa charter for health promotion.* Geneva: World Health Organization; 1986.[18]
[b]Woolf S, Jonas S, Lawrence RS. *Health promotion and disease prevention in clinical practice.* Baltimore: Williams & Wilkins; 2008.[48]
[c]National Wellness Institute. *Defining wellness.* Stevens Point, WI: National Wellness Institute; 2006.[47]

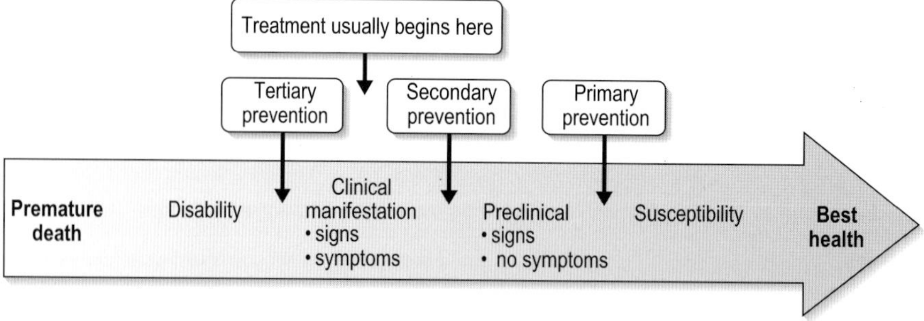

Figure 3.7 • The three phases of prevention in relationship to the continuum of health.

With respect to reimbursement of clinical preventive services, it is especially important that US DCs are familiar with the American Medical Association's Current Procedural Terminology (CPT) codes related to Preventive Medicine Services. The CPT codes are used for billing purposes in the US. Even though it is unlikely at this time that most insurance companies or other payers will reimburse DCs for such services, which include age-appropriate risk assessment, screening and counselling, correct use of these valid billing codes may pave the way for future inclusion as a regular part of chiropractic service coverage.

The model should be relevant to patients' major health heeds

As indicated in Figures 3.4 and 3.5, the major health needs of the public do not seem to be completely reflected by chiropractors' choice of health promotion topics. Certainly, physical activity and diet are very high on the list, but tobacco use, which has a slight edge as the leading cause of death in the US, was considerably lower, with less than 70% of surveyed DCs saying that DCs should provide patients who use tobacco with information on cessation.[46] This is consistent with other surveys of DC practitioners and students as well.[50–54] It could be that, because US chiropractic colleges do not provide standard training on talking to patients about tobacco use,[50,51] students do not have this important type of health promotion counselling in their 'toolbox' of clinical skills.

Also, related to the important concept of patient-centred care[55] is that the doctor should be sensitive to the health issues which the patient identifies as most immediate, while still being sure to call the patient's attention to issues which have the most serious impact, such as tobacco use, even if he or she is not currently ready to deal with that issue.

Based on the actual leading causes of death and disability in the US, as well as on the current identity of the profession as defined by consensus arrived at in 2005 by the Identity Consultation of the World Federation of Chiropractic, 'the spinal health care experts in the health care system',[56] there are key topics which all US chiropractors should be fully prepared to address in their patient populations, at minimum; certainly this does not exclude other topics from their purview as well. These are:

* physical activity and improved function
* healthy diet and weight management
* tobacco cessation
* injury prevention.

These topics will be addressed in more detail later in this chapter.

Wellness model attributes – aspects of the doctor–patient interaction

In order to provide patients with optimal assistance in their wellness process, the DC should develop certain practice attributes closely related to the grounding principles listed in Table 3.1. The chiropractic wellness practice should be patient-centred, holistic, and provide anticipatory as well as episodic care. These attributes will be explained in detail below.

Patient-centred

Although patient-centredness has been described by many authorities in many contexts, it will be interpreted here with respect to a wellness context. A practitioner must help the patient become actively engaged in his or her own wellness pursuit, in order to justifiably claim to be a 'wellness practitioner'. In fact, the term 'wellness coach' is being used with increasing frequency, acknowledging that the practitioner is only providing the patient with the necessary support to reach his or her own goals. Coaching is very much focused on goal setting for the purpose of making positive changes in the 'player's' life; it is much more of an egalitarian relationship than the traditional doctor–patient relationship. The Samueli Institute's 'Wellness Initiative for the Nation' calls for a national programme for training health and wellness coaches.[12] The demand for health coaches appears to be increasing, and the Institute of Alternative Futures recommends that one path the chiropractic profession might take is toward a greater health coaching or wellness coaching position.[42] Another important, and related, aspect of patient-centredness is that the doctor addresses what is important to the patient. This means that care is individualized for each patient, and that the doctor and patient form a partnership.

Holistic

DCs need to be familiar with the epidemiological concept of the 'web of causation' (Figure 3.8), which posits that disease, and health, are not caused by a single factor but by an interactive 'web' of factors. Wellness is multidimensional, and applies to all areas of life. The dimensions of wellness are categorized in several ways; Figure 3.9 uses one of the more common sets of categories. As shown in

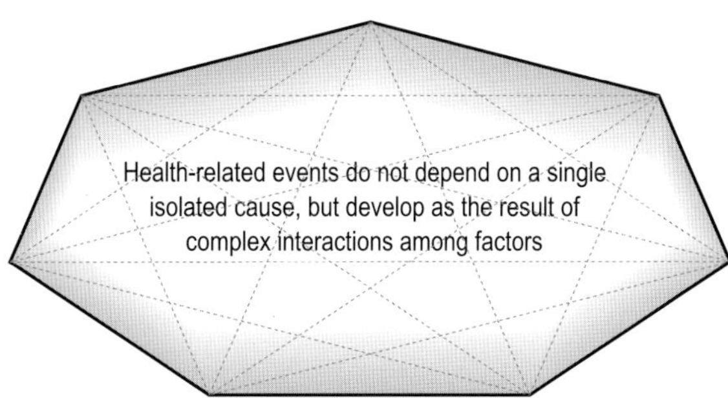

Figure 3.8 • The web of causation.

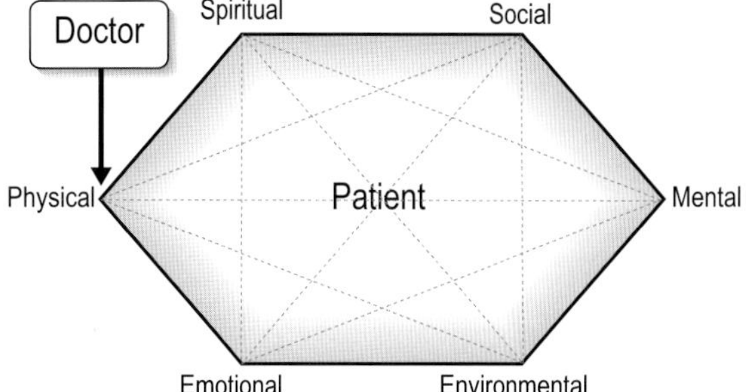

Figure 3.9 • The dimensions of wellness in the clinical encounter.

Figure 3.9, although the doctor may be applying a primarily physical intervention, all the other dimensions present in the patient and in the doctor–patient relationship are interconnected. DCs must understand that, although patients come to their office expecting help with physical problems, these causes are always interlaced with social, emotional, spiritual, mental, and environmental factors. This does not mean the doctor needs to be a psychologist or a minister! It does mean that the doctor appreciates the complexity of this web of interactions and that her or his office has access to appropriate referrals for appropriate additional resources.

Anticipatory as well as symptomatic/episodic focus

Anticipatory care refers to identifying and managing risk factors through early interventions. Referring back to Figure 3.7, anticipatory care would prevent risk factors from progressing into preclinical and clinical manifestation. Thus, it is an extremely cost-saving approach to care. It is always required to be included in the Preventive Medicine service CPT codes. However, patients usually present for symptomatic care – that is, closer to the left side of the continuum of health (Figure 3.7). Thus, it is essential that anticipatory care be included along with symptomatic/episodic care. Another way of conceptualizing this approach is to designate symptomatic/episodic care as 'illness-based thinking', and anticipatory care as 'wellness-based thinking'.

Illness-based thinking is oriented toward the present, and toward the patient's current chief complaint. Wellness-based thinking is oriented toward the future, and toward currently present risk factors that may lead to future negative health events. The key to using these concepts is to remember that the doctor needs to utilize both at the same encounter. Risk factor information must be recorded at the same time as chief complaint findings. This allows prevention and health promotion to be integrated into the care plan. Even though the patient may present with back pain (disability or clinical manifestation), he or she may also have risk factors such as overweight or tobacco use, which affect not only the course of the low back pain, but many other aspects of health as well. The doctor needs to directly address the chief complaint, but also begin to consider ways to help the patient address the accompanying risk factors.[48]

The wellness model in operation

Practising in a wellness model requires very little 'adjustment' for most chiropractors, since it is highly congruent with usual chiropractic practice. However, it enhances the emphasis on promoting and maintaining health, an emphasis lacking in the current climate of symptomatic disease care.

To ensure optimal emphasis on wellness, the chiropractic clinical encounter should be viewed as including three parts: assessment, intervention and integration.

Assessment

In addition to the usual assessment and diagnostic procedures needed for addressing the patient's chief complaint, it is essential the risk factors be assessed also, as explained above. Appropriate screening should also be included to identify early stages of disease. In keeping with the attributes of the wellness model, assessment should be holistic, as well as anticipatory. As detailed in Box 3.3, in general, assessment should include the following factors:

1. Assess lifestyle-related risk factors for disease.

2. Screen for depression, as recommended by the USPSTF.[35,57]

3. Screen for stress.

4. Assess general health status, which can be assessed by questions from the CDC's Behavioral Risk Factor Surveillance System (BRFSS) survey.[58]

5. Assess positive health – wellbeing or vitality.[58,59]

Box 3.3

Basic components of a wellness assessment

1. Risk factors for disease, including but not limited to:
   - Blood pressure
   - BMI
   - Tobacco use (former and current)
   - Physical activity
   - Diet (specific items: fast foods, fruit, vegetables, whole grains)
2. Screen for depression – example from USPSTF:[35]
   - 'Over the past 2 weeks, have you ever felt down, depressed, or hopeless?'
   - 'Over the past 2 weeks, have you felt little interest or pleasure in doing things?'
3. Screen for stress – example of one-page questionnaire giving a stress index score: http://www.themetabolic-institute.com/secure/pdf/life%20Stress%20Questionnaire.pdf
4. General health status – example:
   - 'For how many days during the past 30 days was your physical health not good?' (Source: CDC Behavioral Risk Factor Surveillance Survey[58])
5. Assess positive health – wellbeing or vitality:
   - 'During the past 30 days, for about how many days have you felt very healthy and full of energy?' (Source: CDC Behavioral Risk Factor Surveillance Survey[58])
   - The Global Well-Being Scale measures changes in wellbeing over short or longer intervals. It is a 10 cm visual analog scale anchored by 'the worst you could possibly feel' and 'the best you could possibly feel'.[59]

A separate aspect of assessment is identifying the patient's readiness to make behaviour changes. This will allow the doctor to tailor behaviour change strategies to the individual, which is in keeping with the recommended patient-centred approach. In this 'information age', patients are often overwhelmed with information from various media, and need assistance in actually utilizing the information and resources that are right for them. This not only will be more helpful to the patient, but also will reduce the DC's time spent in health promotion counselling.

One of the most widely used theories of health behaviour is the Trans-theoretical Model, which posits that there are stages of change related to health behaviour.[60,61] These are:

- pre-contemplation
- contemplation
- preparation

- action
- maintenance.

Table 3.4 shows the approach best suited to a patient in each of these stages. Using strategies appropriate for that patient's current stage increases the likelihood of success.[61]

Intervention

Of course, in chiropractic practice, manual procedures, especially adjustments/manipulation, are the primary type of intervention. The proposed wellness model views manual procedures as its centrepiece, for their role in optimizing function and restoring homeostasis. However, the application of manual procedures is not within the scope of this chapter; these are thoroughly covered during chiropractic training and post-graduate programmes.

This chapter deals with the health promotion counselling intervention. The focus of this counselling is determined by the needs indicated by the assessment as well as by the physical examination and history. As indicated in Table 3.4, the patient's stage of change will help the doctor determine what type of information and resources will be most useful, while also considering the patient's age, education, and preferences. For all patients, use of interactive tools to engage them in their process of change is extremely important. Exercise and nutrition diaries, BMI calculators, journals, and calendars are available in hard copy or online format.

Furthermore, the patient's entire experience when visiting the chiropractic office should support successful behaviour change. The clinical encounter should be carefully engineered to support the patient's wellness process. The USPSTF recommends the following components to most fully support successful behaviour change:[35]

- form a therapeutic alliance
- be responsive to patients' needs
- make the behaviour/health connection
- identify barriers to change
- gain commitment to behaviour change
- help patients target risk factors to change
- use multiple strategies
- design a plan for behaviour change
- monitor progress (follow-up contact)
- take a team approach.

Table 3.4 Stages of change

	Precontemplation	Contemplation	Preparation	Action	Maintenance
Characteristic	No intention to change	Aware of need to change	Planning to change in next month	Has taken action toward goal	Has been in action stage at least 6 months
	Lack of awareness	Thinking about change			
	Denial	May not know how to start			
	May feel hopeless				
Strategies	Raise awareness	Engage emotions/ motivation	Help set start date	Positive reinforcement	Continue action strategies
		Provide information	Develop plan/ contract	Engage support system	Positive reinforcement
			Identify support system	Establish rewards	Continue rewards
Tools	Health risk appraisal	Brochures	Diary		
		Websites	Join support group		

Integration with community resources

An aspect of wellness practice that is often overlooked is its potential for integration with community resources. Not only is it helpful to individual patients to be given referrals to local support groups, exercise classes, health-related courses, mall or nature walks and other community activities, but also it is helpful to the chiropractic practice to gain cultural authority and status in the community. Public health departments are required to participate in Healthy People activities, and having local chiropractors volunteer or refer community residents to participate is a mutually beneficial arrangement.

Patients' individual wellness processes can become exponentially more successful when they are connected with others with similar interests. Their chiropractor can be the conduit for helping them with this integration, and in the process gain integration for the chiropractor in the local health care community and community in general.

Putting it all together: management of key wellness topics

To conclude this chapter, examples of how to assist the wellness processes of patients with issues in key topics for the US will be presented, to illustrate the concepts presented throughout the chapter. These are:

- physical activity and improved function
- healthy diet and weight management
- tobacco cessation
- injury prevention.

Counselling on physical activity

It has been documented that advice on physical activity from a physician results in improvements in adult patients' fitness.[62,63] To maximize patients' success, the following components have been found to be necessary:

- Help the patient set a goal. Be sure it is not overly ambitious in order to help her/him succeed.

- Provide a written plan – some call it an exercise prescription, and have 'prescription' pads printed out for this purpose.
- Tailor the exercise regimen to the patient's preferences, access, and fitness level.
- Follow up! Flag patients' charts and ask them about their progress whenever they visit.
- Link patients to community resources such as: mall walks for older adults; YMCAs and other fitness centres for classes, swimming, etc. Community colleges often have a number of physical activity courses such as yoga, Pilates, tai chi, etc.

One useful option for a busy chiropractic practice is to connect patients with America On the Move (americaonthemove.org). This programme is explained in the section below.

Healthy diet and weight management

Although nutrition is a highly complex topic, its practical application for the wellness process of most Americans is very simple: eat whole foods as much as possible. Most people do not eat enough fruits, vegetables and whole grains. An important principle of counselling is that it is easier to do something than to restrict oneself from doing something. Therefore, it is usually more successful to counsel a patient to eat *more* fruits and vegetables than it is to tell them to *stop* eating fast foods and junk foods. Fruit and vegetables are so important to health that the CDC has a 'Fruit and Veggies—More Matters' programme (see Table 3.2 for website).

Thus, it will be beneficial in almost all cases to make the first rule of a wellness diet be to try to eat at least five servings of fruit and vegetables a day. This entails explaining serving size to patients: one small whole piece of fruit, or 1/2 cup of canned or cooked fruit or vegetables, constitutes a serving.

Another very simple recommendation that will benefit almost all patients who need to improve their diet is to increase their intake of pure water. Many Americans think they are hungry when they are actually thirsty. The DC should ask patients who drink large quantities of soft drinks if they are willing to substitute a glass of water for just one of those drinks. Gradually, as they succeed at making this change, they can be weaned away from soft drinks.

These two simple recommendations provide an opportunity for making a small, yet achievable and measurable change most patients can make – and it will give them a feeling of success and willingness to make further changes.

Weight management

Healthy diet and physical activity are the major components of weight management, although certainly overweight and obesity are conditions fraught with psychosocial issues as well. The key, as with any behavioural change, is to provide opportunities for success through planning small, incremental and achievable improvements.

One of the very simplest programmes for weight management, appropriate for even the busiest chiropractic office, is the America on the Move programme (americaonthemove.org). Its main components are:

- increase walking by 2000 steps per day over baseline (this expends 100 kcal)
- decrease dietary intake by 100 kcal per day.

Since one pound equals 3500 calories, this programme will result in observable, if not dramatic, weight loss over time. This exceedingly low-key approach has been shown to be effective in achieving significant permanent weight loss.[64] It is also helpful for arthritis, and can be done by people of any age or level of fitness.

Patients can be referred to the America on the Move website for materials. They can purchase step counters there, or the chiropractic office can purchase them and sell them to patients, thus making them immediately available when they start the programme.

Tobacco cessation

As shown previously in this chapter in Figures 3.5 and 3.6, US DCs do not emphasize tobacco cessation as much as physical activity and diet, even though it is an equally significant cause of death and contributes to decreased quality of life. It is essential that chiropractors join national efforts to decrease tobacco use. It has been documented that personalized advice from their doctor definitely influences patients to quit.[63] The busy chiropractic office can use a systems approach to efficiently integrate tobacco cessation counselling into the practice. These are:[48]

Box 3.4

Tobacco cessation: the 5 A's and the 5 R's*

5 A's: Patients willing to quit	5 R's: Patients unwilling to quit
Ask all patients if they use tobacco	**R**elevance
Advise users to quit	**R**isks
Assess willingness to quit	**R**ewards
Assist in making a quit attempt	**R**oadblocks
Arrange follow-up	**R**epetition

*Source: Fiore MC, Bailey WC, Cohen SJ, et. al. *Treating Tobacco Use and Dependence*. Quick Reference Guide for Clinicians. Rockville, MD: US Department of Health and Human Services, Public Health Service; 2000.[65]

- flag tobacco users' charts
- designate a staff person as coordinator
- use a progress card to keep notes
- post cessation information and make brochures available to show that the office is committed to tobacco cessation.

Concerning individual patients, the DC should follow the 5 A's and 5 R's of tobacco cessation,[65] listed in Box 3.4. The government resources listed in Table 3.2, at a minimum, should be used to provide every tobacco user with information which has been well-documented to be effective in helping users quit.

Injury prevention

Although chiropractors see patients with injuries every day, in the US they have not, to date, emphasized injury prevention as part of their health promotion counselling (Figures 3.5 and 3.6). Injury prevention is a health promotion field which is primarily practised at a community level, but there are some actions private practitioners can take to help decrease the incidence of injuries, which are the leading cause of the death in the US up to age 45.

Two simple actions the DC can take immediately is to ask patients about safety practices such as use of seat belts, child car seats and restraints, and bicycle and motorcycle helmets. Simply asking patients about these items increases their awareness of their importance. Second, safety checklists are readily available for home and playground safety for children, and for home hazards for older adults. These are listed in Table 3.2.

General principles for adapting the practice for wellness

The following principles will facilitate adapting the chiropractic practice for wellness care:

- Formulate goals and set priorities: these should be consistent with the office team's interests but also with the needs of the local population. Example: in a rural area, farm injuries and environmental toxins are priority issues, while in an urban professional area, physical inactivity and stress may predominate.
- Decide on an approach: is the practice oriented toward nutrition? physical activity? children's issues? senior health? If so, make it explicit and emphasize wellness in that context throughout the office.
- Function as a team: every person on the staff can help carry out the wellness message, whether on the phone, behind the desk, treating patients, or participating in local community activities, such as school athletics or local charities.
- Visibly emphasize wellness: using posters and brochures; providing pure water and healthy snacks; or ergonomic seating.
- Use a reminder system: colour code patient charts so you know what stage each patient is in and what his or her wellness interests are.
- Provide resources for patients: at minimum, provide referrals for wellness activities such as exercise classes, cooking courses, websites; or offer classes and lectures on wellness topics in your office.

Taking a holistic approach to wellness throughout the practice not only will provide patients with maximum support for their wellness journey, but also will also enhance not merely the chiropractors' standing in the community but the credibility and value of the profession as a whole.

Conclusion

Following a wellness practice model is more of an issue of organization than of changing a belief system, because chiropractic practice and education have traditionally been oriented toward a healthy lifestyle. Systematically ensuring that appropriate risk factor screening and wellness counselling are included along with manual procedures in every chiropractic clinical encounter is a way to enhance, not radically change, usual and customary chiropractic practice in the US.

References

1. Heron M, Hoyert DL, Murphy SL, Xu J, Kochanek KD, Tejada-Vera B. Deaths: final data for 2006. *Natl Vital Stat Rep.* 2009;57(14):1–134.
2. Kohn K, Corrigan JM, Donaldson MS. *To Err is Human: Building a Safer Health System.* Washington, DC: National Academy Press; 1999.
3. US Department of Health and Human Services. *Healthy People 2010: Understanding and Improving Health.* 2nd ed. Washington, DC: US Government Printing Office; 2000.
4. National Center for Health Statistics. *Health, United States, 2008 with Chartbook.* Hyattsville, MD: National Center for Health Statistics; 2009.
5. Mokdad A, Marks JS, Stroup DF, Gerberding JL. Actual causes of death in the United States, 2000. *JAMA.* 2004;291 (10):1238–1245.
6. United States Bone and Joint Decade. *The Burden of Musculoskeletal Diseases in the United States.* Rosemont, IL: American Academy of Orthopaedic Surgeons; 2008.
7. Rosemann T, Grol R, Herman K, Wensing M, Szecsenyi J. Association between obesity, quality of life, physical activity and health service utilization in primary care patients with osteoarthritis. *Int J Behav Nutr Phys Act.* 2008;5:4.
8. Pincus T, Santos R, Breen A, Burton AK, Underwood M. A review and proposal for a core set of factors for prospective cohorts in low back pain: a consensus statement. *Arthritis Rheum.* 2008;59(1):14–24.
9. World Health Organization. *Integrating prevention into health care.* Geneva: Fact sheet No. 172. WHO; 2002.
10. Center for American Progress. *The health care delivery system: a blueprint for reform* http://www.americanprogress.org; 2008.
11. Porter M. A strategy for health care reform—toward a value-based system. *N Engl J Med.* 2009;361 (2):109–112.
12. Samueli Institute. *A wellness initiative for the nation.* http://www.siib.org
13. Brantingham JW, Globe G, Pollard H, Hicks M, Korporaal C, Hoskins W. Manipulative therapy for lower extremity conditions: expansion of literature review. *J Manipulative Physiol Ther.* 2009;32(1):53–71.
14. Bronfort G, Haas M, Evans R, Kawchuk G, Dagenais S. Evidence-informed management of chronic low back pain with spinal manipulation and mobilization. *Spine J.* 2008;8(1):213–225.
15. Hurwitz EL, Carragee EJ, van der Velde G, et al. Treatment of neck pain: noninvasive interventions. *Spine.* 2008;33(45): S123–S152.

16. Redwood D. The health reform moment: peril and possibility in the Obama era. *J Altern Complement Med.* 2009;15(1):1–3.

17. Leboeuf-Yde C, Hestbaek L. Maintenance care in chiropractic – what do we know? *Chiropr Osteopat.* 2008;16(1):3.

18. World Health Organization. *Ottawa Charter for Health Promotion.* Geneva: WHO; 1986.

19. Cardinal B, Krause JV. *Physical Fitness: The Hub of the Wellness Wheel.* Dubuque, IA: Kendall Hunt; 1989.

20. Council on Chiropractic Education. *Standards for Doctor of Chiropractic Programs and Requirements for Institutional Status.* Scottsdate, AZ: Council on Chiropractic Education; 2007.

21. Evans MW, Rupert R. The Council on Chiropractic Education's new wellness standard: a call to action for the chiropractic profession. *Chiropr Osteopat.* 2006;14:23.

22. Perillo M. A model course for public health education in chiropractic colleges. *J Am Chiropr Assoc.* 2002;6:18–19.

23. Perillo M, Anderson E, Katz DL, et al. *A Model Course for Public Health Education in Chiropractic Colleges: A Users Guide.* ASPH Project H092-04/04. 2002.

24. Borody C, Till H. Curriculum reform in a public health course at a chiropractic college: are we making progress toward improving clinical relevance? *J Chiropr Educ.* 2007;21(1):20–27.

25. Globe GA, Azen SP, Valente T. Improving preventive health services training in chiropractic colleges: a pilot impact evaluation of the introduction of a model public health curriculum. *J Manipulative Physiol Ther.* 2005;28(9):702–707.

26. Killinger LZ, Azad A, Zapotocky B, Morschhauser E. Development of a model curriculum in chiropractic geriatric education: process and content. *JNMS: J Neuromusculoskeletal Sys.* 1998;6(4):146–153.

27. Rose KA, Ayad S. Factors associated with changes in knowledge and attitude towards public health concepts among chiropractic college students enrolled in a community health class. *J Chiropr Educ.* 2008;22(2):127–137.

28. Christensen M, Kollasch M, Ward R, Webb K, Day A, ZumBrunnen J. *Job Analysis of Chiropractic.* Greeley, CO: NBCE; 2005.

29. Redwood D, Globe G. Prevention and health promotion by chiropractors. *Am J Lifestyle Med.* 2008;2(6):537–545.

30. Hawk C, Rupert RL, Hyland JK, Odhwani A. Implementation of a course on wellness concepts into a chiropractic college curriculum. *J Manipulative Physiol Ther.* 2005;28(6):423–428.

31. Jamison J. *Maintaining Health in Primary Care: Guidelines for Wellness in the 21st Century.* London: Churchill Livingstone; 2001.

32. Gatterman MI. *Chiropractic, Health Promotion and Wellness.* Boston: Jones and Bartlett; 2007.

33. Hawk C. The wellness hypothesis. In: Leach RA, ed. *The Chiropractic Theories.* Baltimore: Williams & Wilkins; 2003:399–415.

34. Haneline M, Meeker WC. *Introduction to Public Health in Chiropractic.* Boston: Jones and Bartlett; 2009.

35. USPSTF. *Guide to Clinical Preventive Services.* Washington, DC: Agency for Healthcare Research and Quality (AHRQ); 2008.

36. Coulter I. *The roles of philosophy and belief systems in complementary and alternative health care.* Paper presented at: Conference on Philosophy of Chiropractic Education Toronto; 2000.

37. Coulter ID. A wellness system: the challenge for health professionals. *J Canadian Chiropr Assoc.* 1993;37(2):97–103.

38. Hawk C. Toward a wellness model for chiropractic: the role of prevention and health promotion. *Top Clin Chiropr.* 2001;8(4):1–7.

39. Hawk C. The role of chiropractic in providing clinical preventive services. *Top Clin Chiropr.* 1995;2(1):1–11.

40. Hawk C. The interrelationships of wellness, public health, and chiropractic. *J Chiropr Med.* 2005;4(4):191–194.

41. Hawk C. Are we asking the right questions? *Chiropr J Aust.* 2007;37(1):15–18.

42. Institute for Alternative Futures. *The Future of Chiropractic Revisited: 2005–2015.* Alexandria, VA: Institute for Alternative Futures; 2005.

43. Association of Chiropractic Colleges. *Chiropractic Paradigm.* Bethesda: Association of Chiropractic Colleges; 2008.

44. Rupert RA. Survey of practice patterns and the health promotion and prevention attitudes of US chiropractors. Maintenance care: part I. *J Manipulative Physiol Ther.* 2000;23(1):1–9.

45. Rupert RL, Manello D, Sandefur R. Maintenance care: health promotion services administered to US chiropractic patients aged 65 and older, part II. *J Manipulative Physiol Ther.* 2000;23(1):10–19.

46. Hawk C, Long CR, Perillo M, Boulanger KT. A survey of US chiropractors on clinical preventive services. *J Manipulative Physiol Ther.* 2004;27(5):287–298.

47. National Wellness Institute. *Defining Wellness.* Stevens Point, WI: National Wellness Institute; 2006.

48. Woolf S, Jonas S, Lawrence RS. *Health Promotion and Disease Prevention in Clinical Practice.* Baltimore: Williams & Wilkins; 2008.

49. Hawk C. Is it time to adjust our thinking about subluxation? *J Am Chiropr Assoc.* 2006;43(5):20–22.

50. Evans MW, Hawk C, Strasser S. An educational campaign to increase chiropractic intern advising roles on patient smoking cessation. *Chiropr Osteopat.* 2006;14:24.

51. Hawk C, Evans MW. Does chiropractic clinical training address tobacco use? *J Am Chiropr Assoc.* 2005;42:6–13.

52. Hawk C, Dusio ME. Chiropractors' attitudes toward training in prevention: results of a survey of 492 U.S. chiropractors. *J Manipulative Physiol Ther.* 1995;18(3):135–140.

53. Hawk C, Dusio ME. A survey of 492 U.S. chiropractors on primary care and prevention-related issues. *J Manipulative Physiol Ther.* 1995;18(2):57–64.

54. Hawk C, Baird R. "Chiropractors Against Tobacco" pilot project: a practice-based research study. *J Am Chiropr Assoc*. 2005;42:8–15.

55. Gatterman MI. A patient-centered paradigm: a model for chiropractic education and research. *J Altern Complement Med*. 1995;1(4):371–386.

56. Chapman-Smith D. The spinal experts: the profession reaches agreement on an identity. *The Chiropractic Report*. 2005;19(4):1–7.

57. Whooley MA, Avins AL, Miranda J, Browner WS. Case-finding instruments for depression. Two questions are as good as many. *J Gen Intern Med*. 1997;12(7):439–445.

58. Centers for Disease Control and Prevention (CDC). *Behavioral Risk Factor Surveillance System. Survey Questionnaire*. Atlanta, GA: US Department of Health and Human Services, CDC; 2002.

59. Hawk C, Dusio M, Wallace H, Bernard T, Rexroth C. Development of a patient-centered instrument for the assessment of global well-being: a study of reliability, validity, and clinical responsiveness. *Palmer J Res*. 1995;2(1):15–22.

60. Prochaska JO, Velicer WF. The transtheoretical model of health behavior change. *Am J Health Promot*. 1997;12(1):38–48.

61. Anspaugh D, Hamrick MH, Rosato FD. *Wellness: Concepts and Applications*. 7th ed. Boston: McGraw-Hill; 2009.

62. Bull FC, Jamrozik K. Advice on exercise from a family physician can help sedentary patients to become active. *Am J Prev Med*. 1998;15(2):85–94.

63. Kreuter MW, Chheda SG, Bull FC. How does physician advice influence patient behavior? Evidence for a priming effect. *Arch Fam Med*. 2000;9(5):426–433.

64. Hill JO, Wyatt HR, Reed GW, Peters JC. Obesity and the environment: where do we go from here? *Science*. 2003;299(5608):853–855.

65. Fiore MCBW, Bailey WC, Cohen SJ, et al. *Treating Tobacco Use and Dependence. Quick Reference Guide for Clinicians*. Rockville, MD: US Department of Health and Human Services, Public Health Service; 2000.

Self-care: the mindset

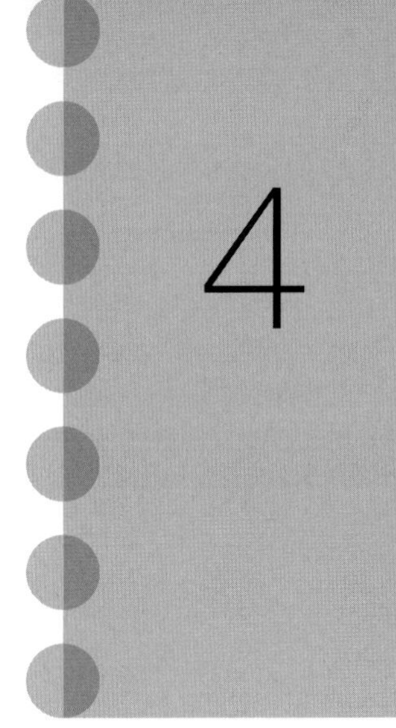

Points to Ponder !

- Wellness is not only a consequence of what one does, but also the result of what one thinks.
- Individuals benefit from self-care because of the way they think and the way they behave.
- Primary practitioners contribute to self-care by helping clients and patients realize their outcome and efficacy expectations.

Cost-effective health-promoting initiatives are urgently needed to offset the escalating health care costs of caring for an ageing population within a technologically advanced health care system. Increased personal responsibility in health care has emerged as a potentially productive option. In fact, Pietroni and Pietroni, in 1996, suggested that 'it is no longer possible to consider self-care as an optional extra in a package of health services. Rather, self-care should be seen as central to all clinical interventions and clinicians should be looking for new ways to involve people in their own health care.'[1]

Self-care encompasses individuals taking responsibility for maintaining a healthy lifestyle, recognizing, monitoring and actively promoting personal wellbeing, and using good professional care as necessary. Effective self-care requires a realistic perception of personal risk. Tobacco is implicated in the death of approximately 450 000 Americans each year and some 8.6 million people in the USA currently suffer from a smoking-caused illness.[2] Despite this, a survey of smokers currently smoking 40 or more cigarettes daily found 49% acknowledged they were at increased risk of cancer; 39% perceived an increased risk of myocardial infarction.[3] In this study, fewer than half of those smokers with hypertension, angina or a family history of myocardial infarction perceived their risk of a heart attack to be higher than average. Primary practitioners have an important role to play in helping their patients acquire realistic self-perceptions while preparing them to undertake appropriate, effective and safe self-care.

In order competently to promote self-care, primary practitioners do, however, require a new model of patient care. The biomedical model successfully promotes a one-dimensional form of health characterized by the absence of disease. Self-care encompasses a more comprehensive notion: it seeks to promote wellness. Wellness is a multidimensional construct that includes physical, psychological, social and spiritual aspects. Primary practitioners offering their patients self-care need to sever the shackles of the biomedical model and embrace a more holistic approach to patient care. The wellness model, with its focus on optimal functional integration, offers a viable alternative. The shift from the notion of biomedical health to wellness is contingent upon a paradigm shift characterized by a profound change in how the relationship between mind and body is viewed (Table 4.1). For a successful paradigm shift, conventional biomedical thinking will need to accept some of the premises upon which complementary and alternative medicine (CAM) is based.

The fundamental shift that has enormous implications for both patients and the clinical consultation relates to the relationship between mind and body.

Table 4.1 Models of health care

Characteristics	Biomedical model	Wellness model
Fundamental principles	Reductionism	Holism
	Dualism	Interactionism
	Determinism	Indeterminant
Valid and valued data	Objective signs	Objective signs and subjective symptoms equally valued
Outcome	Predictable based upon unilinear cause–effect	Unpredictable based upon mutual interaction
Outcome measurement	Pathological change	Functional change
Therapeutic focus	Disease	Patient
Clinical relationship	Contractual	Mutual exchange
	Dominant:submissive	Fiduciary
Patient role	Dependency: a passive recipient	Self-reliance: active self-organization
Practitioner role	Treat the condition with appropriate physical/drug intervention	Offer the patient psycho-emotional support and physical/drug therapy

Four perspectives dominate the ongoing mind–body discussion.[4] The physical monist view denies the existence of mental processes; other perspectives acknowledge mental processes but differ in their interpretation of the relationship between mind and body. Epiphenomenalists recognize mind but deny the possibility that mental processes may trigger behavioural events. Adherents to psychophysical parallelism have a dualist perspective and consider that mind and body do not interact, even though events in one sphere may be associated with corresponding events in the other. In contrast, the interactionist view suggests that mind and body interact and that the body dominates such communication.

The biomedical model takes a dualistic perspective; the wellness model, a monistic one. Recent research demonstrates that mental processes and physical functioning are mutually and bidirectionally interactive.[5] Such findings have contributed both to a re-evaluation of the communication style and patient–practitioner relationship supported by the biomedical model, and to the emergence of the wellness model. It is within this emerging framework that a mindset appropriate for managing patient self-care is developing.

The mindset for promoting patient self-care

The biomedical model has made a profound contribution to our understanding of disease. By separating mind and body, a genre of medicine based upon rationality and scientific method developed. The rules governing the growth of medical science were reductionism, determinism and dualism, the logic of enquiry being guided by the conviction that knowledge of the whole could be derived from an appreciation of the parts. The incomprehensible thus became understandable by exploring each part. Outcome became predictable within a framework of direct cause-and-effect relationships. The separation of mind and body ensured that only objective or measurable findings were pertinent. Signs – objective changes providing evidence of function or dysfunction – became the currency of the clinical encounter and the measure of both disease and therapeutic success.

A repercussion of the dualistic perspective is that the patient came to be viewed not so much as a person but as a disease. The clinical consultation focused on the disease, and therapy was prescribed to change the course of the disease. As thoughts were not deemed to have any causal role in disease within this framework, patients' feelings were considered to be of little importance and were sub-ordinated to biological changes. The biomedical model effectively meets the demands of acute life-threatening situations, but it is not particularly successful when used as a framework for managing chronic conditions and is inadequate when used to promote wellness.

The unquestioned assumptions of the biomedical model do, however, give only a partial explanation of clinical reality. Dissatisfaction with the biomedical model resulted in the search for a new perspective. The infomedical model described by Foss and Rothenberg provides a dynamic framework in which wellness can be more effectively contemplated.[6] At the primary practice level, the mechanistic biomedical model is gradually being supplanted by a dynamic model in which reductionism is replaced by holism, dualism by an interactionist form of monism, and uni-linear causality by the circularity of mutual causality.[6] The responsive and reflective nature of the infomedical framework provides an environment conducive to contemplating wellness and implementing self-care.

Within this evolving wellness model, the patient, rather than the disease, is the central focus. Patients' feelings and expectations are relevant clinical data. Patient thinking, along with physical, chemical and microbial factors, is recognized to influence clinical outcome. Disease and wellness triggers are being revisited: a mutual interplay of somatic and extrasomatic factors is envisaged in the initiation and progression of disease. Thoughts are perceived causally to influence the body. Emotions are conceptualized as interlinking the psyche and soma, social experiences and biochemical events. The system proposed is one of a reflexively and reflectively self-referential organization.[7] Clinical outcome within the wellness model is the probable consequence of numerous interacting events that cannot be viewed in isolation. An inevitable casualty of this transformation is the certainty contingent on a reductionist unilinear cause-and-effect perspective. As clinical outcomes are increasingly recognized as being unpredictable, uncertainty becomes the norm in clinical care. This non-linear or cybernetic circularity of the dynamic systems approach finds support in quantum physics and Jungian psychology.[8–10] Within the context of quantum physics, the distinction between objective and

subjective disappears, and health care becomes a total psychophysiological experience. Mutually causal links between genetic and symbolic factors, between matter and mind, are assumed.

Conventional health care is being reconstructed as an interpretative science in which dynamic inter-communication between the physical and the social body gives meaning to wellness.[11] Self-care extends beyond the confines of the biomedical model. It requires a new mindset in which statistical significance is replaced by substantive importance, in which the boundaries defined in quantitative research are shifted to include recognition of the results of qualitative investigations. CAM thinking, by broadening the horizons of conventional medical care, is changing the nature of the clinical encounter, especially at the primary level of health care.

Self-care: the epitome of mind–body medical practice

Although it provides a potential avenue for containing escalating health care costs, the real relevance of self-care is that it fundamentally enhances wellness. Self-care has the potential to achieve the high-to-low-risk population shift required for a workable health care system. Current research shows that we are not only what we eat, but also what we think. Self-care prepares us for healthy thinking and living. There is increasing scientific evidence to support the biological impact of thoughts and feelings. Medical thinking is evolving from the physiological emphasis on structural–functional explanations, through the analytical dominance of biochemistry and the mind–body dualism of psychosomatic disorders, to psycho-neuroimmunology. Psychoneuroimmunology focuses on the relationship between diverse psychosocial life events and the neuroendocrine and immune systems. It explores how the stresses of modern life can have physiological, behavioural and emotional repercussions. Psychoneuroimmunology studies the interaction between mind and body by focusing on how thoughts, feelings and actions may be linked to immune system activity and consequently to health and disease.[12] In this new monism, the body is construed as a system of intercommunicating processes in which all conditions are of the mind and the body. Chopra suggests that 'subjective reality and objective reality are tightly bound together. When the mind shifts, the body cannot help but follow'.[13]

This is a marked departure from reductive isolation, which stemmed from the notion that nature's order can be conceptualized in terms of universal constants. Where the biomedical model envisaged people as biological machines and patients as diseases, mind–body medicine conceives individuals as having an identity that transcends their material composition.[14] Form takes precedence over matter in a system of dynamic interaction in which the individual is perpetually undergoing self-generation and integration. The critical thinking, analysis and logic that have served technology well are emerging as being too simplistic when applied to such self-organizing systems.[15]

Within the biomedical model, symptoms and signs were interpreted in terms of empirical pathophysiology; therapy was intervention based upon an understanding of the cause. Such an approach is well suited to acute disease and emergency treatment. Within the wellness model, symptoms are interpreted in terms of their meaning to the patient, intervention focusing on reformulating the patient's self-understanding. The therapeutic goal within an infomedical framework is to help patients to achieve an understanding of their illness reality and to transform that reality.[16] This approach lends itself to self-care and the management of chronic conditions. Communication is re-emerging as a vital aspect of the clinical consultation: 'There is no empirical test for the meaning of experience, event or utterance; the only way to establish what an experience means to an individual is to enter into a dialogue with that person from which the meaning gradually emerges.'[17]

An acceptance of the intrinsic and inseparable nature of the dynamic interaction between mind and body implies the need to revisit the clinical consultation.[18] Both the patient's cognitive experience, i.e. the perception and appraisal of the symptom, its cause and the response to therapy, and the patient's emotional response – symptom distress – need to be addressed.[19] Patient care, as exemplified in the proposed management of psoriasis, needs to be expanded so that traditional drug therapy routinely includes stress-reduction strategies such as biofeedback, meditation and self-help approaches.[20] Patient–practitioner bonding that gains access to the core of the mind–body interface is believed to maximize the healing outcome.[21]

A prerequisite for evidence-based medicine is a logical explanation. A biologically satisfactory explanation for mind–body medicine is available (Figure. 4.1).

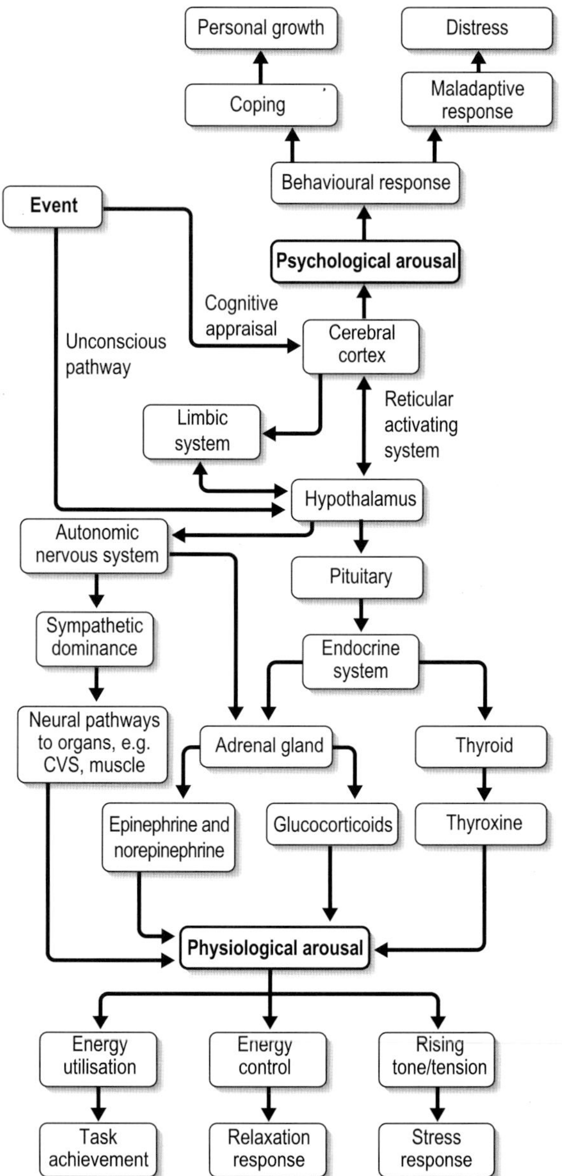

Figure 4.1 • Mind–body interaction.

The current understanding of the mechanism underlying mind–body interaction can be summarized as follows:[22]

The immune system is influenced by central nervous system processes that are shaped by social and psychological factors … we have found an orderly relationship between autonomic, neuroendocrinologic, and immunologic responses to acute psychological stressors, with different mediating roles played by the hypothalamic-pituitary-adrenocortical and sympathetic adrenomedullary systems.

The hypothalamus primes body 'tone' according to the intensity of stimulation from the reticular activating system, which receives motor and sensory information from the body. This basal tone is modified according to the information supplied from the limbic and cortical areas. The level of arousal is determined by physiological, emotional and cognitive information. The hypothalamus sets body tone through its control of the autonomic nervous and endocrine systems. The two major components of the stress response are the corticotrophin-releasing hormone (CRH) and the locus ceruleus–noradrenaline/autonomic sympathetic nervous systems.[23,24] CRH triggers the activation of the pituitary–adrenal axis and sympathetic nervous system. The locus ceruleus–noradrenaline system enhances vigilance and increases anxiety centrally, while the sympathetic arm of the autonomic nervous system acts peripherally through the adrenal medulla and peripheral nerves. The stress systems seem to interact with each other in a positive feedback loop. Stress causes disease when persistent arousal overload results in tonal exhaustion. Adaptation to chronic stimulation by the reticular activating system results in a lowered arousal threshold, and persistent sympathetic dominance tunes the body's arousal homeostat at a level at which the capacity of the individual to adapt to change is severely hampered.

Psychosocial stress provides a useful explanatory model for describing the dynamic interaction between thoughts and biology. Stress-provoking experiences may be routed to the immune system either via central nervous system activation of the sympathetic nervous system or through neuroendocrine pathways.[25] The sympathetic nervous system has adrenergic nerves terminating in lymphoid tissue. Neuroendocrine pathways that may influence the immune system involve, for example, the central nervous system and adrenal medulla, releasing various hormones including catecholamines, growth hormone, prolactin and endogenous opioid peptides produced by the pituitary. The interactive nature of psychoneuroimmunology is exemplified by stress causing the release of CRH, which activates the hypothalamic–pituitary–adrenal axis and the sympathetic nervous system. Cortisol and catecholamines released in response to stress bind to lymphocyte receptors and suppress the immune system. Lymphocytes, in addition to having receptors for CRH, adrenocorticotrophic hormone and endogenous

opioids, are themselves capable of neuropeptide production. Peptide messengers, cytokines and lymphokines produced by immune cells affect the central nervous system. Peripherally generated cytokines signal CRH neurons to activate the pituitary–adrenal counter-regulation of inflammation through increased glucocorticoid production. Immune cytokines act locally and centrally, recruiting central stress-responsive neurotransmitters:

> Peripherally generated cytokines, such as interleukin-1, signal hypothalamic corticotropin-releasing hormone (CRH) neurons to activate pituitary-adrenal counter-regulation of inflammation through the potent antiinflammatory effects of glucocorticoids. Corticotropin-releasing hormone not only activates the pituitary-adrenal axis but also sets in motion a coordinated series of behavioral and physiological responses, suggesting that the central nervous system may coordinate both behavioral and immunologic adaptation during stressful situations.[26]

Research has confirmed that chronic stress and depression can increase the peripheral production of proinflammatory cytokines, such as interleukin (IL)-6. High serum levels of IL-6 have been linked to increased risk for several chronic conditions, including cardiovascular disease, type 2 diabetes, mental health complications, and some cancers.[27] Stress-induced immune dysregulation has been shown to be significant enough to result in health consequences. Links between life's stresses and inflammatory responses have been found to have profound clinical implications.[28]

The phenomenon of neuroimmunomodulation has now been well established.[29] While 20 years ago anecdotal evidence and clinical observations suggested that exposure to psychosocial stress can affect disease outcomes in immune-related disorders such as viral infections, chronic autoimmune diseases and tumours, today research has shown that acute and chronic psychological stress are able to induce pronounced changes in innate and adaptive immune responses.[5] Changes are predominantly mediated via neuroendocrine mediators from the hypothalamic–pituitary–adrenal axis and the sympathetic–adrenal axis. Neuropeptide chemical mediators provide important links in the mind–body communication network. The limbic system, an area particularly rich in neuropeptides, is that portion of the brain especially concerned with emotion and motivation. Neuropeptides produced by the brain affect the immune system. Beta-endorphin, a natural opioid, for example, enhances the activity of natural killer (NK) cells, one of the first lines of defence against cancer and viruses.[30] A higher level of NK cells correlates with positive indicators of quality of life, for example social adjustment, while negative indicators, such as emotional distress, negative self-evaluation and perceived lack of social support, are predictive of a lower NK level and/or activity.[25,31,32]

NK cell function seems to be subject to voluntary modulation. A significant increase can be induced using stress management techniques. Increased NK cell function was detected in 10 healthy subjects who, for 1 hour over 10 days, undertook relaxation and guided imagery.[33] A short-lasting mild psychological stressor induced by unsatisfactory puzzle-solving or by a mental arithmetic challenge increased NK cell number or cytotoxicity, albeit only for a limited period (less than 60 minutes).[34]

Laboratory evidence of the impact of emotion on physical status is reinforced at a clinical level. A randomized trial in patients with mild to moderately severe asthma or rheumatoid arthritis found that those who wrote about stressful life experiences had a clinically relevant improvement in their health status at 4 months compared with those in the control group who wrote about emotionally neutral events.[35] Compelling evidence of brain–immune interactions influencing immunity and of immune system-mediated disease being modulated by psychological factors is growing.[36] It is increasingly accepted that stressors do not act indiscriminately but are filtered and interpreted by the brain. Patients' perceptions may affect wellness through both direct and indirect mechanisms. Concepts such as coping, control, helplessness and hopelessness require investigation in any comprehensive exploration of the mechanisms underlying psychoneuroimmunology.[37]

Behaviour: a mediator of wellness in self-care

Wellness is both directly and indirectly influenced by personal perceptions. Health values and beliefs lead to personal convictions that are a direct determinant of behavioural choice. Behavioural choices in turn influence wellness. A variety of lifestyle choices, such as the decision to smoke, drink alcohol or consume fat, influence macrophage activity.[38]

Macrophages carry receptors on their surface for numerous ligands, including neuroendocrine peptides and hormones. Once activated, macrophages secrete monokines. Excess secretion of tumour necrosis factor, a monokine, can cause myalgia, malaise, anorexia, fatigue and depression.[39] The decision to smoke appears to have wellness repercussions more subtle than an increased risk of cancer or ischaemic heart disease.

Both acute and chronic exposure to a stressful lifestyle has physical repercussions. Persistent exposure to psychosocial stimuli perceived as being stressful may induce a state of chronic anxiety-stress that may cause muscle spasm and present clinically as fibromyalgia and possibly irritable bowel syndrome.[40] Stress increases the risk of cardiovascular problems. Short-term mental stress, including the mental activity of problem-solving, can cause a temporary change in haemodynamic parameters. Mental stress has been shown to induce significant increments in heart rate, systolic and diastolic blood pressure, and platelet aggregation.[41] Haemodynamic parameters and platelet function tests, however, do return to baseline values after about 30 minutes. Studies have shown that individuals who exhibit exaggerated cardiovascular responses to mental stress tasks are at increased risk for developing hypertension in subsequent years.[42] Animal studies support the proposition that the haemodynamic concomitants of sympathetic activation contribute to atherogenesis and that animals exhibiting a heightened cardiac responsiveness to stress do develop extensive coronary lesions.[43] Epidemiological evidence strongly supports the notion that psychosocial data can predict, with considerable accuracy, cardiovascular mortality.[44] Recent reviews have concluded that psychosocial stress is a major independent risk factor for hypertension, coronary artery disease, and cardiovascular mortality.[45] Research also suggests that chronic psychosocial stress contributes to the pathogenesis of insulin resistance syndrome – a documented risk factor for heart disease.[46] Psychosocial stress is increasingly becoming regarded as a risk factor of similar magnitude to traditional cardiovascular disease risk factors for myocardial infarction.[47] Evidence linking psychosocial stress with heart attacks is so compelling that concern has been expressed that current guidelines for reducing the risk of ischaemic heart disease do not give consideration to managing psychosocial stress and depression.[48] Similarly, although hypertension management guidelines fail to include recommendations for patients to reduce stress, the 2007 Canadian Hypertension Education Program recommends considering stress reduction intervention for hypertensive patients.[49] Psychosocial stress is acquiring the status of obesity, diabetes, hypertension and smoking as a risk factor for cardiovascular disease.

Chronic psychosocial stress, in addition to its adverse effect on the cardiovascular system, also downgrades immunoresponsiveness.[50] Today, both subjective and objective stress not only can be associated with altered immune function but also have been shown to be linked to disease onset. Current thinking suggests that behavioural choices can affect immune function, and events that occur as part of immune responses probably modulate behaviour.[51] In addition to health beliefs affecting behavioural choices, there is evidence that perceptions directly affect wellness.

Perceptions: a direct mediator of wellness in self-care

While perceptions may influence health indirectly through lifestyle choices, they may also directly influence wellness through modifying physiological parameters. Popular literature on positive thinking has long ascribed to a mind–body perspective insofar as it has lent credence to how what we chose to believe becomes our reality; the subconscious mind accepts what the imagination conjures up. Research supports this perspective. Independently of standard coronary risk factors, self-reported job strain was significantly associated with ischaemic heart disease whereas objective classification of the components in the job strain model failed to support this hypothesis.[52] The literature suggests that symbolic needs can play a causal role in the production of disease: Foss states that 'not the substance but its meaning to the rat is the pathogenic agent of note' when discussing the finding that rats' conditioned expectation of cyclophosphamide produced the same effect as did the cytotoxic agent itself.[7]

The ability of the mind to influence the body is not a recently discovered phenomenon. The power of the placebo has long been reluctantly acknowledged in health care. Although current definitions of the placebo concept elude logical consistency and are fraught with contradictions,[53] interventions based upon a placebo response are likely to be somewhat effective in a large number of conditions. The generation of advanced medical scientists who rely on double-blind, placebo-controlled trials to reach scientifically acceptable clinical answers free of placebo distortion bear testament, albeit inadvertently, to the potential power of the placebo. It is only relatively recently that infatuation with the biomedical model has waned and the clinical benefits of the placebo acknowledged in conventional medicine. Despite 12% of respondent US physicians studied insisting that placebo use in routine medical care should be categorically prohibited, 96% believed that placebos can have therapeutic effects, with up to 40% of the physicians reporting placebos could benefit patients physiologically for certain health problems.[54] Although 48% of respondents surveyed did report giving at least one type of placebo treatment in a situation where there was no evidence of clinical efficacy, the desirability of a more personalized approach has emerged in conventional health care:

> Both randomization and blinding are intended to prevent patient variability and subjectivity ('placebo effect') from interfering with measurement of the 'true' effectiveness of the procedure. However, 'real life' includes variability and subjectivity, and real people make choices and decisions.[55]

Placebos seem to work best and most often to relieve pain; in disorders of the autonomic nervous or neurohumoral systems such as those regulating blood pressure, bronchial airflow or gastric acidity; and in depression, phobias and psychoneuroses. Most potentially reversible symptoms seem to respond, but there are also cases of diabetes, malignancy and angina that respond to interventions until recently regarded as placebo.

Necessary elements of placebo action appear to be both a dynamic relationship, real or implied, between doctor and patient, and a disease or symptom that varies in intensity in the same patient over time and in different patients.[56] Given this combination, placebo medications or procedures are documented to have a measurable efficacy and potency. Placebo intervention may furthermore have untoward effects (nocebo) in certain circumstances. The placebo response cannot be used to differentiate between organic and functional disorders.[57] In all instances, the process of administering and receiving placebo treatment is embedded in learned expectancies and symbolic meaning.[58]

Expectations are particularly important perceptions from a wellness perspective. Outcome expectancies are the belief that a given behaviour will lead to a particular outcome; efficacy expectancies are the belief that one can successfully execute the behaviour necessary to achieve the desired outcome.[59] Expectancies have even been reported, in certain circumstances, to override pharmacological effects.[60,61] Personal or vicarious experiences that create expectations of mastery; verbal persuasion and feedback from autonomic arousal all influence efficacy expectations. Techniques that practitioners can use to enhance a positive outcome expectancy include correctly predicting changes following intervention, enhancing the patient's awareness of minor positive changes, providing an understandable explanation of the presenting complaint, supplying feedback on how competently the patient is implementing practitioner instructions, and keeping patients informed of their progress.[62] Expectancies can be formed symbolically, and conditioning over a number of trials appears to be an effective technique to form expectancies.[63] What was in the past paraded as a placebo outcome of caring clinical care, in the context of mind–body medicine, can today be considered to be non-specific therapeutic intervention.

Clinical interventions that enhance the patient's psychosocial coping behaviour have been shown to have biochemical consequences. Under experimental conditions, it has been found that coping behaviour leads to the release of endogenous compounds that induce brain and behavioural changes similar to those resulting from benzodiazepine administration.[64] In contrast, when individuals think or talk about upsetting experiences, different coping and defensive psychological mechanisms and biological changes are evoked.[65] Coping gives some sense of personal control and is a powerful mediator of emotion.[66] The appropriateness of a coping strategy depends on the situation. When nothing can be done to change a situation, emotion-focused coping resulting in a change in perception converts a threatening predicament to a bland event. When something can be done to change a situation, task-orientated coping can convert a threat into a challenge and an opportunity. Coping depends on the appraisal of each situation.[67]

A number of phases have been identified in behavioural coping;[68] attention to each of these phases in the clinical situation can enhance health outcome. Particular coping strategies change from one phase of a complex stressful encounter to another. Practitioner support during the various phases of coping consistent with competent clinical care includes:

- establishing realistic health risk perceptions
- creating the belief that the selected approach will help
- providing patients with the information or skills necessary to acquire the belief that the implementation of the chosen approach is possible
- monitoring whether the exercise or mental task is actually being performed
- providing ongoing encouragement
- helping patients actively to record gains such as a reduction in distress level.

Self-care influences health both at a subconscious level and at a conscious level. It shapes wellness both through individuals' belief systems and through their considered lifestyle choices to meet perceived and actual health needs.

Why promote self-care?

Self-care is a powerful wellness trigger. It catapults individuals into a wellness lifestyle dimension that is a 'way of being'. Not only does self-care influence behaviour, it also affects thinking. Individuals practising self-care undergo a fundamental life change which transforms their health status from high to low risk.

Health professionals practising within the framework of the infomedical model create an environment conducive to fostering self-care. They help patients establish and achieve realistic wellness goals. The challenge is to facilitate clients and patients in formulating meaningful wellness outcome expectations and then to provide access to the knowledge and skills required for the successful implementation of the wellness ideals.

Both professionals who serve as successful self-care facilitators and clients who embrace self-care are transformed by their interaction within the wellness model of clinical practice. Professionals promoting and individuals practising self-care underpin a sustainable health care system.

References

1. Pietroni P, Pietroni C, eds. *Innovation in Community Care and Primary Health*. Churchill Livingstone: Singapore; 1996.

2. Campaign for Tobacco Free Kids. *Toll of tobacco in the USA*. www.tobaccofreekids.org/research/factsheets/pdf/0072.pdf. Accessed January 1, 2010.

3. Ayanian JZ, Cleary PD. Perceived risks of heart disease and cancer among cigarette smokers. *JAMA*. 1999;281(11):1019–1021.

4. Farrar MK. *Psychoneuroimmunology: implications for psychology of mind/body indivisibility*. Forrest Grove, Oregon: Pacific University; 1992 PhD dissertation.

5. Kemeny ME, Schedlowski M. Understanding the interaction between psychosocial stress and immune-related diseases: a stepwise progression. *Brain Behav Immun*. 2007;21(8):1009–1018.

6. Foss L, Rothenberg K. *The Second Medical Revolution*. Boston: New Science Library; 1988.

7. Foss L. The challenge to biomedicine: a foundations perspective. *J Med Philos*. 1989;14:165–191.

8. Zohar D. *Through the Time Barrier*. London: Heinemann; 1982.

9. Davies P. *The Mind of God: Science and the Search for Ultimate Meaning*. London: Simon & Schuster; 1992.

10. Chopra D. *Perfect Health*. Moorebank, NSW: Bantam Books; 1990.

11. Levin DM, Solomon GF. The discursive formation of the body in the history of medicine. *J Med Philos*. 1990;15:515–537.

12. Lyon ML. Psychoneuroimmunology: the problem of the situatedness of illness and the conceptualization of healing. *Cult Med Psychiatry*. 1993;17:77–97.

13. Chopra D. *Quantum Healing*. New York: Bantam Books; 1990.

14. Gunderman RB. Rethinking basic concepts. *Acad Med*. 1995;70:676–683.

15. Dugdale C. General practice and the new renaissance. *Aust Fam Phys*. 1995;24:746–749.

16. Good BJ, Good MD. The meaning of symptoms: a cultural hermeneutic model for clinical practice. In: Eisenberg L, Kleinman A, eds. *The Relevance of Social Science for Medicine*. Dordrecht: D Reidel; 1980:165–196.

17. McWhinney IR. Primary care research in the next 20 years. In: Norton PG, et al. ed. *Primary Care Research: Traditional and Innovative Approaches*. London: Sage; 1991:1–11.

18. Weinberg IR. Psychoneuroimmunology: a new concept in holistic health care. *Med Law*. 1994;13:205–211.

19. Rhodes VA, Watson PM. Symptom distress – the concept: past and present. *Sem Oncol Nurs*. 1987;3:242–247.

20. Farber EM, Nall L. Psoriasis: a stress-related disease. *Cutis*. 1993;51(5):322–326.

21. Cassel EJ. *The Healers Art*. Philadelphia: JB Lippincott; 1976.

22. Cacioppo JT. Social neuroscience: autonomic, neuroendocrine, and immune response to stress. *Psychophysiology*. 1994;31:113–128.

23. Chrousos GP, Gold PW. The concepts of stress and stress system disorders. *JAMA*. 1992;267:1244–1252.

24. Johnson EO, Kamilaris TC, Chrousos PW, Gold PW. Mechanisms of stress: a dynamic overview of hormonal and behavioural homeostasis. *Neurosc Biobehav Rev*. 1992;16:115–130.

25. Andersen BL, Kiecolt-Glaser JK, Glaser R. A biobehavioral model of cancer stress and disease course. *Am Psychol*. 1994;49:389–404.

26. Sternberg EM, Chrousos GP, Wilder RL, Gold PW. The stress response and the regulation of inflammatory disease. *Ann Intern Med*. 1992;117:854–866.

27. Godbout JP, Glaser R. Stress-induced immune dysregulation: implications for wound healing, infectious disease and cancer. *J Neuroimmune Pharmacol*. 2006;1(4):421–427.

28. Irwin MR. Human psychoneuroimmunology: 20 years of discovery. *Brain Behav Immun*. 2008;22(2):129–139.

29. Tausk F, Elenkov I, Moynihan J. Psychoneuroimmunology. *Dermatol Ther*. 2008;21(1):22–31.

30. Cohen S, Herbert TB. Health psychology: psychological factors and physical disease from the perspective of human psychoneuroimmunology. *Annu Rev Psychol*. 1996;47:113–142.

31. Birmaher B, Rabin BS, Garcia MR, et al. Cellular immunity in depressed, conduct disorder, and normal adolescents: role of adverse life events. *J Am Acad Child Adolesc Psychiat*. 1994;33(5):671–678.

32. Matsunaga M, Isowa T, Kimura K, et al. Associations among central nervous, endocrine, and immune activities when positive emotions are elicited by looking at a favorite person. *Brain Behav Immun*. 2008;22(3):408–417.

33. Zachariae R, Kristensen JS, Hokland P, Ellegaard J, Metze E, Hokland M. Effect of psychological intervention in the form of relaxation and guided imagery on cellular immune function in normal healthy subjects. An overview. *Psychother Psychosom*. 1990;54(1):32–39.

34. Brosschot JF, Benschop RJ, Godaert GL, et al. Effects of experimental psychological stress on distribution and function of peripheral blood cells. *Psychosom Med*. 1992;54(4):394–406.

35. Smyth JA, Stone AA, Hurewitz A, Kaell A. Effects of writing about stressful experiences on symptom reduction in patients with asthma or rheumatoid arthritis. A randomized trial. *JAMA*. 1999;281:1304–1309.

36. Ziemssen T, Kern S. Psychoneuroimmunologycross-talk between the immune and nervous systems. *J Neurol*. 2007;254(suppl 2): II8–II11.

37. Ursin H. Stress, distress, and immunity. *Ann N Y Acad Sci*. 1994;741:204–211.

38. Adams DO. Molecular biology of macrophage activation: a pathway whereby psychosocial factors can potentially affect health. *Psychosom Med*. 1994;56(4):316–327.

39. Smith RS. The macrophage theory of depression. *Med Hypotheses.* 1991;35:298–306.

40. Yunus MB. Primary fibromyalgia syndrome: current concepts. *Compr Ther.* 1984;10(8):21–28.

41. Grignani G, Pacchiarini L, Zucchella M, et al. Effect of mental stress on platelet function in normal subjects and in patients with coronary artery disease. *Haemostasis.* 1992;22(3):138–146.

42. Moseley JV, Linden W. Predicting blood pressure and heart rate change with cardiovascular reactivity and recovery: results from 3-year and 10-year follow up. *Psychosom Med.* 2006;68:833–843.

43. Manuck SB, Marsland AL, Kaplan JR, Williams JK. The pathogenicity of behavior and its neuroendocrine mediation: an example from coronary artery disease. *Psychosom Med.* 1995;57(3):275–283.

44. Eysenck HJ. Prediction of cancer and coronary heart disease mortality by means of a personality inventory: results of a 15-year follow-up study. *Psychol Rep.* 1993;72(2):499–516.

45. Khan N, Hemmelgarn B, Padwal R, et al. The 2007 Canadian Hypertension Education Program recommendations for the management of hypertension: part 2—therapy. *Can J Cardiol.* 2007;23:539–550.

46. Innes KE, Vincent HK, Taylor AG. Chronic stress and insulin resistance-related indices of cardiovascular disease risk, part I: neurophysiological responses and pathological sequelae. *Altern Ther Health Med.* 2007;13(4):46–52.

47. Rainforth MV, Schneider RH, Nidich SI, Gaylord-King C, Salerno JW, Anderson JW. Stress reduction programs in patients with elevated blood pressure: a systematic review and meta-analysis. *Curr Hypertens Rep.* 2007;96:520–528.

48. Ware WR. Psychological stress, insulin resistance, inflammation and the assessment of heart disease risk. Time for a paradigm shift? *Med Hypotheses.* 2008;71(1):45–52.

49. Khan N, Hemmelgarn B, Padwal R, et al. The 2007 Canadian Hypertension Education Program recommendations for the management of hypertension: part 2—therapy. *Can J Cardiol.* 2007;23:539–550.

50. Kort WJ. The effect of chronic stress on the immune response. *Adv Neuroimmunol.* 1994;4(1):1–11.

51. Riether C, Doenlen R, Pacheco-López G, et al. Behavioural conditioning of immune functions: how the central nervous system controls peripheral immune responses by evoking associative learning processes. *Rev Neurosci.* 2008;19(1):1–17.

52. Netterstrøm B, Kristensen TS, Sjøl A. Psychological job demands increase the risk of ischaemic heart disease: a 14-year cohort study of employed Danish men. *Eur J Cardiovasc Prev Rehabil.* 2006;13(3):414–420.

53. Gotzsche PC. Is there logic in the placebo? *Lancet.* 1994;344:925–926.

54. Sherman R, Hickner J. Academic physicians use placebos in clinical practice and believe in the mind-body connection. *J Gen Intern Med.* 2008;23(1):7–10.

55. Cassidy CM. Social science theory and methods in the study of alternative and complementary medicine. *J Altern Complement Med.* 1995;1:19–40.

56. Oh VMS. Magic or medicine? Clinical pharmacological basis of placebo medication. *Ann Acad Med Singapore.* 1991;20:31–37.

57. Brody H. *Placebos and the Philosophy of Medicine.* Chicago: University of Chicago Press; 1980.

58. Tursky B. The 55% analgesic effect: real or artefact? In: White L, Tursky GE, Schwartz GE, eds. *Placebo: Theory, Research and Mechanisms.* New York: Guilford Press; 1985:229–234.

59. Bandura A. Self-efficacy: towards a unifying theory of behavioral change. *Psychol Rev.* 1977;84:191–215.

60. Wolf S. Effects of suggestion and conditioning on the action of chemical agents in human subjects – the pharmacology of placebos. *J Clin Invest.* 1950;29:100–109.

61. Dinnersteint AJ, Halm J. Modification of placebo effects by means of drugs. *J Abnorm Psychol.* 1970;75:308–314.

62. Jamison JR. The placebo in clinical practice. In: Lawrence D, ed. *Advances in Chiropractic.* 3: Chicago: Mosby Year Book; 1996:319–343.

63. Peck C, Coleman G. Implications of placebo theory for clinical research and practice in pain management. *Theor Med.* 1991;12:247–270.

64. Drugan RC, Basile AS, Ha JH, Ferland RJ. The protective effects of stress control may be mediated by increased brain levels of benzodiazepine agonists. *Brain Res.* 1994;661:127–136.

65. Hughes CF, Uhlmann C, Pennebaker JW. The body's response to processing emotional trauma: linking verbal text with autonomic activity. *J Pers.* 1994;62:565–585.

66. Lazarus A. From psychological stress to the emotions. *Annu Rev Psychol.* 1993;44:1–21.

67. Antonovsky A. Pathways leading to successful coping and health. In: Rosenbaum M, ed. *Learned Resourcefulness: On Coping Skills, Self-Control and Adaptive Behavior.* New York: Springer; 1990:31–63.

68. DeGood DE, Shutty MS. Assessment of pain beliefs, coping and self-efficacy. In: Turk DC, Melzack R, eds. *Handbook of Pain Assessment.* New York: Guilford Press; 1992:214–234.

Communication: first-line wellness intervention

5

Health care in the 21st century is being challenged by changing circumstances. Medical advances have altered prevalence disease patterns. Instead of infectious diseases, non-communicable disorders now dominate. This transformation has fundamentally changed the characteristics of the clinical consultation (see Table 5.1). Instead of the majority of patients requiring acute, short-term medical intervention, they now require long-term care for incurable chronic conditions. Compared with the mid-20th century, the doctor–patient interaction in the 21st century is brief, with doctors viewed as providers and patients as clients.[1] Health care has moreover become commercialized and patients' health needs have become one of many considerations in the clinical consultation. 'As the 20th century ended, both physicians and patients had lost status. Federal reforms in Medicare, the national health insurance program for Americans aged 65 and over, and the exponential growth of managed health care in the 1980s and 1990s drastically changed the roles of both physicians and patients, reinforced the notion that health care is a commodity and it became increasingly unusual to discuss health care without referencing costs. Health care expenses rather than patients became the focus of US health care.'[1] The doctor–patient relationship has become a market transaction in which economic concerns are paramount to the perceived success or failure of the encounter. This has had widespread repercussions at all levels of health care (see Table 5.2).

The physician's authority, undermined by commercialization of the health system, is also being questioned by critical consumers. Instead of the paternalism of yesteryear in which the doctor was trusted to make the best decision in the patient's interest, consumerism drives the modern consultation. While physicians possess technical and medical knowledge, patients hold a definite value system and want more control over their wellbeing. Self-care is one area well suited for consumers to exert control and take personal responsibility. Within the wellness consultation, clients can enhance their autonomy in decision-making. Wellness consultations conducted within the framework of the info-medical model empower patients (see Table 5.3). With chronic conditions now dominating health care, the interest and increasing commitment of consumers to health partnerships provides a golden opportunity to start curtailing health care expenditure.

Levin defines self-care as 'the self-initiated and self-controlled application of knowledge necessary to the promotion of health, reduction of undesired risk, self-diagnosis and treatment of disease'.[2] In order for individuals to take personal responsibility for their health, primary practitioners of the 21st century will need to do more than promote health by merely screening for and diagnosing disease early; they will need to foster wellness. This may be achieved by helping individuals acquire new knowledge, change their behaviours and increase their

Table 5.1 The changing health care scene*

	Mid-20th century	Early 21st century
Changing consultation relationships		
Person seeking care	Patient	Client
Professional providing care	Doctor	Provider
Interaction	Implicit acceptance of doctor's clinical decisions	Questioning doctor's decisions
Consultation characteristics	Intimate: Patient–doctor relationship	Crowded: Patient, doctor, insurance company, government
Ultimate treatment authority	Physician	Insurance company or other third-party payer
Doctors evaluated on	Patient care	Patient turnover
Physician employment opportunities	Private practice/self-employed	Health care team/ Organizational employee
Changing disease typology: the impact and consequences		
Preponderant diseases	Acute, communicable	Chronic, non-communicable
Treatment aim	Reversion to 'normal'	Cope with irreversible condition
Clinical interaction	Brief	Ongoing

*Potter SJ, McKinlay JB. From a relationship to encounter: an examination of longitudinal and lateral dimensions in the doctor–patient relationship. *Soc Sci Med.* 2005;61(2):465-479.[1]

Table 5.2 A comparison of conventional, public and patient-centred care*

	Ambulatory biomedical care	Population disease control	People-centred primary care
Focus	Illness and cure	Prevalent diseases	Person's health needs
Relationship	Limited to consultation programme	Limited to programme implementation	Enduring personal relationship
Care	Episodic curative care	Defined by disease-control interventions	Comprehensive, continuous
Responsibility	Effective and safe advice at the moment of consultation	Disease control in targeted population	Health along the life cycle; tackling determinants of ill-health
Users	Consumers of purchased care	Targets of government disease-control programmes	Partners in self-care management

*Adapted from The World Health Report 2008. Primary health care – now more than ever. Table 3.1, page 42. http://www.who.int/whr/en/ Accessed 02.12.2008.

Table 5.3 The wellness consultation

Communication characteristics	Biomedical model	Wellness model
	Impose practitioner's (medical) reality	Negotiate a shared perspective of the patient's problem
Aim	Convey information to the patient	Facilitate patient understanding
Knowledge	Universal	Personalized
Information	Objective takes precedence	Objective and subjective
Ethos	Scientific appraisal	Empathic understanding
Process	Analysis	Synthesis
Practitioner attitude	Detached observer	Interactive carer
Focus	Disease, condition	Individual, client
Significance	Statistical	Substantive
Information processing	Objective problem-solving	Context-sensitive problem-solving
Dominant power base	Legitimate, expert, coercive	Referent, informational

health competence. Consumers require the knowledge and skills to undertake self-care. The primary practitioner of the 21st century has the dual role of clinician and teacher. Information-sharing becomes a priority. Patients are advising each other to 'educate yourself and ask questions'.[3] Physicians provide advice but patients make decisions. For patients to make informed considered decisions, physicians need to be good communicators. Medical education now includes formal assessment in communication skills.[3] An effective helping relationship consistent with self-care, in addition to empathy, positive regard and congruence, requires power-sharing.[4]

The clinical encounter

The interaction between patient and practitioner has a substantial impact on the clinical outcome. Clinical outcomes have been attributed to the natural history of disease, specific and non-specific interventions. A condition may remit spontaneously or may respond to a therapy that specifically targets the pathogenesis of the presenting complaint. Interventions that do not target the particular problem may, however, enhance overall wellness. It is well accepted that a non-specific therapeutic outcome is maximized when there is a good patient–practitioner relationship. The characteristics of that relationship would seem to include:[5,6]

- the combination of a practitioner who believes in the intervention and a patient with expectations of a positive outcome
- a patient supported by a caring group, the clinical circumstances in which demoralization appears to be counteracted being:[7]
  - a confiding relationship with a helping person
  - a healing setting
  - a rational conceptual scheme or myth
  - a ritual
- a patient–practitioner interaction that results in:
  - a positive modification of the meaning of the illness
  - the patient acquiring a sense of mastery or control over the illness.

The potency of the patient–practitioner relationship is not limited to the illness encounter but is at least as influential in the wellness consultation. An understanding of the dynamics of patient–practitioner interaction can contribute to a successful wellness consultation. The wellness consultation is most effective when the client is empowered by a clinician with referent power who bestows unconditional regard and positive acceptance.[8] Referent power operates when the individual feels valued and liked, and trusts and identifies with the clinician. Individuals are most likely to behave in a manner consistent with a set of norms communicated by those with referent power. Health professionals are most effective at influencing their clients or patients when these individuals identify with their practitioners.

Subjective validity results when the individual behaves in a manner consistent with a view held personally and shared with a reference group or person. Wellness behaviours are most likely to be maintained when they have subjective validity and are perceived to be internally controlled. Empowerment is the process of enabling the client to take control. It is fostered by clearly communicating the knowledge and skills necessary to achieve a rationally considered behaviour change. The successful wellness consultation is a participatory process during which the referent and informational powers of the clinician converge to change the beliefs, attitudes and behaviour of the client.

Modes of patient–practitioner interaction

Parsons, described in Bloom and Wilson, suggests that patient–practitioner relationships are best viewed within the framework of social roles,[9] as neither party can define its role independently of the other. The interaction consequently involves a meshing of viewpoints. The clinical encounter should be viewed in terms of reciprocity dynamics and mutuality. Role reciprocity is seen as a dynamic process with obstructing and facilitating factors. Factors that influence communication and satisfaction include:

* health sophistication: the practitioner needs to speak in lay language
* differences in social status
* discrepancies in cultural/racial/ethnic groups: the practitioner needs to guard against 'universalism', i.e. treating all patients alike
* the asymmetry of the therapeutic relationship: the practitioner has both professional prestige and situational authority; the patient has situational dependency
* the deviant role, sociologically speaking, of the patient. The legitimation of sickness permits individuals to withdraw, without penalty, from their normal work. The practitioner is inevitably an agent of social control.

Parsons suggests that the interaction between patient and practitioner is patterned and shows predictable regularities. In industrialized society, the sick role is institutionalized, the ill person being defined as 'needing help'. The sick person is obliged to accept this help and cooperate with the therapeutic agent. Patients, although relieved of their normal duties without penalty, are required to want to get well and to comply with the proposed therapeutic regimen. Incapacity, defined as illness, is a legitimate basis for exemption from one's normal role and task obligations. The patient is made dependent on the non-sick in society. The legitimation of the sick role, with its secondary benefits, is conditional upon recognition by the sick person that illness is an undesirable state, as well as an acceptance of the obligation actively to attempt to get 'well'. This also implies the requirement that competent professional help be sought.

In the Parsons' model, the practitioner is an authority figure who provides their 'best' care, with patients doing everything in their control to get well. The practitioner role in this relationship is one of support, permissiveness, denial of reciprocity and a manipulation of reward. Support is contingent upon the patient's continuing efforts to get well. Permissiveness encompasses patients being allowed to behave and express feelings not normally permitted in social relationships. Normal responsibility is waived in view of the illness. As a condition of support and permissiveness, the practitioner withholds interpersonal responsiveness: the practitioner has access to the patient's emotions, but the patient is not privy to the practitioner's feelings. The practitioner assumes a stance of 'affective neutrality'. Practitioners exhibit sympathy rather than empathy. They understand the patient's feelings without becoming personally involved. Practitioners also demonstrate 'functional specificity', i.e. they limit their attention and activities to a rigidly circumscribed 'medical' field. The practitioner manipulates reward – leverage ranges from a sick certificate to unconditional regard and approval. The possibility for abuse of power is inherent in any relationships with marked disparities in knowledge and power. This potential for conflict opened the door to medical consumerism. While the Parsons' clinical encounter is largely consistent with practice within the biomedical model, it is neither conducive to self-care nor reflective of primary care in a consumerist health care system.

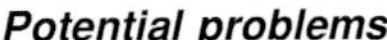

Problems arising in the adversarial mode: When refusing a work release certificate:
- use a cushion statement
- justify the refusal
- identify similar situations
- provide an alternative

Figure 5.1 • Saying 'No'.

Carmichael postulates three distinct modes of patient–practitioner interaction: adversarial, clinical and relational.[10] The adversarial and clinical modes are consistent with the biomedical model, the relational mode with the wellness approach. In the adversarial mode, the patient's primary motive is the legitimation of the sick role. The motive for the clinical consultation is to achieve the secondary benefit of exemption from normal tasks. The practitioner perceives that the patient's goal is a sick certificate, and the practitioner is viewed as a legitimating agent rather than a health professional.

Conflict can arise as a result of the patient's demands and the practitioner's responsibility to society as an agent of social control over illness, patient hostility and practitioner ambivalence being features of such clinical encounters. Figure 5.1 provides some practice tips for dealing with patients in an adversarial mode. An adversarial mode clinical interaction is inconsistent with promoting self-care. Only those modes of clinical consultation in which health care is the primary objective are compatible with the wellness model of health care.

Although disease management – and, by default, health promotion – is the objective of the clinical mode, this consultation is of limited use in promoting self-care. The patient assumes a dependent role and obediently follows the directives of the authority figure (the clinician). The acceptance by the patient of a passive role, instead of a fostering of increased personal responsibility, may result in untoward dependence on the practitioner. Figure 5.2 outlines a strategy to manage this clinical circumstance. An analysis of the patient's locus of control may be helpful in predicting which patients are more likely to become dependent.[11,12] The clinical mode epitomizes the principles of the biomedical model. Depersonalization of the clinical encounter due to objectifying the patient as a disease is exacerbated by the clinician's reliance on sophisticated laboratory investigations rather than patient information. The less harsh version of the clinical model is the paternalistic variant of the Emanuels' model,

Potential problems
Pitfalls for patients in the clinical mode. Patients may:
- feel a degree of dependency
- make frequent 'urgent' demands
- feel angry and rejected when demands are not met
- Pitfalls for practitioners in the clinical mode.

Practitioners may:
- encourage dependency
- feel rewarded when successfully meeting patient's needs
- perceives they are being manipulated – and react with anger and withdrawal

Tips for managing *interaction* in the clinical mode
- ☐ try to develop a tolerance for dependency
- ☐ explore the reason for dependency
- ☐ avoid becoming involved in dependency requests
- ☐ focus on underlying psychosocial problem

Dependency is a symptom of unfulfilled need.

Figure 5.2 • The clinical mode.

which assumes the use of shared objective criteria for determining what is best for the patient.[13] Although there is little or no patient participation, these models provide effective care in the acute emergency medical encounter. Neither lends itself to wellness care.

Wellness care is best achieved using either Carmichael's relational modes of guidance–cooperation and mutual participation, or the informative, interpretative and deliberative variants of the Emanuels' model. All these modes require active patient participation and are conducive to the practice of self-care. The difference between these modes lies in the extent of patient responsibility. In the relational mode, the reciprocal relationship that develops between patient and practitioner ranges from one in which the practitioner provides guidance and the patient selectively cooperates, to one in which patient assumes substantial personal responsibility for his or her health care. The Emanuels' modes fit along the spectrum described by Carmichael.

In the informative mode, the practitioner provides the patient with relevant factual information, and the patient, using personal values, selects the preferred intervention. In the interpretative mode, the practitioner elucidates the patient's values and wants, and then helps with the selection of an intervention. In the deliberative mode, the practitioner provides factual information and clarifies the types of value embodied in each option. There is less patient participation than in the interpretative variant as the practitioner also explains why certain health-related options are more worthy and should be aspired towards. In each of these instances, when the focus is on self-care and the objective is wellness, the helping relationship can, instead of being between patient and practitioner, be between client and health professional.

Elements in the communication game

The currency of patient–practitioner or client–clinician interaction is communication. The power of practitioner communication and the consultation process has long been recognized.[14–16] A study comparing the clinical outcome of four groups of patients found that patients who enjoyed a positive clinical consultation fared better than those who had a negative one, regardless of any associated placebo drug therapy.[14] The practitioner's performance as an information resource is a good predictor of patient satisfaction.

When the practitioner is acting as an information resource, both the content or message and the communication process employed deserve consideration. The results of a study on clinical information exchange suggest that practitioners could sacrifice explanations of aetiology and prognosis with little loss of satisfaction and might achieve greater patient satisfaction by exploring ideas, concerns, expectations and the potential effects of the condition and the intervention.[17] The relevance and quality of information provided appears to be more important than its quantity. Attending to the concepts, perceptions and views of the patient appears to offer a more effective strategy for consultation management than does providing vast amounts of standardized information. By selectively tailoring the message, practitioners can enhance patient compliance and formulate treatment programmes consistent with the patient's lifestyle and expectations.

Practice within the wellness model can also be enhanced by effectively using the communication process. Communication can serve as a wellness trigger, the practitioner's personal communication technique influencing the efficiency of the clinician as an instrument of healing. An understanding of the communication process may therefore prove useful. Two processes, encoding and decoding, are simultaneously undertaken during the clinical encounter. During encoding, a message is being prepared with respect to its factual information and is presented in the context of the speaker's lifeworld. Patients' presenting complaints provide information about their biological state in the context of their socio-cultural belief system, coloured by their emotional experience. During decoding, the message is interpreted by the recipient. The practitioner's message to the patient may be distorted by:

* environmental noise: the patient may find the consultation environment intimidating and be distracted by unspoken fears
* biological variables such as fatigue, pain or emotional distress
* social factors such as a dislike of the patient role
* structural circumstances such as a cultural difference in the meaning of non-verbal cues
* language or vocabulary discrepancies.

Communication is both verbal and non-verbal.[18,19] Verbal questions posed by the practitioner can be categorized into those which seek to ascertain recall, remember facts or provide information, and those which explore the patient or client's expectations and perceptions. The format of the questions asked by the practitioner may be closed, open or multiple. Closed questions are useful for gaining factual information, for example ascertaining the presence or absence of symptoms. With open questions, it is possible to obtain diverse information. Such questions can be used to explore the patient's perceptions, opinion, judgment, evaluation and/or prediction. Open questions may be:

* affective, assessing emotions, attitudes and feelings
* leading, in order to confirm expected clinical data
* probing, to seek clarification, confirm relevance or exemplify.

Questions can also be multiple, patients being offered a structured choice.

Figure 5.3 provides practice tips for listening.

Non-verbal communication used by clinicians includes:[19,20]

* silence: a pause may be used to draw attention or facilitate listening
* proactive listening, which involves paraphrasing the content or feeling and/or reflecting feeling
* eye contact, helpful for achieving emotional connection
* bodily gesture and personal appearance
* space: personal space is less than 30 cm (12 in), family space is 30–60 cm (12–24 in), social space is 60–90 cm (24–36 in) and conference space exceeds 90 cm (36 in). Clinicians, by virtue of their examination procedures, invade personal

Perceptive or active listening is a prerequisite to good communication.

Barriers to listening include:
- preconceptions and prejudices
- being self- rather than other-centred
- being in a hurry
- stress
- wandering attention. The brain thinks faster than we can speak and therefore thoughts may wander

Tips for listening:
- Try to understand the meaning behind the words
- Be open minded
- Don't interrupt – know when to be silent
- Use non-verbal communication to indicate interest/attention
- Ask questions
- Make a mental checklist of what has been said
- Don't react to emotive phrases – respond when the speaker has finished
- Screen out distractions
- Start listening from the first word/sentence
- Don't pretend to listen, actually listen

Figure 5.3 • Listening.

space, which inevitably affects the patient. The psychoemotional impact of the physical examination is greatly influenced by the cultural background of the patient

- physical environment, a comfortable restful environment being conducive to openness

- time.

Figure 5.4 demonstrates how patients or clients can convey information to the practitioner about their

The anxious patient:
- dilated pupils
- trembling dry mouth
- raised eyebrows
- shallow rapid respiration
- erect stance
- fine tremor of the hands
- 'ready for flight'

The grieving/sad patient:
- downcast red eyes
- slow sighing respiration
- soft speech
- slouched posture
- limpness/lack of energy

The angry patient:
- frowning forehead
- knitted brows
- clenched teeth
- tense grin
- loud precise speech outbursts
- clenched hands
- tense muscles
- explosive energy

Figure 5.4 • Non-verbal clues to psychoemotional status.

emotional state using non-verbal cues. Despite culturally mediated differences, useful information about the person's emotional state is mediated through non-verbal information. Careful observation of non-verbal information can give information about:

- the nature of the patient's feelings
- the intensity of the patient's feelings
- the amount of emotional control that the patient has over the feelings.

The particular mannerisms, postures and gestures used to express feelings, however, may differ from culture to culture. The expression of feeling thus occurs against the background of the patient's culture.

The communication process

Both healing and wellness clinical encounters take place in a context of sincerity and respect. Unconditional positive regard provides a psychoemotional environment that helps clients and patients reveal the diverse dimensions of their aspirations and problems. As all aspects of the patient's wellness objectives have implications for management, it is desirable for practitioners to become aware of diverse factors affecting patient health. Practitioners create a milieu conducive to client or patient disclosure by demonstrating genuineness and respect. Genuineness is conveyed by:

- a spontaneous but not uncontrolled relationship
- remaining open even when feeling threatened or being criticized
- being consistent: discrepancies in the practitioner's values, behaviours, thoughts and words should be avoided
- being tactful yet forthright.

Persons perceive that they are respected when the practitioner demonstrates attentive and active listening, is flexible, consistent, spontaneous and open, and is assertive. Respect is characterized by:

- recognizing the patient as unique
- acknowledging the patient's right to self-determination and active participation in the clinical encounter
- being committed to and capable of improving the patient's health status
- maintaining confidentiality.

Individuals are further encouraged to participate when their statements are met with acceptance, when information sources are shared and when social distance is reduced by highlighting similarities.

The basic skills demonstrated by an effective communicator are attending, active listening, empathy and questioning. Non-verbal communication can also convey that the practitioner is listening. Non-verbal listening behaviour is engaged by sitting squarely facing the client, leaning towards the client, assuming a relaxed, open posture and using eye contact. Active listening includes a sensitive appraisal of the client's message. An analysis of client information into the categories of experience, behaviour and feelings provides a useful analytical framework. Experiences, the person's subjective account, are accurately documented as symptoms. An initial working diagnosis is based upon this account, being clarified by actively searching for confirmatory evidence (signs) during the physical examination.

The behaviours or strategy used by the individual to cope with the clinical experience provides information on the client's coping skills and social support system. Both verbal and non-verbal responses provide useful information when making personalized management decisions. In addition to listening, good communicators are observant. Over 90% of the message is conveyed by non-verbal behaviour. Non-verbal behaviour provides information on the nature of the patient's feelings, the intensity with which the feeling is experienced and the amount of emotional control that the person has in relation to the current problem. The emotional environment of the consultation is critical. Empathy, 'walking in the shoes of the patient', fosters a clinical atmosphere conducive to unburdening. By demonstrating an understanding of what the patient is experiencing, the practitioner can achieve an empathic relationship. Communicating an understanding of the patient's core message includes reflecting back the clinical experience of the patient with respect to his or her physical, psychoemotional and social experience. Empathy is a way of being. It involves:

- listening for verbal and non-verbal core messages
- listening to the client's point of view and separating it from one's own
- bringing focus into the consultation
- using responses to encourage patients to discuss their feelings, problems and beliefs.

Questioning and listening complement each other obtaining a comprehensive case history. Direct questions are useful for obtaining confirmatory biological information. These should, in general:

- proceed from the general to the specific
- invite a graded rather than a monosyllabic 'yes' or 'no' response
- not be leading, open questions or those offering many options being preferable.

Non-directive questions are used to discover the impact of patients' psychoemotional state on their wellbeing and verify the preliminary assessment of the person's emotional health status derived from non-verbal cues. Useful non-directive openers include 'What brings you here?', 'What seems to be the trouble?', 'Tell me more about it' and 'Is there anything else you would like to discuss?'. Verbal disclosure is in all cases enhanced when the practitioner demonstrates attending skills and facilitates a response using nodding and/or silence.

Figure 5.5 provides an overview of the pointers to skilled communication.

Refining clinical communication

In addition to creating an environment of unconditional acceptance through both verbal and non-verbal cues, an effective helping relationship empowers patients/clients. Determining the client's locus of control and preferred behavioural style may enable practitioners more accurately to predict their client's responses to various circumstances.

The client's locus of control can be used to ascertain the client–clinician interaction most likely to effect behaviour change.[21,22] Those with an external locus are more likely to attribute control to chance or the clinician, the powerful other. Persons with a high 'powerful other' external locus of control are likely to respond best to a more directive practitioner as they are strongly influenced by expert and legitimate power. Clients with an external locus of control are more likely to:

- be motivated by the desire to please or win approval of the practitioner – the impact of referent and expert power should not be underestimated
- demonstrate practitioner dependency
- be compliant, following instructions without question
- have difficulty linking behaviour with its consequences
- have difficulty predicting the consequence of lifestyle choices

To communicate, you need to connect with the client or patient. This requires that you get the person interested and keep them involved.

Tips:

1. *Use language the patient can understand*
2. *Get their attention:*
   - be empathic and sensitive to the person's overt (spoken) and covert (non-verbal) communication needs. Listen and observe
3. *Understand the person:*
   - ask questions and involve the person in interactive communication
4. *Make the message relevant to the person:*
   - identify what they want
   - identify their fears
   - identify current knowledge and understanding
5. *Get into the person's 'shoes'. View from the person's perspective:*
   - the problem
   - the goals and aspirations
   - the solution
   - the implementation of the solution
   - remain approachable, encourage feedback
6. *Deliver the message:*
   - have your ideas clearly organized before you speak
   - get to the point
   - translate the message in terms of benefits to the person
   - check for misunderstanding
   - remember that people think in images – use models, diagrams, demonstrations
   - be natural and enthusiastic

Reassurance and explanation

- Avoid the negative
   - *I can't find anything wrong* (functional disorders, e.g. IBS)
- Provide an unequivocal positive finding/analysis
   - *I am pleased to say we have found the reason for your problem*
- Specifically mention potentially serious conditions which have been excluded
   - *We have looked carefully for cancer and are certain you have nothing like that*

Figure 5.5 • Skilled communication.

- have difficulty making decisions
- experience feelings of helplessness when confronted by health problems
- make poor or inappropriate choices to avoid the disapproval of others
- have difficulty recognizing and expressing their personal needs.

Persons with an internal locus believe they can personally influence an outcome. They are likely to respond well to information-sharing and taking personal responsibility. Persons with a stronger internal locus of control were found to learn their exercises better and do their exercises more frequently.[23] Those with a high internal locus of control are more amenable to self-care.[24] Clients with an internal locus of control are more likely to:

- be actively involved in health decision-making
- take the initiative in promoting their own health
- recognize the relationship between their habits and health status

- acknowledge the consequences of an unhealthy choice
- be more independent
- question the recommendations of the practitioner
- be cooperative rather than compliant
- express personal needs.

Table 5.4 provides a list of statements derived from the Wallstons' work consistent with various types of locus of control.[12,21,22] While persons with a 'powerful other' locus of control may be most susceptible, both those with an internal locus and those with a 'chance' external locus of control are likely to respond well to the clinician's use of referent power. Figure 5.6 provides a self-check screen to make clinicians aware of the nature of the power being used in the wellness consultation.[5]

In addition to ascertaining the client's locus of control, the clinician's preferred behavioural style may need to be adjusted to meet the needs of particular clients. People fit into four broad behaviour

Table 5.4 Locus of control

Internal locus	External locus – powerful other	External locus – chance
If I take the right actions, I can stay healthy	Health professionals keep me healthy	When I become ill, it's a matter of fate
If I get sick, it is my own behaviour which determines how soon I get well	Other people play a big part in whether I stay healthy or become sick	Often I feel that no matter what I do, if I am going to get sick, I will get sick When I stay healthy, I'm just plain lucky
The main thing which affects my health is what I myself do If I take care of myself, I can avoid illness	Following the doctor's orders to the letter is the best way for me to stay healthy	It seems that my health is greatly influenced by accidental happenings Even when I take care of myself, it's easy to get sick
I am in control of my health When I get sick, I am to blame	The type of care I receive from other people is what is responsible for how well I recover from an illness	When I am sick, I just let nature run its course

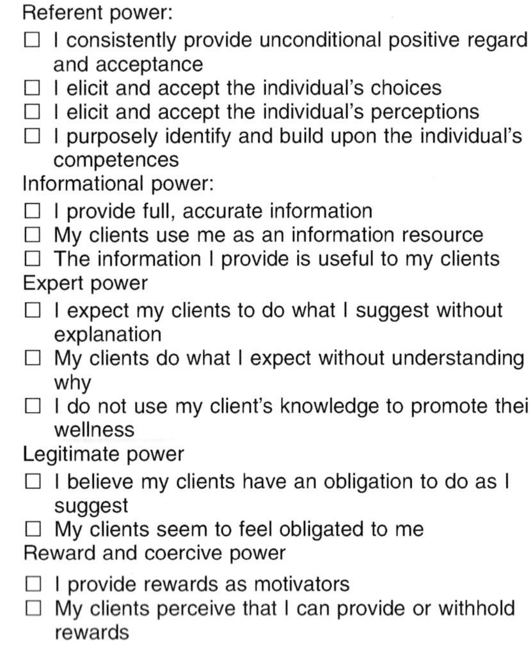

Figure 5.6 • Power and control: the wellness consultation.

styles.[20] Communication is facilitated when the speaker and listener share a similar frame of reference. Health management plans are likely to be more successfully implemented when conveyed in a compatible behaviour style. Practitioners who accurately ascertain their patients' preferred behaviour style can modify their own behaviour to make the consultation process and the treatment plan more acceptable to the patient. Behaviour styles have been categorized as those of the director, thinker, relater and socializer.

Directors are fast paced; they like being in control and getting results. Directors find it stressful to waste time. They make decisions based on end results and rely on past achievements. They do not believe in changing what works. Directors become assertive and seek to take control, especially when stressed. Their health management programme should not be too time-consuming to implement, should give results and should be perceived as being subject to their control.

Thinkers believe in getting things done right, being deliberate and methodical. The thinker plans ahead, likes proof, adheres to rules and is committed to process. It is advisable to allow thinkers generous time for health management projects as they find it stressful to have deadlines. Thinkers withdraw when stressed.

Relaters like to do things together, desiring consensus and valuing congeniality. They operate at a relaxed pace and find conflict stressful. Relaters make decisions based upon the people affected, and a health management programme that takes their family into consideration is more likely to be successful. Relaters become acquiescent when stressed.

Socializers are likeable, creative and hurried. They dislike mundane tasks and, when stressed, become sarcastic. Their health programme works best when they are rewarded for meeting their objectives. They need help with identifying their priorities.

Table 5.5 Meeting patient behaviour style preferences

Preferred clinical style	Director	Thinker	Relater	Socializer
Focus	Task	Task	Relationship	Relationship
Pace	Fast	Slow	Slow	Fast
Priority	Results	Clinical process	Maintain relationship	Interaction
Consultation	Brief	Accurate	Pleasant	Interesting
Avoid	Indecision, inefficiency	Uncertainty	Impatience, insensitivity	Letting patient feel left out
Clinical decisions	Decisive	Deliberate	Considered	Spontaneous

Dealing with vexed clients

1. Listen:
   - Don't interrupt
   - Allow the client to complete their complaint
2. Stay emotionally in tune – never appear indifferent.
3. Write down the complaint – this provides a permanent record and slows the patient down (it is more difficult to be explosively angry at a writing than speaking pace)
4. Respond
   - With a brief statement of regret:
     - apologize if in the wrong
     - empathize if the problem is not of your making.
   - Paraphrase – let the patient know you heard what they were saying
   - Find a point of agreement
   - Generate solutions
   - Take some action

Ask: 'What would you like to have me do for you?'
Conveying a message the client doesn't want to hear:

1. Create a helpful environment:
   - Chose a quiet room with no risk of interruption
   - Be unhurried
   - Have client support persons present if so desired
2. Break the bad news:
   - Slowly in small information bites
   - Be frank and open
   - Keep the message simple
   - Use information brochures where possible
   - Always say something positive
3. Adopt an attitude of empathy

Figure 5.7 • Specific situations.

Step I: **Prepare yourself**
– think about what you are going to say
– when and how you are going to say it
– whether relatives should be present
Step II: **Prepare the patient (?and relatives)**
– give some hints that there are grounds for concern while awaiting confirmatory tests
Step III: **Get to know the patient**
– avoid giving bad news at the first encounter
– review patients support systems
Step IV: **Ensure a correct diagnosis**

Conducting the interview:
- allow time for reasonable discussion
- get to the point but beware of being too blunt
- avoid euphemisms. Call a growth cancer
- encourage questions
- give empathy not sympathy. Allow person to cry. Sitting silently can be helpful
- do not give a precise prognosis. Allow for hope

Understand the patient's feelings of:
- shock, numbness
- inability to comprehend
- anger
- the need to know
- the need for support

Figure 5.8 • Giving bad news.

Table 5.5 provides tips on how practitioners may modify their behaviour to obtain better clinical results when managing patients with any one of these preferred behaviour styles.

While preferred behaviour styles provide a general guide to handling particular types of patients, certain strategies are useful for handling difficult patients or specific situations.[25] Figures 5.7 and 5.8 provides practice tips for handling patients who are upset or angry, or who do not wish to listen. Figure 5.9 provides advice on how to deal with criticism. Figure 5.10 suggests a communication strategy for patients without overt pathology for whom no specific therapy is available.[26,27]

The clinical setting

The wellness care clinic adds a unique dimension to primary care, differing from both outpatient clinics and population targeted screening initiatives

---

Criticizing client behaviour:
- remain calm and relaxed
- assume a helpful attitude – aim to teach
- begin with a positive – identify and encourage what is right
- criticize the harmful behaviour – never the person
- explain the effects of the behaviour on the person's health – physical, psychological and social
- only criticize behaviours the individual can change to enhance their wellbeing
- do not use blaming language
- conclude by expressing confidence that the patient can acquire the health-promoting behaviour

Handling criticism from clients:
- have an attitude 'this may be an opportunity for self-growth'
- don't get defensive
- *listen – DON't start justifying*
- clarify points
- ask what the client would like you to do
- indicate if you are willing to comply with the client's suggestions
- remain calm and friendly
- thank the patient for raising the issue – better to your face than to another practitioner or client!

Figure 5.9 • Dealing with criticism.

Communication as therapy
- ☐ make the patient feel understood
- ☐ establish a positive collaborative relationship
- ☐ correct disease misconceptions
- ☐ give a positive explanation of symptoms
- ☐ avoid unnecessary investigations and treatment
- ☐ negotiate a treatment plan

Communication is a fundamental management tool for functional somatic syndromes.

Communication as reassurance
- ☐ obtain a detailed description of the presenting symptoms
- ☐ elicit the emotional meaning/content of the symptoms
- ☐ perform a detailed relevant examination
- ☐ exclude non-benign disease
- ☐ make a patient-centred diagnosis taking physical and psychosocial factors into consideration
- ☐ explain the significance of the symptoms to the patient
- ☐ conclude with an expression of reassurance and support

Figure 5.10 • Communication: a form of non-specfic therapy.

(see Table 5.3). One major difference is the relationship between patient/client and professional. The establishment of a satisfactory ongoing therapeutic alliance appears to be a characteristic of and prerequisite for a successful wellness consultation. The cognitive and emotional dimensions of a patient–practitioner relationship are the basis for a good therapeutic or working alliance.[28] The emotional and relational aspects of a consultation are considered so important that computer programs to engage patients in dialogue or long-term, repeated interactions are being explicitly designed to accommodate these aspects of an interaction.[29]

A good working alliance appears to explain both a patient's adherence to and satisfaction with treatment. The working alliance has been linked to adherence self-efficacy, the patient's determination and ability to deal with obstacles ranging from side effects of medications to changing habits and acquiring new behaviours. Adherence self-efficacy and the perceived usefulness of treatment are believed to represent psychological determinants of patients' behaviours in health care.

Chiropractors enjoy the reputation of a satisfied patient clientele. Chiropractors' communication skills and empathy are strongly correlated with their patients' overall satisfaction. Overall satisfaction correlated particularly well with chiropractors providing an 'understandable explanation of treatment and choices' and 'concern about me as a person'.[30] Their successful therapeutic alliance is characterized by the development of common goals amidst a strong personal bond. Chiropractors create a therapeutic alliance by:[31,32]

- establishing a personal relationship with their patients, which provides emotional support. Chiropractors provide an empathic understanding of the patient's distress In addition to the specific supportive milieu of the clinical consultation, clinic receptionists are trained to create a generally welcoming and sympathetic clinic environment
- validating the presenting problem: by providing an acceptable explanation for the illness, chiropractors simultaneously legitimate their patients' illnesses and reassure them that someone understands their problem
- creating a clinical reality conducive to wellness. Psychological triggers that enhance patients' sense of control over their illness create a healing environment, the triggers to wellness being the patients' expectations.

Chiropractors create positive outcome expectations by:[33]

- their personal conviction that they can help
- providing information on how they intend to help
- an impressive therapeutic ritual
- predicting outcome with respect to both early muscle aches and subsequent pain relief
- providing an outcome substantially different from that of no therapy
- a track record of personal and a history of professional therapeutic success.

Two particularly important psychological wellness triggers in the clinical encounter appear to be the positive expectations of the practitioner and the patient's growing psychosomatic awareness that the condition can be changed. Medical studies have shown that a physician's expectations of a drug's efficacy can alter the 'outcome of therapy by 25–30% in either direction'.[34] Clinical trials in which a significant benefit was no longer detected when the drug was used by a sceptical physician are as diverse as the use of vitamin E in angina and meprobamate in anxiety.

A prerequisite for successfully triggering wellness by psychoemotional means would therefore seem to be that the practitioner believes the patient can be helped. Such a belief is conveyed to patients by the practitioner's verbal and non-verbal communication. Extrapolation of these clinical findings to the wellness consultation would seem to imply that clients should have the expectation that the behavioural changes negotiated will enhance their health and that the implementation of the proposed changes is both feasible and desirable. Figure 5.11 provides a flow chart for communication in the wellness consultation.

Analysis of diverse publications suggests four common elements of patient centredness are: attention to both the patients' psychosocial and physical needs; disclosure of patients' concerns; conveying a sense of partnership; and active facilitation of patient involvement in decision-making.[35] As disease-specific patient education is quite different in content and intention from chronic disease self-management, patient-centred care needs to be adapted for diverse clinical scenarios. Taking the patients' perspective and activating the patient are two elements of patient centredness that appear associated with different patient outcomes. While the former, discernible as the ability to elicit and discuss patients' beliefs within the consultation, appears sufficient to promote patient satisfaction, it is activating the patient to take control that promotes more general

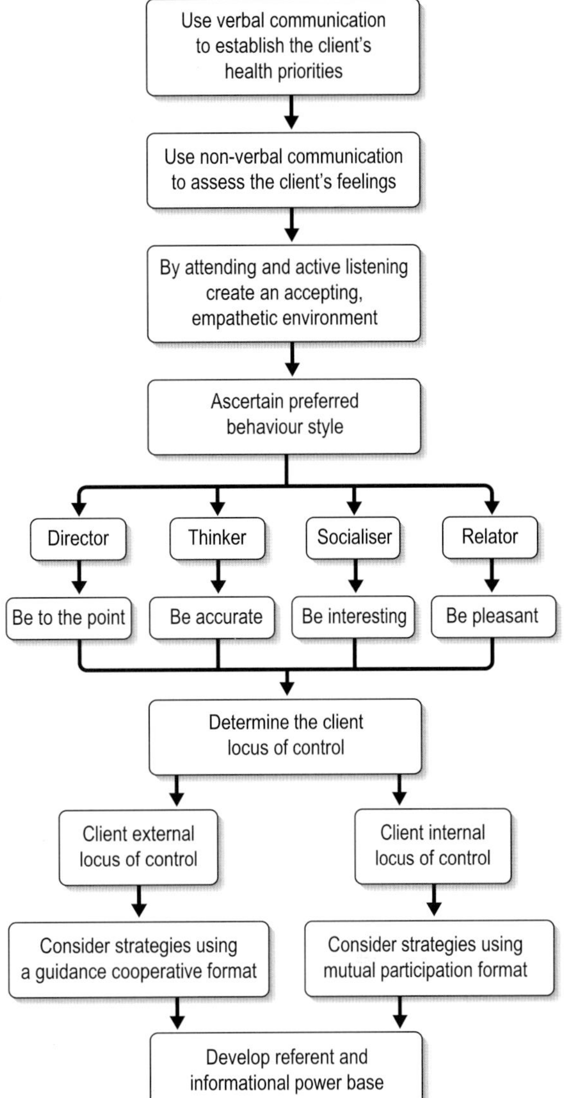

Figure 5.11 • Communication in the wellness consultation.

self-management.[36] Empowerment involves both taking an active part in the consultation and making lifestyle choices. Shared decision-making in wellness-oriented primary care includes agreeing on an agenda for each consultation and recognizing that the patient has diverse sources of technical information that need to be taken into consideration when providing health-promoting information.[37] Health is not a commodity which is collected from the consultation and brought home. Wellbeing arises from interactions between one's genetic composition, the circumstances of an individual's life, lifestyle choices, and interventions from health services. Successful wellness care requires fully engaged patients. This means a shift away from providing knowledge to communicating with patients, moving from decision-making to supporting patients' choices.[38]

The wellness consultation

Within the wellness model, emotions, perceptions and physical states interact, influencing wellness. The wellness consultation addresses all aspects contributing to health and disease. Good patient management, in addition to providing any required physical or drug intervention, actively enhances the patient's desire to achieve wellness, creates the expectation of a satisfactory health outcome and induces a personal sense of coping with the presenting problem. Good wellness care requires skilled communication in the clinical encounter. It has been predicted that health care that involves active patient participation and reorders the patient's experience, increasing self-understanding, will be in great demand in the future.[39]

References

1. Potter SJ, McKinlay JB. From a relationship to encounter: an examination of longitudinal and lateral dimensions in the doctor–patient relationship. *Soc Sci Med.* 2005;61(2): 465–479.

2. Levin L. Self-care: an emerging component of the health care system. *Hosp H Serv Admin.* 1978; Winter: 17–25.

3. Teutsch C. Patient-doctor communication. *Med Clin North Am.* 2003;87(5):1115–1145.

4. Northouse PG. Effective helping relationships: the role of power and control. *Health Educ Behav.* 1997;24:703–706.

5. Benson H, Friedman R. Harnessing the power of the placebo effect and renaming it 'remembered wellness'. *Annu Rev Med.* 1996;47:193–199.

6. Brody H, Waters DB. Diagnosis is treatment. *J Fam Pract.* 1980;10:445–449.

7. Frank JD. The placebo is psychotherapy. *Behav Brain Sci.* 1983;6:291–292.

8. Van Ryn M, Heaney CA. Developing effective helping relationships in health education practice. *Health Educ Behav.* 1997;24:683–702.

9. Bloom SW, Wilson RN. Patient–practitioner relationships. In: Freeman S, Levine S, Reeder LG, eds. *Handbook of Medical Sociology.* Englewood Cliffs, NJ: Prentice-Hall; 1972:315–339.

10. Carmichael LP. The relational model: a paradigm for family medicine. *J Florida Med Assoc.* 1980;67:860.

11. Jamison JR. Locus of control – an aid to clinical care. *J Aust Chiropr Assoc.* 1987;17:25–27.

12. Wallston WA, Wallston BS. Development of the multidimensional health locus of control scales. *Health Educ Monogr.* 1978;6:160–170.

13. Emanuel EJ, Emanuel LL. Four models of physician–patient relationship. *JAMA.* 1992;267:2221–2226.

14. Thomas K. General practice consultation. *Lancet.* 1987;294:1200.

15. Vernon H. Chiropractic: a model of incorporating the illness behavior model in the management of low back pain patients. *J Manipulative Physiol Ther.* 1991;14:379.

16. Thomas K. The placebo in general practice. *Lancet.* 1994;244:1067.

17. Frederickson LG. Exploring information-exchange in consultation: the patients' view of performance and outcomes. *Patient Educ Counsel.* 1995;25:237–246.

18. Hargie O, Saunders C, Dickson D. *Social Skills in Interpersonal Communication.* Guildford: Billing; 1981.

19. Pease A. *Body Language.* Australia: William Collins; 1987.

20. Pease A, Alessandra T, Cathcart J. The four personality styles. Alessandra T: Relationship strategies. Audio cassette training courses.

21. Wallston BS, Wallston KA, Kaplan SA, Maides SA. Development and validation of the Health Locus of Control Scale. *J Consult Clin Psychol.* 1976;44:580–585.

22. Wallston BS, Wallston KA. Locus of control and health. A review of the literature. *Health Educ Monogr.* 1978; Spring:107–117.

23. Harkapaa K, Jarvikoski A, Mellin H, Hurri H, Luoma J. Health locus of control beliefs and psychological distress as predictors for treatment outcome in low-back pain patients: results of a 3 month follow-up of a controlled intervention study. *Pain.* 1991;46:35–41.

24. Mclean J, Pietroni P. Self-care – who does best? In: Pietroni P, Pietroni C, eds. *Innovation in Community Care and Primary Health.* Singapore: Churchill Livingstone; 1996:88–95.

25. Schwenk TL, Romano SE. Managing the difficult physician–patient relationship. *Am Fam Physician.* 1992;46:1503–1509.

26. Sharpe M, Wessely S. Non-specific ill health: a mind–body approach to functional somatic symptoms. In: Watkins A, ed. *Mind–Body Medicine.* New York:

Churchill Livingstone; 1997:169–186.

27. Sapira JD. Reassurance therapy. What to say to symptomatic patients with benign disease. *Ann Intern Med*. 1972;77:603–604.

28. Fuertes JN, Mislowack A, Bennett J, et al. The physician-patient working alliance. *Patient Educ Couns*. 2007;66(1):29–36.

29. Bickmore T, Gruber A, Picard R. Establishing the computer–patient working alliance in automated health behavior change interventions. *Patient Educ Couns*. 2005;59:21–30.

30. Gaumer G. Factors associated with patient satisfaction with chiropractic care: survey and review of the literature. *J Manipulative Physiol Ther*. 2006;29(6):455–62.

31. Jamison JR. An interactive model of chiropractic practice: reconstructing clinical reality. *J Manipulative Physiol Ther*. 1997;20:382–388.

32. Jamison JR. The chiropractic practice model: an observational study. *Chiro Tech*. 1997;9(3):115–119.

33. Jamison JR. Non-specific interventions in chiropractic care. *J Manipulative Physiol Ther*. 1998;21:423–425.

34. Luskin F, Newell K. Mind–body approaches to successful aging. In: Watkins A, ed. *Mind–Body Medicine*. New York: Churchill Livingstone; 1997:251–268.

35. de Haes H. Dilemmas in patient centeredness and shared decision making: a case for vulnerability. *Patient Educ Couns*. 2006;62(3):291–298.

36. Michie S, Miles J, Weinman J. Patient centredness in chronic illness: what it is and does it matter? *Patient Educ Couns*. 2003;51(3):197–206.

37. Murray E, Charles C, Gafni A. Shared decision-making in primary care: tailoring the Charles et al. model to fit the context of general practice. *Patient Educ Couns*. 2006;62(2):205–211.

38. Cayton H. The flat-pack patient? Creating health together. *Patient Educ Couns*. 2006;62(3):288–290.

39. Pietroni P. Holistic medicine – new map, old territory. In: Pietroni C, Pietroni C, eds. *Innovation in Community Care and Primary Health*. Singapore: Churchill Livingstone; 1996:4–14.

Self-care: a framework for action

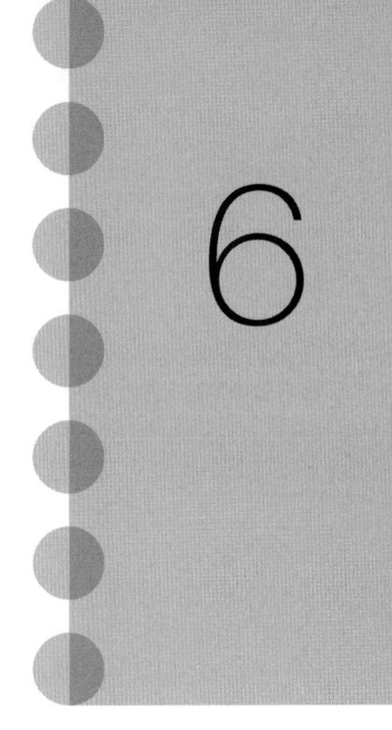

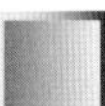

- A lifetime of self-care improves the quality of life in old age.
- Lifestyle choices influence your health – and that of your future progeny.
- Although self-care can be initiated at any age, the younger the start date the greater the personal gain.

Wellness care requires a discrete set of skills, different to those required to manage disease. Exploring the dimensions of wellness and monitoring progression along the health–disease spectrum provides insight into the levels of intervention possible in primary practice.

The dimensions of wellness

Health has traditionally been defined as the absence of disease. Although this definition has been useful in diagnosing disease, it has done little to promote health. The World Health Organization recognized this limitation and proposed a definition for health that encompassed physical, psychological, social and spiritual wellbeing. As shown in Table 6.1, various dimensions of health and disease are recognized in the everyday vocabulary of the health care system. In addition to the realization that wellbeing has diverse dimensions, each of which contributes to wellness, nomenclature in the health care system recognizes the importance of discriminating between reversible and irreversible change. The notion of

health promotion through disease prevention relies upon identifying risk factors and detecting biological changes early so as to intervene at a stage when a condition is reversible. In contrast, the wellness construct, in addition to promoting health and preventing disease, seeks to improve the function of healthy people. It seeks to achieve optimal wellbeing through the use of biological, psychological and social wellness triggers.

Recognizing individual limitations

Health and disease are not discrete entities; rather, they are relative states on a sliding scale. People inherit the genetic potential for both health and disease. The expression of health or disease is ultimately determined by the interaction of an individual's genetic composition with the total environment. The capacity of chromosomes to duplicate determines lifespan. Based on the number of chromosomal duplications determined by telomere length, the ultimate human lifespan appears to be around 122 years. Actual life expectancy is closer to 80 years. The cellular environment to which genes are exposed is deemed to account for this discrepancy. Lifestyle choices can alter genetic exposure. Whilst genes can be damaged by radiation or certain viruses, genetic expression can be modified by dietary excesses, deficiencies or toxin ingestion. Nutrigenomics is a field which aims to modify genetic expression by nutritional means. Nutrigenomics suggests bioactive nutrients, functional foods

Table 6.1 Terminology in health care

Functional state	Optimal function	Reversible dysfunction		Irreversible dysfunction
Biological	Health	Dis-ease	Disease	Impairment
Psychological	Well	Illness		Disabled
Social	Well	Sickness		Handicapped

and designer diets provide a key to preventing chronic disease.[1] The tenets of nutritional genomics hold that:

- dietary chemicals alter gene expression or structure
- diet-regulated genes play a role in the onset, incidence, progression and severity of various chronic diseases
- inappropriate dietary choices are a serious risk factor.

Being healthy is not necessarily a matter of chance – we can choose to be more or less healthy within the confines of our genetic inheritance.

Technological advances have made it possible to sometimes insert normal genes into chromosomes with aberrant gene sequences. This approach conforms to the 'one gene–one disease' theory that arises from the unilinear cause–effect thinking of the biomedical model. Phenylketonuria is an example of a genetic aberration that results in the absence of a single enzyme. It would theoretically be possible to cure this condition by supplying sufferers with the gene that codes for the missing enzyme. On the other hand, screening infants' urine for phenylacetic acid and eliminating one amino acid, phenylalanine, from the diet can neutralize the phenotypic effects of this condition. As illustrated in Figure 6.1, environmental

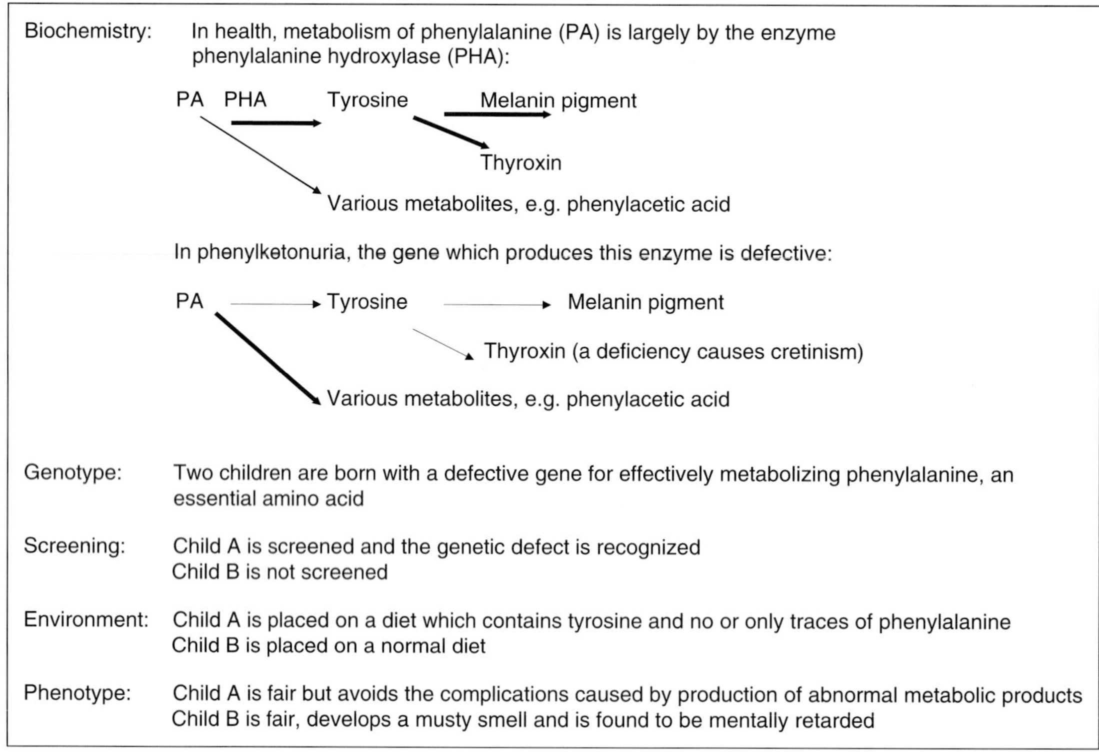

Figure 6.1 • A phenylketonuric case study.

modification can alter gene expression. In-utero screening to detect genetic defects is currently available for a number of conditions.

In reality, diseases are more often associated with polygenic inheritance than with a single dominant gene. Osteoporosis provides a good example of how multiple genes impact on the clinical expression of a condition. Bone mass is determined by a number of genes with multiple common polymorphic alleles interacting with each other and environmental factors. Although occasionally unusually high bone mass can occur as the result of mutations in a single gene, susceptibility to osteoporosis is essentially mediated by multiple genes, most having only a small effect.[2] The vitamin D receptor gene, the collagen type I alpha 1 gene and oestrogen receptor gene alpha all play a role in regulating bone mineral density, but the effects are modest and together probably account for less than 5% of the heritable contribution.[3] The contribution inheritance makes to bone mineral density furthermore varies by anatomical site; it lies between 70% and 85% in the spine and hip and between 50% and 60% at the wrist. Some understanding of the extent to which particular genetically determined processes are involved in bone formation and resorption has been achieved. Genetic factors influencing serum PTH and 1,25-dihydroxyvitamin D levels may influence up to 65% of bone mass. The genetic contribution, as judged by bone formation markers, is up to 29% for serum osteocalcin and 74% for bone-specific alkaline phosphatase. From a clinical perspective,

however, the critical consideration is not bone mass but rather the fracturing of an osteoporotic bone. The heritability of fractures is estimated to lie between 25% and 35%. The impact of inherited skeletal phenotypes that predispose to breakage is diluted by fall-related factors determining fracture risk.[2] To modify fracture risk by gene replacement is unworkable; on the other hand, to reduce the risk by making dietary lifestyle choices that enhance bone mass and exercising regularly is realistic.

While many of the genetic determinants of osteoporosis have been identified, the genetic blueprint for essential hypertension is less well defined. While lifestyle management of essential hypertension is well defined, the causes of essential hypertension remain obscure. As essential hypertension is due to a multitude of interacting factors, and a relatively small number of people are salt-sensitive, sodium restriction only benefits a subgroup of people with raised blood pressure. Nonetheless, as demonstrated in Figure 6.2, in this subgroup of people decreasing salt intake does benefit the condition.

Although replacing a single gene is no longer impossible, replacing multiple genes is impractical – even when most of the genes involved have been identified! On the other hand, much can be achieved by providing an environment that favours the expression of healthy genes and suppresses the penetrance of defective genes. Polygenic inheritance makes it possible to modulate disease pathogenesis by multiple diverse interventions. Consistent with the multifactorial causation of the infomedical model,

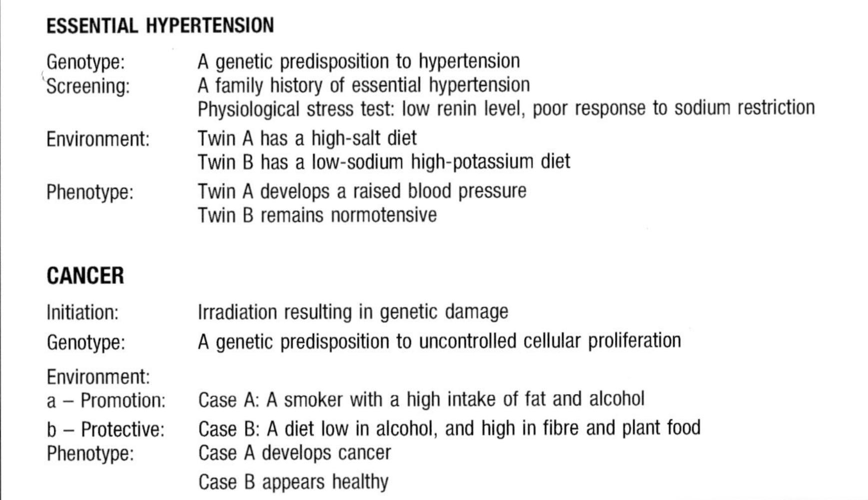

Figure 6.2 • Two postulates.

phenotypes are determined by the combined effects of several genes and environmental influences. The potential for lifestyle choices to impact on health has become even more important with the emergence of epigenetics.

It was originally supposed that sequencing and identifying man's genetic complement would explain all heritable differences. However, unmasking the human genetic code alone does not explain the diversity of disease phenotypes within a population. While classic genetics is unable to explain differences observed between identical twins, epigenetics can.[4] Epigenetics is defined as heritable changes that can alter gene expression without affecting the corresponding DNA sequence. Environmental exposures early in development play a role in susceptibility to disease in later life – and some of these environmental effects seem to be passed on through subsequent generations. Heritable environmentally induced epigenetic modifications underlie reversible transgenerational alterations in phenotype.[5] Heritable changes in gene expression, not due to alterations in DNA sequence, can be passed on both mitotically and transgenerationally due to epigenetic mediators such as posttranslational modification of histone proteins in chromatin, DNA methylation, and non-coding RNAs.[6] Epigenetic modifications of chromatin and DNA permit and suppress genome expression via gene transcription.[7] Emerging evidence suggests a key role for epigenetics in human pathology. The epigenetic state is a central regulator of cellular development and activation. Epigenetic reprogramming is the process by which an organism's genotype interacts with the environment to produce its phenotype. The epigenome is influenced by environmental factors throughout life.

Creation of an environment in which genetic expression is optimized is the rationale for health promotion. Gene function may be altered by a change in the sequence of the DNA or a change in epigenetic programming of a gene. Bioactive dietary components can alter the phenotype through diverse mechanisms ranging from modulating the pattern of gene expression through organization of chromatin to modification of cells' protein and/or metabolite profiles. Nutrients are considered to be 'signalling' molecules that, through appropriate cellular sensing mechanisms, change gene, protein, and metabolite expression.[8] Development of epigenetic drugs makes it possible to contemplate reversing aberrant gene expression profiles associated with different disease states.[9] Cancer is as much an epigenetic disease as

it is a genetic disease, and epigenetic alterations in cancer often serve as potent surrogates for genetic mutations.[10] The risk of cancer can be reduced by lifestyle choice. Early recognition of homeostatic strain provides opportunities for intervention at a stage when conditions are reversible. In the case of cancer, the first stage of the disease involves changes to the genetic code (see Figure 6.2). Progress to cancer after exposure to the initiating factor is not inevitable. Healthy lifestyle choices, i.e. avoidance of cancer-promoting factors, can prevent the phenotypic expression of the disease.

Health promotion is a general endeavour and disease prevention is the specific attempt to create such an environment. Phenotypic changes, once established, may be irreversible. It is therefore important to:

- promote health by creating an environment conducive to a healthy phenotype
- prevent disease by recognizing health risks early and specifically avoiding potential health hazards
- diagnose covert disease by actively screening for metabolic and functional dysfunction – early diagnosis and treatment are believed to give the best results.

Wellness results when individuals achieve their full health potential. Wellness is the greatest degree of wellbeing possible given a particular genetic composition. Wellness, the objective of health promotion and disease prevention, is optimal health given one's genetic potential. It is the rationale for actively encouraging patients to pursue self-care. Its achievement is only possible when patients, with the help of their practitioners, participate in striving towards a shared goal.

The health–disease spectrum

As individuals move from wellness to death, they move through a number of phases. Each of these phases has particular implications for the clinical consultation, the nature of the assessment and intervention required (see Figure 6.3). The patient–practitioner relationship varies depending on the health status of the presenting patient. As individuals move through this spectrum, their presentation varies, with reciprocal changes occurring in their life-world and total being. Changes can be detected and monitored in various dimensions, including social, psychological, biological, spiritual and occupational/economic.

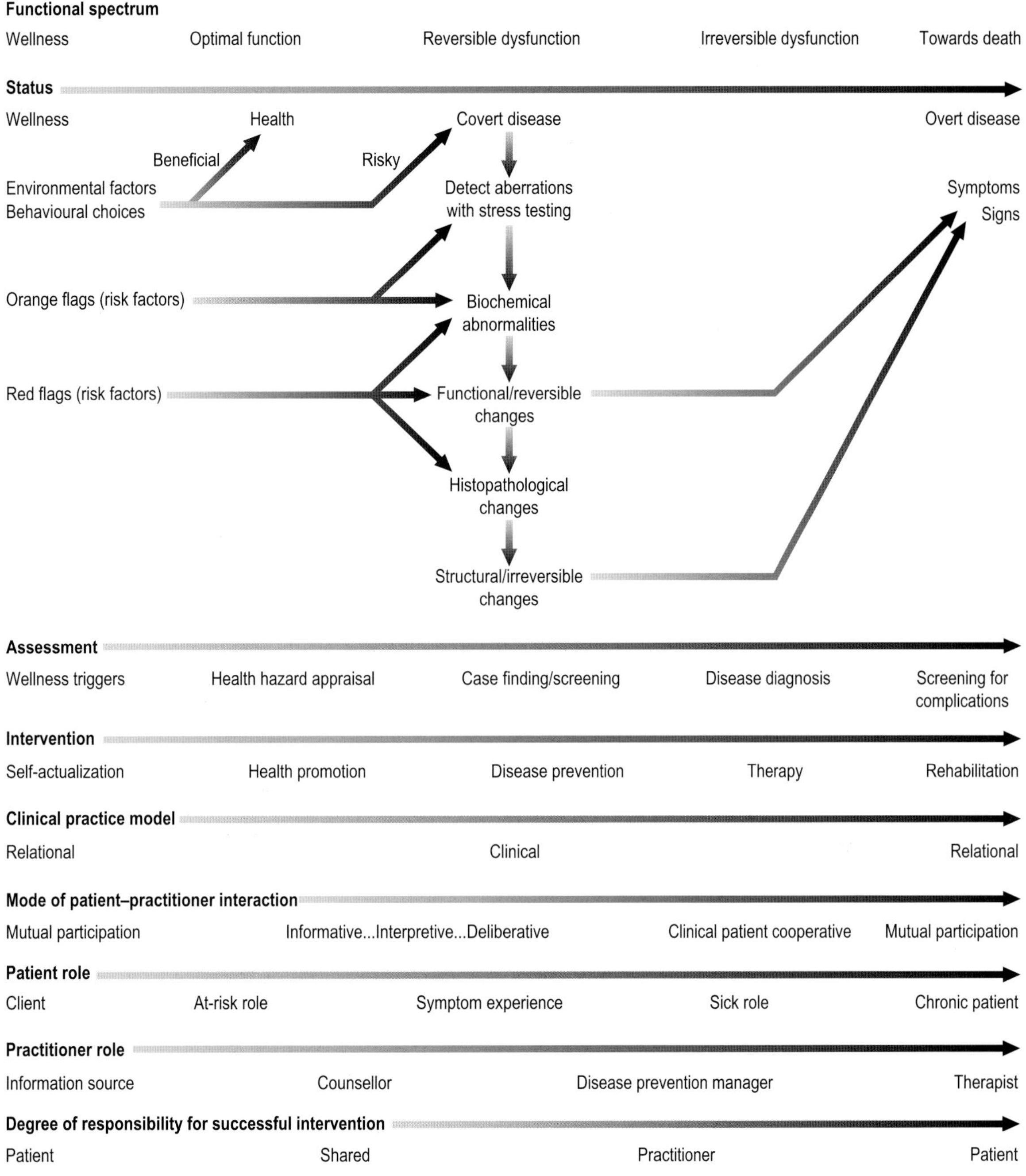

Figure 6.3 • The spectrum of health care.

The social dimension

Suchman has described sickness from a sociological perspective.[11] Stage 1 is the stage of symptom experience. The individual becomes aware of a change in health status. The perception that 'something is wrong' may result from a sensation of pain or unusual fatigue or it may be based upon observation of a skin rash or difficulty with carrying out routine tasks. The severity of the psychophysical experience is evaluated by the individual. Both the physical and emotional impact and expression of the symptom experience are influenced by the individual's sociocultural background. The realization that 'something is wrong' results in a decision to take action. At this early stage, the action taken is usually either self-medication or application of folk medicine. The outcome of this intervention may be:

* resolution of the symptoms and a return to baseline health status
* denial of the changed health status (a flight into health): this response delays entry into stage 2 until the individual can no longer ignore persisting, and often worsening, symptoms
* acceptance: the individual enters stage 2.

Stage 2 is assumption of the sick role. With persistence of symptoms, the individual assumes a sick role and seeks validation for the sick role. Endorsement of the sick role is initially sought from significant others (family, peers, friends, workmates). At this stage, individuals seek to relinquish their normal role. Rejection by others of the individual's claim to a sick role results in the individual being obliged either to resume normal duties or to present with more convincing symptoms. Acceptance by others that the individual is sick implies agreement that the individual be excused from their usual duties. During this period of 'provisional validation', further home remedies, including patent medicines, traditional cures and lay referral to unconventional health care practitioners, may be attempted.

The outcome of stage 2 is:

* rejection of the individual's claim to the sick role or
* provisional validation of the sick role. Individuals who have achieved provisional validation of their sick role undergo a period of assisted self-treatment which results in one of the following:
  ○ recovery
  ○ failure of the underlying condition to respond, with delay in diagnosis and initiation of appropriate therapy
  ○ acceptance of the illness and progression to stage 3.

Stage 3 involves interaction with the conventional health care system. With the decision to seek professional advice, individuals move beyond lay health care to seek authoritative validation of their sick role. Sanction of the sick role by health professionals both formalizes release from duties and provides an explanation of the malady. Symptom explanation may range from reassurance to a detailed elucidation of a pathophysiological mechanism. The outcome of this professional encounter may be:

* the individual is declared well and a return to normal duties follows
* the individual is declared well by the clinician but the individual rejects this assessment and seeks another opinion: the individual often seeks other opinions and goes 'shopping' until satisfied with the diagnosis
* confirmation of the sick role and the individual assumes the status of a patient.

Agreement that the individual is ill results in entry to stage 4.

In stage 4, the individual assumes the dependent-patient role. This stage potentially involves:

* intrapersonal conflict between the patient's childlike dependence on the clinician and their adult state of independence
* the meaning of symptoms within the context of the patient's sociocultural background, the pathophysiological implications and the likely physical and economic outcome
* conflict between the therapy prescribed by the clinician and that acceptable to the patient. This impacts on patient compliance and may result in 'shopping'
* the patient seeking secondary gains from the illness experience. Some patients enjoy the benefits of a 'dependent role' and do not strive to get well; they welcome the security of a protected dependency.

The outcome of this stage of illness behaviour is either acceptance of the sick role and development of a chronic sick role or compliance with therapy, i.e. movement to stage 5.

Stage 5 is the phase of recovery and rehabilitation. Stage 5 may lead to:

* relinquishing the sick role, with restoration of baseline health status and a return to normal duties
* reluctance, indeed refusal, to relinquish the sick role. Enjoyment of the secondary gains may require re-categorization of the patient as a malingerer
* the inability to relinquish the sick role and assumption of a chronic sick role.

Suchman's description of the illness experience illustrates the importance of the patient's perceptions and decisions in health care.

The psychological dimension

Paralleling the social changes in the illness experience are the psychological changes associated with loss. Kübler-Ross originally described these changes with respect to death and bereavement but later recognized that these phases apply to any loss, including the loss of good health.[12] The individual may progress through consecutive phases or may skip certain stages and duplicate others. The psychological stages associated with loss are:

- Denial. The initial response to a perceived change in health status is often denial. The duration of the denial stage will vary depending on the individual involved. Individuals whose habitual response is prolonged denial are more likely to seek professional help at a late stage, a stage at which irreversible change has occurred. Persons who pass rapidly through the denial period are capable of employing a more problem-oriented approach and are more likely to gain early access to health care. The mind has an impact on the stage at which the body is permitted to access health care intervention.

- Bargaining. As the patient realizes that the symptom is persisting and acknowledges illness, a phase of questioning ('why me?') and bargaining may be manifest. With reversible disease, the bargaining position is appropriate for the clinical model of health care. Patients relinquish control of their health, acquiescing to the clinician's instructions. This dependency role is acceptable to the patient; it is part of the covert pact entered into between patient and clinician.

- Anger. The patient rebels against a loss of health. Anger may serve to spur the patient to greater health-restoration efforts. In cases of irreversible disease in which a permanent impairment is inevitable, mastery becomes the objective; this implies the striving to maximize physical, psychological, and social independence given the constraints of the patient's condition. It is particularly important that the anger experienced by these patients be channelled into health-promoting activities.

- Depression. Both acutely and chronically ill patients are subject to periods of depression. This response is part of the anticipated reaction to loss. Depression may recur at various stages of the illness.

- Acceptance. Acceptance in the sense of giving up is not conducive to health; acceptance in the sense of acknowledging the reality of the situation and resolving to achieve the best possible health status, given current circumstances, demonstrates psychological health. Such individuals may demonstrate optimal psychological and social health despite being physically impaired.

The physical dimension

The biological dimension of the health–disease spectrum is described by the natural history of the condition. An understanding of the natural history of disease is the key to early diagnosis and health promotion through disease prevention. The natural history or pathogenesis of a disease describes progressive biological changes that result from exposure to disease-causing or aetiological agents. A study of the natural history of a disease considers changes occurring in response to exposure to aetiological factors as the condition progresses from covert to overt disease, from reversible dysfunction to the irreversible structural changes associated with disability or death.

Variables associated with disease states may be categorized as causal, non-causal, confounding or modifying. Risk factors are variables which, if present, increase the individual's susceptibility to a particular disease. They are the orange and red flags that draw attention to problems ahead. Disease prevention is theoretically achieved by eliminating recognized risk factors. However, whilst some risk factors have a direct *causal* relationship with a particular disease, others serve as markers suggesting the presence of an underlying pathological process. When the exact nature of the association between particular variables and disease remains undetermined, the clinical validity of a particular health promotion is problematic. A statistically significant association between a variable (risk factor) and disease reduces the likelihood that the association is attributable to chance.

Epidemiological investigations demonstrate a correlation between a variable and the disease under investigation. Smoking causes cancer of both the lung and bladder. Any increased incidence of bladder cancer in patients with lung cancer who smoke is attributable to smoking, not lung cancer. There is a *non-causal* association between lung and bladder cancer. Variables that are not recognized may further complicate the identification and quantification of risk factors. A study of lung cancer in smokers employed in asbestos mines can be distorted because asbestos, itself a cause of lung cancer, can function as a *confounding* variable. If vitamin C does, as postulated, protect smokers against lung cancer, then vitamin C intake would be regarded as a *modifying* variable in any studies examining the relationship between smoking and lung cancer.

Validated causes may themselves be essential but insufficient to solely precipitate the disease. *Mycobacterium tuberculosis* is necessary before a patient can develop tuberculosis; the presence of this acid-fast bacillus, however, does not inevitably result in tuberculosis. Identification of risk factors and subsequent confirmation of these variables as causes of disease remain problematic. Seldom is there a one-to-one relationship between the suspected causal agent and disease; however, lack of such specificity does not rule out a causal relationship. In fact, such specificity is seldom, if ever, encountered in chronic disease. Chronic diseases are often attributable to multiple factors and associated with a prolonged natural history. In such cases, risk factors are most likely to have a causal relationship with a disease when:[13]

- they are consistently present simultaneously
- there is an appropriate temporal relationship, i.e. the risk factor must precede the disease
- there is a dose–response curve between the risk factor and the disease
- the risk factor has a strong association with the disease, i.e. even minor exposure to the variable results in the disease.

Furthermore, the hypothesized relationship should be biologically plausible; not conflict with already established data about the disease's natural history; at least be analogous with other models of pathogenesis; and at best be confirmed by experimentation.

Exposure of a susceptible individual to a pathogen may result in the development of covert disease. The stage of covert disease is characterized by the presence of subclinical, pathophysiological changes detectable at a biochemical or histological level. Change at this stage of disease pathogenesis may be reversible. Therefore, it is important that potentially reversible conditions be recognized early. Hazard may be suspected when risky choices are made, alerting health professionals to the presence of 'orange flags' for particular diseases. Screening tests, capable of detecting subclinical changes,

may act as 'red flags' confirming the early stage of disease pathogenesis. Case finding in primary practice enables disease prevention at this stage of pathogenesis. Criteria used by Frame and Carlson[14] to justify active case finding in their critical review of periodic health screening include the requirement that:

- the disease have a significant effect on the quality and quantity of life
- acceptable methods of treatment are available
- the natural history of the disease incorporate an asymptomatic period during which intervention significantly reduces mortality or morbidity
- intervention during the asymptomatic period yields a result that is superior to that obtained by delaying treatment until the onset of symptoms
- tests enabling recognition of the asymptomatic condition are available at reasonable cost
- the incidence of the condition justifies the cost of case finding.

An analysis of a condition according to these criteria ideally requires:

- a knowledge of the natural history of the condition: more specifically, adequate decision-making requires data pertinent to the incidence and prevalence of the disease, to the risk factors associated with the aetiology and pathogenesis of the disorder, and to the prognosis of the untreated condition
- objective data on the outcome of therapeutic intervention at various stages of the disease process, i.e. information about the potential for early intervention to positively influence disease prognosis
- a financial costing of treatment of symptomatic disease as compared with the expense of screening in an asymptomatic population.

Whereas it is not always practical to meet all these theoretical prerequisites, implementation of this approach does provide a rational guideline in clinical practice.

If the disease is not detected by case finding, the patient may present with symptoms. Symptoms are the patients' complaints or subjective experience of 'something wrong'. Signs are the clinically or objectively detectable structural or functional changes. Clinical or overt disease presents with the ongoing evolution of the signs and symptoms characteristic of particular disease syndromes. Early recognition of clinical signs and symptoms facilitates timely interruption of the natural history of the disease process and increases the likelihood of restoring the individual to health. The earlier the patient presents, the more poorly defined and diffuse the presenting signs and symptoms and the greater the diagnostic challenge.

Prognosis is the predicted outcome of a disease. The prognosis of a disease varies according to its aetiology and pathogenesis. In certain cases, disease prognosis is good and, even in the absence of intervention, the patient's health will return to normal. In other cases, specific intervention is required.

In certain conditions, the natural history of the disease includes exacerbations and remissions; in these circumstances, it is difficult to differentiate between clinically effective intervention and the natural progression of disease. When the natural history of a disease is attended by complications with irreversible sequelae leading to disability and/or death, the effectiveness of diverse clinical intervention is more easily demonstrated. The majority of conditions for which primary practitioners are called upon to intervene are not irreversible organic diseases. Adequate scientific proof of the clinical effectiveness of interventions at the primary level of health care may consequently be somewhat elusive. Cause–effect validation is further complicated by polygenic inheritance ensuring that multiple environmental factors interact to determine health status.

Intervention in primary practice

Health and disease are dynamic concepts; individuals are continually modifying their health status along the health–disease continuum. When the individual is healthy, personal responsibility in health care is emphasized; when disease supervenes, dependence on professional care increases. The objective of self-care and professional health care is to maximize health. Wellness triggers include those at the:

- Physical level. Physical interventions range from self-care interventions such as exercise to learned skills such as massage.
- Chemical level. Body chemistry may be modified by nutrients in self-care or drugs in professional practice.
- Microbial level. The body flora may be changed. The use of lactobacilli to recolonize the gut after a bout of diarrhoea or the vagina after a candida infection represents the use of microbial health triggers.

- Psychological level. Psychological intervention may be task-orientated at the cognitive level or defence-orientated at the emotional level. Development of a problem-solving strategy in the former or changing one's attitude to the problem in the latter are reputable approaches to promoting wellness. Clinicians can help patients reconstruct their health reality and adapt their wellness/disease status construct.
- Social level. Social acceptance and peer support are conducive to health. Social isolation is a health risk. Social capital represents the degree of social cohesion in communities.
- Spiritual level. Spiritual wellbeing is the belief that one's life has meaning and purpose.

Intervention at the wellness pole of the spectrum is undertaken by individuals who have no overt susceptibility to disease. Persons functioning at this level actively seek to implement healthy lifestyle options, whether this be through dietary choices, exercise regimens, self-improvement courses and/or spiritual growth. At this level, the objective is self-actualization, physical fitness, social creativity, and spiritual evolution. Health at this stage is a personal prerogative with individuals taking full responsibility for their wellbeing.

Shifting from the extreme of the wellness pole, the next level of intervention in the health care spectrum is at the phase of risk exposure. The precursors of disease are present in the individual's environment. Only probability separates the individual from initiation of the disease process. Intervention at this stage aims to reduce the individual's vulnerability to initiation and development of the disease process. Identification of disorders suffered by the person's ancestors gives a clue to the diseases to which the individual is more likely to be genetically predisposed. Wise lifestyle choices can modify the phenotypic expression of aberrant genes. Analysis of harmful lifestyle choices provide insight into how risk to the individual may be minimized. A number of internet-based tools are available for undertaking health risk assessments and learning about risk-reducing lifestyle choices.[15–17] Any decision to change unhealthy habits at the level of health hazard appraisal will be influenced by the individual's perception of the risk to their health status and the perceived benefits of intervention weighed against any perceived barriers to action. While health hazard appraisal and intervention can be undertaken by motivated individuals without practitioner guidance, those deemed at risk would benefit from motivation provided by health professionals.

Questionnaire analysis of lifestyle risks provides a useful guideline to orange flags, especially with respect to identifying where lifestyle changes are needed. Detection of biochemical risk markers more precisely detects red flags heralding early evidence of stress or homeostatic strain. For example, the presence of raised C-reactive protein indicates subclinical inflammation. High-sensitivity C-reactive protein is elevated years in advance of the first-ever myocardial infarction or thrombotic stroke and is highly predictive of recurrent heart attacks, recurrent stroke, diabetes, and cardiovascular death.[18] Levels of high-sensitivity C-reactive protein <1, 1 to 3, and >3 mg/L denote lower, average, and higher relative risk for future vascular events. Monitoring decreasing levels of high-sensitivity C-reactive protein can be used to evaluate how an individual's risk is being reduced by implementing dietary, exercise and tobacco-quitting lifestyle changes. The inflammatory process has emerged as a major pathway in the pathogenesis of chronic lifestyle-related diseases.

Another useful risk marker is vitamin D deficiency. In adults, vitamin D deficiency has been linked to a large number of disorders. It may precipitate or exacerbate osteopenia, osteoporosis, muscle weakness, fractures, many cancers, and autoimmune, infectious and cardiovascular diseases. A population study found that compared to those with high levels of vitamin D, persons in the lowest quartile (25[OH]D levels <17.8 ng/mL) had a 26% increased rate of all-cause mortality.[19] The Third National Health and Nutritional Examination Survey (NHANES III) suggested the optimum blood level of 25[OH]D is 30 ng/mL or higher. However, in the US, about 41% of men and 53% of women have levels lower than 28 ng/mL. Diabetics, current smokers and overweight persons appear to be prone to vitamin D deficiency. Whereas the practitioner's role is largely that of wellness counsellor, formulation of a personalized wellness programme is appropriate at this level of clinical intervention. A wellness programme is even more important for patients identified to be at risk through periodic health examination.

The next level of the health–disease spectrum is characterized by subclinical or asymptomatic disease. Screening for biological changes can be undertaken at a population level through government-sponsored case-finding initiatives or when individuals present for a periodic health examination. Diagnosis of covert disease depends on the appropriate use of special investigations, knowledge of epidemiology, and disease pathogenesis. The practitioner's role is to actively screen for subclinical evidence of disease. Early recognition and treatment increases the likelihood of reversing pathophysiological changes. A health-literate and engaged population increases the chances of successful primary prevention. Motivated informed women reduce their risk of breast and cervical cancer by presenting for mammography and Pap smears at case-finding centres. Men reduce their risk of cardiovascular disease by presenting for a periodic health examination offering screening for hypertension and hypercholesterolaemia.

The next level of intervention in the health–disease spectrum is diagnosis of overt or clinical disease. The focus shifts to secondary prevention. The earlier pathological changes are detected, the greater the success of secondary disease prevention. The earlier the natural history of disease is interrupted, the greater the likelihood of limiting the disease process and reversing pathological changes. Whereas intervention at this level of health care is largely the prerogative of trained health professionals, the first person to detect a change in health status is the patient. Recognition of the importance of early diagnosis by the community has led to clients actively acquiring the knowledge necessary to act appropriately when they first experience symptoms. In the absence of successful intervention, the next level of intervention occurs once disease has progressed to a point of irreversible change. At this late stage, tertiary intervention depends on rehabilitation of the patient. It is particularly important to distinguish between the various dimensions of health status when the disease process results in permanent sequelae. Enhancing daily functioning and wellbeing is increasingly being advocated in the management of patients with chronic conditions. Compared to individuals with no chronic disorders, persons with chronic conditions show markedly worse physical and social functioning, mental health and bodily pain perceptions. Yet wellness is possible in the presence of disease. The paraplegic whose expectations have been shattered by a motor vehicle accident need not be psychologically, socially, and/or spiritually crippled. Clinical intervention requires a multidimensional approach.

The final stage of life and disease is death. This is the extreme pole of the health–disease spectrum. It is the only absolute dimension on the physical spectrum; all other stages of the spectrum are subject to ongoing modification.

Self-care: a task for all age groups

The objective of self-care is to enhance the quality of life and delay the onset of conditions that lead to death. In the US, the six major causes of death are heart disease, stroke, cancer, chronic obstructive pulmonary disease, accidents and diabetes mellitus.[20] Lifestyle choices can reduce an individual's risk of dying from any one of these conditions.

Between 1970 and 1990, death rates for chronic obstructive pulmonary disease doubled in the US. Not smoking can reduce the risk of chronic obstructive airways disease. Exercise, dietary care and taking low-dose aspirin can reduce the risk of a heart attack. Maintaining an ideal body weight can reduce the risk of adult-onset diabetes – a condition for which the death rate has doubled since 1987![20] By controlling for risk factors such as tobacco use and sun exposure, the risk of developing cancer can be reduced. By screening to ensure early diagnosis, the risk of dying of breast, colon, skin, prostate, uterine and oral cancer can be lowered. Health care problems confronting modern society cannot be resolved by governments alone, individuals need to take increased personal responsibility for promoting their own wellbeing and minimizing their lifestyle risks.

Self-care contributes to successful primary, secondary and tertiary prevention.

In perspective

Sensible lifestyle choices reduce the risk of healthy people becoming sick. Screening, leading to early detection, can limit progression of covert disease. Intervention to limit complications and restore function in the chronically sick enriches life. Health promotion, disease prevention and rehabilitation require active participation on the part of the individual. Self-care is a rewarding initiative for everybody, regardless of age. Furthermore, epigenetics has shown that wise lifestyle choices not only enhance personal wellbeing but also provide future offspring with a more life-enhancing blueprint. Self-care is emerging as an imperative for one's own wellbeing and an obligation for enabling wellness in future generations.

References

1. Gillies PJ. Preemptive nutrition of pro-inflammatory states: a nutrigenomic model. *Nutr Rev.* 2007;65(12 Pt 2):S217–S220.

2. Ralston SH. Genetic control of susceptibility to osteoporosis. *J Clin Endocrinol Metab.* 2002;87(6): 2460–2466.

3. Williams FM, Spector TD. Recent advances in the genetics of osteoporosis. *J Musculoskelet Neuronal Interact.* 2006;6(1): 27–35.

4. Ezzat S. Chromatin remodeling: the interface between extrinsic cues and the genetic code? *Clin Invest Med.* 2008;31(5):E272–E281.

5. Jirtle RL, Skinner MK. Environmental epigenomics and disease susceptibility. *Nat Rev Genet.* 2007;8(4):253–262.

6. Tang WY, Ho SM. Epigenetic reprogramming and imprinting in origins of disease. *Rev Endocr Metab Disord.* 2007;8(2):173–182.

7. Wilson AG. Epigenetic regulation of gene expression in the inflammatory response and relevance to common diseases. *J Periodontol.* 2008; 79(suppl 8):1514–1519.

8. Afman L, Müller M. Nutrigenomics: from molecular nutrition to prevention of disease. *J Am Diet Assoc.* 2006;106 (4):569–576.

9. Szyf M. Epigenetics, DNA methylation, and chromatin modifying drugs. *Annu Rev Pharmacol Toxicol.* 2009;49:243–263.

10. Iacobuzio-Donahue CA. Epigenetic changes in cancer. *Annu Rev Pathol.* 2009;4:229–249.

11. Suchman EA. Stages of illness and medical care. *J Health Hum Behav.* 1965;6:293–299.

12. Kubler-Ross E. *On Death and Dying.* London: Tavistock Publications; 1969.

13. Gordis L. *Epidemiology.* Philadelphia: WB Saunders; 2008.

14. Frame PS, Carlson SJ. A critical review of periodic health screening using specific screening criteria. *J Fam Pract.* 1975;2:29–34.

15. Health status assessment. http:// www.healthstatus.com/ Accessed 14.11.08.

16. Revolution Health. http://www. revolutionhealth.com/trackers Accessed 31.03.09.

17. HealthCheck USA. http://www. healthcheckusa.com/ Accessed 14.11.08.

18. Ridker PM, Silvertown JD. Inflammation, C-reactive protein, and atherothrombosis. *J Periodontol.* 2008;79(suppl 8):1544–1551.

19. Melamed ML, Michos ED, Post W, Astor B. 25-hydroxyvitamin D levels and the risk of mortality in the general population. *Arch Intern Med.* 2008;168 (15):1629–1637.

20. Jemal A, Ward E, Hao Y, Thun M. Trends in the leading causes of death in the United States, 1970– 2002. *JAMA.* 2005;294(10): 1255–1259.

Safe self-care

Points to Ponder !

- Optimal self-care requires a lifelong commitment to choosing a healthy lifestyle options.
- Safe self-care is only possible when individuals know when to seek a professional opinion.

For self-care to enhance wellbeing effectively, it is not enough to acquire healthy habits and avoid unhealthy habits: it is also necessary to recognize the onset of disease. Safe self-care therefore requires screening for early evidence of dysfunction and disease. Screening is undertaken at the level of both the practitioner and the individual.

Self-assessment

Patients have the ability to judge their own health status. It is unclear whether such judgments are based on concerns about risky lifestyle choices, specific health problems, or both. A number of cross-sectional studies have confirmed that risky lifestyle choices are associated with poor self-rated health. Smoking, alcohol excess, physical inactivity and low intakes of vegetables have all been shown to be associated with poor self-rated health. A longitudinal cohort study of elderly people found regular exercise improved mobility, achieved better functional status, protected against poor self-rated health and decreased mortality 4–6 years later.[1] A population-based cohort study confirmed an association between eating a less prudent diet and the

prevalence of poor self-rated health; it also demonstrated independent associations between mortality and both poor self-rated health and a low prudent food intake score.[2] Self-rated health in women and a positive attitude towards health in men have been shown to predict mortality patterns.[3] It has even been reported that patients' self-reports are better able to predict health outcome than information gained from laboratory tests, physician health reports or risk factor analysis.[4] Whereas people who smoke are twice as likely to die during the next 12 years as non-smokers, people who considered themselves to be in 'poor health' were seven times as likely to die as those who considered themselves in 'excellent health'. Regardless of their relative importance, both personal health status assessment and risk factor analysis deserve consideration when formulating a self-care package.

Self-care resources

The opportunities for primary practitioners to deliver the wellness message are limited. Practitioners can deliver a self-care message during illness and periodic health examination encounters. However, individuals who enjoy robust health are prone to ignore advice to have an annual check-up. Consequently, despite current clinical practice guidelines to deliver clinical preventive services during illness encounters, dissemination of the wellness message by primary practitioners is severely restricted. The only exposure many consumers may have to self-care messages may be through mandates from insurance companies, pre-employment health checks, workplace health promotion, or public education initiatives via the lay press, television or the internet.[5] Sources such as these ensure that health information is readily available to interested consumers. Some of internet sites focus on one health dimension, e.g. Heart Foundations in America, Australia and Britain all spread the healthy heart message on the internet. Similarly, each of these countries has an organization that focuses on cancer.[6] Government health authorities tend to be more constrained in their recommendations for routine screening than are various disease-specific organizations. Cancer societies favour annual pelvic examinations for all women over 40 years of age; governments restrict this to high-risk patients. Health messages are also spread by private profit-making organizations that provide public access to more esoteric screening tests. Self-check personal screening tests for heavy metals, free radicals and metabolic typing are available for purchase.[7] While government, not-for profit organizations and health care businesses all use the internet to spread their health information message,[6–12] the quality of health information is variable and critical appraisal of information is desirable.

Variability in the quality of information accessed is one difficulty consumers face when independently formulating a wellness plan; another is that access to resources does not necessarily result in behaviour change. Motivation to implement advice is needed. One study found that supplementary reinforcement, involving contact by health professionals over and above routine clinical encounters, may be a prerequisite for effective use of technology-based delivery of health promotion information in older people.[13] Another report found that for health risk appraisals questionnaires to be effective they should be combined with follow-up interventions, ranging from information and support to referral.[14] Health risk appraisal questionnaires systematically collect information to identify personal risk factors. When used alone or with one-time feedback, the health risk appraisal questionnaire is not an effective health promotion strategy. On the other hand, when used as part of an interactive health promotion programme, health risk appraisal has been shown to promote healthy lifestyle behaviours particularly with respect to exercise and control of blood pressure and weight control.

In addition to motivating and helping consumers obtain validated information, health professionals can guide individuals in their choice of screening test. The US Preventative Services Taskforce and the Canadian Task Force on Preventive Health Care list a comprehensive range of possible screening tests and make sound recommendations on their use.[8,11] These authorities *strongly* recommend a screening test when good-quality evidence exists which demonstrates substantial net benefit over harm, and the intervention is perceived to be cost-effective and acceptable to nearly all patients. They also recommend use of services when there is fair evidence that the service improves important health outcomes and benefit outweighs harm. No recommendation for or against routine population-based provision of a service is made when there is insufficient evidence of benefit or the cost–benefit ratio is too close to call. It is in such instances that professional guidance assumes greatest importance. Similarly, there are age-specific periods during the lifecycle when certain screening tests become appropriate[10] (see Table 7.1). Health professionals can alert consumers and enable timely screening. Consumers benefit from professional guidance.

Self-screening

Self-care requires taking increased personal responsibility for one's wellbeing. Successful self-care requires a three-pronged approach: those of being aware of and willing to implement healthy lifestyle choices, knowing how to detect covert changes that require investigation, and recognizing overt signs of disease that require professional assessment. At the wellness pole, consumers need to be aware whether their lifestyle choices are healthy or risky. Safe self-care necessitates knowing when professional intervention is indicated. It requires consumers to recognize change at a stage when the outcome of treatment is likely to be most successful. The very earliest suggestion of disturbed homeostasis is the presence of risk markers. **Handout 7.1** identifies some healthy and unhealthy lifestyle choices. Unhealthy lifestyle choices are orange flags indicating hazards ahead. The next phase is early recognition of ominous body changes. Population screening programmes have been developed to detect red flags. Individuals also need to be aware of certain signs and symptoms that may herald serious disease. Women need to know to request professional assessment of any abnormal gynaecological bleeding prior to menopause or any vaginal blood loss after menopause. Some red flags indicating the need for professional guidance are listed in **Handout 7.2**. Despite no official recommendations, it is also helpful for patients to be aware when common symptoms, such as a headache, fever, a cough or chest pain, should not be ignored. **Handouts 7.3–7.6** provide some referral guidelines for symptomatic persons who are committed to self-care.

In addition to knowing how to evaluate symptom experiences, safe self-care encompasses actively searching for evidence of covert disease. Detecting the early signs of disease may require routine self-examination of the breast or testis, skin and mouth. In addition to body awareness, successful self-screening requires acquisition of palpatory skills to detect relevant changes. Self-screening based on the practitioner education of healthy patients is recommended for:[15,16]

- all women, who should perform breast self-examination at monthly intervals
- all males, who should palpate for testicular lumps at monthly intervals
- all persons discovering any oral lesions that persist for more than 1 week
- all those finding a new or changing skin lesion.

The timing of self-examination may be important: menstruating woman should perform breast self-examination a few days after the end of their menstrual period; in postmenopausal women, any day of the month that is easy to remember will suffice. **Handout 25.3** provides details on the technique used in breast self-examination. Video breast examination is demonstrated on the internet,[17] as are guidelines from the American Cancer Society.[18] **Handout 7.7** lists findings on breast self-examination that suggest the need for professional evaluation.

Despite health authorities disagreeing about the usefulness of routine periodic testicular examination, it may be prudent for testicular self-examination to be initiated at puberty. Testicular cancer is the most common malignancy in men aged 15–35 years. Monthly self-examination is certainly recommended for men with a family history of testicular cancer or a personal history of undescended testes. Men who carry out regular testicular self-examination are advised to examine their testicles after a warm bath or shower. **Handout 13.14** provides information on the technique used in testicular self-examination. **Handout 7.8** identifies findings on testicular self-examination that suggest the need to consult a doctor. All suspect masses should be biopsied and a definitive diagnosis made. In addition to

information regarding testis palpation, the Office of Men's Health provides clear self-check guidelines to enable men to recognize early evidence of skin, oral and breast cancer.[12] While internet-based instructions are helpful, it may nonetheless be sensible for primary practitioners to check that their patients are implementing the technique effectively. Videos demonstrating how to do various cancer self-screening techniques are also available on the internet.[17]

In addition to routine gender-specific self-examination, both the skin and mouth should be regularly checked. There are three important types of skin cancer, each type having unique findings suggestive of malignancy. While a knowledge of the presentation of each type of cancer may refine an individual's self-screening, a more simplistic guide to dermatological changes indicating a need for immediate professional investigation may suffice (see **Handout 7.9**). A video on skin self-examination is available on the internet.[19] Those suffering from prolonged sun exposure also have an increased risk of lip cancer. Tobacco-chewing or any chronic mechanical or chemical irritation of the buccal mucosa also increases the risk of malignant change. **Handout 7.10** provides hints on oral lesions that require professional assessment.

Self-screening is not restricted to the detection of physical findings: effective self-care includes screening for evidence of mental distress. Although population self-screening for stress is not recommended by health authorities, a strategy to identify the emotional, cognitive and physical impact of stress may be appropriate in the periodic health examination or illness encounter. As the impact of stress is more a function of individuals' perceptions of, and ability to cope with, their life stresses than any objective measure of exposure to stressful stimuli, it may be helpful to become aware of the need to improve one's personal stress management. **Handout 7.11** can be used to screen for evidence of stress. The more items checked, the greater the necessity to acquire an effective stress management strategy.

Professional screening

To ensure that population-based screening programmes are cost-effective, they need to conform to a number of criteria, ranging from a more successful clinical outcome when a condition is detected and treated during the asymptomatic stage to the diagnostic and therapeutic intervention being acceptable to the patient. The lag time between an individual choosing an unhealthy lifestyle and experiencing symptoms or developing signs of disease provides an opportunity for professional intervention. Case finding is a strategy for active disease prevention in primary practice. Case finding takes two forms: that of the annual check-up and the periodic health examination. The annual check-up or 'physical' involves a battery of tests to screen an asymptomatic individual for subclinical evidence of pathological changes. Multiphasic screening does detect pathology in apparently well patients; however, the statistical inevitability of occasional false-positive results, uncertainty about the implications of abnormal tests in healthy people, and the reluctance of people who feel well to implement change all mitigate against the usefulness of this disease prevention initiative. Annual check-ups, criticized as being non-specific and time-wasting, are now recommended only for those over 65 years of age. In younger people, it has been largely superseded by the more specific periodic health examination. Early and Periodic Screening, Diagnosis, and Treatment (EPSDT) examinations are increasingly being included in Medicaid managed care plans.[20]

The periodic health examination becomes a more acceptable, cost-effective use of resources when it is based upon age- and sex-specific disease screening schedules. It can be further refined in primary practice by focusing on health risks resulting from a particular patient's genetic or lifestyle predisposition to disease. Active case finding is limited to those conditions with a substantial morbidity or mortality in which the clinical outcome is improved by intervention during the covert stage of the disease. Cost-effective and reliable methods of diagnosis and treatment must also be available. To determine the usefulness of detecting a disease marker in an asymptomatic individual, information is needed about the cause, pathogenesis and prognosis of the untreated condition. To decide whether and when intervention in a 'well' individual is indicated, objective data on the outcome of therapeutic intervention at various stages of disease progression are required.

Periodic health examination schedules are embedded in public health programmes.[10,11,21] Major risk markers such as hypertension, hyperlipidaemia, overweight/obesity and, where indicated, hyperglycaemia are recommended with greatest frequency (see **Professional Poster 7.1**). The frequency recommended for physician screening varies according to the condition. In general, it is suggested that, every 4 years, adults should be screened for:

- **an elevated serum cholesterol level:** screening involves determining the total serum cholesterol level, except in those over the age of 50, who should also have a high-density lipoprotein cholesterol determination. Men should be screened for lipids disorders from the age of 35, women from the age of 45
- **obesity**, which may be determined by either using the body mass index or comparing actual and ideal body weight
- **hypertension**, a blood pressure reading above 140/90 mmHg on three or more serial readings being diagnostic of hypertension in healthy adults of 25–40 years of age. Older adults require more frequent blood pressure assessment.

Every 2 years, adults should be screened for:
- **hypertension:** blood pressure should be checked every 2 years in healthy adults between 40 and 60 years of age
- **breast cancer:** a professional breast examination of women aged 20–50 years should be performed, mammography being recommended for high-risk patients under the age of 50
- **cervical cancer:** Papanicolaou smears should be taken for sexually active women until the age of 70. The first two smears should be performed yearly. All sexually active women aged 18 and above are advised to have Pap smears every 2 years.[22]

In older or high-risk adults, annual screening is recommended to check for:

- **breast cancer:** annual professional breast examination should be performed in high-risk women under the age of 50, annual professional breast examination and mammography being recommended for all women over the age of 50 years
- **coronary artery disease:** blood pressure and serum cholesterol level should be checked in high-risk patients
- **hypertension,** annual blood pressure checks being advocated for patients over the age of 60 years.

The age at which screening should commence varies. Periodic questioning about hearing loss and Snellen chart screening for visual impairment is recommended from the age of 65 years (see **Professional**

Posters 7.2 and 7.3). Screening for colorectal cancer is strongly recommended from the age of 55 years. Counselling at-risk adults regarding the benefits ands risks of aspirin prophylaxis and making all, especially parents, aware of the risks of tobacco smoke is also strongly recommended for persons 18 years and over.[21] This is also the age at which screening for overweight, the risk of sexually transmitted diseases and depression is recommended. **Handout 13.5** lists some orange and red flags indicating the need for a professional opinion and **Handout 13.7** describes the clinical presentation of prevalent sexually transmitted diseases. Detection (see **Handout 14.11**) and treatment of depression in primary practice can offer substantial benefit to patients and the community. In childhood, screening for immunization status, obesity and hypertension is suggested. The American Academy of Pediatrics provides up-to-date immunization schedules.[23]

Not all practitioners agree with the stringency with which inclusion criteria are applied, and some would question the use of various procedures. Examples include obesity and aspects of cancer screening. Disputed cancer screening procedures include:

- rectal examination for prostatic carcinoma in asymptomatic men over the age of 40 years
- screening for colorectal carcinoma by an annual digital rectal examination from the age of 40 years
- annual faecal occult blood tests in asymptomatic patients over the age of 50 years
- one flexible proctosigmoidoscopy examination at age 55 years.

Despite controversy, some authoritative bodies such as the American Cancer Society not only would agree with these prostatic and colorectal carcinoma screening procedures but also would recommend annual pelvic examinations for all women over 40 years of age. In the case of obesity, while the Canadian Task Force considers there is insufficient evidence of short-term or long-term benefits from screening for or treatment of childhood obesity to make any recommendations,[24] excess weight is regarded as a critical and increasing health problem in Canada.[25]

Screening recommendations that fulfil listed criteria have been subject to critical scrutiny. These recommendations should therefore be regarded as the minimal population-based periodic health examination procedures for examining asymptomatic adults. Primary practitioners have the opportunity to exercise their clinical judgment to promote wellness in their clients/patients. In addition to disease-specific screening procedures, general health status screening such as a full blood count and urine dipstick may be included. **Professional Poster 7.4** demonstrates how much information can be obtained from a non-invasive test such as urinalysis.

The frequency with which testing is recommended increases with age and personal risk. Table 7.1 outlines the recommendations of the American Medical Association. When risk factors are present, more extensive examination is indicated. On average, young people should be seen by a health professional every 3–5 years; middle-aged persons, every 2–3 years; and elderly persons, every year.[26] These visits should be viewed as opportunities to promote self-care.

In perspective

After considering the work of the Canadian Task Force on the Periodic Health Examination, Battista concluded: 'The achievable health benefits through clinical preventive care may be unavoidably limited and a broadly based approach to preventive care combining clinical and population strategies needs to be considered.'[27] A combination of consumer education, self-screening and professional case finding provides a sound approach to developing self-care programmes. Furthermore, self-assessment of risk, whether this be through self-screening for lifestyle risks, detecting abnormality by self-palpation or awareness of bodily dysfunction, is but one aspect of self-care. Successful self-care is based upon realistic self-assessment and effective intervention. When the recommended intervention requires behaviours that involve making lifestyle choices that eliminate a harmful behaviour, there is little concern for untoward effects. There is no downside to quitting tobacco use or cutting alcohol intake to safe levels. When the recommended intervention requires pharmaceutical or neutraceutical interventions, more care is needed. Megadose mineral or vitamin intake can have harmful side effects. Similarly, injudicious use of over-the-counter or prescription drugs can create, rather than resolve, health problems. It is at this level of health care that consultation with discerning health professionals, although not obligatory, is prudent.

Table 7.1 Recommended frequency for performing screening test

Test recommended by the AMA	General group*			High-risk group*		
Age group (years)	13–30	30–50	>50	13–30	30–50	>50
Eye examination	2	2	2	1	1	1
Dental check-up	0.5–1	1	1–2	On dentist advice		
PAP smear[†]	1	1–3	3–5	1	1	1
Blood pressure[‡]	3–5	1–3	1	1	1	1
Blood cholesterol[‡]	5	3–5	3–5	On doctor advice		
Mammography	0	1–2	1	0	1–2	1
Rectal examination	0	Aft 40	1	Aft 20	1	1
Occult blood stool	0	1	1	0	1	1
Sigmoidoscopy	0	0	3–5	0	0	3–5

*Frequency test should be performed (years).
[†]start once sexually active
[‡]start from 20 years of age
Aft – annually after the age of
Patients can do a self-check at: http://www.mayoclinic.com/health/health-screening/WO000112

References

1. Fillenbaum GG, Burchett BM, Kuchibhatla MN, Cohen HJ, Blazer DG. Effect of cancer screening and desirable health behaviors on functional status, self-rated health, health service use and mortality. *J Am Geriatr Soc*. 2007;55(1):66–74.

2. Osler M, Heitmann BL, Høidrup S, Jørgensen LM, Schroll M. Food intake patterns, self rated health and mortality in Danish men and women. A prospective observational study. *J Epidemiol Community Health*. 2001;55:399–403.

3. Tobiasz-Adamczyk B, Brzyski P, Kopacz MS. Health attitudes and behaviour as predictors of self-rated health in relation to mortality patterns (17-year follow-up in a Polish elderly population—Cracow study). *Cent Eur J Public Health*. 2008;16(2):47–53.

4. Luskin F, Newell K. Mind–body approaches to successful aging. In: Watkins A, ed. *Mind–Body Medicine*. New York: Churchill Livingstone; 1997:251–268.

5. Cherrington A, Corbie-Smith G, Pathman DE. Do adults who believe in periodic health examinations receive more clinical preventive services? *Prev Med*. 2007;45(4): 282–289.

6. National Cancer Institute. http://prevention.cancer.gov/ prevention-detection/cancers Accessed 19.11.08.

7. http://www. worldwidehealthcenter.net/ category.php?cat=SK Accessed 19.11.08.

8. The US Preventative Services Taskforce. *Guide to Clinical Preventive Services 2007*. http:// www.ahrq.gov/clinic/pocketgd07/; Accessed 11.19.08.

9. British Heart Foundation. http://www.bhf.org.uk/ keeping_your_heart_healthy/ default.aspx; Accessed 19.11.08.

10. Medline plus. http://www.nlm.nih. gov/medlineplus/healthscreening. html; Accessed 19.11.08.

11. Canadian Task Force on Preventive Health Care. http://www.ctfphc. org/; Accessed 20.11.08.

12. Office of Men's Health. http:// www.illinois.gov/menshealth/ selfscreening.cfm; Accessed 19.11.08.

13. Harari D, Iliffe S, Kharicha K, et al. Promotion of health in older people:

a randomised controlled trial of health risk appraisal in British general practice. *Age Ageing.* 2008;37(5):565–571.

14. Shekelle P, Tucker J, Maglione M, et al. *Evidence Report, and Evidence-Based Recommendations.* Baltimore, MD: Prepared for the US Department of Health and Human Services, Health Care Financing Administration; Sept 2003. (Also available as RAND RP-1225.)

15. Frame PS. A critical review of adult health maintenance. *J Fam Pract.* 1986;22:341–346, 417–422, 511–520; see also 23: 29–39.

16. Lindberg SC. Adult preventive health screening: 1987 update. *Nurse Pract.* 1987;12:19–29.

17. Self-examination. http://www.videojug.com/tag/cancer; Accessed 19.11.08.

18. American Cancer Society. Breast self-examination. http://www.cancer.org/docroot/CRI/content/CRI_2_6x_How_to_perform_a_breast_self_exam_5.asp. Accessed 19.11.08.

19. Skin cancer. http://www.videojug.com/film/how-to-check-for-skin-cancer; Accessed 19.11.08.

20. Millar JS, Mitchell L, McCauley D, Winston T, Hays C. Early and periodic screening, diagnosis, and treatment examination completion rates for Oklahoma Medicaid managed care: 1995–1998. *J Okla State Med Assoc.* 2001;94 (5):151–154.

21. The Commission on Public Health and Scientific Affairs. AAFP age charts for periodic health examinations. *Am Fam Physician.* 1991;43(5):1845–1847; for 65 years and over 1992;45(5):2391–2394; for 40 to 64 years 1992;45(4):1917–1920; for 19 to 39 years 1992;45 (3):1367–1370; for 7–12 years 1992;45(1):267–268; for 19 months to 6 years 1991;44(6):2241–2242; from birth to 18 months 1991;44 (5):1882–1884.

22. Waxman AG, Zsemlye MM. Preventing cervical cancer: the Pap test and the HPV vaccine. *Med Clin North Am.* 2008;92 (5):1059–1082.

23. American Academy of Pediatrics. http://www.cispimmunize.org/; Accessed 21.11.08.

24. Canadian Task Force on the Periodic Health Examination. 1994 update: 1. Obesity in childhood. *CMAJ.* 1994;150(6):871–879.

25. Bélanger-Ducharme F, Tremblay A. Prevalence of obesity in Canada. *Obes Rev.* 2005;6 (3):183–186.

26. Branch WT, Crouch M. Periodic health exams: what really matters? *Patient Care.* 1998;32:21–47.

27. Battista RN. Practice guidelines for preventive care: the Canadian experience. Canadian Task Force on the Periodic Health Exami006Eation. *Br J Gen Pract.* 1993;43(372):301–304.

Strategies for promoting self-care

- Successful wellness promotion is tailored to meet the needs of the client.
- Self-care programmes inform, motivate and empower clients.
- The practitioner's role is that of a reliable information resource, facilitator and motivator.
- Health literacy and self-efficacy are crucial attributes in wellness self-care.

Leading a healthy lifestyle improves survival and reduces the incidence of disease.[1] In fact, 'A few key lifestyle components – smoke- and tobacco-free living, a diet that emphasizes: fruits and vegetables with only lean meats and low-fat dairy products, 30 minutes of physical activity a day, and control of blood pressure and serum cholesterol – have a significant impact on life expectancy.'[2] However, the opportunity for substantial public health benefit comes about only when behaviour-change interventions are embraced by large numbers of people. At a population level, overall risk factors typically change only 1% to 20%, yet these 'modest' impacts translate to significant benefits to the health of the population.[3] A low-risk population is the foundation upon which a sustainable health care system can be built.

Delivering the message

Social marketing is used to motivate populations to change. In contrast to commercial marketing where the aim is financial gain, social marketing uses marketing principles to achieve specific behaviour goals for social good. The aim is to sell ideas, attitudes and behaviours. Aided by supporting government policy and environmental changes, social marketing aims to bring about voluntary healthy behavioural changes in individuals.[4] As targeted clients have the power to ensure success or failure of population-based health promotion programmes, the message needs to be couched in culturally sensitive terms. In successful campaigns, the primary focus is on what the consumer wants and needs. Social marketing is an integral part of community health promotion. Various health-promoting campaigns, e.g. Sunsmart to prevent skin cancer, are marketed in Australia, Canada, New Zealand, the UK and the US.[5–7]

Media-based communication channels vary from Internet programs and computer-assisted interventions to video viewing and self-help guides.[3] Fully automated low-cost intervention such as Alive! have been shown to effect significant improvements in important health parameters.[8] Alive! is an email-based intervention to increase physical activity, fruit and vegetable consumption and to reduce added sugars, and saturated and trans fats. Intervention strategies include assessments followed by individualized feedback, weekly goal-setting, individually tailored goals and tips, reminders, and promotion of social support. With this public health trend towards self-care, 'primary care providers are increasingly being called upon to transfer some of their present functions to patients, but they will then undertake alternative or supplementary functions including education'.[9] Health professionals are well positioned to provide patients with quality evidence-based information. However, regardless of its validity, poorly packaged information may confuse rather than enlighten, and information overload may discourage rather than motivate. A literature review found no evidence supporting approaches based on information/knowledge alone with or without brief values clarification.[10] Quality education goes beyond having access to health information. Although knowledge is essential, alone it does not lead to change.[11] In order to achieve change, whether delivered through the mass media or in the clinical consultation, the message must be modified to suit the patient.

A number of models have been proposed to provide insights into the drivers of current behaviour patterns. Each of these models emphasizes various considerations in preparing a patient-centred health message. The Health Belief Model focuses on individuals' perceived vulnerability to a disorder, both with respect to contracting the condition and the overall impact of having the disease. Concerns arising from these perceived risks are then measured against the benefits from, and barriers to, undertaking protective health behaviours.[11] Table 8.1 lists some obstacles that must be overcome to achieve change. Research has confirmed that people are only willing to change if they believe they are susceptible to a serious condition which can be avoided if they take certain actions – provided the benefit of such action outweighs the costs.[10] The Explanatory Model emphasizes the cultural context of illness.[11] It suggests change is influenced by how societies and individuals in those societies explain illness with respect to its cause, natural history, severity and treatment options. Research has confirmed that patients are more likely to change when provided with personalized normative feedback.[10] The Theory of Planned Behaviour expands the constructs of the Explanatory Model by including the notion of perceived behavioural control, i.e. believing one can control a causal chain of events, alters attitudes and drives behavioural intentions.[12] Given this framework, persons with an internal locus of control would be good candidates for behavioural change programmes as they believe they can exercise control over the cause and progression of a condition. The Theory of Planned Behavior assumes the most important determinants of behaviour are intention, influenced by a person's attitude toward performing a behaviour, and beliefs about whether significant others approve or disapprove of the behaviour. When others approve of behavioural choices, the individual is afforded social support, buffering the individual against some of the stresses associated with change. In all these models, the primary focus is the patient/client; in each case, change is the result of an ongoing process.

The Self-Regulation Model recognizes that self-care is essentially an exercise in problem solving in which a plan is generated to control a potential problem given the individual's beliefs about a possible health threat and their appraisal of intervention options.[11] Table 8.2 lists some prerequisites that must be met before lifestyle changes are likely to be made. The Social Cognitive Theory sees problem solving as a dynamic, ongoing process. In this model, the main factors influencing successful change are goals, outcome expectancies and self-efficacy.[12] Outcome expectations are the results an individual anticipates from taking action. Self-efficacy is the ability to reach one's goals. It is an individual's level of confidence in their own skills

Table 8.1 Obstacles to behaviour change

Obstacles	Solutions
Health a low priority	Enhance awareness of personal health risk and advantages of wellness
Poorly informed, lack resources and skills	Provide relevant knowledge and skills
Deny personal risks	Self-assessment of personal risk
Lack commitment	Ownership of wellness protocol/lifestyle script

Table 8.2 Prerequisites for achieving change

Prerequisites	Meeting prerequisites
Motivation Knowledge and skills Self-efficacy/personal control	Relevant education selected by client-personalized, active participation
Acceptable lifestyle change	Select interventions least disruptive
Expect and achieve a positive outcome	Monitor progress and change as needed

and persistence to accomplish a desired goal. Self-efficacy predicts future behaviour across a wide variety of lifestyle risk factors. Practitioners can increase their patients' self-efficacy by breaking goals into interim targets, negotiating behavioural plans that specify goals and rewards, and by monitoring progress and reinforcing success through feedback. The '5A's' offers a practical approach for implementing change by assessing, advising, agreeing, assisting, and arranging follow-up. This programme provides a useful framework for delivering behavioural risk factor interventions in primary care settings.[13]

When combined with the Transtheoretical Model, the '5 A's' offers a comprehensive approach to change. The Transtheoretical Model describes an individual's motivation and readiness to change a behaviour through the stages of pre-contemplation, contemplation, preparation, action, and maintenance.[12] The model is circular, allowing for relapse. Table 8.3 demonstrates how these models can be applied in clinical practice. Self-care programmes based on the principles of adult learning that use interactive, sequential learning opportunities appear to have the best outcome regardless of whether the target audience is the general population or the individual patient.

The role of the practitioner

Self-care is most successful when undertaken as a joint venture between patient and practitioner. Practitioners can provide patients with evidence-based information and motivation in small group workshops or as part of a clinical consultation. In fact, brief interventions integrated into routine primary care have been shown to effectively address the most common and important risk behaviours.[3] Brief motivational interventions are short therapeutic encounters that typically combine motivational interviewing with personalized feedback. Brief motivational interventions usually involve at least two components: those of assessing the nature/quality, frequency, and consequences of a behaviour and of tailoring motivational strategies, most commonly through personalized feedback and normative comparisons. Other strategies that are useful, but only when combined with the brief motivational interviews, are 'timeline followback' and 'decisional balancing'.[14,15] In the case of the former, requesting a patient to complete a retrospective record of the hazardous behaviour prior to the consultation raises awareness and encourages movement from pre-contemplation to the contemplation stages of change.[14] Weighing up the costs and benefits of behaviours has a similar motivational impact.[15] Counselling, defined as a cooperative interaction between the clinician and an actively participating patient, aims to help patients cope and take independent initiatives.[16] Engaging patients actively in the self-management practices needed to change and maintain healthy behaviours is a central component of effective behavioural counselling. A single counselling session embedded in a routine motivational clinical consultation can be beneficial. Spending 5 to 10 minutes in motivational counselling, with or without the aid of a self-help booklet and/or physical assessment, has been shown to successfully decrease alcohol use.[17]

Table 8.3 Wellness: an ongoing process		
Change	**The practitioner**	**The client/patient**
Step 1	ASSESS: data-gathering to establish health need	PRE-CONTEMPLATION: no intention to change
Step 2	ADVISE: motivate by enhancing awareness of risks, benefits of change, outcomes, identify health need	CONTEMPLATION: weighing up pros and cons
Step 3	AGREE: negotiate a programme tailored to individual to encourage adherence by agreeing on priorities and outlining range of strategies	PREPARATION: agree on priorities, choose effective strategies least disruptive to lifestyle, initiate programme
Step 4	ASSIST: implement programme, agree deadlines, monitoring	ACTION: implement changed behaviours, perform progression self-checks
Step 5	ACTION: follow-up to detect relapses and identify changing needs, modify as required	MAINTENANCE: Healthy behaviour becomes a habit, ongoing review of changing health needs

Unlike disease management, in which pain or discomfort provides strong motivation to implement a treatment programme, a self-care programme requires behavioural change by those who feel well. Motivation to change has emerged as a stronger predictor of successful change than any demographic variable.[18] Patients are more likely to be motivated when they are provided with information of immediate relevance that leads to an outcome that is significant to the patient's physical, psychological and/or social wellbeing. A major task for practitioners is to motivate clients/patients to commit to a lifetime of self-care. Empathic practitioners who ask patient-centred questions and provide congruent verbal and non-verbal messages are most likely to be successful.[19] The four habit coding scheme can be translated to provide a useful framework in which to conduct self-care education.[20] The practitioner role is that of facilitator. A therapeutic climate conducive to self-care is one in which:

- suggestions are open for negotiation rather than presented as recommendations
- information is casually supplied and open to informal discussion
- client proposals for change are supported
- independence and self-care are encouraged.

Practitioners who treat their patients as independent adults with a wealth of useful previous experience fare best. Tips on motivational interviewing are available.[21] Patients/clients who demonstrate a cognitive and affective acceptance of a health need, who assume ownership of a health programme and take responsibility for the implementation of personally selected health strategies are most likely to comply with their self-care wellness programme.

Patient literacy: a skill set

Major sources of health information include health professionals, laypersons and the media. Laypersons, particularly family and friends, are an influential source of information and possibly misinformation. Some individuals rely on health professionals and peer opinion for much of their health information, others depend on the electronic and print media. Self-help materials are readily available – and useful. One study even suggested that clinical intervention using the McKenzie method of physical therapy and chiropractic manipulation might have achieved only a marginally better outcome than did an educational booklet.[22] Use of the media requires consumer literacy, whether it be electronic – television, video, radio, the Internet – or print media, such as books, booklets, pamphlets or brochures.

Six core skills or literacies have been identified as essential for effective use of health information. These are categorized as: traditional, health, information, scientific, media, and computer literacy.[23] Analytic ability is required for effective traditional, media and information literacy. Analytic ability combines cognitive processes and critical thinking skills. Critical appraisal is the process of assessing and interpreting evidence by systematically considering its validity, results and relevance to the individual. Media literacy, for example, is a means of critically thinking about media content that enables people to place information in a social and political context and to consider issues such as the marketplace, audience relations, and how media forms in themselves shape the message that is conveyed.

Context-specific, or more situation-specific, understanding is required for computer, scientific and health literacy. Health literacy requires that the person have the ability to read, understand, and act on health care information. Computer literacy is the ability to use computers to solve problems. Scientific literacy requires an understanding of the nature, aims, methods, application, limitations, and politics of creating knowledge in a systematic manner. Lay people who lack scientific literacy may find it helpful to scrutinize the speaker or author's qualifications and affiliations. As a rule of thumb, the content should be regarded more critically when the messenger lacks relevant training in the topic area. A balanced view of the topic, in which both the benefits and the costs, the advantages and the disadvantages, are considered, probably gives a more realistic picture than one promoting a one-sided opinion. With respect to print media, the source of the information may also allow the reader some safeguards. Provided that it is accurately presented, material derived from work published in recognized peer-reviewed scientific journals usually reflects current thought in professional circles. Work that faithfully reflects information from referenced, relevant, recent and reputable publications is more deserving of respect. The data upon which the author's conclusions are based are highly relevant. Where it is available, information on the method used to generate the information provides a fundamentally meaningful comment on content.

Preparing the message

An ability to comprehend and determine the accuracy and relevance of content are paramount to successful self-use of information resources. Health messages should provide accurate, verifiable information. Three important types of evidence-based information resources are recognized. Information can be derived from anecdote, expert consensus, or scientifically validated studies. *Anecdote* is based upon, at worst, hearsay and, at best, personal experience. In any event, anecdote is probably an important source of misinformation. *Expert consensus*, as the name implies, is an agreement between experts in the field. This traditional form of consensus appears as a consensus statement, usually following a conference. Meta-analysis is emerging as a modern form of consensus. This technique combines information from separate sources to yield a summary of the available evidence. It uses a statistical technique to combine data from a number of studies to produce an overall estimate of the size of an effect. Studies used range from observational to randomized controlled clinical trials. Meta-analysis provides strong qualitative evidence for whether a treatment works, and robust but conservative quantitative evidence on how well it does so.[24] The data upon which meta-analysis is based can also be analysed. At this level, the quality of the science used to produce the information is evaluated.

The final type of information is that arising from scientifically validated studies. The most persuasive data are produced from studies that use double-blind, placebo-controlled, randomized clinical trials. Cause-and-effect relationships are best demonstrated using randomized clinical trials. The probability of a cause-and-effect relationship is increased when there is:[25]

- substantiating evidence from 'experiments' on humans
- consistency between different studies, supporting a relationship between intervention and outcome
- an appropriate temporal relationship, cause consistently preceding effect
- a dose–response relationship
- a strong relationship between intervention and outcome
- biological plausibility
- an identifiable analogous situation.

Ranked in order of decreasing merit, other less stringent research methodologies that suggest an association include:

- the analytic epidemiological trial: cohort/ prospective longitudinal, or case series
- descriptive epidemiology: prevalence/survey/ cross-sectional studies
- case studies
- case reports, a single case report being a close relative of the anecdote.

Health information messages need to be understandable. As over 40% of adults in the US and Canada appear to have basic (or prose) literacy levels below that which is needed to optimally participate in civil society, unless health education material is tailored to patients' literacy levels, it may even fail to inform.[23] A study of patient information on websites found the readability level to be higher than that regarded as comprehensible to the majority of patients.[26] Another study recommended simplifying hospital material to no higher than a grade five level to enable comprehension by the majority of hospital patients.[27] Text simplicity and comprehension influence the usefulness of health information material. Strategies are available for analysing the readability and appropriateness of printed material. Readability is determined by the patient's reading level, comprehension depending on language, logic and experience. Poor readers tire easily, take words literally, read slowly, missing the meaning, and skip over words, thus missing the context.

When assessing the readability of text, a number of formulae can be applied to ascertain the reading level (Figure 8.1). The simplicity of printed material is determined by the length of the sentences and size of the words. The Flesch Reading Ease formula measures the average sentence length in words (sl) and the number of syllables per 100 words (wl).[28] Reading ease is equivalent to:

$$206.835 - 0.846(\text{wl}) - 1.015(\text{sl})$$

On a scale of zero to 100, the lower the number, the more difficult the material is to read.

The Gunning Fog Index measures the average sentence length and the number of words of three syllables or more per 100 words.[28,29] A reading grade is obtained by totalling these two measurements and multiplying their sum by 0.4. Easy reading is any grade between 6 and 10. Patient information graded at 13 or over is probably unsuitable as this is equivalent to the reading level of a college freshman.

The Reading Score or SMOG grade is the reading grade a person must have reached to fully understand the assessed text.

Fog Reading Score
- Choose a passage of about 100 words ending in a full stop
- Find average sentence length by dividing 100 by the number of sentences
- Find number of long words, defined as those of three syllables or more. Exclude:
  - proper nouns
  - combinations of easy words, like photocopy
  - verbs that become three syllables when '-es', '-ing' or '-ed' is added, e.g. committed
  - jargon that the reader will know
- Add the average sentence length to the number of long words
- Multiply by 0.4 to get the 'reading score'

Select material with a Fog Reading score of 10 and under. Reject material at 13 and over as unsuitable.

SMOG Grade
- Count 10 consecutive sentences near the beginning, the middle and end of the text. A sentence is any string of words ending with a full stop, question mark or exclamation.
- Count every word of three or more syllables in the 30 sentences selected. Any string of letters or numbers is counted if ended with a space or punctuation mark and if at least three syllables are present when read aloud. If a polysyllabic word is repeated, count each repetition.
- Estimate the square root of the number of polysyllabic words counted. Choose the square root of the nearest square, e.g. for 95 use square root of 100. Choose the lower number if the count is midway.
- Add 3 to the approximate square root to get the SMOG grade.

Select material with lower SMOG grades. Reject material with SMOG grades >13.

RIX
- Analyse whole text – exclude captions and headings
- Count the number of sentences.
- Count the number of long words, i.e. words of seven or more characters after excluding:
  - hyphens
  - brackets
  - punctuation marks
- Determine RIX by dividing the number of long words by the number of sentences (to 2 decimal places)

Figure 8.1 • Patient education materials: readability assessment.

McLaughlin's SMOG grade formula also counts words of three or more syllables but restricts itself to 30 sentences.[28,30] A figure of 3 is added to the square root of the polysyllable count. A SMOG readability grade of 3–8 is equivalent to the reading ability of those with a primary level education, 9–12 to that of a secondary level and 13–16 to a college education. To understand material with a SMOG grade of 17–18, graduate training is required, while material with a grade of 19 and over is best understood by individuals with a higher professional qualification.

The Australian Rix readability formula also assesses the frequency of long words per sentence.[31,32] It is calculated by counting the number of words with more than six characters and dividing the total by the number of sentences, 'WHO' and '1999–2000', for example, both counting as a single word. The score can then be transferred to a grade of reading difficulty. A Rix score of less than 2.9 is recommended for patient materials; this equates to grade 7. A Rix score of 7.2 and over requires a college qualification.

The results of the 1989 Australian literacy survey found that 45% of those assessed were not functioning at a reading grade of 7 with respect to correctly identifying the dosage on an analgesic packet.[31] The aforementioned American study of hospital patients supported targeting patient education material at a grade 5 level. It may therefore be more realistic to distribute health information in print form with a Rix score of less than 2.3 (grade 6). Readability is enhanced by using short sentences and short words, avoiding any unnecessary words.

Comprehension can be enhanced by conceptually organizing the material. A message is successfully communicated by the logical arrangement of material relevant to the reader's experience. As short-term linguistic memory holds four to six unrelated items, simple, concise messages that arouse the reader's interest are best remembered. The efficacy of print media as an information source is enhanced

- The purpose of the brochures should be clearly stated in the title or introduction
- Content focuses on how the health problem can be solved, i.e. on the *behaviours* that need to be changed to improve health. Provide information on a 'need to know' basis
- The scope of the message is restricted to essential information. For triggering the patient's short-term memory:
  - gain the individual's attention
  - present 7 or fewer items at a time
  - get to the point
  For triggering the patient's long-term memory:
  - associate new information with prior knowledge
  - involve the patient in interaction with the information
  - repeat or review
- Provide a summary that repeats important points
- Use understandable language
- Encourage interaction – questions, actions, tasks
- Motivate by providing clear instructions for attainable behavioural changes
- Produce messages consistent with individual's life world – culture, age, gender, experience

Figure 8.2 • Principles for preparing health information messages.

by using the active rather than passive voice and by being personal, for example 'we believe', 'you should', 'please'. Figure 8.2 provides guidelines for structuring the message. Helpful design features that increase the user-friendliness of print material include:[29,33,34,35]

- a layout with a large type size (at least 12 point)
- clear headlines: excess bold typeface and italics should be avoided, as should unnecessary capitals
- white space to frame the text, but avoid glossy paper
- illustrations to convey relevant information, as pictures are easier to remember than words.

Figure 8.3 provides tips for preparing written material.

Slaytor and Ward's paper[36] on the risks and benefits of mammographic screening provides an example of how pamphlets can be analysed for information or content rather than just readability. While readable and comprehensible health information material may convey the message effectively, it is ultimately the content of the message that will determine the health information value of a brochure or booklet.

Electronic media provide an information resource with potential that outstrips print media. However, use of such resources requires additional consumer skills. To enhance wellness or solve a health problem, consumers using electronic sources need to be able to seek out, find, evaluate, appraise,

I Apply the fundamental principles listed in Figure 8.2
II Consider:
- the patient's reading level. Provide information in a form that is easy to understand. Use simple short sentences
- the writing style. This should be conversational, in active voice. Use simple sentences with a friendly tone. Write the way you talk
- the vocabulary used. Common explicit words should be used. Avoid technical jargon, categories, concepts or value judgments. Be specific. Give examples
- the sentence construction. Present content before new information. *To assess your fitness* (content/context), *please walk on the treadmill* (new information)
- layout. Organize material using clear headings. Topic captions provide a road map
- presentation. Present key messages using illustrations. Single line drawings promote realism without distracting details
- focusing aids. Use explanatory captions with figures and graphs to help the reader focus on pertinent points

III Apply these layout tips for written material:
- Place illustrations adjacent to text
- Facilitate flow by having a consistent layout and sequence of information
- Use visual cues to direct attention, e.g. arrows
- Reduce clutter with adequate white spaces
- Any colour supports should not distract from the message
- Limit line length to 30–50 characters/spaces
- Have a high contrast between paper and type
- Use non- or low-gloss paper
- Chunk information – limit message to three or four main points
- Typography tips for written material:
  - For text, use serif type in upper and lower case
  - Use type size of at least 12 point
  - Avoid long headings in all upper case
  - Use typographical cues to emphasize key points – italics, bold, size

Figure 8.3 • Tips for producing written health information materials.

integrate, and apply that information. The eHEALS, a self-report tool that can be administered by a health professional, provides a means of assessing the likelihood a patient will cope with information provided through the electronic media. The instrument is designed to provide a general estimate of consumer eHealth-related skills; it is based on an individual's perception of her or his own skills and knowledge within each measured domain.[37] This eight-item measure of eHealth literacy can be used to inform clinical decision making and health promotion planning with individuals or specific populations. It measures consumers' combined knowledge, comfort, and perceived skills at finding, evaluating, and applying electronic health information to health problems by asking consumers the following questions:[37]

> How useful do you feel the Internet is in helping you make decisions about your health?
>
> How important is it for you to be able to access health resources on the Internet?
>
> Do you know:
> - what health resources are available on the Internet?
> - where to find helpful health resources on the Internet?
> - how to find helpful health resources on the Internet?
> - how to use the Internet to answer your questions about health?
> - how to use the health information you find on the Internet to help you?
>
> Do you have the skills you need to evaluate the health resources you find on the Internet?

A study of 4000 US postal workers found that, despite an increase in the knowledge of safe behaviour, the prevalence of back injury appeared to be unchanged.[38] This failure to translate information into action demonstrates that knowledge alone does not necessarily achieve behaviour change. Self-care requires a more structured approach.

The motivational consultation

Successful self-care programmes utilize wellness education strategies to promote long-term behavioural changes conducive to wellness. They engender critical-thinking processes that result in routine selection of wellness-promoting lifestyle choices.

Programme formulation based on a problem-solving approach favours this outcome. The problem-solving process sequentially involves:

- defining the problem
- identifying alternative solutions
- selecting a preferred course of action based on a ranking of possible solutions
- implementing the selected solution
- evaluating the outcome, i.e. the result of having implemented the solution
- testing alternative solutions as necessary.

Translating these general principles into a wellness format involves:

- identifying the individual's health need
- describing diverse strategies for achieving the health goal
- selecting and implementing an effective strategy that is acceptable to the individual
- monitoring the individual's health status for a detectable improvement
- modifying or maintaining the intervention strategy to achieve the health goal.

The development of a wellness programme in the clinical consultation involves five distinct phases. Before describing these stages it is necessary to review the dimensions of wellness. Wellness is a dynamic, unique, relative, multidimensional, measurable state. As wellness is a *dynamic state*, health actualization requires a lifelong commitment. Wellness is subject to both voluntary and involuntary fluctuation. Wellness is *unique* within the context of each individual's genetic composition and environmental exposure. Successful health promotion implies improving the individual's personal health status rather than attaining some population health status equivalent. Wellness is *relative* rather than absolute, placing any particular individual anywhere along the spectrum that extends from optimal health to disease. Professional and personal intervention can shift the patient's health status towards health, but the reverse is also true. Wellness is *multidimensional*: it is possible to be psychologically, socially and spiritually healthy in the presence of devastating physical disease. Finally, wellness is *measurable*. Objective assessment is usually performed by health professionals and expressed on a scale ranging from the absence of disease to the presence of healthy lifestyle choices. Subjective assessment is best performed by the individual and is expressed in functional terms. Self-rated health has been prognostically linked to the development of adverse clinical effects.[39] In fact, persons with 'poor' self-rated health had a twofold higher mortality risk compared with persons with 'excellent' self-rated health.[40] The greater the organic change, the more important the objective professional assessment of the situation; the healthier the individual, the greater the role of the individual in subjective self-assessment and care.

Wellness is the health experienced at the extreme pole of the health–disease spectrum; the wellness programme aims to shift the individual's health status towards this 'healthy' position. A three-pronged approach is recommended. The first consideration is the good management of any disease already present. The second focus is risk-screening, the identification of red flags, and control of any pathological processes to which the individual is predisposed. The final objective is to analyse health-relevant behaviours, to detect orange flags, and modify risky choices, thereby optimizing health.

It is helpful to conceptualize health as a multi-dimensional construct that includes physical, psychological, sociocultural and spiritual aspects. At a physical level, health may imply the absence of pain and discomfort, or it may suggest an abundance of energy. At a psychological level, wellness may constitute self-esteem and quiet contentment or it may mean vigorously pursuing self-actualization. Social wellbeing may for one person constitute financial security and peer acceptance; for another, it may mean the freedom to disagree in a context of unconditional regard and acceptance. Wellness is the best health outcome that can be achieved by any individual within the constraints of his or her genetic composition. Within this framework, rather than being an often-unattainable absolute, optimal health becomes achieving one's personal best.

Development of a self-care programme in clinical practice passes through five phases. The framework for the brief motivational intervention is as follows:

Stage 1: ASSESS: Identification of personal health needs

Consumers are not necessarily aware of the risks associated with certain behaviours – in fact, a telephone survey of 9058 adult smokers in the US,

the UK, Canada and Australia found significant gaps in their knowledge of the risks of smoking.[41] It is therefore important that individuals be made aware of how their current lifestyle choices may impact on their long-term health. Personal health awareness can be heightened by comparing the individual's actual behaviour with health-promoting behaviours recommended by health experts. The client's 'health need' is the discrepancy between ideal wellness and the individual's actual health status and behaviour. At the wellness pole, health actualization targets are identified by screening for the presence of risky and the absence of healthy lifestyle choices. The composite of health needs for each individual is unique; the personal identification of health needs is the first stage of self-motivation.

Stage 2: ADVISE: Problem selection

Professional advice on how to change has been shown to be associated with greater readiness to amend risky choices such as smoking, physical inactivity and unhealthy dietary behaviours.[42] Practitioners can give clear, specific, and personalized behaviour change advice. They can help patients to determine the potential costs of continuing with their current lifestyle choices and the likely benefits of change. Brochures in the form of clinic handouts may aid patient decision. Not only can such handouts serve as a reminder of verbal information provided, they can also be used to enhance awareness and motivate patients to acquire health-promoting behaviours. Figure 8.4 is an example of the 170 patient handouts provided. In addition to alerting patients to current health needs, anticipatory advice prior to the onset of risky behaviours is recommended. Anticipatory advice is, for example, appropriate for preventing risky sexual activity and tobacco, alcohol and/or illicit drug use by adolescents. Greater cooperation and less resistance are achieved when advice is delivered in a warm, empathetic, non-judgmental style. Communications that emphasize positive, rather than negative, restrictive messages are more effective.[43]

Step 3: AGREE: Prioritize health goals and intervention strategies

A hallmark of shared decision making is that patients and providers have different, but equally valuable,

Diabetes is a major health concern. Up to 50% of people with type 2 diabetes (non-insulin-dependent diabetes) are thought to be undiagnosed and untreated. By the time they are diagnosed, 1 in 5 may already have nerve, eye, kidney and heart damage due to their diabetes. More than 4 out of 5 diabetics die from some form of heart disease. Each year in the United States almost 6000 new cases of blindness are due to diabetes and about half the non-traumatic amputations involve diabetic patients.

Are you at risk of type 2 diabetes?

Type 2 diabetics are usually obese and often have a family history of diabetes. They are usually over 40 years of age and present with excessive tiredness. As there are many different causes of tiredness it is necessary to screen for diabetes.

Specific risk factors for type 2 diabetes include:
- having a family history of diabetes
- belonging to a high-risk ethnic group, e.g. Aboriginal, Polynesian, Indian, Maltese
- being over 65 years of age
- giving birth to babies of 4.5 kg or more
- having a low birth weight
- being overweight (BMI $=$ wt(kg)/ht(m)^2 $=$ 28 or greater)
- gaining over 5 kg in weight after 18 years of age
- having an adult abdominal girth of over 94 cm (males) or 80 cm (females)
- having a waist:hip ratio of over 1.0 (in males) or 0.9 (in females)
- leading a sedentary lifestyle, especially if over 45 years of age
- eating a high-fat diet
- smoking

If you tick two or more boxes, ask your doctor to check your blood sugar
If you tick one box, be sure to make healthy lifestyle choices

For further risk assessment see:
http://www.healthcalculators.org/calculators/diabetes.asp
http://www.yourdiseaserisk.siteman.wustl.edu/hccpquiz.pl?lang=english&func=home&quiz=diabetes
Lifestyle choices to reduce your risk

Risk is reduced by:
- losing weight. Loss of 4.5 kg reduces the risk by 30%
- eating fish in preference to meat
- eating a low-fat diet that favours monounsaturated fat. Eat:
    - olive or canola oil
    - avocado, mustard seeds
    - nuts, e.g. almonds, pecans, almonds, macadamias, pistachios
- a diet rich in fruit and vegetable
- a diet rich in soluble fibre: legumes, oatmeal
- foods with a low glycaemic index: legumes, pasta, wholegrain bread
- eating less than 1.5 teaspoons of salt a day
- exercising regularly
- a low alcohol intake, and only with meals

Each healthy choice made reduces your risk of diabetes

For more information on how to prevent diabetes see
http://www.diabetes.org/diabetes-prevention.jsp

Figure 8.4 • Diabetes mellitus.

perspectives and roles.[44] Shared decision making in self-care requires that practitioners elicit and respond to patients' views. Open-ended exchange can engage even marginally interested patients in a non-threatening way that may increase knowledge, self-confidence and motivation. In negotiating a self-care programme, practitioners and patients should both suggest and review various interventions. Both parties should discuss the pros and cons of options raised, particularly as they may have different perspectives on the relative importance of benefits, risks, and costs, be they financial, convenience or opportunity. The patients' perspectives are determined by clarifying their values and preferences and by exploring their ideas, concerns, and outcome expectations. Both parties should periodically check facts and confirm perspectives are shared. Further elucidation is provided as needed. Resistance to changing a behaviour is reduced when the parties collaborate and explore how best to proceed. The collaborative approach emphasizes patient choice and autonomy. The ultimate control rests with the patient.

Self-efficacy for specific behavioural change is a fundamental determinant of success.[45] Efficacy expectations are beliefs about how capable one is of performing a behaviour that leads to a particular outcome. Efficacy expectations are heightened in competently negotiated programmes, as clients select strategies they perceive themselves to be most capable of implementing. Discussion of patients' ability to follow through with a plan is therefore critical. Self-efficacy predicts the likelihood of initiating communication, engaging in recommended health behaviours and adhering to self-care programmes. It is a consistent predictor of short- and long-term success in health promotion programmes.

Success requires clinician–patient agreement with respect to:

- Health needs. Both patient and practitioner should rank the health needs from their own perspective. The professional's prioritization of health needs is based upon their knowledge of health risks and disease prognosis; the patient's is derived from their self-knowledge. Both parties negotiate and agree on a joint ranking of health needs.
- Intervention options. Multiple intervention options should be canvassed. Figure 8.5 provides an example of different strategies, all of which contribute to a successful outcome. While any one strategy contributes to dental hygiene, implementing a combination of strategies achieves a better outcome. Giving the patient choices generates a sense of freedom of choice and permits the generation of a programme that causes minimal lifestyle disruption. Simple language listing concrete, specific recommendations avoids confusion. Verbal advice should be accompanied by written recommendations and practical demonstrations to minimize misunderstandings.
- Selecting a health plan. A wellness programme is most likely to be successful when the patient believes they are capable of implementing and adhering to proposed lifestyle changes. Compliance is enhanced when the intended health changes implement strategies compatible with the individual's lifestyle. Motivation is increased when the programme focuses on self-perceived health needs.

Stage 4: ASSIST Programme formulation and implementation

Good wellness programmes empower patients. Empowerment refers to the ability of individuals to gain understanding, make decisions and have personal control over improving their life situation. It combines self-efficacy and competence with a sense of mastery and control in the process of participatory decision-making. The mutually agreed upon health needs and intervention strategies form the basis for developing the wellness programme. The major consideration now is identifying the criteria to be used to monitor progress and measure a successful outcome. Useful programme formulation strategies are to

---

See Oral health a window to wellness
http://www.mayoclinic.com/health/dental/DE00001
From Dental Health to Disease
Dental plaque is a major culprit in the development of caries. Plaque, composed of food and bacteria, concentrates in the crevices of individual teeth and is trapped between teeth and gums. Refined carbohydrates, e.g. sugar and foods made from white flour, are particularly prone to encourage plaque formation. Starch, often eaten as cakes and buns, sticks to teeth and is bathed in saliva. Amylase, an enzyme in saliva, breaks down the starch molecules into smaller units, polysaccharides and disaccharides. These smaller units are used by bacteria in the mouth for growth and multiplication. Bacteria digest food, producing acidic end-products. These end-products bathe the tooth in a more acidic environment. The minerals in the tooth matrix are leeched out of the tooth by acid. It has been shown that plaque becomes strongly acidic within 10 minutes of rinsing the mouth with a sugar solution. To neutralize or restore the oral pH to 7 with saliva takes about 1 hour. Prolonged exposure of teeth to an acid medium results in the formation of dental caries. Prolonged exposure of gums to an acid medium results in gum irritation (gingivitis) with exposure of a 'sensitive' tooth margin.

To get rid of bacteria in the mouth is impossible; however, it is possible to deprive bacteria of their sugar and starch diet. It is possible to prevent sugars and starches sticking to the surface of teeth. Adequate and regular brushing can prevent dental caries. The secret of success in dental hygiene is to prevent creation of an acid environment and to never permit plaque to accumulate. You can achieve these goals by avoiding refined carbohydrates (the major plaque-forming foods) and cleaning teeth after eating (remove food before it becomes plaque).

Figure 8.5 • Dental health care information guide.

Continued

Intervention Strategies for Dental Hygiene
There are four easy strategies for improving dental health.
Strategy 1: Healthy Eating
☐ Avoid sticky, sugary food, e.g. sweet buns, cakes, and toffees
☐ Avoid acidic drinks, e.g. carbonated beverages, grape and lemon juice
☐ Drink fruit juice and sweet or carbonated drinks using a straw, do not sip
☐ Only drink juices or sweet drinks at mealtimes
☐ Avoid eating between meals; if snacks are necessary, eat fruit, nuts, or chips
☐ Chew fibrous foods regularly, e.g. raw carrots, lettuce, cabbage, or celery
☐ Drink milk; it is a good source of calcium with some limited ability to act as an oral buffer and reduce pH changes
☐ Always clean your teeth after eating
☐ Remove plaque from all dental surfaces within 10 minutes of eating sugary foods or drink

Strategy 2: Toothbrushing
Food can be trapped between teeth or in tooth crevices, and mucopolysaccharides in saliva can be deposited on teeth as an adherent film or pellicle. Bacterial action then creates an acidic plaque. Brushing can help to remove surface plaque.
☐ Position your toothbrush horizontally on your teeth
☐ Brush using short vertical strokes(scrub) the outer, inner, and biting surfaces of all teeth
☐ Position the toothbrush at an angle to tooth-gum margin
☐ Brush in a short rotary motion over the margin between gum and teeth and brush back and forth gently to clean the teeth and massage the gums
☐ Use a toothpaste with fluoride. Fluoride combines with the tooth enamel to reduce dental susceptibility to acid; rinse thoroughly and avoid swallowing the toothpaste
☐ Use a toothbrush with soft end-rounded or polished bristles to massage the gums and harder bristles to remove dental plaque
☐ Replace your toothbrush three to four times a year. Don't rely on a toothbrush with splayed bristles
☐ Brush after eating – not only after meals
Brushing does not eliminate plaque at points of contact between teeth; brushing alone is not adequate for cleaning teeth.

Strategy 3: Floss Teeth
☐ Clean between teeth using dental floss
☐ Use waxed or unwaxed floss of more than 45 cm in length
☐ Wrap floss around one middle finger and control a 'working strip' of over 5 cm in length between the index and thumb of each hand
☐ Position floss over the thumb of one hand and the forefinger of the other to floss upper teeth. Insert floss between teeth using a thumb to hold back the cheek
☐ Wrap floss around both forefingers and insert between lower teeth
☐ Holding the floss tightly, move floss up and down between teeth, removing debris
☐ When floss reaches the gum line, curve it into a 'C' around the tooth and scrape dental plaque off the tooth
☐ Avoid snapping floss against the gums
☐ Wind floss around the finger, exposing a fresh section, and move to the next tooth
☐ Floss teeth after eating
☐ Balsa wood sticks may also be used by people with gum recession
Neither flossing nor brushing removes plaque from fissures or pits.

Strategy 4: Dental Hygiene – Quality Control
☐ Check the efficacy of your brushing and flossing techniques. Plaque detecting or disclosing tablets turn invisible plaque red
☐ Have a professional dental check up at 6-month intervals
☐ Public health authorities recommend that drinking water supplies have a fluoride content of one part per million.
See http://www.mayoclinic.com/health/dental/DE00003Chosing a toothbrushhttp://www.mayoclinic.com/health/electric-toothbrush/AN01705

Figure 8.5—Cont'd

specify dates by which particular health objectives should be met, provide regular feedback and reward interim successes.[46] Assistance techniques vary according to the health need, but enhancing problem-solving skills to replace problem behaviours is always helpful. Barriers to successful implementation include the individual's perception of obstacles to implementing the intervention, a lack of positive feedback, and feelings of helplessness.[47]

Programmes are most successful when:

* written in simple language
* health goals are clearly specified and broken into interim manageable sub-goals
* deadlines are specified
* a self-monitoring system is included. A diary comparing current, intended and actual behaviour is a useful self-evaluation tool. Figures 8.6 and 8.7

Step 1: Complete the following questionnaire, indicating your usual behaviour in the CURRENT column. Insert today's date.

Step 2: Identify risks that you are prepared to change. Select a date by which you will have changed your behaviour. Note this date in the INTENDED column.

Step 3: Monitor the outcome at the specified date by which the goal should have been achieved. Note your finding in the ACHIEVED column.

The more of the following behaviours you demonstrate, the smaller your risk of dying or being injured in a motor vehicle accident.

	CURRENT	INTENDED	ACHIEVED
I always wear a seat belt			
I always adhere to speed limits in speed zones			
I always adhere to speed limits on the open road			
I always indicate when I am changing lanes			
I always indicate when I am turning			
I always indicate when I am passing another vehicle			
I always obey traffic signals			
I only cross green traffic lights			
I never drink alcohol when I intend to drive			
I refuse to be driven by friends who have been drinking			
I only cross busy roads at traffic lights			
I only drive roadworthy vehicles			

Figure 8.6 • A motor vehicle accident risk reduction programme.

Step 1: Complete the following questionnaire, indicating your usual behaviour in the CURRENT column. Insert today's date.

Step 2: Identify risks that you are prepared to change. Select a date by which you will have changed your behaviour. Note this date in the INTENDED column.

Step 3: Monitor the outcome at the specified date by which the goal should have been achieved. Note your finding in the ACHIEVED column.

The more of the following behaviours you demonstrate, the smaller your risk of dental caries.

	CURRENT	INTENDED	ACHIEVED
I brush my teeth after each meal. (maximum score 3)			
I brush my teeth after nibbling			
I brush my teeth correctly*			
I floss my teeth*			
I avoid sugary confections			
I avoid starchy sticky snacks			
I clean my teeth immediately after eating refined carbohydrate treats			
I use plaque disclosing tablets daily			
My plaque disclosing tablets show 'no plaque present' when used			
I snack on fresh produce, e.g. carrots			

*see Figure 8.5

Figure 8.7 • Dental wellbeing: a self–assessment tool.

provide examples of how recording the current, intended and actual behaviour can serve as a useful behaviour-monitoring tool. Lifestyle diaries provide a record of success and help patients maintain healthy behaviours.[48] Self-monitoring, in addition to ensuring patient involvement, helps patients actively to reconstruct their wellness experience, enhancing independent self-care and increasing personal awareness of the health impact of their behavioural choices

- a reward system is included. Pavlovian-induced reward expectancies can change both performance and brain processes aiding behaviour change.[49]

Stage 5: ARRANGE Monitor progress and correct shortfalls

Self-monitoring and modification of the programme to accommodate lifestyle preferences without compromising long-term goals is the basis of a realistic self-care programme. Monitoring is a useful tool for reinforcing adherence to a wellness lifestyle and reviewing programme objectives and strategies in the light of changing needs. Ongoing involvement and monitoring by the practitioner adds incentive for the patient to adhere to the programme. Follow-up contacts, in person or by telephone, to provide ongoing assistance/support and adjust the wellness plan as required are scheduled. When targets are not met, explanations for such failures are identified and alternative strategies to meet the health promotion objectives explored. Strategies are modified until a more acceptable approach is substituted. Wellness is a lifelong endeavour and behavioural risk factors need to be reassessed as health challenges change over time.

Figure 8.8 identifies nodal decision points in formulating the five-stage wellness programme.

Successful self-care programmes are owned by the patient. Ownership is achieved by actively involving clients in formulating their own programme. The underlying premise shared by the practitioner and client in contract formulation is that health is a valued attribute and health improvement an attainable goal. The client/patient is involved in all phases of programme formulation, including the determination of goals, the selection of implementation strategies and the progress monitoring schedule. Each phase is influenced by the client's current physical, psychological, socio-cultural and economic environment. Only individuals themselves can ascertain which lifestyle changes are acceptable and which interventions require modification.

Ownership also derives from involving significant others in the programme. Family and friends can help to motivate and serve as an additional source for clarifying obscure guidelines. Involvement in the individual's health care programme can encourage the family's acceptance of the patient's health promotion programme.

In perspective

Self-care is a potentially potent tool for creating a new level of community wellness. The patient role is that of active participant, the practitioner that of facilitator. The interventions used are not therapist dependent. From the patients' perspective, programmes that provide information and are integrated into their lifestyles are likely to be more productive. From the practitioners' perspective, the promotion of wellness, although including the early discovery of functional change, focuses on detecting risk exposure and encouraging acquisition of healthy behaviours. Strategies such as goal-setting, imagery, self-monitoring, self-instruction

---

Step 1: Describe the optimal or ideal situation
Step 2: Ascertain the 'needs', i.e. the discrepancy between the individual's health status and the ideal circumstance
Step 3: Rank the health needs
Step 4: Explore diverse strategies for meeting each health need
Step 5: Define each health need as a wellness objective and specify when and how each objective will be met
Step 6: Implement and monitor the wellness programme
Step 7: Identify failures and modify the programme to meet achievable interim goals

Figure 8.8 • The framework for programme formulation.

and cognitive restructuring have been found to support behavioural changes that enhance sports performance.[50] Packaged programmes are suitable for boosting diverse self-care initiatives. A lifelong lifestyle commitment to self-care is a prerequisite for a successful wellness programme. Successful self-care requires the re-evaluation of priorities and a clear understanding of self. It also requires that lifestyle changes be founded upon evidence-based information.

References

1. Ebrahim S, Wannamethee SG, Whincup P, Walker M, Shaper AG. Locomotor disability in a cohort of British men: the impact of lifestyle and disease. *Int J Epidemiol*. 2000;29(3):478–486.

2. Preventing cardiovascular disease through personal commitment and community action. http://www.cardiovision2020.org/; Accessed 07.06.08.

3. Whitlock EP, Orleans CT, Pender N, Allan J. Evaluating primary care behavioral counseling interventions: an evidence-based approach. *Am J Prev Med*. 2002; 22(4):267–284.

4. Cairns G, Stead M. Symposium on "The challenge of translating nutrition research into public health". Session 5: Nutrition communication. Obesity and social marketing: works in progress. *Proc Nutr Soc*. 2009;68(1):11–16.

5. Sunsmart. http://www.sunsmart. com.au/; Accessed 25.11.08.

6. Social marketing campaigns Canada. http://www.hc-sc.gc.ca/ahc-asc/ activit/marketsoc/camp/index-eng. php; Accessed 25.11.08.

7. Social marketing campaigns UK. http://www.nsms.org.uk/public/ default; Accessed 25.11.08.

8. Block G, Sternfeld B, Block CH, et al. Development of Alive! (a lifestyle intervention via email), and its effect on health-related quality of life, presenteeism, and other behavioral outcomes: randomized controlled trial. *J Med Internet Res*. 2008;10(4):e43.

9. Faber MM. Sharing responsibility: a new health care partnership. In: Faber MM, Reinhardt AM, eds. *Promoting Health through Risk Reduction*. New York: Macmillan; 1982:336–351.

10. Larimer ME, Cronce JM. Identification, prevention, and treatment revisited: individual-focused college drinking prevention strategies 1999–2006. *Addict Behav*. 2007;32(11):2439–2468.

11. Haller DM, Sanci LA, Sawyer SM, Patton G. Do young people's illness beliefs affect healthcare? A systematic review. *J Adolesc Health*. 2008;42(5):436–449.

12. National Cancer Institute. *Theory at a Glance. A Guide for Health Promotion Practice*. 2nd ed. Washington, DC: US Department of Health and Human Services, NIH; 2005. *http://www.cancer.gov/ theory; Accessed 24.11.08*.

13. Goldstein MG, Whitlock EP, DePue J. Planning Committee of the Addressing Multiple Behavioral Risk Factors in Primary Care Project. Multiple behavioral risk factor interventions in primary care. Summary of research evidence. *Am J Prev Med*. 2004;27(suppl 2): 61–79.

14. Carey KB, Carey MP, Maisto SA, Henson JM. Brief motivational interventions for heavy college drinkers: a randomized controlled trial. *J Consult Clin Psychol*. 2006;74(5):943–954.

15. Collins SE, Carey KB. Lack of effect for decisional balance as a brief motivational intervention for at-risk college drinkers. *Addict Behav*. 2005;30(7):1425–1430.

16. Nupponen R. What is counseling all about—basics in the counseling of health-related physical activity. *Patient Educ Couns*. 1998;33 (suppl 1):S61–S67.

17. Barnes HN, Samet JH. Brief interventions with substance-abusing patients. *Med Clin North Am*. 1997;81:867–879.

18. Kelly RB. Controlled trial of a time-efficient method of health promotion. *Am J Prev Med*. 1988;4:200–207.

19. Grossberg PM, Brown DD, Fleming MF. Brief physician advice for high-risk drinking among young adults. *Ann Fam Med*. 2004;2(5): 474–480.

20. Krupat E, Frankel R, Stein T, Irish J. The Four Habits Coding Scheme: validation of an instrument to assess clinicians' communication behavior. *Patient Educ Couns*. 2006; 62(1):38–45.

21. Anthea Williams Motivational Interviewing. http://som.flinders. edu.au/FUSA/CCTU/; Accessed 11.11.07.

22. Cherkin DC, Deyo RA, Battie M, et al. A comparison of physical therapy, chiropractic manipulation, and provision of an educational booklet for the treatment of patients with low back pain. *New Engl J Med*. 1998;339:1021–1029.

23. Norman CD, Skinner HA. eHealth literacy: essential skills for consumer health in a networked world. *J Med Internet Res*. 2006;8(2):e9.

24. Stockler M, Coates A. What have we learned from meta-analysis? *Med J Aust*. 1993;159:291–293.

25. Sackett DL, Haynes RB, Tugwell P. *Clinical Epidemiology*. Boston: Little Brown; 1988:298.

26. Graber MA, Roller CM, Kaeble B. Readability levels of patient education material on the world wide web. *J Fam Pract*. 1999;48:58–61.

27. Estey A, Musseau A, Keehn L. Patients' understanding of health information: a multihospital comparison. *Patient Educ Couns*. 1994;24:73–78.

28. Mumford ME. A descriptive study of the readability of patient information leaflets designed by nurses. *J Adv Nurs*. 1997;26:985–991.

29. Albert T, Chadwick T. How readable are practice leaflets? *BMJ*. 1992;305:1266–1268.

30. McLaughlin GH. SMOG grading – a new readability formula. *J Reading*. 1969;12(May):639–646.

31. Sarma M, Alpers JH, Prideaux DJ, Kroemer DJ. The comprehensibility

of Australian educational literature for patients with asthma. *Med J Aust*. 1995;162(7):360–363.

32. Anderson J. Lix and Rix: variations on a little known readability index. *J Reading*. 1983;26:490–496.

33. Bastian H. Health literacy and patient information: developing the methodology for a national evidence-based health website. *Patient Educ Couns*. 2008; 73(3):551–556.

34. Hussey LC. Strategies for effective patient education material design. *J Cardiovasc Nurs*. 1997;11:37–46.

35. Doak CC, Doak LG, Root JH. *Teaching Patients with Low Literacy Skills*. Philadelphia: JB Lippincott; 1996.

36. Slaytor EK, Ward JE. How risks of breast cancer and benefits of screening are communicated to women: analysis of 58 pamphlets. *BMJ*. 1998;317:263–264.

37. Norman CD, Skinner HA. eHEALS: the eHealth literacy scale. *J Med Internet Res*. 2006;8(4):e27.

38. Daltroy LH, Iversen MD, Larson MG, et al. A controlled trial of an education program to prevent low back injuries. *N Engl J Med*. 1997;37:322–328.

39. Ried LD, Tueth MJ, Handberg E, Nyanteh H. Validating a self-report measure of global subjective well-being to predict adverse clinical outcomes. *Qual Life Res*. 2006; 15(4):675–686.

40. DeSalvo KB, Bloser N, Reynolds K, He J, Muntner P. Mortality prediction with a single general self-rated health question. A meta-analysis. *J Gen Intern Med*. 2006; 21(3):267–275.

41. Hammond D, Fong GT, McNeill A, Borland R, Cummings KM. Effectiveness of cigarette warning labels in informing smokers about the risks of smoking: findings from the International Tobacco Control (ITC) Four Country Survey. *Tob Control*. 2006;15(suppl 3): iii19–iii25.

42. O'Connor PJ, Rush WA, Prochaska JO, Pronk NP, Boyle RG. Professional advice and readiness to change behavioral risk factors among members of a managed care organization. *Am J Manag Care*. 2001;7(2):125–130.

43. Rolls BJ, Ello-Martin JA, Tohill BC. What can intervention studies tell us about the relationship between fruit and vegetable consumption and weight management? *Nutr Rev*. 2004;62(1):1–17.

44. Makoul G, Clayman ML. An integrative model of shared decision making in medical encounters. *Patient Educ Couns*. 2006;60(3): 301–312.

45. Krummel DA, Semmens E, Boury J, Gordon PM, Larkin KT. Stages of change for weight management in postpartum women. *J Am Diet Assoc*. 2004;104(7): 1102–1108.

46. Kok G, van den Borne B, Mullen PD. Effectiveness of health education and health promotion: meta-analyses of effect studies and determinants of effectiveness. *Patient Educ Couns*. 1997;30(1):19–27.

47. Sluijs EM, Kok GJ, van der Zee J. Correlates of exercise compliance in physical therapy. *Phys Ther*. 1993;73:771–782.

48. Reynolds LR, Anderson JW. Practical office strategies for weight management of the obese diabetic individual. *Endocr Pract*. 2004; 10(2):153–159.

49. Savage LM, Ramos RL. Reward expectation alters learning and memory: the impact of the amygdala on appetitive-driven behaviors. *Behav Brain Res*. 2009;198(1):1–12.

50. Meyers AW, Whelan JP, Murphy SM. Cognitive behavioral strategies in athletic performance enhancement. *Prog Behav Modif*. 1996;30:137–164.

PART 2

Green flags: highways to wellness

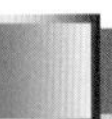

Points to Ponder !

- Healthy habits are the currency of good health.
- It is never too late to develop good habits – but the younger you start, the longer you enjoy the benefits of good health.
- Motivate by delivering messages in terms of health gains.

The single greatest opportunity to improve health and reduce premature deaths lies in personal behaviour. Unhealthy behaviours account for almost 4 in 10 deaths in the US.[1] Making healthy lifestyle choices reduces the risk of disease. Yet, during the 30 days before the national Youth Risk Behavior Surveillance system survey in 2007, one in three youths had watched television for at least 3 hours on an average school day. During the 7 days before the survey, two in three had not met recommended levels of physical activity and almost four in five had failed to eat five or more fruits and vegetables daily. Furthermore, almost half the students surveyed had had sexual intercourse, one in three high school students were currently sexually active, and almost two in three currently sexually active high school students had not used a condom during the last act of sexual intercourse.[2] Physical inactivity, a lack of fruit and vegetables, and unsafe sex are listed amongst the top 10 health risks faced by Australians in 2006.[3] Failure to make healthy lifestyle choices is not a problem confined to the US and Australia.

In 2006 in England, only 4 in 10 men and 3 in 10 women exercised for at least 30 minutes on each of 5 days of the week.[4] They also failed to meet the minimum recommendations for fruit and vegetable intake. Nonetheless, attempts to encourage populations to acquire health-promoting habits are meeting with some success. The proportion of men and women achieving current physical activity recommendations in England has significantly increased, as has fruit and vegetable consumption. However, there remains much room for improvement. In 2006, only one in three Britons were eating five or more portions of fruit and vegetables daily.[4] Furthermore, those eating more than the recommended fat intake has increased rather than declined.[4]

Diet and nutrition, exercise, and attitude and behavior are established modifiable causes of the major chronic diseases prevalent in older age groups.[5] Until such time as health-promoting behaviours are established societal norms, making prudent lifestyle decisions is a matter of individual choice.

The principles underlying the development of good habits are:

- an appreciation of the nature and rationale for healthy behaviour. It is necessary to know which behaviours promote health. Understanding why particular behaviours are effective helps with the day-to-day implementation of the activity

- self-awareness of current behaviour patterns. Unless one is aware of current behaviours, it is difficult to know what to change

- freedom to select from a smorgasbord of potential lifestyle options to enhance behaviour change. Once the health goal has been identified, it is usually possible to choose more than one activity that will achieve the goal.

Figure P2.1 lists a number of fundamental lifestyle changes conducive to acquiring health promoting habits. **Handout P2.0.1** can be used to identify personal values. It can be used as a yardstick for selecting strategies most suited to the individual's goals. Figure P2.2 identifies stages in the overall process of acquiring healthy habits. Figure P2.3 pinpoints important steps en route to acquiring good habits.

When developing good habits, a balanced approach to any possible wellness initiatives should be used. This includes analysing the idea with respect to:[6]

- its pluses. The benefits to be derived from the behaviour should be noted

---

Clarify values and beliefs.
Build on strengths
Recognize weaknesses
Adapt lifestyle to minimize the impact of weaknesses
Persistently look for agreeable options for achieving
   change
Keep self-talk positive
Learn from failures
Make laughter a habit

Figure P2.1 • Tips for making successful lifestyle changes

The overall process of acquiring healthy habits is one of:
- identification of and utilization of stimuli to trigger desired behaviour.
- development of techniques to implement the desired behaviour.
- reinforcement of the healthy behaviour by rewarding adherence to the desired habit
- continued conscious performance of the desired behaviour
- self monitoring. This provides a record of progress.
- automatic performance and establishment of a healthy habit.

Figure P2.2 • Acquiring healthy habits: the process

Step 1: The dimensions of good habits
To enhance wellness behaviour, it is necessary to have a sound knowledge of behaviours conducive to wellness. This includes:
- dispelling 'health' myths
- establishing criteria for healthy behaviours

Step 2: Awareness of personal behaviour patterns
Prepare a personal diary documenting health relevant behaviours
Assess your healthy lifestyle score
See https://data.webmd.com/sdclive/SdcForm.aspx?formid=kAssessPg1

Step 3: Identify health behaviour needs
Determine the healthy habits that are needed by comparing actual behaviour with healthy behaviours

Step 4: Rank habits to be acquired
Rank desirable habits according to their potential health benefit

Step 5: Explore strategies for change
Explore diverse strategies for acquiring each health-promoting behaviour

Step 6: Specify objectives
Define each healthy habit as a wellness objective and specify when and how each objective will be met

Step 7: Implement the proposed habits
Implement the healthy habits and monitor progress

Step 8: Monitor progress
Identify failures and modify the programme to meet achievable interim goals

---

Figure P2.3 • Step to acquiring good habits.

- its minuses. Nothing is perfect. Identify the downside. A good habit may carry financial and/or personal costs

- the possibilities. The opportunities created by developing the healthy behaviour should be identified. This includes potential physical, emotional and social outcomes

- other people's views. Attitudes and beliefs of family and friends towards the behaviour can enhance or diminish the likelihood of success

- possible consequences: the likely impact of the behaviour on one's lifestyle and significant others.

It has been suggested that people are risk-averse when they consider gains. When persuading people to make healthy lifestyle choices, the message should be framed in terms of potential wellbeing gains. Gain-framed messages are thought to be more effective for influencing decisions regarding behaviours with low-risk and certain outcomes.[7] Gain-framed messages are ideally suited for motivating health-promoting behaviours.[7] Wellness is based upon making healthy lifestyle choices. Accumulating green flags, the trademark of healthy behaviours, is a sound lifelong investment.

References

1. Schroeder SA. Shattuck Lecture. We can do better—improving the health of the American people. *N Engl J Med*. 2007;357(12):1221–1228.

2. Eaton DK, Kann L, Kinchen S, et al. Centers for Disease Control and Prevention (CDC). Youth risk behavior surveillance—United States, 2007. *MMWR Surveill Summ*. 2008;57(4):1–131.

3. Australian Institute of Health and Welfare (AIHW). Australia's health 2006. http://www.AIHW.gov.au/publications/index.CFM/title/10321 Accessed 11.12.07.

4. NHS The Information Centre. Health Survey for England 2006. http://www.ic.nhs.uk/statistics-and-data-collections/health-and-lifestyles-related-surveys/health-survey-for-england/health-survey-for-england-2006:-cvd-and-risk-factors-adults-obesity-and-risk-factors-children Accessed 01.02.09.

5. Hazzard WR, Larson EB, Perls TT. Preventive gerontology: strategies for optimal aging. *Patient Care*. 1998;32:198–203.

6. De Bono E. *Serious Creativity*. London: Harper Collins; 1992.

7. Werch CC. The Behavior-Image Model: a paradigm for integrating prevention and health promotion in brief interventions. *Health Educ Res*. 2007;22(5):677–690.

Healthy dietary choices

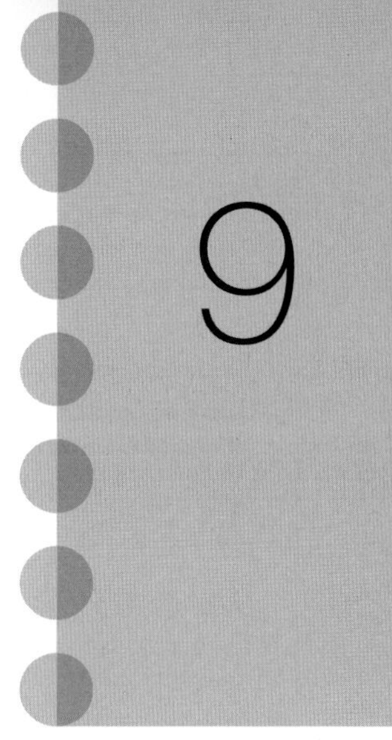

The U.S. Preventive Services Task Force found insufficient evidence to recommend for or against routine behavioural counselling to promote a healthy diet in unselected patients in primary care settings.[1] Nonetheless, dietary intake has been clearly linked with mortality and disease risk. A 20-year longitudinal study of men aged 50–70 found dietary intake correlates with all-cause mortality in different cultures.[2] Another study concluded that dietary habits are associated with around 60% of cancers in women and 40% of cancers in men.[3] Major dietary patterns have been shown to predict the risk of ischaemic heart disease independent of other lifestyle variables.[4]

Particular dietary patterns have been associated with heightened or diminished risk. The 'Western pattern' is characterized by a higher intake of red meat, processed meat, refined grains, sweets and dessert, French fries, and high-fat dairy products; the 'prudent pattern' is characterized by higher intake of plant foods, fish, and poultry. The American-healthy pattern is characterized by high intakes of green, leafy vegetables; salad dressings; tomatoes; other vegetables (e.g. peppers, green beans, corn, and peas); cruciferous vegetables; and tea. The Western pattern correlates directly with increased levels of markers of inflammation and endothelial dysfunction; the prudent pattern is inversely associated with plasma concentrations of C-reactive protein and E-selectin.[5] Another study, which confirmed the Western pattern was associated with increased levels of serum C-peptide, also reported increased levels of serum insulin and glycated haemoglobin.[6] In contrast to the Western diet, the American-healthy pattern has no linear relation with any of the biomarkers examined. Dietary patterns may influence pathological processes underlying many chronic diseases prevalent in modern society.

Standard recommendations

Standard recommendations for healthy eating are to:

1. *Eat a variety of foods.* Eating from the five major food groups provides a balanced intake of nutrients – however, care must be taken not to consume too many calories (see Figure 9.1). There are also particular considerations for eating from each of the food groups and for nutrient requirements at various stages of the life cycle.

2. *Maintain a normal body weight.* A BMI between 20 and 25 is suggested, with small-framed individuals at the lower end of the scale. Food consumption or energy intake should be balanced by activity or energy expenditure. Low-energy nutritionally adequate diets can be formulated by limiting energy-dense and eating generously from

See
http://www.webmd.com/video.following-food-pyramid
http://www.mayoclinic.com/health/healthy-diet/NU00190
A nutritionally balanced diet requires food from all of the food groups.

RECOMMENDED SERVINGS

FOOD GROUP	OLD	NEW
Meat/legumes/nuts	☐ 1–4 male, 3 female	☐ 2–3
Bread/cereals/rice/pasta	☐ 4–8 male, 6 female	☐ 6–11
Vegetables/fruit	☐ 4–8 male, 6 female	☐ 5–11
Milk/dairy products	☐ 1–4 male, 3 female	☐ 2–3
Fat	☐ 15–30 g	☐ sparingly

Serving size

The following represent one serve from the respective food group;
15–30 g margarine (1 tablespoon = 20 g)

Fruit: 1 medium apple, banana, orange; ½ cup of chopped, cooked, or canned fruit; ¾ cup of fruit juice

Vegetables: 1 cup of raw leafy vegetables; ½ cup of other vegetables – cooked or chopped raw; ¾ cup of vegetable juice

Grains: 1 slice bread; ½ cup of cereal, pasta or rice

Meat/Beans: 75–100 g lean meat, poultry or fish; ½ cup of cooked dry beans or 1 egg or 2 tablespoons of peanut butter or 1/3 cup of nuts = 40g of lean meat

Dairy: 300 mL milk, 30 g cheese, 1 cup of milk or yoghurt

It is also useful to know that:
1 mEq sodium = 23 mg; 1 mEq chloride = 35.5 mg; 1 mmol sodium chloride = 58.5 mg 2400 mg per day for sodium or 6 g of sodium chloride (salt) = one level teaspoon of salt

IN PERSPECTIVE
☐ Choose most foods from the grain products and vegetable/fruit groups
☐ Eat moderate amounts of foods from the milk and meat/beans groups
☐ Choose sparingly foods that provide few nutrients and are high in fat and sugars

Figure 9.1 • Guidelines for a balanced diet.

nutrient-dense foods. Nutrient-dense foods include eggs, green leafy and yellow vegetables, liver, milk and oysters. Butter, sugar, alcohol and soft drinks have a low nutrient density. Energy-dense foods include butter, oil and nuts; moderately energy-dense foods, boiled egg or rice, grilled lean meat, bread and fried fish; and low energy-dense foods are pumpkin, broccoli, carrot, skimmed milk and clear soup. The nutrient density of foods is modified by harvesting, processing, home storage, preparation and cooking. Foods should be eaten fresh or with as little processing as possible. Cook food for as short a period as palatable and avoid salt- or fat-rich processed foods. Minimize nutrient losses. See **Handout 9.1**.

3. *Choose a diet low in total fat, saturated fat and cholesterol.* Derive approximately 25%, certainly less than 30%, of dietary energy from fat. At low intakes of fat, the type of fat appears to be less significant; however, total daily cholesterol should be restricted to less than 300 mg and saturated fat should be reduced to less than 10%

of total calories. Avoid roasting and frying; grilling or steaming is a healthier option. Decrease consumption of foods rich in saturated fat and cholesterol, including red meat, butter and cream. Replacing full-cream dairy products with low fat milks, yoghurts and cheeses is a helpful strategy. Read food labels and avoid processed food. See **Handout 9.2**.

4. *Choose a diet rich in grain products, vegetables and fruits.* Include 25 g of fibre each day. The relative proportions of various types of fibre within these limits have yet to be clarified. However, at least five servings of fruit and vegetables and at least six servings of breads, cereals or legumes each day are recommended.

5. *Choose a diet moderate in sugars.* Avoid processed foods. Fruits and vegetables are a better dietary source of sweetness than refined sugar. Sweeteners may be an option (see Table 9.1).

6. *Choose a diet moderate in salt and sodium.* A sodium intake of less than 2.5 g or 100 mmol per day requires that no salt be added during

Table 9.1 Artifical sweeteners

Sweetener	Sweetness quality	Sweetness relative to sucrose = 1
Saccharin	Sweet Bitter metallic aftertaste	300
Cyclamate	'Chemical sweetness' No aftertaste	30
Aspartame	Clean sweetness Sweet aftertaste Unstable heating and in solution pH <4 – not useful for cooking	180
Acesulphame K	Sweet Bitter aftertaste (less bitter than saccharin)	130
Thaumatin	Slow onset of sweetness Lingering licorice aftertaste	2500
Sucralose	Derived from sugar but does not contribute energy	600

See also:

http://www.mayoclinic.com/health/artificial-sweeteners/MY00073

http://www.medicinenet.com/artificial_sweeteners/article.htm

or after food preparation and that heavily or visibly salted items are excluded. Most processed foods also need to be avoided (see Figure 9.2). Companies are adjusting their products to improve dietary standards. Food labels provide useful information. See **Handout 9.2**.

7. *Only drink alcoholic beverages in moderation or not at all*. The consumption of alcohol by men should not exceed 4 units or 40 g of absolute alcohol per day on a regular basis, or 28 units per week. The safe level is lower in women and abstinence during pregnancy is highly desirable.

8. *Ensure an adequate intake of minerals*. Zinc, calcium and iron are minerals of particular note. Zinc is deficient in the soil of many countries. Exclusion or limitation of dairy products jeopardizes calcium consumption. The RDA for calcium is under continuous review. At least 1000 mg per day is prudent. Calcium intake up to 2000 mg/day appears safe for most individuals. Menstruation challenges the iron status of many females. Although there is insufficient evidence to recommend for or against routine screening for iron deficiency anaemia in asymptomatic persons, screening for iron deficiency anaemia using a haemoglobin or haematocrit test is recommended for pregnant women and high-risk infants. An adequate iron intake is

Read food labels http://www.mayoclinic.com/health/food-labels/DA00129
Nutrition profile for Foods USA http://www.ars.usda.gov/services/does.htm?docid=17032
Fats: what you need to know
http://www.mayoclinic.com/health/fat/NU00262
http://www.mayoclinic.com/health/trans-fat/CL00032

FAT CONTENT OF FOODS
The fat content of McDonalds foods http://www.weightlossforall.com/fat-mcdonalds.htm
Restaurant choices: check the fat and fibre content of dishes
http://ww.webmd.com/diet/features/healthy-restaurant-lunches
Sodium: get perspective
http://ww.mayoclinic.com/health/sodium/NU00284

SODIUM CONTENT OF FOODS
Sodium content of common foods
http://www.collectivewizdom.com/SodiumInCommonFoods.html
Check your restaurant for salt
http://ww.thesun.co.uk/sol/homepage/woman/health/health/article2187941.ece
Sodium surprises
http://www.thesun.co.uk/sol/homepage/woman/health/health/article2206020.ece
Beware 'Junk Food' http://pediatrics.about.com/od/nutrition/a/0308_junk_food.htm

Figure 9.2 • Processed food and eating out.

Compared to cow's milk. Human milk has:

- less protein. Human milk protein (1.1 g/100 mL) is rich in lactalbumin and sulphur-containing amino acids. Cow's milk protein (3.5 g/100 mL) is 80% casein and less digestible
- more carbohydrate (7.3 g compared with 5.0 g per 100 mL). Lactose provides one-third of the infant's energy and enhances calcium and magnesium absorption and the intestinal growth of lactobacilli
- less sodium. Human milk has 0.7 mmol of sodium per 100 mL; Cow's milk has 2.2 mmol per 100 mL. The solute load of cow's milk requires that it is diluted for infants.
- less calcium (35 mg compared with 120 mg per 100 mL) and phosphate (15 mg compared with 95 mg per 100 mL). The high phosphate load of cow's milk may lead to calcium resorption from bone
- double the iron. The iron content is relatively low but well absorbed. Breast milk is an adequate source of minerals for no more than 4–6 months.
- double the vitamin C
- more than 5 times the vitamin D
- slightly more fat (4 g/100 mL compared with 3.7 g/100 mL) but with a concentration of only 46% saturated fatty acids (compared to 66%) and a concentration of up to 11% of linoleic acid (cow's milk – 3% linoleic acid). Acid-resistant lipases in human milk enhance digestion. Infants absorb monoglycerides, triglycerides with palmitic acid in position 2, and short- and medium-chain fatty acids best

See also

http://blissful-baby.blogspot.com/2007/08/breast-milk-vs-cows-milk.html
http://www.helium.com/items/272267-breastfeeding-baby-wet-nurse-breast-milk-vs-cow-milk

Figure 9.3 • Human versus cow's milk.

particularly important for girls, women, vegetarians and athletes.

9. *Encourage breastfeeding.* Breastfeeding has emotional, nutritional, microbial and immunological benefits for the infant. Figure 9.3 compares human with cow's milk. In general, the metabolic needs of an infant can be met by breastfeeding for the first 4–6 months of life; after this period, semi-solid and later solid food should be introduced.

Dietary choices affect health status. Diet has been implicated in the pathogenesis of those conditions mainly responsible for death and disability in developed society. The challenge is to find and eat a healthy diet.

The Palaeolithic diet

The Palaeolithic diet is the diet on which we evolved and our genetic profile was programmed. Accumulating evidence suggests that a mismatch between our modern diet and lifestyle and our Palaeolithic genome is contributing to obesity, hypertension, diabetes, and atherosclerotic cardiovascular disease.[7] Our ancestors' diet was rich in lean protein, polyunsaturated and monounsaturated fats, fibre, vitamins, minerals, antioxidants, and phytochemicals.[8] Meat from grass-fed animals and nutrient-dense, fibre-loaded low glycaemic index foods were plentiful in the Palaeolithic diet. In contrast, the Western diet is energy-dense, rich in refined higher glycaemic index foods and meat from grain-fed animals.[5] The dietary fats of these two diets are dramatically different.[8,9] The saturated:polyunsaturated fatty acid ratio of the Palaeolithic diet was <4:1; the Western dietary ratio is >40:1. The omega-6:omega-3 fatty acid ratio has changed from <4:1 in the Palaeolithic diet to >11:1 in the Western diet. Excessive amounts of omega-6 polyunsaturated fatty acids (PUFA) promote the pathogenesis of cardiovascular disease, cancer, and inflammatory and autoimmune diseases. Increased levels of omega-3 PUFA exert suppressive effects.[10] An omega-6: omega-3 ratio of no more than 10:1 is recommended. While this represents an improvement of the reported 16.7:1 ratio,[10] at 10:1 the physiological balance still favours vasospasm, vasoconstriction and increased blood viscosity, and, in asthmatics, bronchospasm! In the secondary prevention of cardiovascular disease, a ratio of 4:1 was associated with a 70% decrease in total mortality.[10] A ratio of 2.5:1 reduced rectal cell proliferation in patients with colorectal cancer; a ratio of 2–3:1 suppressed inflammation in patients with rheumatoid arthritis; and a ratio of 5:1 benefited patients with asthma.[10]

The balanced diet

Health authorities recommend a dietary approach less radical than that of the Palaeolithic diet. They recommend 'counseling adults and children over the age of 2 to limit dietary intake of fat (especially saturated fat) and cholesterol, maintain caloric balance in their diet, and emphasize foods containing fibre (i.e. fruits, vegetables, grain products)'.[11] More particularly, they are guided by the food pyramid.[12,13] Standard dietary recommendations are to maintain an ideal body weight and select 6–11 serves from the bread, cereal, rice, pasta group; 3–5 serves of vegetables and 2–4 serves of fruit; 2–3 serves of meat, poultry, fish, beans, eggs and nuts; 2–3 serves of dairy products; and to use fats, oils and sweets sparingly. Serving size is important. One serve is the equivalent of 1 medium-size piece of fruit or ½ cup of chopped/cooked/canned fruit; ½ cup of vegetable, 1 cup of raw leafy vegetable or ¾ cup of vegetable juice; 1 slice of bread, or ½ cup of cooked cereal, rice or pasta; 2 ounces of cooked lean meat, poultry or fish or ½ cup cooked dry beans; 1 cup of milk or yoghurt or 1.5–2 ounces of cheese.[13] See **Handout 9.3**.

Dairy products

Dairy products are an important source of calcium, riboflavin and protein. Almost 75% of calcium in the Western diet is derived from dairy products. Clinical trials indicate that the consumption of recommended levels of dairy products reduces the risk of low bone mass, contributes to lower blood pressure and can have a beneficial effect on body weight and fat loss.[14] Compared to diets low in dairy products, consuming dairy products at recommended levels does not contribute to weight gain.[15] The 2005 Dietary Guidelines for Americans recommend three servings of milk products per day. The dairy product chosen is important – low-fat varieties are recommended. Dairy products, but milk in particular, have been found to be inversely associated with risk of colorectal adenoma recurrence.[16] Two servings of yoghurt per day can reduce the risk of developing bladder cancer by up to 40%. Total dairy intake was not significantly associated with risk of bladder cancer, but sour milk and yoghurt had a statistically significant inverse association with this disease.[17]

The meat, poultry, fish, beans, eggs and nuts group

The biological value of animal protein is higher than that from vegetables. The biological value for egg is 100; for milk, 93; for beef and/or fish, 75; and for corn, 72. Animal protein provides first-class proteins containing the full complement of amino acids required for health; vegetable protein sources are often deficient in one or more essential amino acids. Vegetarians need to combine foods to ensure adequate nutrition (see Figure 9.4). Meat is an important source of iron, B12 and niacin. Although present in vegetables (see Figure 9.5), iron is better

---

When evaluating foods as a source of protein intake it is necessary to consider:

- The concentration of protein
- The digestibility/availability of the protein. The protein in eggs and chicken is more digestible than that in milk and peas
- The amino acid composition of the protein. Unlike animals, plants provide incomplete protein. The biological value of plant protein can be improved by combining foods at any meal

PLANTS SOURCES	LIMITING AMINO ACID
Sesame & sunflower seeds	Lysine
Wheat, rice, barley, millet	Lysine, threonine
Corn	Lysine, threonine, tryptophan
Peanuts	Lysine, threonine, methionine
Green peas, soybeans	Methionine
Beans:	Methionine, cystine
Lima, navy, pinto, white, kidney	

The biological value of proteins, i.e. the amount of protein nitrogen retained for growth and maintenance expressed as a percentage of the protein nitrogen digested and absorbed, varies for different proteins. The biological value for egg is 100, for milk 93, for beef and/or fish 75, and for corn 72. the protein efficiency ratio also measures the quality of protein and is expressed as the grams of weight gained by animals per weight of dietary protein eaten.

See also
Sources http://www.hsph.harvard.edu/nutritionsource/what-should-you-eat/protein/
For vegans http://www.vrg.org/nutrition/protein.htm
Protein overview http://www.hsph.harvard.edu/nutritionsource/what-should-you-eat/protein-full-story/index.html

Figure 9.4 • Protein.

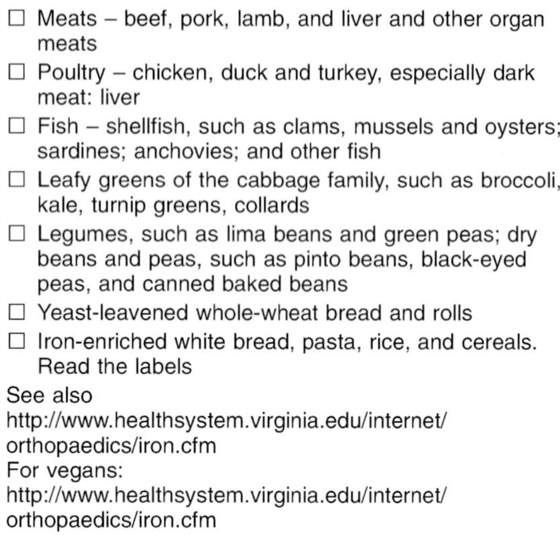

Figure 9.5 • Some good sources of iron.

absorbed in its organic form, i.e. as found in meat. Inadequate meat intake may result in low serum protein, iron deficiency and vitamin B12 deficiency; overconsumption, an increased risk of obesity and hyperlipidaemia. See http://www.webmd.com/video/healthy-meat-choices.

Fish is important in the diet. It provides first-class protein and is the major dietary source of omega-3 fatty acids. Coldwater fish are a rich source of omega-3 fatty acids. These include kippers, mackerel, pilchards, Atlantic salmon, trout, blue grenadier, herring, sardines, albacore tuna, yellowtail and perch. At least two servings of oily fish each week are recommended. For optimal health, fish can be broiled, steamed, baked or raw, but not fried.[18,19] In the elderly, a diet high in fish and fish products is associated with better cognitive performance in a dose-dependent manner.[20] Eating one portion of an omega-3 fatty acid-rich fish per week may halve the risk of age-related macular degeneration![21] Eating coldwater fish particularly benefits cardiovascular health. Benefits include improved lipoprotein metabolism; inhibition of smooth muscle cell proliferation in the arterial wall, decreasing subclinical atherosclerosis; a reduced coagulation tendency through both platelet and vessel wall interactions; an antiarrhythmic effect; and a lower risk of death, especially from heart failure.[19,22,23]

Eggs are an excellent source of first-class protein. Among egg consumers in the US, although eggs contributed less than 10% of the daily energy intake, they provided 20% to 30% of vitamins A, E and B12, and 10% to 20% of the folate, and total, saturated and polyunsaturated fat consumed. See www.webmd.com/food-recipes/features/eggs-friend-or-foe. There has also been a rethink regarding the risk posed by eggs with respect to ischaemic heart disease. It now appears that one egg daily does not enhance the risk of coronary heart disease in non-diabetic men and women.[24] In fact, a study involving 56 healthy adults found that eating one egg daily improved the lipoprotein profile, raising HDL and decreasing the ratio of total to HDL-cholesterol.[25] Concerns about egg intake arose from the high cholesterol content of eggs – 210 mg cholesterol per egg. However, it is oxidized rather than native cholesterol that is thought to enhance atherosclerosis. The risk of consuming oxidized cholesterol when eating eggs can be reduced by only eating raw eggs or eggs with runny yolks, avoiding spray-dried eggs, or eating eggs from hens with 80 IU vitamin E added to each kilogram of feed.[26] Eggs are a source of selenium. Selenium boosts the antioxidant immune system and may reduce the risk of some types of cancer and cardiovascular disease. Eggs provide an important source of selenium for populations in countries with selenium-depleted soil.

Nuts are energy- and nutrient-rich foods. They are a source of minerals: 50 g of cashews contains 3 mg of iron; 50 g of almonds contains 240 mg of calcium, a similar amount to 200 mL of milk; while one Brazil nut supplies twice the RDA of selenium. Eating two Brazil nuts daily effectively increases selenium status.[27] Walnuts are rich in omega-3 fatty acids. Eating peanuts increases dietary vitamin A, vitamin E, folate, calcium, magnesium, zinc and iron, and dietary fibre.[28] Nuts are a rich source of monounsaturated fatty acids and fibre. Nuts favourably affect serum lipids and endothelial function; they enhance insulin sensitivity and have anti-inflammatory properties. They have been shown to decrease the risk of cardiovascular disease and type 2 diabetes mellitus.[29,30] As nuts are energy-dense they may contribute to positive energy balance and weight gain. However, current knowledge suggests moderate nut consumption does not pose a threat for weight gain.[31] This may be due to its satiety effect, promotion of energy expenditure and/or inefficient energy utilization. In fact, nuts, when included as part of an energy-controlled diet, may assist weight loss![32] Two tablespoons of peanut butter or 1/3 cup of nuts is considered equivalent to a serve of 40 g of lean meat.

Legumes are low in fat and an excellent source of protein, dietary fibre, various micronutrients and phytochemicals.[33] Legumes include peas, lentils, peanuts, and beans, including soybeans. The protein content of beans is generally between 20% and 30% of energy. A serving of beans (90 g or ½ cup cooked beans) provides 7–8 g of protein or 15% of the RDA for protein for a 70-kg adult. Bean proteins are relatively low in sulphur amino acids, which compromises their status as first-class proteins but provides an advantage in terms of calcium retention. Except for chickpeas and soybeans, which contain 15% and 47% fat, respectively, most beans are very low in fat, generally containing 5% of energy as fat. The dietary ratio of omega-6 to omega-3 fatty acids among vegetarians is 10:1. Beans are an excellent source of folate – one serving of beans provides more than half of the current RDA. Beans are rich in iron; one serving provides 2 mg. However, iron bioavailability from legumes is poor. Zinc and calcium bioavailability from legumes is relatively good, at 20–25%. Beans are an excellent source of dietary fibre; one serving provides 2–4 g of a mix of soluble and insoluble fibre. High-fibre, high-bean diets have been shown to lower serum cholesterol and have very low glycaemic indices. Beans are a rich source of oligosaccharides – markedly increasing flatulence.

Soybeans are unique legumes offering a concentrated source of isoflavones. Isoflavones have weak oestrogenic properties and the isoflavone genistein influences signal transduction. Soybeans are rich sources of polyunsaturated fat (20%) compared to other beans (1%). The ratio of linoleic (omega-6) to alpha-linolenic acid (omega-3) is around 7:1. The concentration of iron is around 16 mg/100 g dry weight; of zinc, 4.8 mg/100 g dry weight; and of calcium, 276 mg/100 g dry weight. Soybeans contains around 138 mg of calcium per 90-g serve (½ cup boiled soybeans) and bioavailability is largely equivalent to that in milk. Soy foods and isoflavones have a potential role in preventing and treating cancer and osteoporosis. The UK and USA governments recommend 25 g of soy protein per day to help reduce serum cholesterol. One serve supplies 6–10 g. This means consuming about 3 cups of soymilk or 200–300 g of tofu daily. It has been suggested that less than two serves of soy, i.e. 200 g of tofu and 2 cups of soy milk or 1 cup of soy flour, may decrease cholesterol and increase vasodilatation, decreasing blood pressure.[34] However, it should be noted that soy protein loses the ability to reduce serum cholesterol if ultra heat treated or pasteurized.[35]

Grains/cereals/bread/pasta

Breads, pasta and cereals are a source of energy, carbohydrate, protein, thiamine, and, potentially, niacin. The health impact of whole grain and refined foods is vastly different. Processing reduces the nutrient value of this group. Refining grains removes many biologically active agents, including, amongst others, fibre, vitamins, minerals, lignans and phytosterols. If maize flour is processed under alkaline conditions, niacin forms complexes and becomes biologically available; dietary fibre and thiamine are lost when wheat is used to produce white flour. Health may be compromised by nutrient lost and sodium added during processing.

While simple sugars should be used sparingly, consuming three or more servings per day of whole grain foods is desirable. Cereal grains and their products provide around 30% of total energy intake of British adults, much more than any of the other major food groups.[36]

There is strong evidence to suggest that eating a variety of whole grain foods is beneficial in the prevention and management of type 2 diabetes and ischaemic heart disease. Whole grains, like legumes, potentially benefit glycaemic control. Prospective studies consistently show a reduced risk for developing type 2 diabetes by a high intake of whole grain foods (27% to 30%) or cereal fibre (28% to 37%).[37] Habitually eating whole grain foods may reduce the risk of ischaemic heart disease by as much as 40%.[38] Consumption of at least 2.5 g of whole grains every day may lead to a 21% lower risk of heart attacks and strokes.[39] Health authorities such as the US FDA now regard it as valid to make health claims that whole grain cereal foods and oatmeal or bran may reduce the risk of ischaemic heart disease.[40] Whole grain intake may contribute to a healthy body weight in adult women. In fact, eating about three servings per day of whole grains is associated with a lower BMI and less central adiposity.[41] It appears that a higher intake of whole grains can increase fibre intake by 9 g, while total and saturated fat intake may decrease by 11 and 3.9 g, respectively. For maximum benefit, carbohydrate-rich foods should be whole grain.

Fruits and vegetables

Fruits and vegetables are an important source of antioxidants, vitamins and minerals. The old dietary recommendations of two fruits and three vegetables have been increased to three to five serves of 60–90 g of vegetables and two to four serves of 120–150-g pieces of fruit daily. Higher intakes of fruits and vegetables are associated with a lower risk of the metabolic syndrome.[42] The metabolic syndrome increases the risk both of ischaemic heart disease and of type 2 diabetes. Compared to eating less than one piece of fruit daily, eating five or more pieces of fruit per day reduces the risk of coronary heart disease by 44%.[43] Compared to a vegetable-free diet, eating more than three vegetable items per day reduces the risk of coronary heart disease by 75%.[43] A prospective study found that greater consumption of green leafy vegetables and whole fruit may be associated with a lower risk of type 2 diabetes mellitus, whereas greater consumption of fruit juices may be associated with a higher risk.[44] An increase of one serving per day in fruit juice consumption was associated with an 18% increased risk of diabetes.

Case-control, cohort, and ecologic observational studies have consistently associated increased consumption of fruits and vegetables with a decreased risk for a wide variety of epithelial cancers.[45] While it is likely that the protective effect of fruits and vegetables against cancer is linked to multiple interacting regulatory molecules, certain compounds are of particular interest. Cruciferous and Allium vegetables have been shown to be chemoprotective; potato, carrot, tomato and lettuce are generally ineffective.[46] The anticancer effects of Allium vegetables, e.g. garlic, is linked to organosulphur compounds, while that of cruciferous vegetables, such as broccoli and cauliflower, to isothiocyanates.[47] Unlike cancer chemotherapy drugs, many bioactive food components selectively target cancer cells.[48]

All coloured phytochemicals that absorb light in the visible spectrum have antioxidant properties. To get maximum benefit from fruits and vegetables it is advisable to eat a wide range of colours. The greater the range of colours chosen, the more comprehensive the antioxidant cover provided. Eat at least one food from each of the seven colour groups:[49]

- red – e.g. tomatoes
- yellow–green – e.g. corn, leafy greens, avocado
- red–purple – e.g. red apples, grapes, berries, wine
- orange – e.g. carrots, mango, pumpkin
- orange–yellow – e.g. oranges, lemons, peaches, cantaloupe
- green – e.g. broccoli, Brussels sprouts, kale
- white–green – e.g. onion, garlic, leeks.

The colour code ensures a broad spectrum of different antioxidants; however, individual fruits and vegetables have varying concentrations of antioxidant activity. Wild blueberries were found to have the highest cellular antioxidant activity, while bananas and melons were found to have the lowest.[50] Pomegranates and other berries (blackberry, raspberry, and blueberry) were also found to have high levels of cellular antioxidant activity. Each serving of salad consumed increases levels of folic acid, vitamins C and E, lycopene, and alpha- and beta-carotene to above that of the RDA.[51]

In addition to disease protection, higher intakes of fruits and vegetables have been associated with higher academic performance.[52]

Fats and oils

Owing to its high energy concentration, dietary fat should be limited. The daily energy intake from fat should be 30% or less; 10% or less from saturated and 20% from mono- and polyunsaturated fats (largely vegetable oils). Animal products are the major dietary sources of cholesterol, saturated fatty acids and arachidonic acid. Plants are cholesterol-free and an important dietary source of polyunsaturated fatty acids. Polyunsaturated fatty acids are needed for cell membrane function and structure.

Fats are the most energy-dense of all foods. The body uses adipose tissue and glycerol to store long- and short-term energy supplies. Body fat stored as triglyceride is readily synthesized from dietary fats and carbohydrates. Hepatic synthesis of triglycerides is enhanced after a meal rich in simple sugars. Ironically, fruit juices and other fructose-rich beverage stimulate lipogenesis even more strongly than sucrose.[53] Dietary saturated fatty acids stimulate cholesterol synthesis, an important precursor of hormones and vitamin D. Hepatic synthesis of cholesterol is reduced as dietary cholesterol increases.

Although saturated fatty acids and cholesterol can be synthesized by the body, some essential polyunsaturated fatty acids can only be obtained from the diet. Neither linoleic, an omega-6 fatty acid, nor alpha-linolenic acid, from the omega-3 series, can be synthesized. Dietary intake is essential.

Linoleic acid is the precursor of longer-chain polyunsaturated fatty acids such as arachidonic; alpha-linolenic acid is the substrate for eicosapentaenoic acid (EPA) and docosahexaenoic acid (DHA). The long-chain polyunsaturated fatty acids of the omega-3 family have anti-inflammatory, antithrombotic, antiarrhythmic, hypolipidaemic, and vasodilatory properties. These fatty acids are needed for normal cellular function, including eicosanoid synthesis. Eicosanoids are important in cell regulation. In addition to being synthesized from essential fatty acids, long-chain polyunsaturated fatty acids are derived from the diet. Marine sources, particularly coldwater fish, are the major dietary source of EPA and DHA, while meat and eggs are rich sources of arachidonic acid. While seafood is the major source, land animals are not devoid of omega-3 fatty acids. Whereas one or two portions of seafood weekly can contribute 200 mg/day DHA, 100 g cooked lean red meat can provide up to 30 mg DHA, and a standard egg generally contains 45 mg DHA.

The form in which fats are eaten is important. When plant fats are consumed as oils, they are rich in polyunsaturated fats; when these oils are processed, many of the unsaturated bonds are hydrogenated and the saturated fatty acid content is increased. Heating also isomerizes fats, creating *trans* fatty acids. Spreadable vegetable oils, although cholesterol-free, with their increased saturated fat and *trans* fatty acid content offer little, if any, health advantage over animal fats. The results of a recent study suggest that consuming foods prepared with and/or cooking with partially hydrogenated vegetable oils may increase inflammation in the body, thereby increasing the risk of a plethora of diseases associated with increased inflammation.[54]

The dietary pyramid is a well-established guide to achieving dietary balance. Food-based dietary indices are also available. One such index consists of 15 items reflecting the dietary guidelines, including dietary indicators of vegetables and legumes, fruit, total cereals, meat and alternatives, total dairy, beverages, sodium, saturated fat, alcoholic beverages, and added sugars.[55] Diet quality is incorporated using indicators relating to whole grain cereals, lean meat, reduced-/low-fat dairy, and dietary variety. Higher dietary guideline index scores were associated with lower intakes of energy, total fat and saturated fat and higher intakes of fibre, beta-carotene, vitamin C, folate, calcium and iron.

Dietary quality can be more broadly ascertained by considering the dietary patterns selected by various population groups.

The Mediterranean diet

Although different regions in the Mediterranean basin have unique characteristics, the consumption pattern of the Mediterranean diet tends to consist of:[56]

- non-refined cereals daily – whole grain bread, pasta, brown rice etc.
- vegetables (2–3 serves daily)
- fruits (6 daily)
- olive oil daily
- dairy products (1–2 serves daily, particularly cheese and yoghurt)
- fish (4–5 serves weekly)
- poultry (3–4 serves weekly)
- olives, pulses and nuts (3 serves weekly)
- potatoes, eggs and sweets (3–4 serves weekly)
- red meat/meat products (4–5 serves monthly).

The diet is also characterized by moderate consumption of wine (1–2 wineglasses/day) and a monounsaturated:saturated fat ratio in excess of 2. Mediterranean diet indices provide a summary of the diet by means of a single score based on a function of different components, such as food, food groups or a combination of foods and nutrients.[57] Recent reports of the Mediterranean diet confirmed favourable effects on lipoprotein levels, endothelium vasodilatation, insulin resistance, metabolic syndrome, antioxidant capacity, cancer incidence in obese patients, and myocardial and cardiovascular mortality in those with previous myocardial infarction.[58–60] The consumption of certain typical Mediterranean foods is associated with lower serum concentrations of inflammatory markers, especially those related to endothelial function.[61] It is probably the combination of fruits, cereals, virgin olive oil and nuts that creates a healthy cellular environment. Certainly, a cumulative analysis evaluating overall mortality in relation to adherence to a Mediterranean diet showed that a two point increase in the adherence score is significantly associated with a reduced risk of mortality.[62] This study reported that greater adherence to a Mediterranean diet is associated with a significant improvement in health status, as seen by a significant reduction in overall mortality (9%), mortality from cardiovascular diseases (9%), incidence of or mortality from cancer (6%), and incidence of Parkinson's disease and Alzheimer's disease (13%).[62] The Mediterranean diet is a healthy diet.

The vegetarian diet

Diets with generous amounts of plant foods and limited quantities of animal foods are increasingly being recommended.[63] The American Institute for Cancer Research and the World Cancer Research Fund support predominantly plant-based diets rich in a variety of legumes, vegetables and fruits, with minimally processed starchy staple foods and limited quantities of red meat; the American Cancer Society recommends choosing most food from plant sources; the American Heart Association advocates a balanced diet with an emphasis on vegetables, grains, and fruits; and the Heart and Stroke Foundation of Canada recommends using grains and vegetables instead of meat as the focus of meals. The American Dietetic Association and Dietitians of Canada have concluded that appropriately planned vegetarian diets are healthful, nutritionally adequate, and provide health benefits in the prevention and treatment of certain diseases.[63]

Vegetarians exclude meat, fish and poultry from their diet. An extreme option is the fruitarian diet consisting largely of fruit. This dietary variation is fraught with difficulties and persons cannot survive for prolonged periods on a diet solely of fruit. The vegan diet is plant based and includes grains, vegetables, fruits, legumes, seeds and nuts. The lacto-vegetarian diet includes dairy products. The lacto-ovo-vegetarian eating pattern is plant based and incorporates dairy products and eggs. The semi-vegetarian diet includes occasional meat or fish but is largely similar to the lacto-ovo-vegetarian. People choosing macrobiotic diets follow a largely vegetarian diet; eating grains, legumes and vegetables and using fruits, nuts and seeds to a lesser extent. The vegetarian diet contains more antioxidant vitamins (vitamin C, vitamin E, and beta-carotene) and copper but less bioavailable zinc than does the omnivorous diet.[64] Dietary intake of selenium depends on the selenium content of the soil. Vegetarian diets benefit health due to their lower levels of saturated fat, cholesterol and animal protein; and higher levels of carbohydrates, fibre, magnesium, boron, folate, antioxidants such as vitamins C and E,

carotenoids and phytochemicals. Scientific evidence suggests a positive association between the vegetarian diet and reduced risk for several chronic disorders, including obesity, coronary artery disease, hypertension, diabetes, some types of cancer, and possibly dementia.[65] A vegetarian diet is not obligatory – compared to health-conscious omnivores from the same population, cohort studies of vegetarians have shown the additional health advantage is limited to a moderate reduction in death from ischaemic heart disease.[66] The health benefits of a vegetarian diet can furthermore be seriously compromised unless a well-balanced diet is chosen.

The vegetarian diet pyramid provides a food guide to healthy eating.[67] It recommends multiple daily servings of foods from the three mini-pyramids 'fruit and vegetables', 'whole grains' and 'legumes and beans'; daily servings from the three mini-pyramids 'nuts and seeds', 'plant oils' and 'egg whites, soy milk and dairy'; and occasional or small-quantity servings from the 'eggs and sweets' mini-pyramid. Moderate regular intake of alcoholic beverages such as wine, beer or spirits is optional. Unrefined plant oils should be used daily and dietary supplements should be considered, depending on personal variables. The major dietary hazard of a vegetarian diet is perhaps an inadequate intake of omega-3 fatty acids. The vegetarian diet does not have a direct source of eicosapentaenoic acid and docosahexaenoic acid and relies on the ability of the desaturase enzyme system to convert alpha-linolenic acid to the long-chain omega-3 polyunsaturated fatty acids. Alpha-linolenic acid is not equivalent in its biological effects to the long-chain omega-3 fatty acids found in marine oils. With the exception of fruitarians, whose diet predictably leads to undernutrition, vegans are at greatest risk of deficiency. Unless cautious, vegans risk deficiency of omega-3 fatty acids, vitamin B12, vitamin D, calcium, zinc, and occasionally riboflavin. Vitamin B12 may be obtained from fortified cereals, 'veggie' meats, soymilk or nutritional yeast. Vitamin D is best obtained from fortified foods or sun exposure. Calcium is present in many plant foods and fortified foods but bioavailability may be a problem. Low-oxalate greens, bok choy, broccoli, Chinese cabbage, collards, kale, okra and turnip are plant sources with bioavailability between 49% and 61%. The bioavailability in calcium-set tofu, fortified fruit juices, and cow's milk is 31%, while that in soymilk, sesame seeds, almonds, and red and white beans drops to around 23%. Zinc bioavailability can be increased by food preparation techniques that reduce binding of zinc by phytate. Vegans should soak beans and sprouting beans, grains, and seeds and opt for leavened bread. Mushrooms, almonds, fortified cereals and soymilk are sources of riboflavin. Careful dietary selection can successfully overcome any potential deficiencies in the vegan diet.[63]

The popularity of vegetarianism is growing. Reasons for choosing a vegetarian diet are varied and include health considerations, concern for the environment, animal welfare factors, economic issues, ethical considerations, world hunger issues, and religious beliefs. Vegetarian diets are a healthful option, not only because of their exclusions but also because of their high intake of plant foods rich in fibre, antioxidants and phytonutrients. Vegan diets, however, do require increased vigilance in dietary selection. The health of vegetarians is related to their propensity to make informed dietary choices. See **Handout 9.4**.

Dietary prevention of disease

The U.S. Preventive Services Task Force recommends intensive behavioural dietary counselling for adult patients with hyperlipidaemia and other known risk factors for cardiovascular and diet-related chronic disease.[1] Although a balanced diet provides a rough guide to preventing most nutritional deficiencies, prevention of certain diseases requires that the minimal dietary health standard be adapted. **Handout 9.3** provides a template for general dietary health, additional changes are recommended to specifically target prevention of particular diet-related diseases.

Dietary prevention of cardiovascular disease

Dietary changes to promote cardiovascular wellness focus largely on hyperlipidaemia as a risk factor and recommend:

- no more than 30% of total energy be derived from fat
- daily cholesterol intake not to exceed 300 mg
- total saturated fat to contribute 7% or less of total energy
- polyunsaturated fat intake be increased but to no more than 7% of total energy

- monounsaturated fat intake be increased to 16%
- *trans* fatty acids be avoided
- at least 50% of energy be derived from carbohydrate, especially complex carbohydrates
- sodium intake not to exceed 3 g per day
- alcohol consumption not to exceed 30–60 mL per day.

Handout 9.5 provides dietary guidelines consistent with these recommendations.

Dietary prevention of diabetes

The risk of type 2 diabetes is reduced by:

- maintaining an ideal body weight
- getting 50–60% of energy from carbohydrates:
  - select foods with a low glycaemic index (<55), e.g. whole grains, vegetables and fruit
  - eat carbohydrates rich in soluble fibre (40 g/ day), e.g. peanuts, kidney and white beans, fresh pears, peas, green beans
  - limit refined carbohydrates and sugars
- getting no more than 40% of energy from fat, and half of this should be from monounsaturated fats, e.g. avocado, nuts, olive oil
- getting 12–20% of energy from protein – fish is preferable to meat.

See **Handout 9.6**.

Dietary prevention of osteoporosis

Recommendations to improve or maintain skeletal mineralization include:

- ensuring an adequate intake of calcium and vitamin D – dairy products are a good source
- decreasing animal proteins and increasing vegetables as a source of protein – moving towards the alkaline pole of the acid–base balance
- avoiding excess sodium consumption, thereby reducing obligatory calciuria
- reducing alcohol and caffeine intake
- increasing consumption of food sources rich in phytoestrogens which may prevent bone resorption and increase bone density
- regular weight-bearing exercise.

Handout 9.7 provides dietary guidelines consistent with these recommendations.

Dietary prevention of cancer

Dietary changes to reduce the personal risk of cancer include:

- maintaining a healthy body weight. Weight gain should be limited to less than 5 kg during adulthood
- a low-energy diet
- a reduction of fat consumption to 25% of energy intake. The composition of the fat in the diet should be low in saturated fat, limited in omega-6 polyunsaturated fat and permit moderate omega-3 polyunsaturated and monounsaturated fats. Avoid *trans* fatty acids
- getting at least 25 g of fibre each day from a diet rich in vegetables and fruit, particularly cruciferous vegetables and yellow/orange fruit. Eat five or more serves (400–800 g) per day of fruit and vegetables. A diet based upon plant products is recommended
- increasing consumption of food rich in resistant starch
- increasing the intake of isoflavones, and other phytoestrogens. Soy products and to a lesser extent peas and beans are good sources of isoflavones. Lignans are found in cereals, vegetables and fruit
- eating fish and poultry in preference to red meat. Limit red meat to less than 89 g daily
- avoiding sources of carcinogens such as:
  - cigarette smoke
  - charred, burnt, smoked, cured or pickled foods
- moderation in alcohol consumption: fewer than two drinks a day for men and one for women
- reading food labels to identify and exclude any potential carcinogens or mutagens in food substances
- restricting total salt consumption to less than 6 g per day
- food storage and preparation:
  - perishable foods should be consumed promptly when fresh
  - perishable foods should be kept frozen or refrigerated
  - foods should be stored at low temperatures
  - food should be boiled or steamed rather than fried or grilled.

Handout 9.8 provides dietary guidelines consistent with these recommendations.

Dietary requirements during the life cycle

While the balanced, Mediterranean and lacto-ovo-vegetarian diets are all health promoting, there are certain phases of the life cycle with additional dietary demands.[68]

Diet during childhood and adolescence

The American Heart Association has published guidelines for healthy eating in infancy, childhood and adolescence.[69] Modification of general dietary recommendations encompasses the following. Children need to eat a wide variety of nutritious foods. Their diet should include eating lots of bread, cereals (preferably whole grain), vegetables (including legumes) and fruits. Adequate dietary fibre should be consumed. The recommendation for children is to achieve the 'age plus five' rule by 3 years of age. The rule is: eat 8 g of fibre per day (3+5) from the age of 3 years and increase the daily fibre intake by 1 g each year until the adult recommendation is reached (25–35 g/day). A low-fat diet is not suitable for children. A gradual reduction in fat intake is advocated from around 35% of total energy at age 5 years to 30% by age 15 years. Whole rather than skimmed milk is recommended for children under the age of 5 years. Drinking water is to be encouraged and alcohol is unsuitable. Low-salt foods and sparing use of salt is advocated. Similarly, only a moderate amount of sugar and foods with added sugar should be eaten. Childhood obesity is of concern. Unacceptable adiposity should be avoided.

For 2–2.5 years during the ages of about 10 to 16, adolescents undergo a growth spurt, during which time boys gain about 20 cm in height and 20 kg in weight. The peak velocity for increased height precedes the weight gain by about 3 months. The increased energy requirement during this time provides some protection against the types of foods (energy-dense rather than nutrient-dense) often selected by adolescents. Foods containing iron and calcium need to be specifically selected. Peak bone mass now appears to be reached in the late teens rather than the early 30s as previously supposed. An adequate intake of calcium in 9- to 14-year-olds is vital for development of adequate bone mass. Prepubescent females should have a particularly rich calcium diet.

Guidelines for a good diet during childhood are outlined in **Handout 9.9**.

As children reach adolescence, their eating habits often cause concern. Dietary behaviours that may potentially cause later problems include:

- missed meals, especially breakfast. Cereal intake at breakfast time is associated with greater physical activity throughout the day.[70] Compared to non-cereal breakfast, a cereal-based breakfast leads to greater intakes of fibre, iron, folic acid and zinc, and lesser intakes of fat, sodium, sugar and cholesterol.[70] Cereal at breakfast displaces consumption of fat-, sugar- and sodium-rich foods

- excessive reliance on 'fast' or takeaway foods. These are often rich in cholesterol, saturated fat, energy and sodium. Fast foods, although usually having adequate amounts of protein, B vitamins and iron, are often deficient in calcium, fibre, folate, and vitamins E, C and carotene. This may be aggravated by the frequent consumption of snacks that are energy-dense and nutrient-poor

- adolescent dieting. Obesity is regarded as socially unacceptable in this group and nutritionally unacceptable dieting may be a problem. Diet is also popularly believed to aggravate acne. Zinc, polyunsaturated fatty acids and vitamin A are reported to improve acne; chocolate, confectionery and fatty foods are suspected of exacerbating the condition.

Eating family meals has also been found to enhance the health and wellbeing of adolescents. Frequency of family meals was inversely associated with tobacco, alcohol, and marijuana use; low grade point average; depressive symptoms; and suicide involvement after controlling for family connectedness.[71] See **Handout 9.9**.

A prudent diet when contemplating pregnancy

It is increasingly recognized that the nutritional and drug-related behaviour of both parents around the time of conception influences fertility and fetal development. A healthy diet not only is likely to increase the likelihood of conception, it also favours development of a healthy fetus.

For 3 months before desired conception, it is wise to build up body stores in anticipation of pregnancy. Eating at least two serves of calcium-rich low-fat foods, seven serves of fruit and vegetables, two serves of iron-rich lean meat and six serves of whole grains per day is a good start. The strongest evidence supporting nutritional supplementation in the periconceptual period relates to folic acid. Folic acid can prevent neural tube defects if taken periconceptually in doses of 4–5 mg/day by women who have a personal or family history of spina bifida or in doses of at least 0.4 mg/day by women at low risk. The time when folate deficiency may have greatest clinical effect is around 28 days after conception. Folate, in view of its importance in DNA replication, may also be important in preventing diverse congenital defects including cleft palate and cleft lip. Good dietary sources of folate include: dry beans, lentils, chickpeas, cowpeas, and peanuts; many vegetables, especially leafy greens, and fruits, particularly the berries and kiwifruit.

Social drugs, including tobacco and alcohol, should be avoided. Not only may drugs taken by the mother affect the fertilized ovum, but also drugs such as cocaine may reach the conceptus in the ejaculate. Epigenetics emphasizes the importance of dietary care during pregnancy. Environmental exposures early in development play a role in susceptibility to disease in later life. Somewhat paradoxically, as demonstrated by a recent study, mothers who received folic acid during the first trimester produced children at increased risk of wheezing and lower respiratory infections during their first 18 months of life.[72] Some dietary guidelines for women contemplating pregnancy are provided in **Handout 9.10**.

Diet during pregnancy

In pregnancy, the RDA for energy increases only 17%, while the RDA for vitamins and minerals increases 20% to 100%. Careful selection of nutrient-dense foods is therefore important. During pregnancy women would benefit from:

- increasing their daily protein intake from 54 to 60 g. Meat supplies iron and protein; milk is a good source of calcium and protein, fish supplies omega-3 fatty acids. Omega-3 fatty acids are important for fetal development

- doubling their folic acid intake to 400 µg/day. Good sources of folate include yeast, Marmite, Bovril, liver, bran, endive, nuts, broccoli, spinach, peas, Brussels sprouts and kidneys

- increasing their iron intake from 12 to 30 mg/day. Meat, fish and poultry contain haem iron, which is readily absorbed. Non-haem iron, found in plants, is poorly absorbed. Citrus fruit, tomatoes, pawpaw, broccoli, pumpkin and cabbage are among the better plant sources of iron
- doubling their calcium intake to at least 1200 mg/day. Dairy products, sesame seeds, dark green vegetables, dried legumes, sardines, tuna and salmon are good sources
- increasing their zinc intake by 25% to 19.5 mg/day. Good sources are oysters, red meat, liver, whole grain cereals, nuts, cheese and crustaceans
- increasing their iodine intake by 20% to 150 µg/day. Kelp, seafood, dairy products and iodized salt are useful sources. Goitrogens such as cabbage, turnips, Brussels sprouts, cauliflower and mustard may impair utilization
- eliminating alcohol from their diet
- vitamin A. In doses of less than 10 000 IU during the first trimester, vitamin A is protective against birth defects; higher doses later in pregnancy are safe, i.e. not teratogenic.

Handout 9.11 provides some dietary guidelines for pregnant women.

Maternal diet during breastfeeding

While maternal milk yields vary, many women are capable of breastfeeding. Regular and frequent suckling is a well-established stimulus to lactation. The major stimulus to prolactin production is stimulation of the nipple by sucking. As the neonate's rooting and sucking reflexes are strongest 20–30 minutes after birth, placing the baby on the breast shortly after birth facilitates lactogenesis.

There is little evidence that dietary energy, protein, fat, water or other nutrients have a consistent effect on milk volume in adequately nourished communities. Maternal diets that are deficient in energy, however, may lead to a reduction in the volume of milk produced. In situations in which severe malnutrition is encountered, the fat content of milk may also be reduced. Mothers producing over 600 mL of milk per day can supply their infants with sufficient energy. Human milk supplies 289 kJ per 100 mL.

Extra considerations for lactating mothers are:

- an additional 700 mg of calcium, 100 µg of folate, and 10 µg of vitamin D per day

- an additional 2500 kJ (600 kcal) and 850 mL of water per day; both may be supplied by milk rich in calcium
- avoiding drugs that are concentrated in breast milk (e.g. cannabis, opiates) or which may cause allergy or toxicity to the infant (e.g. chloramphenicol, reserpine, diazepam, indometacin).

Breastfeeding is associated with significant maternal bone loss (4% lumbar spine) during the first 3 months of lactation. This bone loss is offset by a comparable gain of bone within 6 months of weaning.

Handout 9.12 provides some dietary guidelines for breastfeeding mothers.

Infant diet during breastfeeding and weaning

From birth until 3 months of age, an infant's daily requirement is 485 kJ/kg body weight; from 3 months to 1 year, this requirement varies between 415 and 420 kJ/kg. Energy requirement is least between 6 and 9 months, when metabolic rate slows before infant activity increases. Mothers producing between 600 and 1000 mL of milk per day can supply their infants with sufficient energy.

Breast milk is subject to alteration by:

- maternal physiology. The composition of human milk varies with the stage of lactation, between individuals and with maternal nutrition
- environmental pollution, e.g. DDT
- maternal drug ingestion. Maternal ingestion of alcohol, valium or phenobarbital can cause sedation in the infant. Maternal ingestion of rhubarb or laxatives, e.g. senna, aloe or cascara, can increase bowel activity in the infant. Lactating mothers smoking more than 20 cigarettes a day can cause restlessness, vomiting and tachycardia in their babies. Smoking may also reduce the volume of milk produced.

The advantages of breastfeeding include:

- the nutritional value of breast milk. In addition to its adequate quantity of energy and nutrients, breast milk, with its whey:casein ratio, is easily digestible and contains the necessary essential amino acids, it contains fat in an easily digestible form and has a relatively low solute load. Breastfed babies appear to be at less risk of overfeeding and obesity
- emotional benefits of infant–maternal contact and bonding

- immunological protection. Immunoglobulins (especially IgA), particularly high in colostrum, are present in breast milk. Lysozyme, active against the cell walls of Gram-positive bacteria, complement, and cells of the lymphocyte, leukocyte and macrophage series are all present in breast milk. Lactoferrin, an iron-binding protein, limits the amount of iron available for *E. coli* growth; while lactose enhances the growth of commensal lactobacilli in the infant's intestine
- encouraging proper development of the jaw and teeth by sucking
- weight loss in the lactating mother; some protection against further pregnancies and better uterine involution in the presence of oxytocin stimulation
- convenience. A temperature-controlled, microbiologically safe feed is instantly available
- allergy prevention or minimization. The risk of allergy is reduced but not eliminated in breastfed infants. Maternal ingestion of foods, e.g. cow's milk, wheat or egg, may result in the respective antigen being transmitted in breast milk. Removing the allergenic food from the mother's diet may ease symptoms in the infant. Early weaning may also be considered.

Early weaning, with introduction of wheat products, however, may precipitate coeliac disease in infants at risk of gluten sensitivity. It has therefore been recommended that potentially allergic infants be exclusively breastfed for at least 4 and preferably 6 months. It is important that the baby is frequently fed and the mother has an adequate fluid and nutritional intake.

Babies should be breastfed or given a milk-based formula for at least the first 4–6 months of life. Milk formula preparations tend to more closely approximate human than cow's milk. Milk formulas may be richer in vitamin C, vitamin D and linoleic acid than are human or cow's milk. Breast milk is richer in cholesterol and omega-3 and omega-6 polyunsaturated fatty acids than are commercial formulas. The types of formula feeds available include:

- whey-dominated cow's milk formulas, e.g. Nan, S26. These are most similar to human milk
- casein-dominated cow's milk formulas, e.g. Lactogen, SMA. Gastric emptying is slower, casein is more difficult to digest and hence more satiety is reported
- lactose-free cow's milk modified formulas e.g. Digesta-Lac, O-Lac

- soy-modified formulas, e.g. ProSobee, Isomil. Four out of 10 infants with cow's milk allergy are also allergic to soy
- hydrolysed protein formulas, e.g. Pregestimil (fat mainly medium-chain triglycerides), Alfaré (butterfat, which is well absorbed). Protein is hydrolysed and resulting amino acids are less antigenic. The main carbohydrate source is glucose rather than lactose.

The time to start feeding solid foods is when energy derived from milk becomes insufficient. This occurs anywhere between 3 and 8 months. When the infant still seems hungry after a good feed, then the time to consider the introduction of solids has arrived. Furthermore, by 6 months, in exclusively milk-fed infants, body stores of iron, zinc and vitamin C may be becoming depleted. The concern in converting from breast milk to solid foods is food sensitivity. Suspect food allergy if the child develops a red, itchy skin, a loose offensive stool or colic. Solids should be introduced one at a time, at weekly intervals. Infant cereals, usually iron enriched, are typically selected first. **Handout 9.13** provides some guidelines for weaning.

Diet during old age

The elderly tend to lose lean body mass, muscle bulk and skeletal mass, while body fat increases. This conundrum is explained by decreased physical activity and decreased metabolism with ageing. Despite the increase in obesity that occurs with ageing, there is a linear decrease in food intake over the life span. Older persons fail to adequately regulate food intake and develop a physiological anorexia of ageing.[73]

Recent findings emphasize the importance of an adequate diet in old age. Better cognitive function in the elderly has been linked with diet. In a study of 260 elderly persons aged 65–90 years, those who had no errors on the Pfeiffer's Mental Status Questionnaire had higher dietary intakes of total food, vegetables, fruit, carbohydrate, fibre, folate, vitamin C, beta-carotene, iron and zinc, and lower intakes of saturated fatty acids, compared with those who made errors.[74] The authors suggest that a diet with less fat, saturated fat, and cholesterol, and more carbohydrate, fibre, vitamins (especially folate, vitamins C and E, and beta-carotene), and minerals (zinc and iron) may improve cognitive function as well as general health.

In general, older persons should avoid big meals but take care not to miss any meals. Inadequate protein and energy intake can become a problem unless three nutritious meals are eaten daily. Nutrients most likely to be deficient in the elderly include:

- potassium. Eat sufficient whole cell foods, e.g. bananas and other fruits. Deficiency can present with confusion, constipation, muscle weakness and arrhythmias. Potassium deficiency is potentiated by diuretic and purgative use
- iron. Deficiency may result from dietary inadequacy or blood loss exacerbated by aspirin ingestion
- B vitamins. Folate, B12 and B6 all are important for homocysteine metabolism. Increased levels of the amino acid homocysteine have been shown to double the risk of dementia or cognitive impairment[75]
- omega-3 fatty acids. Elderly people's cognition and general health benefit from eating at least 10 g of oily fish daily – maximum benefit is achieved at 75 g daily[20]
- zinc. Loss of taste and smell and cold extremities suggest zinc deficiency.

Dietary advice for the elderly includes an adequate intake of fruit (two serves) and vegetables (five serves) each day and at least two serves of dairy products daily to meet vitamin D, calcium and magnesium requirements. Supplementation with calcium and calcitriol is prudent, especially for housebound individuals. Coffee and tea in the evening may contribute to insomnia.

Handout 9.14 provides some dietary guidelines for elderly persons.

In perspective

While a plant-based diet would seem to offer a good basis for dietary health, specification of optimal dietary guidelines remains elusive. Discrepancies in the nutrient content of fresh produce due to plant species diversity, cultivation techniques and processing practices permits only determination of generalized guidelines. Metabolic uniqueness, with respect to both nutrient absorption and metabolism, ensures that correlations between dietary intake and disease pathogenesis vary between individuals. Actual dietary requirements due to individual differences in physiological requirement are further modified by activity levels and sociocultural preferences for particular foods and food combinations. The bioavailability of both iron and zinc is greater in omnivorous than vegetarian diets. Vitamin E requirements are influenced by the polyunsaturated fatty acid content of the diet. The RDA for vitamin C for adult non-smoking men and women is 60 mg/day. This is based on a mean requirement of 46 mg/day to prevent the deficiency disease scurvy. The optimal intake of vitamin C to enhance immune function, avoid DNA damage, and decrease the risk of various cancers and degenerative and chronic diseases would seem to require a daily vitamin C supplement of 1000 mg accompanied by a diet rich in fruits and vegetables.[76] Unconventional diets attempt to take some of these variables into consideration through food selection. See **Handout 9.15**.

While fine-tuning is needed to achieve the 'perfect' diet, general guidelines for healthy eating are well established. Certainly, diets that provide nutrients, but not energy, beyond the RDA promote health.

References

1. U.S. Preventive Services Task Force (USPSTF). Counseling to promote a healthy diet. In: *Guide to Clinical Preventive Services*. 3rd ed. Rockville, MD: Agency for Health Care Research and Quality; 2003. http://www.ahrq.gov/Clinic/uspstf/uspsdiet.htm. Accessed 12.02.08.
2. Huijbregts P, Feskens E, Räsänen L, et al. Dietary pattern and 20 year mortality in elderly men in Finland, Italy, and The Netherlands: longitudinal cohort study. *BMJ*. 1997;315(7099):13–17.
3. Wynder EL, Gori GB. Contribution of the environment to cancer incidence. *J Natl Cancer Inst*. 1977;58:825–832.
4. Hu FB, Rimm EB, Stampfer MJ, Ascherio A, Spiegelman D, Willett WC. Prospective study of major dietary patterns and risk of coronary heart disease in men. *Am J Clin Nutr*. 2000;72(4):912–921.
5. Lopez-Garcia E, Schulze MB, Fung TT, et al. Major dietary patterns are related to plasma concentrations of markers of inflammation and endothelial dysfunction. *Am J Clin Nutr*. 2004;80(4):1029–1035.
6. Kerver JM, Yang EJ, Bianchi L, Song WO. Dietary patterns associated with risk factors for cardiovascular disease in healthy US adults. *Am J Clin Nutr*. 2003;78(6):1103–1110.

7. O'Keefe Jr JH, Cordain L. Cardiovascular disease resulting from a diet and lifestyle at odds with our Paleolithic genome: how to become a 21st-century hunter-gatherer. *Mayo Clin Proc.* 2004;79 (1):101–108.

8. Simopoulos AP. Evolutionary aspects of omega-3 fatty acids in the food supply. *Prostaglandins Leukot Essent Fatty Acids.* 1999;60 (5–6):421–429.

9. Eaton SB, Eaton 3rd SB, Sinclair AJ, Cordain L, Mann NJ. Dietary intake of long-chain polyunsaturated fatty acids during the paleolithic. *World Rev Nutr Diet.* 1998;83:12–23.

10. Simopoulos AP. The importance of the omega-6/omega-3 fatty acid ratio in cardiovascular disease and other chronic diseases. *Exp Biol Med (Maywood).* 2008;233 (6):674–688.

11. Truswell AS. Practical and realistic approaches to healthier diet modifications. *Am J Clin Nutr.* 1998;67:583S–590S.

12. The Food Pyramid. http://mypyramid.gov/ Accessed 02.12.08.

13. A Guide to Daily Food Choices. http://www.nal.usda.gov/fnic/Fpyr/pmap.htm Accessed 02.12.08.

14. Huth PJ, DiRienzo DB, Miller GD. Major scientific advances with dairy foods in nutrition and health. *J Dairy Sci.* 2006;89(4):1207–1221.

15. Zemel MB, Donnelly JE, Smith BK, et al. Effects of dairy intake on weight maintenance. *Nutr Metab (Lond).* 2008;5:28.

16. Hubner RA, Muir KR, Liu JF, et al. Members of UKCAP Consortium. Dairy products, polymorphisms in the vitamin D receptor gene and colorectal adenoma recurrence. *Int J Cancer.* 2008;123(3):586–593.

17. Larsson S, Andersson S, Johansson J, Wolk A. Cultured milk, yogurt, and dairy intake in relation to bladder cancer risk in a prospective study of Swedish women and men. *Am J Clin Nutr.* 2008;88:1083–1087.

18. Chung H, Nettleton JA, Lemaitre RN, et al. Frequency and type of seafood consumed influence plasma (n-3) fatty acid concentrations. *J Nutr.* 2008;138 (12):2422–2427.

19. He K, Liu K, Daviglus ML, et al. Intakes of long-chain n-3 polyunsaturated fatty acids and fish in relation to measurements of subclinical atherosclerosis. *Am J Clin Nutr.* 2008;88(4):1111–1118.

20. Nurk E, Drevon CA, Refsum H, et al. Cognitive performance among the elderly and dietary fish intake: the Hordaland Health Study. *Am J Clin Nutr.* 2007;86(5):1470–1478.

21. Augood C, Chakravarthy U, Young I, et al. Oily fish consumption, dietary docosahexaenoic acid and eicosapentaenoic acid intakes, and associations with neovascular age-related macular degeneration. *Am J Clin Nutr.* 2008;88:398–406.

22. Yamagishi K, Iso H, Date C, et al. Fish, omega-3 polyunsaturated fatty acids, and mortality from cardiovascular diseases in a nationwide community-based cohort of Japanese men and women the JACC (Japan Collaborative Cohort Study for Evaluation of Cancer Risk) Study. *J Am Coll Cardiol.* 2008;52(12):988–996.

23. Abeywardena MY, Head RJ. Longchain n-3 polyunsaturated fatty acids and blood vessel function. *Cardiovasc Res.* 2001;52 (3):361–371.

24. Kritchevsky SB, Kritchevsky D. Egg consumption and coronary heart disease: an epidemiologic overview. *J Am Coll Nutr.* 2000;19(suppl 5): 549S–555S.

25. Mayurasakorn K, Srisura W, Sitphahul P, Hongto PO. High-density lipoprotein cholesterol changes after continuous egg consumption in healthy adults. *J Med Assoc Thai.* 2008;91 (3):400–407.

26. Grune T, Krämer K, Hoppe PP, Siems W. Enrichment of eggs with n-3 polyunsaturated fatty acids: effects of vitamin E supplementation. *Lipids.* 2001;36 (8):833–838.

27. Thomson CD, Chisholm A, McLachlan SK, Campbell JM. Brazil nuts: an effective way to improve selenium status. *Am J Clin Nutr.* 2008;87(2):379–384.

28. Griel AE, Eissenstat B, Juturu V, Hsieh G, Kris-Etherton PM. Improved diet quality with peanut consumption. *J Am Coll Nutr.* 2004;23(6):660–668.

29. Nash SD, Nash DT. Nuts as part of a healthy cardiovascular diet. *Curr Atheroscler Rep.* 2008;10 (6):529–535.

30. Salas-Salvadó J, Casas-Agustench P, Murphy MM, López-Uriarte P, Bulló M. The effect of nuts on inflammation. *Asia Pac J Clin Nutr.* 2008;17(suppl 1):333–336.

31. Mattes RD. The energetics of nut consumption. *Asia Pac J Clin Nutr.* 2008;17(suppl 1):337–339.

32. Natoli S, McCoy P. A review of the evidence: nuts and body weight. *Asia Pac J Clin Nutr.* 2007;16 (4):588–597.

33. Messina MJ. Legumes and soybeans: overview of their nutritional profiles and health effects. *Am J Clin Nutr.* 1999;70(suppl 3):439S–450S.

34. Hermansen K, Dinesen B, Hoie LH, Morgenstern E, Gruenwald J. Effects of soy and other natural products on LDL:HDL ratio and other lipid parameters: a literature review. *Adv Ther.* 2003;20 (1):50–78.

35. Hoie LH, Sjoholm A, Guldstrand M, et al. Ultra heat treatment destroys cholesterol-lowering effect of soy protein. *Int J Food Sci Nutr.* 2006;57(7–8):512–519.

36. Truswell AS. Cereal grains and coronary heart disease. *Eur J Clin Nutr.* 2002;56(1):1–14.

37. Priebe MG, van Binsbergen JJ, de Vos R, Vonk RJ. Whole grain foods for the prevention of type 2 diabetes mellitus. *Cochrane Database Syst Rev.* 2008;(1) CD006061.

38. Flight I, Clifton P. Cereal grains and legumes in the prevention of coronary heart disease and stroke: a review of the literature. *Eur J Clin Nutr.* 2006;60(10):1145–1159.

39. Mellen PB, Walsh TF, Herrington DM. Whole grain intake and cardiovascular disease: a meta-analysis. *Nutr Metab Cardiovasc Dis.* 2008;18:283–290.

40. Good CK, Holschuh N, Albertson AM, Eldridge AL. Whole grain consumption and body mass index in adult women: an analysis of NHANES 1999–2000 and the USDA pyramid servings database. *J Am Coll Nutr.* 2008;27(1):80–87.

41. Harland JI, Garton LE. Whole-grain intake as a marker of healthy body

weight and adiposity. *Public Health Nutr.* 2008;11(6):554–563.

42. Esmaillzadeh A, Kimiagar M, Mehrabi Y, Azadbakht L, Hu FB, Willett WC. Fruit and vegetable intakes, C-reactive protein, and the metabolic syndrome. *Am J Clin Nutr.* 2006;84(6):1489–1497.

43. Nikolic M, Nikic D, Petrovic B. Fruit and vegetable intake and the risk for developing coronary heart disease. *Cent Eur J Public Health.* 2008;16(1):17–20.

44. Bazzano LA, Li TY, Joshipura KJ, Hu FB. Intake of fruit, vegetables, and fruit juices and risk of diabetes in women. *Diabetes Care.* 2008;31(7):1311–1317.

45. Meyskens Jr FL, Szabo E. Diet and cancer: the disconnect between epidemiology and randomized clinical trials. *Cancer Epidemiol Biomarkers Prev.* 2005;14(6):1366–1369.

46. Boivin D, Lamy S, Lord-Dufour S, et al. Antiproliferative and antioxidant activities of common vegetables: a comparative study. *Food Chem.* 2008;112(2):374–380.

47. Antosiewicz J, Ziolkowski W, Kar S, Powolny AA, Singh SV. Role of reactive oxygen intermediates in cellular responses to dietary cancer chemopreventive agents. *Planta Med.* 2008;74(13):1570–1579.

48. Stan SD, Kar S, Stoner GD, Singh SV. Bioactive food components and cancer risk reduction. *J Cell Biochem.* 2008;104(1):339–356.

49. Heber D, Bowerman S. Applying science to changing dietary patterns. *J Nutr.* 2001;131(suppl 11):3078S–3081S.

50. Wolfe KL, Kang X, He X, et al. Cellular antioxidant activity of common fruits. *J Agric Food Chem.* 2008;24(56):8418–8426.

51. Su LJ, Arab L. Salad and raw vegetable consumption and nutritional status in the adult US population: results from the Third National Health and Nutrition Examination Survey. *J Am Diet Assoc.* 2006;106(9):1394–1404.

52. MacLellan D, Taylor J, Wood K. Food intake and academic performance among adolescents. *Can J Diet Pract Res.* 2008;69(3):141–144.

53. Parks EJ, Skokan LE, Timlin MT, Dingfelder CS. Dietary sugars stimulate fatty acid synthesis in adults. *J Nutr.* 2008;138(6):1039–1046.

54. Esmaillzadeh A, Azadbakht L. Home use of vegetable oils, markers of systemic inflammation, and endothelial dysfunction among women. *Am J Clin Nutr.* 2008;88(4):913–921.

55. McNaughton SA, Ball K, Crawford D, Mishra GD. An index of diet and eating patterns is a valid measure of diet quality in an Australian population. *J Nutr.* 2008;138(1):86–93.

56. Panagiotakos DB, Polychronopoulos E. The role of Mediterranean diet in the epidemiology of metabolic syndrome; converting epidemiology to clinical practice. *Lipids Health Dis.* 2005;4(1):7.

57. Bach A, Serra-Majem L, Carrasco JL, et al. The use of indexes evaluating the adherence to the Mediterranean diet in epidemiological studies: a review. *Public Health Nutr.* 2006;9(1A):132–146.

58. Panagiotakos DB, Pitsavos C, Arvaniti F, Stefanadis C. Adherence to the Mediterranean food pattern predicts the prevalence of hypertension, hypercholesterolemia, diabetes and obesity, among healthy adults; the accuracy of the MedDietScore. *Prev Med.* 2007;44(4):335–340.

59. Serra-Majem L, Roman B, Estruch R. Scientific evidence of interventions using the Mediterranean diet: a systematic review. *Nutr Rev.* 2006;64(2 Pt 2):S27–S47.

60. Roman B, Carta L, Martínez-González MA, Serra-Majem L. Effectiveness of the Mediterranean diet in the elderly. *Clin Interv Aging.* 2008;3(1):97–109.

61. Salas-Salvadó J, Garcia-Arellano A, Estruch R, et al. Components of the Mediterranean-type food pattern and serum inflammatory markers among patients at high risk for cardiovascular disease. *Eur J Clin Nutr.* 2008;62(5):651–659.

62. Sofi F, Cesari F, Abbate R, Gensini GF, Casini A. Adherence to Mediterranean diet and health status: meta-analysis. *BMJ.* 2008;a1344:337 doi:10.1136/bmj.a1344.

63. American Dietetic Association; Dietitians of Canada. Position of the American Dietetic Association and Dietitians of Canada: Vegetarian diets. *J Am Diet Assoc.* 2003;103(6):748–765.

64. Rauma AL, Mykkänen H. Antioxidant status in vegetarians versus omnivores. *Nutrition.* 2000;16(2):111–119.

65. Rajaram S, Sabaté J. Health benefits of a vegetarian diet. *Nutrition.* 2000;16(7–8):531–533.

66. Key TJ, Appleby PN, Rosell MS. Health effects of vegetarian and vegan diets. *Proc Nutr Soc.* 2006;65(1):35–41.

67. The Vegetarian Diet Pyramid. http://www.oldwayspt.org/vegetarian_pyramid.html Accessed 12.06.08.

68. Healthy eating at various lifestages. http://www.healthyactive.gov.au/internet/healthyactive/publishing.nsf/Content/healthy-eating Accessed 12.08.08.

69. The AHA dietary recommendation for healthy children. http://www.americanheart.org/presenter.jhtml?identifier=4575 Accessed 12.07.08.

70. Albertson AM, Thompson D, Franko DC, et al. Consumption of breakfast cereal is associated with positive health outcomes: evidence from the National Heart, Lung, and Blood Institute Growth and Health Study. *Nutr Res.* 2008;28(11):744–752.

71. Eisenberg ME, Olson RE, Neumark-Sztainer D, Story M, Bearinger LH. Correlations between family meals and psychosocial well-being among adolescents. *Arch Pediatr Adolesc Med.* 2004;158(8):792–796.

72. Haberg SE, London SJ, Stigum H, et al. Folic acid supplements in pregnancy and early childhood respiratory health. *Arch Dis Child.* 2009;94(3):180–184. Erratum in: *Arch Dis Child.* 2009;94(6)485.

73. Morley JE. Anorexia of aging: physiologic and pathologic. *Am J Clin Nutr.* 1997;66: 760–773.

74. Ortega RM, Requejo AM, Andres P, et al. Dietary intake and cognitive function in a group of elderly people. *Am J Clin Nutr.* 1997;66 (4):803–809.

75. Vogiatzoglou A, Refsum H, Johnston C, et al. Vitamin B12 status and rate of brain volume loss in community-dwelling elderly. *Neurology.* 2008;71:826–832.

76. Deruelle F, Baron B. Vitamin C: is supplementation necessary for optimal health? *J Altern Complement Med.* 2008;14 (10):1291–1298.

Spinal health

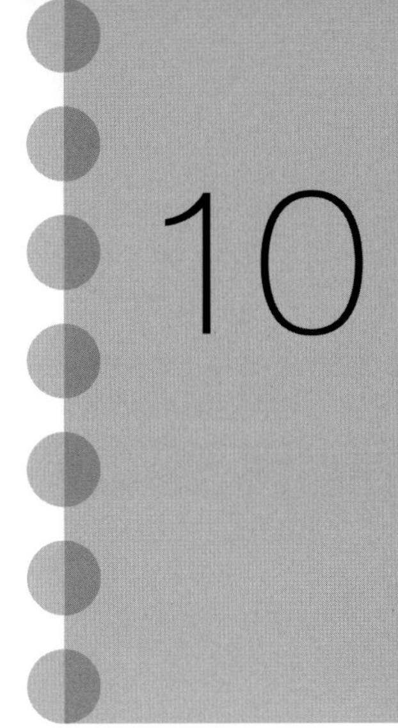

Spinal health: an overview

Low back pain is a prevalent complaint.[1] It affects up to 80% of US adults during their lifetime and as many as every second person may experience backache in any 1 year. Although symptoms are usually acute and self-limited, back symptoms are among the 10 leading reasons patients seek professional health care. Low back pain often recurs, with 5–10% of patients developing chronic backache. Back symptoms top the list of common causes of disability for persons under the age of 45! However, although recommendations for regular physical activity can be made based on other proven benefits, there is insufficient evidence for the U.S. Preventive Services Task Force to recommend for or against counselling patients to exercise to prevent low back pain.[1] There is also insufficient evidence to recommend for or against the routine use of educational interventions, mechanical supports, or risk factor modification to prevent low back pain. While specific strategies to prevent backache are elusive, it is believed that a healthy posture predisposes to a healthy spine.

Posture and muscle tone

Posture is maintained by the interaction of muscles. Maintaining the natural curves of the spine reduces the risk of postural deformity. Regular movement promotes joint integrity and muscle tone. Muscle tone is determined by muscle innervation. Damage to the brain, spinal cord or peripheral nerves modifies muscle tone. Brain damage causes an upper motor neuron lesion and increases muscle tone. If the cerebral cortex is damaged, spasticity results, as seen in a stroke. If damage occurs in the basal ganglion, rigidity results, as seen in Parkinson's disease. Damage to the spinal cord, nerve roots or peripheral nerves causes a lower motor neuron lesion with decreased muscle tone. Muscles become weak and wasted. For good postural tone, in addition to muscles requiring an intact nerve supply, balanced innervation between various muscle groups is required. The cerebellum plays an important role in muscle coordination. Muscle coordination, and therefore balance, can be enhanced by doing cross–laterality exercises, i.e. using the right leg with the left arm and vice versa.

Muscle strength and bulk increase with use. Physical activity is required to maintain muscle strength and size. Isometric exercise programmes increase the size and strength of particular muscle groups. Various exercises strengthen particular muscles. By exercising the muscles of the pelvic floor, the risk of urinary incontinence can be reduced in later life. By strengthening spine and stomach muscles, the risk of back problems may be minimized. By exercising, bone mass can be increased and the future risk of osteoporosis decreased. The pull

Push-ups are useful for improving abdominal, arm, and shoulder muscle strength.

☐ Vertical push-ups for elderly and unfit persons
1. Place your hands flat on the wall
2. Stand straight with arms outstretched at 90 degrees to your body with feet fixed in place
3. Slant your body so that your chin rests on your hands
4. Push away from the wall using arms and shoulders

The degree of difficulty is increased by increasing the distance between your feet and the wall.

Different muscle groups can be exercised by rotating your hands internally and externally.

☐ Horizontal push-ups for the young and fit
1. Lie facedown on the floor with arms bent at the elbow and palms on the floor
2. Lift your body on your hands and toes
3. Gradually lower yourself back onto the floor, keeping your body straight at all times

A variation for people who are a little less fit is lifting their body on their hands and knees.

See http://www.wikihow.com/Do-a-Push-Up

Figure 10.1 • Push-ups for different age groups.

muscles exert on bones, rather than body weight, determines bone strength.[2] Exercise may be prescribed for the young and the old, the fit and unfit.[3–7] Exercises may be adapted to the individual (see Figure 10.1). Exercise increases strength and maintains flexibility. Moving all joints through their full range of motion each day enhances musculoskeletal flexibility. Certain joints are capable of flexion and extension, abduction and adduction, and/or internal and external rotation. Activities that involve the use of many joints include swimming, gardening, and tennis. Exercise need not be strenuous to be beneficial. e.g. breathing exercises. Breathing exercises exercise the diaphragm while helping tense patients to relax. A simple tip for stressed patients is to silently count four and observe their abdomen distend while slowly inhaling. This is followed by slowly exhaling to the count of four. Exercises that cause pain should be avoided. It is always a good idea to check with a health professional to ensure that exercises are within physiological parameters. Exercises should be repeated from 5–30 times each day.

Towards spinal health

Good posture is fundamental to spinal health. Healthy postures should be assumed when standing, lying, sitting, and bending. Good posture reflects

and reinforces the normal curvature of the spine. The spine is a flexible column composed of 26 vertebral segments. The vertebral column is curved in order to facilitate balance and increase carrying strength in the upright position. The normal curves of the spine are in the anteroposterior direction, with a concavity in the lumbar area and a convexity in the thoracic area. An abnormally curved back when standing, sitting, lying, walking, and bending is the basis of a bad posture.[8] **Handout 10.1** provides a quick postural self-screening. The gravity line should fall through the centre of the head – a slouched posture moves the head forward, shoulders drop and breathing becomes more difficult.[4] Another common problem is rounded shoulders – internet resources demonstrating a simple exercise to correct this postural fault are available.[9] Lateral curving of the spine causes a scoliosis. Exaggerated concavity in the lumbar area results in a lordosis; exaggerated convexity in the thoracic area, kyphosis (hunchback). Women with a more pronounced forward inclination of the trunk, more marked thoracic kyphosis and a smaller degree of lumbar lordosis are at increased risk of falling.[10] Poor posture may predispose to falling in the elderly.

The rules of protective body mechanics revolve around an upright back, tightened stomach muscles, buttocks tucked under, and bent knees. Firm strong stomach muscles support the back from the front. Tight buttocks bring the lower spine into a straight-line position. Bent knees serve as spinal shock absorbers. A good erect posture holds the ear, shoulder tip, mid-hip, back of the kneecap, and front of the ankle in the same vertical plane. The belly button is pulled in towards the spine. The weight is carried across the soles of the feet, particularly on the balls of the feet. If prolonged standing is necessary, flexing the hip and knee of one leg and placing the foot on a footrest may rest the back. The footrest need only be 1.5 cm in height. Feet should be alternated. **Handout 10.2** provides tips on how to assume a healthy posture in various positions while **Handout 10.3** gives tips on correcting three common poor postures.

Exercises for spinal health

Appropriate exercises can improve posture. However, although there is some evidence that exercise (flexion, extension, aerobic, or fitness) protects against the development of low back pain, the effect is modest and of unknown duration.[1,4] Exercise, nonetheless, facilitates maintenance of adequate spinal mobility. Spinal mobility not only is essential for movement, but also is important in nutrition of intervertebral discs. Disc nutrition and waste removal depend on passive diffusion, a mechanical process promoted by spinal movement. Adequate muscle strength and flexibility aid spinal movement; and a self-selected exercise programme can enhance muscle strength and flexibility. For example, the lower back is protected by four major muscle groups: the gluteal/buttock, quadriceps/ thigh, abdominal/stomach, and paraspinal muscles. Strengthening these muscles is tantamount to strengthening the lower back.

A number of exercises assist in maintaining the level of strength and flexibility required for moving the body against gravity. Stretching maintains flexibility; isometric exercises increase muscle strength. **Handouts 10.4** and **10.5** provide exercises for a strong healthy spine.

Backache

It has been estimated that three out of four adults will experience at least one episode of back pain during their lifetime. While degenerative changes to the lumbar disc may be a major cause of low back pain, lifestyles that promote excessive sitting, insufficient spinal mobility, and inappropriate lifting of loads contribute to this natural ageing process. Mechanical low back pain is a benign, self-limiting condition; 90% of persons recover within 6 weeks.[11] The annual prevalence of low backache is between 15% and 45%; the lifetime prevalence lies between 56% and 80%.[9–13] Up to 7% of persons have back pain that persists for 3 or more months. These chronic low back pain sufferers account for 75–85% of total worker absenteeism and workers' compensation costs.[12] With low back pain ranking second only to upper respiratory infections as a cause of lost work time, prevention of this condition assumes industrial relevance. It is useful to distinguish between low back pain, impairment, and disability.[14] Pain is an unpleasant symptom experience, while impairment and disability imply some loss of normal function. The mismatch between complaints and pathological lesions and between impairment and disability underscores the importance of non-physical factors in pain management.

The onset of back pain has been related to: lifting heavy weights, bending and twisting, working in the same position for long periods, repetitive movements and vibration.[15–17] Tasks involving lifting, pulling or pushing objects of 25 lb (11 kg) or more are particularly risky.[16] Lifting loads away from the body, twisting while lifting, and lifting with straight legs are especially hazardous. A number of studies have been performed in order to identify the effects of various lifting techniques. One study deduced that the effects on low back loading depended on the task context;[18] another concluded that no single lifting technique can be advised for all lifting conditions.[19] Although it remains unclear which technique should be favoured, squat lifting is generally recommended.[20]

When lifting, the extensor erector spinae muscles, exerting their force about 5 cm posterior to the centre of rotation in the spinal discs, combine with the anterior stabilizing force of the abdominal musculature to resist the external load imposed upon the lumbar spine. The torso muscles provide most of the spinal stability required for heavy lifting. Spinal ligaments and discs, while capable of resisting some of the strain imposed by heavy lifting, should not be exposed to excessive stress. Reduced dynamic strength of flexor muscles has been found to be a consistent predictor for persistence and/or recurrence of back pain. Analysis of spinal ligaments shows that the risk of strain is maximized when lifting with an extremely flexed or rounded back. The biomechanical message is to lift with a straight back. This does not mean bending over at right angles! Because the motion of each spinal segment is controlled by the coordinated function of some 22 different muscles, working with fatigued muscles or with very fast torso motions, as occurs with slipping or tripping, can result in an inappropriate muscle response with consequent ligament or spinal column injury. Biomechanically, it is unwise to attempt to lift excessively heavy or awkward unmanageable loads. **Handout 10.6** provides a screen for patients to check their lifting technique and **Handout 10.7** provides guidelines for developing a safe lifting style.

Prolonged standing or walking for more than 2 hours or driving for more than 10 hours each week increases the risk of back pain.[16] The most important factor in the prevention of initial low back trouble in men is having back muscles with good isometric endurance.[21] Obesity is a risk factor. Weight gain predisposes to postural faults; this is particularly critical when weight exceeds the 80th percentile. Excessive weight encourages anterior weight bearing. At a lumbosacral angle of 30°, the sheer stress between L5 and the sacral base is 50% of the superimposed weight. At a 50° angle, the sheer stress is increased to 75% of the superimposed weight. Weight gain increases the shear stress between L5 and the sacrum, increasing the likelihood of spondylosis, spondylolysis, spondylolisthesis, and facet degeneration. In addition to assuming a good posture and ensuring good muscle flexibility and strength, it is prudent to avoid high-risk behaviours.

Handout 10.8 provides a self-screen for factors increasing the personal risk of backache and **Handout 10.3** provides tips on how to reduce this risk when it is due to poor posture.

Handout 10.9 provides a protocol for implementing a spinal self-care programme.

Orange flags for low back pain of musculoskeletal origin

Injuries and disorders caused by overexertion and repetitive motion are the leading causes of compensable lost-time cases in the US.[22] A number of risk factors have been linked both to low back pain[22] and to upper extremity disorders.[23] Risk factors influence the maximum acceptable physiological and mechanical strain to which the body can reasonably be subject. Risk factors have been divided into the work situation, the actual working method, and worker's characteristics.[24] Preplacement screening, task analysis and workplaces design are strategies used to reduce the risk of injury.

Preplacement assessment, while not specifically selecting persons suited to heavy manual tasks, does help to identify those at particular risk. Although not providing information about who is suited to high-risk tasks, it does identify those who should not be exposed to spinal stress. Screening is holistic, incorporating physical and psychosocial risk factors. Significant risk factors that suggest unsuitability for high-risk jobs include more than two episodes of back pain, a history of 35 or more days' absence from work attributable to low back pain, short intervals between episodes, an aggravated course of low back pain, an acute onset, and truly accident-related causes, such as falls.[25]

Prevention focuses on good manual handling procedures, avoiding certain body movements and an appropriate environment design. The National Institute for Occupational Safety and Health's review of over 600 epidemiological studies in 1997 concluded there was evidence of a causal relationship between low back problems and workplace exposures to forceful exertions, awkward posture, and vibration.[22] Lifting, along with pushing, pulling and carrying, are high-risk activities, especially when excessive twisting, bending or reaching is involved. Other risks are moving excessive loads, prolonged sitting, and falling. Being aware of at-risk postures and activities and designing the job to fit the worker can reduce the prevalence of industrial back injuries. Environmental design can reduce both muscular and spinal problems.[26] Formulas have been developed by the National Institute of Occupational Safety and Health for analysing material handling areas. By adjusting work areas according to formula guidelines, an environment may be created in which 99% of men and 75% of women are able to lift without risk. Ergonomically arranged workstations can position loads that need to be lifted. Loads should be lifted from within the power lift range, i.e. between 30 cm from the floor and shoulder height; the safest lift is knuckle height. Non-slip floors are also part of the ergonomically sound occupational environment. Effective pushing depends on good traction. This requires a suitable floor surface and a rubber or cork shoe sole. Pushing and pulling should be in line with the body; legs, rather than arms, should provide the necessary push. Avoidance of repetitive forward bending can be achieved when unloading of cartons is done from angled platforms; workplace design permits use of a neutral spine by angling the workplace. Other ergonomic interventions include hoists and cranes to lift, carts and manually powered trucks with precisely positioned handles and pivoted tyres to move loads, and specially designed containers to carry loads. Asymmetric loads should be avoided or carried by two persons.

Industrial work situations may enhance back problems. An awkward sitting or standing posture promotes muscle fatigue, increasing the load on intervertebral discs. Work situations that cause whole body vibration, such as truck driving, cause similar problems. Vibration in the 5 Hz range, the dominant frequency of many vehicles and industrial devices (e.g. jackhammers), is associated with energy transfer increasing the risk of mechanical damage to resonating structures. Persons driving heavy machinery, in addition to prolonged sitting, are subject to constant vibration. In trucks, this is in the 2–15 Hz range. Vibration of the spine induces vibriocreep – a phenomenon defined as the acceleration of creep under a compressive bias and an additionally imposed vibratory load.[27] Creep is the reversible loss in stature associated with the erect posture and aggravated by loading. Studies have found that a reduction in stature continues for 20 minutes after loading the shoulder; height is regained within 10 minutes of removing the load. Vibration accelerates this process, particularly when vibration is at the natural frequency of the human trunk, the 4–8 Hz range. The 4–8 Hz range is most harmful to discs, the 16 Hz vibration most affects the head, the 32 Hz vibration affects the lower body, and the 64 Hz the ischial tuberosities. Prolonged sitting also presents potential spinal problems; lumbar spinal pressure is greater when sitting than when standing or lying. Seats with a backrest inclination of 110° or more and curved support for the spine with an apex level with the third lumbar vertebrae will reduce postural stress; firm cushions and shock-absorbing seats with a natural frequency of 1.5 Hz can help to minimize vibratory stress. Seat belts are recommended to stabilize and provide upper body support.

Preventing work-related back problems

Work-related back problems can be reduced by creating a physically safe and emotionally supportive work environment. Working in an ergonomically sound environment is protective. Anthropometric criteria can be used to structure the work environment. In the case of chair manufacture, the following ergonomic norms deserve consideration:[26]

- Seat height should allow both feet to be firmly placed on the ground. A fixed seat height of 48.26 cm or variable height from 40.64 to 57.15 cm is recommended. A 90° knee angle is considered desirable and periodic movement can further reduce leg swelling due to inactivity.
- Seat pan angle is best selected between 5° and 15° forward and 5° backwards. As seated postures are stressful on the spine, the best solution is often permitting the user to select their own angle.
- Seat pan depth of 42 cm, if fixed, or between 35.5 and 47 cm, if adjustable, is recommended. A compromise between thigh support and freedom of body movement is required; excessively deep seats may contribute to venous thrombosis.
- Cushioning of 3.8–5 cm of relatively firm foam is suggested. The body weight should be supported on the ischial tuberosities.

- A backrest angle of 20–30° from the horizontal is proposed, as this can partially relieve stress on the spine.
- Backrest contours that provide a lumbar support depth of 2.5 cm and height of 23 cm at peak plus a thoracic angle of 10° are recommended.
- Armrests should be cantilevered, be 20–25 cm from the seat top, and not extend more than 25 cm from the back of the seat.

Industries may provide ergonomically designed workplaces, offer sophisticated worker instruction programmes, and undertake preplacement screening;[28] however, individuals need to actively practise good body mechanics in order to reduce back problems. Lifting instructions, along with workplace analysis, exercise, and relaxation therapy are the most frequent intervention strategies for the management of low back problems.[29] However, a study on 4000 US postal workers found that despite increased knowledge of safe behaviour, the prevalence of back injury appeared unchanged.[30] Practising adequate body mechanics, although not sufficient to prevent back injury, nonetheless makes a valuable contribution to reducing the prevalence of low back problems.[31] Furthermore, good spinal self-care may reduce the risk of acute low back pain becoming chronic. Low levels of psychological distress, higher than average levels of physical activity, being employed and being satisfied with one's current work status are associated with a quick improvement in symptoms.[13] **Handout 10.10** provides a protocol for reducing industrial back problems.

Red flags predicting backache

The strongest predictors for a chronic back problem are psychosocial. Predictors include: depression, a history of job change due to prior low back pain, a history of back contusion, poor self-rated health, lack of social support, failure of family legitimation of the pain, dissatisfaction with first office visit, family history of low back or other chronic pain, coping style, and unemployment.[32–34] Fear-avoidance has emerged as an important predictor of chronic back pain. Fear should be addressed, and awareness that positions conducive to pain exacerbation can be avoided, enhanced. Persons with low back pain may minimize the discomfort of getting out of bed by rolling onto one side, tightening their abdominal muscles, and pushing to a sitting position as they slip their legs over the edge of the bed. When lying in bed, intradiscal pressure is lowest when in the semi-Fowler position (trunk supported 45–65° from the horizontal). Getting into or out of the seated position may be facilitated by tightening the abdomen to immobilize the spine, doing a pelvic tilt, and using the arms and legs to position the trunk so that no lumbar movement is necessary. Contrary to the normal way of bending, in which lumbar segment movement is used prior to hip joint movement, bending at the hip joints avoids bending at the lumbar segments. Persons with low back pain should also avoid sitting; intradiscal pressure measurements are 140–180% higher when sitting than when standing. Straight-backed chairs may aggravate back pain as these fail to provide enough lumbar support. Pain associated with moving from sitting in flexion to standing can be prevented by not sitting in the fully flexed position, using lumbar support, maintaining the contour position and substituting hip flexion for lumbar flexion. Physical activity and light mobilization programmes are conducive to back wellness; inactivity has a detrimental effect.[35]

Physical predictors of chronic back pain are smoking and factors related to the episode of low back pain, such as duration of symptoms, pain radiating to the leg, widespread pain, and restriction in spinal mobility.[33] The nature of the relationship of predictors to chronic back pain is sometimes difficult to explain. Increased coughing only partially explains the prevalence of back pain in chronic heavy smokers; nicotine is postulated to impair vertebral blood flow and disc metabolism and correlates with degenerative disc disease. Certainly, the intensity, frequency, and duration of episodes of back pain have been found to increase with the number of cigarettes smoked.[36] Another study confirmed the link between smoking and low back pain but suggested that it was unlikely to be a causal association.[37] Although there is a dose–response relationship between daily cigarette consumption, the prevalence of chronic low back pain and chronic widespread musculoskeletal pain, there is no conclusive decrease in pain prevalence after quitting smoking.[38]

When low back pain persists, a condition of low back disability may result. Self-perceived disability and pain severity are directly related to prolonged disability.[39] Low back disability, a condition of musculoskeletal origin, implies the inability to perform one's normal job. It is characterized by pain and impaired work performance. Disability is the most reliable indicator of severity for clinically assessing an individual with low back pain of musculoskeletal origin. The challenge of accurately assessing disability is currently being addressed and minimal meaningful clinical outcomes evaluated.[40,41]

In perspective

Backache is a common complaint. Good posture, regular exercise to increase core strength and maintain spinal flexibility, along with a correct lifting technique currently provides the best preventative approach.

Back strain needs to be differentiated from disc disease. Typically, minor injury is followed by immediate or delayed low back pain in the former. Any movement of the back causes pain but pain is not exacerbated by coughing and sneezing. Analgesics, muscle relaxants, heat or ice and cautious activity help relieve the initial spasm. Low back strain is usually self-limiting. In contrast, persons with disc disease suffer chronic pain. Severe backache, usually on one side and radiating down the buttocks, legs, and feet, suggests disc disease. Pain is aggravated by coughing, sneezing, bending, or car travel. Professional assistance is recommended.

References

1. U.S. Preventive Services Task Force. *Counseling to prevent low back pain*. Chap 60. http://www.ahrq.gov/clinic/2ndcps/backpain/pdf; Accessed 12.08.08.

2. Frost HM. On our age-related bone loss: insights from a new paradigm. *J Bone Miner Res*. 1997;12 (10):153915–153946.

3. Havlin B, Mathn RL, Patterson NJ, Scott RC. *Corrective chiropractic exercises*. Sydney: Australian Chiropractors' Association Council on Sports Injuries; 1983.

4. Gatterman MI. *Chiropractic, Health Promotion and Wellness*. Sudbury, MA: Jones and Bartlett; 2007.

5. Mulry RC, White AH, Klein EA. *The Portable Back School*. St Louis: Mosby; 1981.

6. White AH, White LA, Mattmiller AW. *Back School and Other Conservative Approaches to Low Back Pain*. St Louis: Mosby; 1983.

7. Donovan G, McNamara J, Gianoli P. *Exercise Danger*. Floreat Park, WA: Wellness Australian Publications; 1988.

8. *Look at your posture*. http://www.chiropracticwellness.ca/chiropractic/posture.html; Accessed 12.08.08.

9. *How to improve your posture.* http://www.wikihow.com/Improve-Your-Posture; Accessed 12.08.08.

10. Ostrowska B, Giemza C, Wojna D, Skrzek A. Postural stability and body posture in older women: comparison between fallers and non-fallers. *Ortop Traumatol Rehabil.* 2008;10(5):481–490.

11. Jayson MIV. Why does acute back pain become chronic? *Spine.* 1997;22:1053–1056.

12. Van Tulder MW, Koes BW, Bouter LM, Metsemakers JFM. Management of chronic nonspecific low back pain in primary care: a descriptive study. *Spine.* 1997;22:76–82.

13. Macfarlane GJ, Thomas E, Croft PR, Papageorgiou AC, Jayson MI, Silman AJ. Predictors of early improvement in low back pain amongst consulters to general practice: the influence of pre-morbid and episode-related factors. *Pain.* 1999;80(1–2):113–119.

14. Himmelstein JA, Andersson GBJ. Low back pain: risk evaluation and preplacement screening. *Occup Med.* 1988;3:255–269.

15. Andersson GBJ. Epidemiological aspects of low back pain in industry. *Spine.* 1981;6:53–60.

16. Macfarlane GJ, Thomas E, Papageorgiou AC, Croft PR, Jayson MI, Silman AJ. Employment and physical work activities as predictors of future low back pain. *Spine.* 1997;22(10):1143–1149.

17. Levangie PK. Association of low back pain with self-reported risk factors among patients seeking physical therapy services. *Phys Ther.* 1999;79(8):757–766.

18. Kingma I, Bosch T, Bruins L, van Dieën JH. Foot positioning instruction, initial vertical load position and lifting technique: effects on low back loading. *Ergonomics.* 2004;47(13):1365–1385.

19. Kingma I, Faber GS, Bakker AJ, van Dieën JH. Can low back loading during lifting be reduced by placing one leg beside the object to be lifted? *Phys Ther.* 2006;86(8):1091–1105.

20. Straker LM. A review of research on techniques for lifting low-lying objects: 2. Evidence for a correct technique. *Work.* 2003;20(2):83–96.

21. Biering-Sorensen F. Physical measurements as risk indicators for low back trouble over a one year period. *Spine.* 1984;9:106–117.

22. Keyserling WM. Workplace risk factors and occupational musculoskeletal disorders, Part 1: A review of biomechanical and psychophysical research on risk factors associated with low-back pain. *AIHAJ.* 2000;61(1):39–50.

23. Keyserling WM. Workplace risk factors and occupational musculoskeletal disorders, Part 2: A review of biomechanical and psychophysical research on risk factors associated with upper extremity disorders. *AIHAJ.* 2000;61(2):231–243.

24. Hoozemans MJ, van der Beek AJ, Frings-Dresen MH, van Dijk FJ, van der Woude LH. Pushing and pulling in relation to musculoskeletal disorders: a review of risk factors. *Ergonomics.* 1998;41(6):757–781.

25. Boachie-Adjei O. Conservative management of low back pain. *Postgrad Med.* 1988;84:127–131.

26. Silby H. Conservative management of lumbar disc disability. *Clin Orthop.* 1987;221:121–130.

27. Bigos SJ, Battie MC. Acute care to prevent back disability. *Clin Orthop.* 1987;221:121–130.

28. Stede KM, Hoefner VC. Preplacement low–back screening for high risk areas. *J Am Osteo Assoc.* 1988;88:499–505.

29. Lawlis PG, McCoy CE. Psychological evaluation: patients with chronic pain. *Orthop Clin North Am.* 1983;14:527–538.

30. Daltroy LH, Iversen MD, Larson MG, et al. A controlled trial of an education program to prevent low back injuries. *N Engl J Med.* 1997;37:322–328.

31. Frymoyer JW, Cats-Baril W. Predictions of low back pain disability. *Clin Orthop.* 1987;221:89–98.

32. Reis S, Hermoni D, Borkan JM, Biderman A, Tabenkin C, Porat A. A new look at low back complaints in primary care: a RAMBAM Israeli Family Practice Research Network study. *J Fam Pract.* 1999;48(4):299–303.

33. Thomas E, Silman AJ, Croft PR, Papageorgiou AC, Jayson MI, Macfarlane GJ. Predicting who develops chronic low back pain in primary care: a prospective study. *BMJ.* 1999;318(7199):1662–1667.

34. Klenerman L, Slade PD, Stanley IM, et al. The prediction of chronicity in patients with an acute attack of low back pain in a general practice setting. *Spine.* 1995;20(4):478–484.

35. Haldorsen EM, Indahl A, Ursin H. Patients with low back pain not returning to work. A 12-month follow-up study. *Spine.* 1998;23(11):1202–1207.

36. Scott SC, Goldberg MS, Mayo NE, Stock SR, Poitras B. The association between cigarette smoking and back pain in adults. *Spine.* 1999;24(11):1090–1098.

37. Leboeuf-Yde C, Kyvik KO, Bruun NH. Low back pain and lifestyle. Part I: Smoking. Information from a population-based sample of 29,424 twins. *Spine.* 1998;23(20):2207–2213.

38. Andersson H, Ejlertsson G, Leden I. Widespread musculoskeletal chronic pain associated with smoking. An epidemiological study in a general rural population. *Scand J Rehabil Med.* 1998;30(3):185–191.

39. Gatchel RJ, Polatin PB, Mayer TG. The dominant role of psychosocial risk factors in the development of chronic low back pain disability. *Spine.* 1995;20(24):2702–2709.

40. Farasyn A, Meeusen R. Validity of the new Backache Index (BAI) in patients with low back pain. *Spine J.* 2006;6(5):565–571.

41. Ostelo RW, Deyo RA, Stratford P, et al. Interpreting change scores for pain and functional status in low back pain: towards international consensus regarding minimal important change. *Spine.* 2008;33(1):90–94.

Healthy sleep

Healthy sleep: an overview

Normal sleep is required for optimal functioning. The physiological need for sleep is largely determined by two sleep-regulating mechanisms, i.e. the total quantity of sleep and the daily circadian rhythm. An individual's circadian rhythm is strongly influenced by exposure to light. Melatonin is produced in the human pineal gland, particularly at night. Light exposure at night severely compromises the circadian production of melatonin. Total sleep time and sleep efficiency correlate with the timing of the endogenous melatonin rhythm. The circadian rhythm of sleepiness and alertness promotes a daily cycle of night-time sleep and daytime alertness. In general, sleepiness occurs during the hours between midnight and 7 a.m. and for a brief period in the mid-afternoon, between 1 p.m. and 4 p.m. This physiological mid-afternoon dip in alertness, conducive to napping, is commonly experienced. Normal wakefulness is effortless and free of unintended sleep episodes.

The physiological need for sleep changes through the lifecycle. The duration, overall quality and efficiency of sleep decreases with normal ageing.[1,2]

Efficiency is determined by the total sleep time divided by the time spent in bed. Normal sleep efficiency in young people is about 90–95%. This decreases with ageing, the elderly waking more often and having longer wakeful periods. Total sleep time decreases from around 18 hours in neonates to 11 hours in young children, 9 hours in adolescents, and 7.5 hours in adulthood. From mid-life until 80 years of age, sleep time decreases a further 27 minutes per decade – more so for males than females. There is also a change in the quality of sleep. For optimal daytime alertness, most adults require about 8 hours of sleep per 24-hour day. Sleep deprivation causes increased sleepiness and may cause cognitive impairment.

Unfavourable alteration to the amount and/or quality of sleep raises an orange health hazard flag. Insomnia is associated with significant morbidity in terms of health problems, health care utilization, and work performance.[3] Insomniacs score lower on quality of life and higher on measures of depression, anxiety, neuroticism, extraversion, arousal predisposition, stress perception, and emotion-oriented coping.[4] Individuals with insomnia are more emotionally reactive, more alert and vigilant, and experience more intrusive thoughts than good sleepers. Compared with good sleepers, poor sleepers are more likely to have consulted a health professional in the last year and have used prescription medication, over-the-counter products and/or alcohol as a sleep aid.[3] Although no differences were found for hospitalizations or motor-vehicle accidents, persons with insomnia suffered impaired daytime function, had more non-motor-vehicle accidents, were absent from work more frequently and had reduced productivity.[3] During the 4 years up to June 30, 2003, the average direct and indirect costs in the US for younger adults with insomnia were about $1253 greater than for patients without insomnia; among the elderly, direct costs were about $1143 greater for insomniacs.[5]

Healthy sleep patterns

Normal sleep progresses through a number of stages during each sleep period. The sleeper experiences two forms of sleep. Rapid eye movement (REM) or paradoxical sleep and non-rapid eye movement (NREM) sleep. During a night, REM sleep occurs mostly in the last third of the night, while NREM sleep dominates the first third of the night. A sleep cycle lasts for about 90 minutes. A cycle of NREM followed by REM sleep repeats itself four to six times a night. An episode of REM sleep occurs in each cycle and the duration of each episode tends to increase as the night progresses.

NREM sleep is subdivided into four stages of increasing depth. During normal NREM sleep, the first two phases are periods of light sleep, and the latter two phases are deep sleep. The electrical activity of the brain in each of these phases is different and NREM sleep consequently displays four distinct phases on an electroencephalogram (EEG). When preparing for sleep, individuals enter a state of relaxed wakefulness with alpha waves in a regular rhythm of 8–12 Hz. When dozing or entering the first phase of sleep, the EEG records a slow desynchronous pattern. Environmental disturbances easily wake the sleeper during this phase of light sleep. The second phase is one of moderately deep sleep characterized by spindly waves on the EEG. The third phase, with irregular, pointed waves of 12–16 Hz, is a phase of deep sleep. The final and deepest phase of sleep as recorded by EEG patterns is one of tall, slow waves (1–3 Hz). It is most difficult to rouse an individual during this phase of sleep. The deepest NREM sleep generally occurs in the early part of the night. During NREM sleep, body functions remain relatively stable.

After 70–100 minutes of passing through phases 1–4 of NREM sleep, the individual enters REM sleep. It is more difficult to rouse the sleeper during this sleep phase. REM sleep takes up 15–25% of the total amount of sleep and is associated with dreaming and physiological changes. Heart rate, blood pressure, and respiration fluctuate. During REM sleep, the brain uses as much oxygen and glucose as it does during waking and the EEG pattern approximates wakefulness. The EEG of wakefulness has high frequency and low amplitude waves and displays desynchronized activity. Vivid dreams, including nightmares, encountered during REM sleep are not physically enacted due to marked inhibition of motor activity. Sleepwalking and talking are believed to take place during the more transient and less emotionally stimulating NREM sleep. A lack of REM sleep has a detrimental effect on the psychosocial health of the individual. After sleep deprivation, there is a rebound of REM sleep. REM sleep is affected by antidepressants.

Sleep patterns change with age. Newborns have highest levels of REM sleep. REM sleep is involved in brain plasticity and associated with learning and establishing connections. People require less sleep as they grow older and REM sleep is greatly decreased in the elderly. NREM sleep also decreases with age. Elderly persons have more fragmented sleep and a shorter duration of stage 3 and stage 4 NREM sleep than young adults. In the elderly, the fourth stage of NREM sleep is virtually absent. Typical symptoms of sleep problems in the elderly include difficulty falling asleep and maintaining sleep, early-morning waking, less total sleep time and excessive daytime sleepiness.[6] Daytime wakefulness is interrupted by naps. Refreshing sleep requires both sufficient total sleep time as well as sleep in synchrony with the individual's circadian rhythm.

Handout 11.1 provides a self-screen for patients who suspect they have a sleep problem and **Handout 11.2** provides guidelines for formulating a sleep diary to identify the nature of the problem. Some correlation of symptoms with prevalent causes is also provided.

Sleep disorders

Insomnia, defined as an inability to obtain adequate sleep, is a subjective experience of having too little or poor-quality sleep The diagnostic criteria for insomnia include both a dissatisfactory sleep pattern on at least three nights a week for a minimum duration of 1 month and psychological distress or daytime impairment related to sleep difficulties. Insomniacs suffer delayed sleep onset, poor sleep maintenance, and/or early-morning waking with an inability to return to sleep. Persons with insomnia complain of difficulty falling and staying asleep, waking early, and interrupted or non-restorative sleep. When an individual with symptoms of insomnia uses prescribed medication as a sleep-promoting agent on at least three nights per week, insomnia syndrome is diagnosed. Insomnia may be arbitrarily divided into subjective, short-term and chronic varieties.

Subjective insomnia is a matter of perception. Subjective insomnia is diagnosed when there is disparity between the degree of sleep disturbance reported by the patient and that detected on polysomnography. Typically, such patients complain of taking an hour to fall asleep and then sleeping only 3 hours. Their report contradicts findings on their sleep study, which may provide physiological evidence of falling asleep within 30 minutes and sleeping for 6 hours. The absence of evidence of the effects of insomnia may help to discriminate between subjective and objective insomnia (see **Handout 11.2**).

Acute insomnia usually results from a stressful event or other temporary lifestyle disruption. Chronic insomnia may be pathophysiological or psychophysiological in origin. The management of acute and chronic insomnia is vastly different.

Management of acute insomnia

Acute stress, environmental disturbances and a change in the sleep schedule are the most common causes of transient and short-term insomnia.

Sleep deprivation over two or three nights results in fatigue, irritability, disorientation, feelings of persecution, and ultimately visual and/or tactile hallucinations. If insomnia persists, sleep debt can accumulate and problem sleepiness results.[7] Problem sleepiness is frequent sleepiness at inappropriate times. It often resolves when sleep duration increases, but takes at least two nights to do so. Short-term use of sedative-hypnotics is effective in the management of acute insomnia.

If problem sleepiness does not resolve, causes of chronic insomnia need to be considered. These range from a primary sleep disorder to medical and psychiatric conditions. Drugs and poor sleep hygiene should always be excluded before genetic factors, disease or ageing are blamed. Chronic insomnia can be conveniently considered with respect to its management.

Pharmacological management of chronic insomnia

Drugs may be required as treatment for patients with chronic insomnia; they may also be causes of sleeplessness. Chronic insomnia may result from pathophysiological conditions or specific primary physiological sleep disorders. Intrinsic sleep disorders include obstructive sleep apnoea, narcolepsy, nocturnal myoclonus and restless legs syndrome. The management of insomnia secondary to medical conditions, e.g. cardiorespiratory disorders, or to psychiatric disorders, e.g. depression or anxiety is, initially, through treatment of the primary condition. Ironically, medications used to treat these medical conditions may disturb sleep. Diuretics, antihypertensives and even sedative-hypnotics may cause chronic insomnia. In fact, sleep medications are a major culprit.

Barbiturates and anxiolytic agents such as meprobamate induce tolerance. After only 2 weeks of use, night-time withdrawal of these drugs worsens insomnia. The risk of drug misuse, dependency, withdrawal and rebound insomnia have resulted in recommendations that use of these drugs be limited to a maximum of 6 weeks.[8] Rebound insomnia may also occur following termination of therapy with short- and intermediate-acting benzodiazepines. In addition to drug withdrawal causing rebound insomnia, drug dose and the half-life of sleep medications may cause a sleepiness problem. The half-life of a drug is the time it takes for the serum level of that drug to reach 50% of its peak plasma concentration. Drugs with a long half-life accumulate if taken too frequently. In order to avoid daytime sleepiness, a drug with a short or medium half-life should be used to treat insomnia. Drugs with a half-life of more than about 6 hours are likely to accumulate and cause daytime drowsiness. Other side effects are poor motor coordination and cognitive impairments.

While pain, medical or psychiatric conditions may initially trigger insomnia, as sleep difficulties persist, individuals become conditioned to negative expectations about sleep.[8] Although pharmacologic agents are more reliably in the short term, psychological approaches have greater safety and long-term efficacy. Both approaches are effective in reducing sleep onset latency by 15 to 30 minutes and reducing the number of awakenings by one to three episodes per night.[8] The role of sedative-hypnotics in the management of chronic insomnia is unclear. Intervention to manage sleeping problems associated with pathophysiological changes needs to look beyond drug therapy.

Non-pharmacological management of insomnia

When chronic insomnia is the result of misuse of social drugs or due to psychophysiological conditions, behavioural modification offers the best long-term solution.

Chronic insomnia may be secondary to abuse of social drugs. Alcohol, caffeine and nicotine have all been linked with disturbed sleep.[9] As little as one cup of coffee or two cans of caffeinated soda (10 mg caffeine) slightly increases sleep latency, while alcohol increases sleep fragmentation.[10] Alcohol, although a depressant that initially reduces sleep latency and decreases arousals, causes increased waking in the second half of the night.[11] In a crossover trial, healthy subjects received alcohol to raise their blood alcohol to either 0.03% or 0.1% at bedtime for three consecutive nights. Following an evening blood alcohol level of 0.1%, sleep latency was shortened and there was a reduction in both the number of wake periods and stage 1 sleep in the first half of the night; however, signs of rebound effects were evident in the latter half of the night, with increased stage 1 sleep and lighter sleep. Short-term moderate alcohol consumption to blood levels of 0.03% did not significantly alter objective or subjective parameters of sleep. Prenatal alcohol exposure has been shown to disrupt postnatal sleep organization, suppressing spontaneous movements during sleep, increasing sleep fragmentation and promoting sleep deprivation.[12] Nicotine increases vigilance and decreases sleeping time. Cigarette smoking is associated with difficulty both initiating and maintaining sleep.[13] Nicotine withdrawal disrupts sleep. Polysomnographic recordings performed during the week following nicotine withdrawal in heavy cigarette smokers have shown increased sleep fragmentation and an increased number of awakenings.[14]

Chronic psychophysiological primary insomnia has been hypothesized to result from conditioned arousal or the inability to initiate normal sleep processes. Individuals suffering from psychophysiological insomnia show attention biases, quickly detecting changes in sleep-related stimuli and delayed sleep phase syndrome.[15] Chronic psychophysiological or conditioned insomnia has been linked to hyperarousal, circadian dysrhythmia, and homeostatic dysregulation.[16]

Hyperarousal

Hyperarousal, presenting either as an elevated basal level of arousal or as a failure to down-regulate arousal at night, may be expressed in somatic/physiologic, cognitive, and cortical terms. Somatic evidence of psychophysiological insomnia includes an elevated heart rate, galvanic skin response, sympathetic arousal, and increased hypothalamic–pituitary–adrenal (HPA) axis activity. Cognitive arousal is expressed as a tendency to worry, particularly in relation to sleep. Greater cortical arousal, particularly on waking, results in difficulties in disengaging from wake processes and initiating normal sleep processes. Patients selectively attend to, and monitor, insomnia symptoms in such a way as to perpetually fuel sleep-related worry. The neurocognitive model suggests these insomniacs develop conditioned cortical arousal from the association of sleep-related stimuli with sleep difficulties. Conditioned arousal plays a central role in sleep complaints becoming chronic.[17]

The behavioural model of insomnia posits that trait and precipitating factors result in acute insomnia, which in turn becomes subacute because of the reinforcement of maladaptive coping strategies. Most cases of conditioned insomnia develop initially in response to a medical or psychosocial stressor. Negative associations and anxiety about falling asleep combine to maintain insomnia following this acutely stressful event. As sleeplessness persists, the bed becomes associated with wakefulness and heightened arousal rather than sleep. Despite falling asleep easily when sitting in front of the television, sleep is elusive when lying in bed. The individual may spend excessive time in bed trying to sleep. In order to ensure 6 hours of sleep, some 9 hours may be spent in bed. Insomnia can be learned. The development of conditioned insomnia relates in part to these psychological conditioning processes.[18] Two of the following must be present for a diagnosis of conditioned insomnia:

* excessive worry regarding sleep
* a significant effort to fall asleep
* the ability to fall asleep when not in the bedroom, e.g. in front of television

- paradoxical improvement away from home, i.e. away from the usual anxiety-provoking sleep setting
- difficulty with sleeping begins at time of stress but persists after the stress has abated.

Preventive self-care involves shortening the time spent in bed, taking no naps 6–8 hours before going to bed, and avoiding coffee, caffeine and alcohol 8–10 hours before going to bed. Cognitive–behavioural therapy offers a preferable approach to the symptom-focused approach provided by medications.[19]

Circadian dysrhythmia

With respect to circadian dysregulation, a smaller body of research suggests that chronobiologic abnormalities may be related to sleep initiation or maintenance problems.[16] Initial insomnia occurs in association with a phase delay, and early-morning awakenings occur in association with a phase advance of the core body temperature rhythm. While similar to what occurs with delayed and advanced sleep phase syndrome, the phase shifts are of a smaller magnitude than those seen in circadian rhythm disorders and are not thought to be the sole precipitants of primary insomnia. Primary insomnia only results when the circadian dysregulation is coupled with compensatory strategies attempted by patients.[16] Patients who change their sleep schedule and wake-time activities dramatically altering the timing of their exposure to bright light may inadvertently reset the 'biological clock'. Once altered, the phase shifts may serve to perpetuate the insomnia.

The insomnia associated with shift work, altered sleep phase and jet lag are prime examples of altered sleep rhythms syndromes resulting from disruption to the circadian rhythm. Sleepiness in shift workers is due to both insufficient sleep and displaced timing of sleep wakefulness.[20] Most shift workers complain of problem sleepiness and difficulty falling or staying asleep. Disruption of the circadian rhythm can be minimized by rotating shifts in a clockwise direction and not more than once in 3 days. When workers get off work they should use very dark glasses when outdoors and sleep in darkened, quiet surroundings. The working environment should be brightly lit. Exposure to bright light can help shift the circadian rhythm. Younger workers cope better than older persons.[21]

Altered sleep phase can be delayed or advanced. A significant proportion of young people report symptoms of problem sleepiness including difficulty getting up for school, falling asleep in school or struggling to stay awake while doing homework.[22] Delayed sleep phase syndrome, which has a typical onset during the second decade of life, may be an extreme manifestation of homeostatic and circadian changes in adolescence.[23] The circadian timing system changes during puberty, resulting in a tendency for adolescents to stay up later and sleep in later.[23–25] Adolescents with delayed sleep phase syndrome complain of:

- chronic tiredness
- a delay in sleep onset (going to sleep very late)
- a normal quantity and quality of sleep (society permitting)
- a delay in wake-up time (waking up very late).

Late sleep onset and late awakening in the morning may be helped by regular exposure to bright light at an early-morning hour. This may help to shift the sleep–wake rhythm to an earlier time for sleep at night and waking in the morning.

The elderly also have an altered sleep phase.[7] Older persons' sleep–wake cycle changes so that they get sleepy earlier in the evening and wake up earlier in the morning. Advanced sleep phase syndrome is characterized by:

- early bedtime
- early waking
- late-afternoon fatigue.

Exposure to bright light for 30 to 60 minutes in the evening may benefit patients with early bedtimes who complain of early-morning waking.[26] The essence of asynchronization is a disturbance in various aspects – such as cycle, amplitude, phase and interrelationship – of the biological rhythms that normally exhibit circadian oscillation, presumably involving decreased activity of the serotonergic system.[27] The major trigger of asynchronization is hypothesized to be a combination of light exposure during the night and a lack of light exposure in the morning.

Jet lag results from light exposure at night, or rapid transmeridian travel, which severely compromises the circadian production of melatonin. The disturbed melatonin rhythm contributes to jet lag and sleep inefficiency. Jet lag is the physical, psychological, and physiological derangement associated with a desynchronization of biological rhythms following a rapid change of time zones.[28]

The world is divided into 24 time zones; when travelling westward, time is 'lost'; when travelling eastward, time is 'gained'. Biological rhythms are either circadian (with approximately a 24-hour cycle, e.g. sleep/wakefulness, serum corticosteroid levels); infradian (with cycles longer than 24 hours, e.g. the menstrual cycle); or ultradian (with cycles shorter than 24 hours, e.g. REM sleep patterns). Within each of these cycles, rhythms have peak values or acrophase periods. When a normal relationship exists between the acrophase of a rhythm and real clock-time, then the rhythm is said to be externally synchronized. When a normal temporal relationship exists between the acrophase of two physiological systems, then the rhythms are internally synchronized. A time-zone change causes external desynchronization. Adaptation of an external synchronization system to such change occurs more rapidly than adaptation of the internal synchronization systems. The different rates of readaptation of these systems is believed to be a major contributor to jet lag. Other variables believed to contribute to this phenomenon are travel stress (separation from familiar people and surroundings); flight stress (loss of sleep coupled with anxiety); and destination stress (including dietary, language, and sociocultural change). The clinical manifestations of jet lag include lassitude, fatigue, insomnia, an inability to concentrate, nocturia, anorexia, nausea, headache, ocular irritation, excessive sweating, and menstrual irregularity.

The effects of jet lag may be reduced by breaking long journeys. This gives the traveller an opportunity to adjust to intermediate time changes. It is also advisable to eat sparingly. Attempts should be made to fit into the day/night rhythm of the destination as rapidly as possible by rising at a reasonable time in the morning. It is usually easier to adapt to phase-delay travel (westward) than phase-advance travel (eastward). It is easier to delay the time of settling to sleep than to advance it. It is easier to wake earlier (reduce the hours of sleep) than to delay the time of waking. Adaptation can take up to 2 weeks after changing a time zone.

Handout 11.3 provides guidelines for reducing the effects of jet lag. Melatonin is useful for decreasing sleep latency in travellers but fails to improve sleep maintenance, total sleep time, or subjective self-reports of night-time sleep and day-time alertness.[29] In addition to its sleep-inducing benefit, melatonin offers air travellers the added advantage of being a highly effective direct free radical scavenger and antioxidant.[30]

Cognitive–behavioural management of insomnia

While chronic insomnia is the result of diverse causes and intervention is influenced by the cause, elements of conditioned or primary psychophysiological insomnia overlay diverse varieties of chronic insomnia. While primary or psychophysiological insomnia alone only accounts for 12–15% of patients with chronic insomnia,[31] elements of conditioned sleeplessness complicate other causes of this problem. Although sedative-hypnotic medications are the most often used intervention for insomnia, they carry the risk of adverse effects and dependence while failing to address underlying perpetuating mechanisms. In contrast, non-pharmacological treatment options have few, if any, adverse effects and carry no risk of dependence. Conditioned insomnia is responsive to non-pharmacological intervention and lifestyle modification. As aspects of psychophysiological insomnia are superimposed upon other causes of chronic insomnia, cognitive–behavioural therapies have emerged as a treatment of choice for all cases of chronic insomnia.[19]

Under the general rubric of cognitive–behavioural therapy, commonly used methods include education and sleep hygiene, stimulus control, sleep restriction, relaxation training, biofeedback, paradoxical intention, and cognitive therapy.[8] Of these, stimulus control and sleep restriction have proved most effective for controlling conditioned aspects of insomnia and are associated with durable long-term improvement in sleep.[8]

The purpose of stimulus control therapy is to re-establish the connection between the bed and sleep by prohibiting the patient from engaging in non-sleep activities while in bed. It requires individuals only to go to bed when sleepy; maintain a regular schedule; avoid daytime naps and use the bed solely for sleep. If unable to sleep within 20 minutes, instead of being frustrated, the strategy is to get up and commence a relaxing activity, returning to bed when drowsy.

Sleep restriction therapy involves limiting the amount of time spent in bed to the actual time usually spent sleeping. This requires keeping a sleep log to determine both mean total sleep time and time spent in bed. Sleep efficiency, the total sleep time divided by the time in bed, is ideally over 90%. If sleep efficiency falls below 80%, time in bed is reduced by 15 minutes; if it goes above 90%, time in bed is increased by 15 minutes. The sleep pattern is adjusted over 5–7 days. Time in bed should never fall below 4.5 hours. For example, if the patient normally spends 5 hours in bed but only sleeps for 3.5 hours, then sleep efficiency is 70%. The total time in bed is reduced to 4.75 hours over 5 days to accumulate a sleep debt. This results in more rapid sleep onset on subsequent nights. When sleep efficiency is 90%, the allowable time spent in bed is increased.

Paradoxical intention requires the patient deliberately attempt to remain awake, thereby reducing the performance anxiety believed to interfere with the ability to initiate sleep. Progressive muscle relaxation seeks to enhance relaxation by alternate tensing and relaxing of the muscles. Cognitive therapy attempts to identify maladaptive thoughts such as 'I can't sleep without medication' and replace them with helpful thoughts such as 'I feel drowsy and ready to drop off'.

Meta-analysis of cognitive–behavioural therapy suggests these non-pharmacological approaches have a large effect on reducing sleep latency and improving sleep quality; and a moderate effect for waking after sleep onset, frequency of awakening, and for total sleep time.[8] Mean changes reported were: reduction of sleep latency from about 65 minutes to 35 minutes; reduction in wake time after sleep onset from 70 minutes to 38 minutes; and an increase in total sleep time of about 30 minutes. Subjective measures of sleep quality show greater improvement than the significant but more modest improvements in polysomnographic variables.

Cognitive–behavioural therapies target the behaviours, thought processes and conditioning factors underlying insomnia, thereby restoring normal sleep–wake functioning. The long-term success of cognitive–behavioural intervention makes this the preferred option.

Sleep hygiene: a self-care approach

Sleeping difficulty is a prevalent complaint. A recent study found 25.3% of respondents were dissatisfied with their sleep, 29.9% reported insomnia symptoms, and 9.5% met criteria for an insomnia syndrome; 48% complained of daytime fatigue, 40% of psychological distress and 22% of physical discomfort.[32]

Chronic insomnia has dire consequences. A community-based study found sleep problems were a risk factor for deterioration of general health-related quality of life; more specifically, disturbed sleep and associated daytime fatigue, impaired cognition and increased emotional lability causing personal distress and functional impairment in social and occupational areas.[33] Sleepiness in the workplace and on the highways contributes significantly to errors that increase the risk of accidents.[3] Performance impairment caused by sleepiness is comparable to that caused by alcohol intoxication.[34]

There are a number of self-help measures individuals can use to cope with sleep problems. Self-help measures range from reading, listening to music and relaxation,[32] to attempts to counter sleepiness using cold air or drinking coffee. Drinking coffee (about 150–200 mg caffeine) can temporarily enhance alertness, but may have little benefit as nights of inadequate sleep build up a severe sleep debt.[35] The only solution is sleep; even a short nap has a positive effect on alertness.[36] Self-help measures should therefore seek to improve sleep.

A sleep diary is a good first step. A sleep diary is a questionnaire completed each morning to describe the previous night's sleep. As shown in **Handout 11.2**, the sleep diary records the time of going to bed and waking up, sleep latency (i.e. the time lapse between 'lights out' and falling asleep) and nocturnal arousals or sleep interruptions. It is also helpful to include a subjective rating, on a scale of 1 to 5, to monitor the restfulness of the previous night's sleep. Insomniacs usually underestimate total sleep duration and overestimate sleep latency and nocturnal arousals. A sleep diary can be used not only to monitor the duration and quality of sleep but also to identify factors impairing a good night's rest. A record can be kept of sleep habits, psychological stress, physical problems, disturbed circadian rhythm, and social and medicinal drug use. Variables such as time and quantity of coffee drunk, cigarettes smoked or alcohol consumed can be noted. Environmental factors such as temperature excesses, noise or the comfort of the bed may also influence the quality of sleep. More than 4 hours of sleep per night may prevent frank daytime sleepiness. However, fibromyalgia or nocturnal myoclonus may result in feeling tired on waking in the morning.

When attempting to successfully intervene in insomnia, it is helpful to formulate a sleep regimen that embraces:[37,38]

- creating an environment conducive to sleep. This usually involves eliminating disturbing factors. This includes getting rid of noise, unwanted light and creating a comfortable temperature. The bedroom should be cool, dark and quiet. The bed should be comfortable and the bedding and nightwear appropriate. The bedroom should be prepared for maximum comfort and minimum distraction. Changes may include avoiding eating, reading, television viewing, bill paying, and undertaking other mind-stimulating activities in bed

- relaxing the sleeper both physically and psychologically. This means avoiding physical, chemical amd mental stimulation before retiring. It includes such measures as a warm bath rather than a jog, a glass of warm milk rather than coffee, and a focus on phrases inducing mental tranquillity rather than a dispute before bedtime (see Figure 11.1). Other measures that deserve consideration are sexual intercourse,

progressive muscle relaxation exercises, breathing exercises, relaxation tapes, and meditation. Exercise during the day, but not before going to bed, is to be encouraged.[39] While steady daily exercise probably deepens sleep, occasional exercise does not necessarily improve sleep that night. Check Chapter 10 for a healthy sleep posture

- entraining the circadian sleep–wake rhythm. This means sleeping at night and avoiding daytime naps. Sleep only as long as is needed to be refreshed the next day. Longer than 8 hours in bed may lessen the quality of sleep. Arising at the same time each day appears helpful. Light may disturb sleep. A morning-type behavioural lifestyle is recommended as a way to reduce behavioural/emotional problems, and to lessen the likelihood of falling into asynchronization.[26]

Sleep hygiene involves creating a good sleep environment, assuming a healthy sleep posture; avoiding stimulants such as coffee and other caffeine-rich substances, alcohol, cigarette smoking, and heavy or spicy meals, and not drinking excessive fluids in the evening. It means creating a routine conducive to sleep. **Handout 11.4** provides a screening tool for patients to identify factors that contribute to their sleeping problem. **Handout 11.5** uses sleep hygiene and stimulus control strategies to get a better night's rest. Sleep hygiene education, although typically a component of treatment, has however not been thoroughly investigated as an individual intervention.[8] It may therefore be desirable to combine it with other measures.

A survey found 15% of respondents had used at least once herbal/dietary products to facilitate sleep in the preceding year.[32] Although randomized, placebo-controlled studies have been performed for a few compounds, rigorous scientific data supporting a beneficial effect for the majority of herbal supplements, and dietary and other nutritional supplements used for treating insomnia are lacking.[40]

Nonetheless, one potentially useful nutrient is tryptophan.[41] Tryptophan is the precursor of serotonin, a sleep-regulating neurotransmitter. Tryptophan supplementation (1–2 g at night) has been used with some success in the treatment of insomnia, particularly with respect to normalizing the sleep pattern. The sleep patterns of insomniacs on tryptophan more closely resemble those of normal sleepers than those of untreated insomniacs or persons on sleeping tablets.

- 'Then did the turmoil in me cease for in acceptance lieth peace'

- 'God grant me the courage to change the things I can, the serenity to accept the things I cannot change, and the wisdom to recognize the difference between the two'

- 'When I come to the end of my tether I find God at the other end'

- 'I can and will do my very best'

- 'May we forget our hours of distress, but not what they have taught us'

- 'God grant me the supreme gift of serenity'

- 'Life's greatest personal battles are either won or lost in the quiet place of intrapersonal dialogue'

- 'Struggle is good; it makes one strong; adversity can make me bitter or sweet – would that I achieve the latter'

- 'I know that I am in the right place at the right time experiencing the right circumstances for my eternal evolution'

- 'May I learn to live one day at a time'

- 'They also serve who only stand and wait – I can serve by being, not only by doing'

For more tips see: http://www.webmd.com/video/breus-turn-off-mind

Figure 11.1 • Phrases conducive to mental tranquillity.

Milk is a good dietary source of tryptophan. A glass of milk in the evening is a good substitute for coffee! Another natural alternative is valerian. A systematic review of randomized, placebo-controlled trials of valerian concluded valerian might improve sleep quality without producing side effects.[42] A double-blind, placebo-controlled, crossover study suggested a single 5-mg dose of melatonin appeared as effective as temazepam with less side effects.[43] Despite some herbs and nutritional supplements possibly improving sleep continuity and efficiency, it is worth remembering that sleep improvements are better sustained over time with behavioural treatment.

Figure 11.2 provides a template for practitioners to use the patient handouts provided for helping patients identify and manage behavioural sleep problems.

In perspective

Acute and chronic insomnia are vastly different conditions. The NIH regards chronic insomnia as a major public health problem affecting millions of individuals, along with their families and communities.[44]

While drug therapy is effective for acute insomnia, its use for chronic insomnia is problematic.

Much has yet to be learnt about the mechanisms, causes, clinical course, comorbidities, and consequences of chronic insomnia. Nonetheless, cognitive–behavioural therapy and benzodiazepine receptor agonists are effective in the treatment of chronic insomnia in the short term.[44] Conditioning influences chronic insomnia, whether it be primarily psychophysiological in nature or secondary to drugs, or medical or psychiatric conditions. Management of chronic insomnia, regardless of the cause, should include cognitive–behavioural intervention.

Behavioural management improves sleep continuity and efficiency; improvements are better sustained over time than with other interventions.[45] Although improved sleep may not inevitably lead to clinically meaningful changes in daytime fatigue, it does reduce psychological symptoms and subjective distress.[45] Furthermore, although very little evidence supports the efficacy of other treatments, a lifestyle management approach does attempt to give control back to the patient. As subjective insomnia is itself a recognized condition, the potential benefit of such intervention should not be overlooked.

Step I: Screen for a sleep problem
Provide the patient with Handout 11.1 and let them self-assess their sleep pattern and identify a possible problem

Step II: Confirm and analyse the type
Provide the patient with Handout 11.2 to determine the exact nature of the problem and make them aware of various possible causes and solutions

Step III: Motivate behaviour change
Make the patient aware of the benefits of sleep
If you sleep well, you:

- look younger. See http://www.webmd.com/video/breus-younger-sleep

- have better weight control. See http://www.webmd.com/video/breus-weight-loss

- solve problems better. See http://www.webmd.com/video/breus-nap-benefits

- enhance your memory. See http://www.webmd.com/video/how-sleep-aids-your-memory

- may solve a chronic headache problem. See http://www.webmd.com/video/sleep-and-headaches

Step IV: Search for diverse factors that may be contributing to or aggravating the sleeping problems
Provide all patients with Handout 11.4
Provide travellers, especially those crossing time zones, with Handout 11.3

Step V: Suggest solutions
Provide patients with Handout 11.5. Encourage them to exhaust behavioural measures before resorting to drug management
See http://www.nhlbi.nih.gov/health/public/sleep/index.htm

Figure 11.2 • The practitioner's roadmap.

References

1. Nau SD, McCrae CS, Cook KG, Lichstein KL. Treatment of insomnia in older adults. *Clin Psychol Rev*. 2005;25(5):645–672.

2. Petit L, Azad N, Byszewski A, Sarazan FF, Power B. Non-pharmacological management of primary and secondary insomnia among older people: review of assessment tools and treatments. *Age Ageing*. 2003;32(1):19–25.

3. Daley M, Morin CM, Leblanc M, Grégoire JP, Savard J, Baillargeon L. Insomnia and its relationship to health-care utilization, work absenteeism, productivity and accidents. *Sleep Med*. 2009;10(4): 427–438.

4. LeBlanc M, Beaulieu-Bonneau S, Mérette C, Savard J, Ivers H, Morin CM. Psychological and health-related quality of life factors associated with insomnia in a population-based sample. *J Psychosom Res*. 2007;63(2): 157–166.

5. Ozminkowski RJ, Wang S, Walsh JK. The direct and indirect costs of untreated insomnia in adults in the United States. *Sleep*. 2007; 30(3):263–273.

6. Neubauer DN. Sleep problems in the elderly. *Am Fam Physician*. 1999;59(9):2551–2560.

7. Dinges DF, Pack F, Williams K, et al. Cumulative sleepiness, mood disturbance, and psychomotor vigilance performance decrements during a week of sleep restricted to 4–5 hours per night. *Sleep*. 1997;20:267–277.

8. Sateia MJ, Nowell PD. Insomnia. *Lancet*. 2004;364 (9449):1959–1973.

9. National Centre on Sleep Disorders Research Working Group. Recognizing problem sleepiness in your patients. *Am Fam Physician*. 1999;59:937–944.

10. Stepanski EJ, Wyatt JK. Use of sleep hygiene in the treatment of insomnia. *Sleep Med Rev*. 2003; 7(3):215–225.

11. Feige B, Gann H, Brueck R, et al. Effects of alcohol on polysomnographically recorded sleep in healthy subjects. *Alcohol Clin Exp Res*. 2006;30(9): 1527–1537.

12. Troese M, Fukumizu M, Sallinen BJ, et al. Sleep fragmentation and evidence for sleep debt in alcohol-exposed infants. *Early Hum Dev*. 2008;84(9):577–585.

13. Underner M, Paquereau J, Meurice JC. [Cigarette smoking and sleep disturbance.] *Rev Mal Respir*. 2006;23(3 suppl):6S67–6S77.

14. Staner L, Luthringer R, Dupont C, Aubin HJ, Lagrue G. Sleep effects of a 24-h versus a 16-h nicotine patch: a polysomnographic study during smoking cessation. *Sleep Med*. 2006;7(2):147–154.

15. Bastien CH, St-Jean G, Morin CM, Turcotte I, Carrier J. Chronic psychophysiological insomnia: hyperarousal and/or inhibition deficits? An ERPs investigation. *Sleep*. 2008;31(6):887–898.

16. Pigeon WR, Perlis ML. Sleep homeostasis in primary insomnia. *Sleep Med Rev*. 2006;10(4): 247–254.

17. Cortoos A, Verstraeten E, Cluydts R. Neurophysiological aspects of primary insomnia: implications for its treatment. *Sleep Med Rev*. 2006;10 (4):255–266.

18. Lichstein KL, Riedel BW. Behavioral assessment and treatment of insomnia: a review with an emphasis on clinical application. *Behav Ther*. 1994;25:659–688.

19. Means MK, Lineberger MD, Edinger JD. Nonpharmacologic treatment of insomnia. *Curr Treat Options Neurol*. 2008;10(5): 342–349.

20. Monk TH, Folkard S, Wedderburn AI. Maintaining safety and high performance on shiftwork. *Appl Ergonomics*. 1996;27:17–23.

21. Härmä M. Sleepiness and shiftwork: individual differences. *J Sleep Res*. 1995;4(suppl 2):57–61.

22. Carskadon MA, Mancuso J, Rosekind MR. Impact of part-time employment on adolescent sleep patterns. *Sleep Res*. 1989;18:114.

23. Crowley SJ, Acebo C, Carskadon MA. Sleep, circadian rhythms, and delayed phase in adolescence. *Sleep Med*. 2007; 8(6):602–612.

24. Okawa M, Uchiyama M. Circadian rhythm sleep disorders: characteristics and entrainment pathology in delayed sleep phase and non-24-h sleep-wake syndrome. *Sleep Med Rev*. 2007;11(6): 485–496.

25. Park YM, Matsumoto K, Shinkoda H, Nagashima H, Kang MJ, Seo YJ. Age and gender difference in habitual sleep-wake rhythm. *Psychiatry Clin Neurosci*. 2001;55(3):201–202.

26. Campbell SS, Terman M, Lewy AJ, Dijk DJ, Eastman CI, Boulos Z. Light treatment for sleep disorders: consensus report. V. Age-related disturbances. *J Biol Rhythms*. 1995;10:151–154.

27. Kohyama J. A newly proposed disease condition produced by light exposure during night: asynchronization. *Brain Dev*. 2009;31(4):255–273.

28. Bellamy N. The jet lag phenomenon: pathogenesis, aetiology, clinical features, management. *Mod Med Aust*. 1988;31:45–55.

29. Hughes RJ, Sack RL, Lewy AJ. The role of melatonin and circadian phase in age-related sleep-maintenance insomnia: assessment in a clinical trial of melatonin replacement. *Sleep*. 1998;21(1): 52–68.

30. Reiter RJ, Korkmaz A. Clinical aspects of melatonin. *Saudi Med J*. 2008;29(11):1537–1547.

31. Sateia MJ, Doghramji K, Hauri PJ, Morin CM. Evaluation of chronic insomnia. An American Academy of Sleep Medicine review. *Sleep*. 2000;23(2):243–308.

32. Morin CM, LeBlanc M, Daley M, Gregoire JP, Mérette C. Epidemiology of insomnia: prevalence, self-help treatments, consultations, and determinants of help-seeking behaviors. *Sleep Med*. 2006;7(2):123–130.

33. Yoshimura K, Oka Y, Kamoto T, et al. Night-time frequency, sleep disturbance and general health-related quality of life: is there a relation? *Int J Urol*. 2009;16(1): 96–100.

34. Dawson D, Reid K. Fatigue, alcohol and performance impairment (letter). *Nature*. 1997;388:235.

35. Gregory JM. Sleep: a good investment in health and safety. *J Agromedicine*. 2008;13(2): 119–131.

36. Gillberg M, Kecklund G, Axelsson J, Akerstedt T. The effects of a short daytime nap after restricted night sleep. *Sleep*. 1996; 19(7):570–575.

37. Floyd JA. Sleep promotion in adults. *Annu Rev Nurs Res*. 1999; 17:27–56.

38. Williams A. An effective strategy for sleep. *Practitioner*. 1997;241:606–609.

39. Youngstedt SD, O'Connor PJ, Dishman RK. The effects of acute exercise on sleep: a quantitative synthesis. *Sleep*. 1997;20(3): 203–214.

40. Meolie AL, Rosen C, Kristo D, et al. Clinical Practice Review Committee; American Academy of Sleep Medicine. Oral nonprescription treatment for insomnia: an evaluation of products with limited evidence. *J Clin Sleep Med*. 2005;1(2):173–187.

41. Jamison JR. *Clinical Guide to Nutrition and Dietary Supplements in Disease Management*. Edinburgh: Churchill Livingstone; 2003.

42. Bent S, Padula A, Moore D, Patterson M, Mehling W. Valerian for sleep: a systematic review and meta-analysis. *Am J Med*. 2006; 119(12):1005–1012.

43. Rogers NL, Kennaway DJ, Dawson D. Neurobehavioural performance effects of daytime melatonin and temazepam administration. *J Sleep Res*. 2003;12(3):207–212.

44. NIH State-of-the-Science Conference Statement on manifestations and management of chronic insomnia in adults. *NIH Consens State Sci Statements*. 2005;22(2):1–30.

45. Morin CM, Bootzin RR, Buysse DJ, Edinger JD, Espie CA, Lichstein KL. Psychological and behavioral treatment of insomnia: update of the recent evidence (1998–2004). *Sleep*. 2006;29(11): 1398–1414.

Exercise

12

Physical activity is any bodily movement produced by musculoskeletal activity that results in energy expenditure. Exercise is a subset of physical activity defined as planned, structured and usually repetitive bodily movement that aims to improve or maintain one or more components of physical fitness. Physical fitness encompasses cardiovascular fitness, muscle strength, muscle endurance, flexibility and body composition.

Physical activity requirements

Sufficient movement for health is 30 minutes of physical activity at moderate intensity on at least 5 days of the week.[1] Both a total of 150 minutes each week plus five sessions are considered important. In energy terms, a minimum level of energy expenditure of about 1000 kcal (4200 kJ) weekly is required.[2] Expending 1000 kcal weekly can be achieved by walking for an hour at moderate intensity on 5 days a week. Although health benefits start with energy expenditures as low as 700 kcal (2940 kJ) a week, greater benefits occur at higher activity levels. The recommended daily energy expenditure for health is currently 150–400 kcal (630–1680 kJ) each day. A sedentary person, by increasing their physical activity by 1000 kcal (4200 kJ) per week or 1 metabolic equivalent task (MET), may reduce their risk of an early death by as much as 20%.[2] Walking at an average pace of 2 to 2.9 mph for 1 hour is equivalent to expending 3 MET.

Both aerobic and anaerobic activity contribute to wellness. Adults under the age of 65 years should do 8–10 strength training exercises with 8–12 repetitions of each exercise twice a week plus either moderately intense aerobic exercise for 30 minutes on 5 days or vigorously intense cardio exercise for 20 minutes on 3 days of the week.[3] For older adults, 8–10 strength training exercises doing 10–15 repetitions of each exercise two to three times a week coupled with either moderately intense aerobic exercise 30 minutes/day, 5 days a week, or vigorous aerobic exercise 20 minutes/day on 3 days a week are recommended.[3] A good rule of thumb for adults is to do continuous or intermittent exercise for 20–60 minutes, 3–5 days each week, at 55–90% of maximum heart rate. Intermittent exercise should be made up of bouts of 10 or more minutes.

The majority of adults in developed countries do not get sufficient exercise. The recommendations in the *2008 Physical Activity Guidelines for Americans*, issued by the U.S. Department of Health and Human Services, of at least 150 minutes per week of moderate activity or 75 minutes per week of vigorous activity for adults were not met by one in three Americans.[4] The guidelines outlined in the federal government's *Healthy People 2010*, which called for adults to engage in at least 30 minutes of moderate-intensity activity 5 days per week or 20 minutes of vigorous activity 3 days per week, were not met by more than half of those surveyed.[4] In England, only 21% of the adult population takes part regularly in sport and active recreation.[5] Regular participation in sport and recreation was defined as, over 4 weeks, taking part on at least 3 days each week in moderate-intensity sport and active recreation for at least 30 minutes continuously in any one session. Walking was the most popular recreational activity, followed by swimming and going to the gym. The 2004-05 National Health Survey found 66.9% of Australian males and 73.6% of females were sedentary or spent less than 3.8 hours a week exercising.[6] **Handout 12.1** provides a physical activity self-check.

The benefits

Physically active people are healthier, live longer and decrease their risk of various disorders. Physically active people enjoy many health benefits (see **Handout 12.2**). A randomized trial of moderate- to vigorous-intensity physical activity in middle-aged, sedentary women found doing at least 45 minutes of moderate-intensity aerobic exercise 5 days per week for 12 months improved mental health, general health perceptions, and physical functioning.[7] These changes were most pronounced at the 3-month follow-up. They persisted at the 12-month follow-up for general health perceptions and to a lesser extent for physical and mental health values. No negative effects on functioning were detected. Physical activity is independently related to all-cause mortality.[8] Compared with being inactive, being moderately active (at least 30 minutes on most days of the week) or doing vigorous exercise (at least 20 minutes three times per week) decreased the risk of dying by 27% and 32% respectively.[9] These benefits extended to smokers, the overweight, and persons who watched television for more than 2 hours daily. Fitness and fatness are both associated with mortality from all causes and being fit does not completely reverse the increased risk associated with excess adiposity.[10] Nonetheless, physically active overweight and obese persons significantly reduce their all-cause mortality compared with their sedentary counterparts.[7]

The benefits of an active lifestyle are independent of body weight.

Physical inactivity is an independent risk factor for a plethora of conditions. There is strong evidence that exercise can be used to either reduce the risk of developing and/or contribute to the management of metabolic syndrome-related disorders, type 2 diabetes, dyslipidaemia, hypertension, obesity, chronic obstructive pulmonary disease, coronary heart disease, osteoarthritis, osteoporosis and depression.[11] A prospective follow-up study found physically active subjects have significantly lower age-adjusted mortality from cardiovascular, cancer and all causes compared with sedentary ones. Further adjustment for smoking, systolic blood pressure, cholesterol, BMI, diabetes and education affected the results only slightly.[12] Adhering to physical activity guidelines both lowers the risk of dying and promotes musculoskeletal, cardiovascular, metabolic and mental health.

Musculoskeletal health

To build and maintain strong bones, a dynamic exercise schedule is desirable. Exercise that intermittently and relatively briefly imposes an unusual load that exceeds both an intensity threshold and strain frequency is most beneficial. Bone health is maximized when exercise is supported by adequate nutrition, including but not limited to calcium and vitamin D.[13] A study that examined the effects of exercise, oral contraceptive use and calcium intake during adolescence concluded only exercise was significantly associated with increased bone mineral density and bone bending strength.[14] Exercise appears to be the predominant lifestyle determinant of bone strength in the young. As most bone mass is accrued well before the age of 30, the importance of adequate exercise in young people cannot be overemphasized.

Physical activity reduces the risk of osteoporotic fractures. The risk of an osteoporotic fracture is determined both by bone mineral density and by falling. A 3-month exercise programme to improve muscular strength, coordination, balance and endurance, accompanied by appropriate nutrition, showed significant reductions of risk for falling, an increase in muscle strength, and increased activity.[15] In addition to improving balance, exercise programmes with special emphasis on bone density can significantly improve strength and endurance and reduce bone loss and back pain in osteopenic women during the critical early postmenopausal years.[16] This study also demonstrated that exercise reduces lipid levels.

Cardiovascular health

Regular exercise improves the lipid profile and reduces blood pressure. Hyperlipidaemia and hypertension, two of the major modifiable risk factors for cardiovascular disease, respond to intervention with physical activity. Dose–response relationships between exercise training volume and blood lipid changes suggest that exercise can favourably alter blood lipids. One study reported this could be achieved at low training volumes, with improvements in blood lipids occurring once the threshold for adaptations of 1200 to 2200 kcal/week had been met.[17] Another study confirmed that improvements in the lipoprotein profile, rather than being related to the intensity of exercise or fitness level, were related to the amount of activity.[18] One study found the effects upon blood lipid profiles to be greatest for walks in excess of 20-minute bouts.[19] Another reported most of the changes were associated with distances of 7 to 14 miles per week.[20] A gradual increase in high-density lipoprotein cholesterol (HDL) level was observed with increased miles. HDL increased by 0.008 mmol/L (0.308 mg/dL) per mile. Levels of low-density lipoprotein cholesterol, triglycerides, and the ratio of total cholesterol to HDL also improved with weekly mileage.

A study which reported a significant reduction in the 10-year risk of ischaemic heart disease in a walking group detected no significant changes in lipid levels.[21] This study detected significant decreases in systolic and diastolic blood pressure when mature adults walked briskly for 30 minutes on 5 days a week. Physical activity of moderate intensity involving rhythmic movements with the lower limbs for 50–60 minutes, three or four times per week, reduces blood pressure and appears to be more effective than vigorous exercise.[22] Compared with sedentary persons, 8 weeks of aerobic exercise of more than 30 minutes a week reduced systolic and diastolic blood pressure in patients with untreated stage 1 or 2 essential hypertension.[23] Exercising 61 to 90 minutes a week resulted in maximal reduction of systolic blood pressure. Regular aerobic exercise training attenuates age-related reduction in central arterial compliance, an independent risk factor of cardiovascular disease. The improvement of central arterial compliance by aerobic exercise training appears to be achieved even with low-intensity exercise training, i.e. at a 40% heart rate reserve.[24] Another study found that a 6-month programme of aerobic and resistance training lowered diastolic blood pressure but did not improve aortic stiffness in older adults with mild hypertension more than in controls.[25]

Physical activity benefits the lipid profile and lowers blood pressure. The mechanism whereby this is achieved is unclear but probably involves interacting pathways. There is clear evidence of an inverse linear dose–response relation between the volume of physical activity and death from all causes, including cardiovascular disease, in adults regardless of age;[26] however, the amount of physical activity required is unclear. The minimal exercise intensity, frequency and duration required to achieve a health benefit requires further investigation, particularly as it appears that engaging in physical activity at levels less than those generally recommended also reduces the risk of dying prematurely.[9]

Metabolic health

A constellation of interrelated metabolic risk factors, collectively called the metabolic syndrome, appear to directly promote the development of diabetes and cardiovascular disease. The metabolic syndrome is characterized by insulin resistance and is linked to genetic factors, abdominal obesity and physical inactivity. Elderly individuals who complete a 6-month programme of aerobic and resistance training significantly improve their aerobic and strength fitness, increase lean mass, and reduce general and abdominal obesity.[25] Exercise such as brisk walking results in reduced body weight and body fat.[27] Exercise, even without weight loss, is associated with a substantial reduction in total and abdominal obesity.[28] In fact, weight loss associated with a period of intense physical training preferentially reduces abdominal fat without decreasing fat-free mass.[29] Physical activity reduces abdominal obesity – at worst, a cause, and at best, a risk marker, of the metabolic syndrome.

In certain individuals, visceral obesity may be a marker of a dysmetabolic state causally linked with the metabolic syndrome.[30] In such instances, visceral obesity may be viewed as a clinical intermediate phenotype in which subcutaneous adipose tissue fails to adequately act as a protective metabolic sink for the clearance and storage of extra energy derived from dietary triglycerides. The metabolic syndrome can be viewed as a discrete adipose tissue disease characterized by insulin resistance and inflammation, clinically detectable through systemic inflammatory markers such as high-sensitivity C-reactive protein.[31] In vivo insulin resistance is a key abnormality associated with the atherogenic, prothrombotic inflammatory profile of the metabolic syndrome. Markers of the metabolic syndrome include a large waist circumference, raised triglycerides, blood pressure and fasting plasma glucose, and low levels of HDL.[32] Exercise has a marked effect on the metabolic syndrome and its sequelae.

Independent of the duration of a sedentary lifestyle, moderate to vigorous leisure-time physical activity is inversely associated with the risk of developing the metabolic syndrome in men and women over 44 years of age.[33] Men engaging in more than 3 hours of moderate or vigorous leisure-time physical activity weekly are half as likely as sedentary men to have the metabolic syndrome.[34] Vigorous leisure-time physical activity has an even stronger inverse association. Exercise modifies metabolic changes that occur in the metabolic syndrome. Exercise regulates endothelial genes mediating oxidative metabolism, inflammation, apoptosis, cellular growth and proliferation.[35] It increases vascular endothelial nitric oxide synthetase expression and alters vascular smooth muscle function. It enhances antioxidant systems and reduces serum inflammatory cytokines. Aerobic, but not resistance, exercises can significantly reduce serum inflammatory mediators.[36]

Exercise modifies the postprandial metabolic response. Sixty minutes of endurance exercise performed 17 hours before consuming high-sugar food attenuates the negative effects of glucose on endothelial function. Consumption of a candy bar and soft drink significantly decreases flow-mediated dilation, an indicator of endothelial function.[37] Compared with no exercise in inactive, normolipidaemic individuals, a single bout of intermittent exercise proved more effective than continuous exercise for lowering postprandial lipaemia.[38] Intermittent exercise comprised a single session of three bouts, each lasting 10 minutes and separated by a 20-minute rest period. A more recent study confirmed that walking briskly in 3-minute bouts, 10 times per day, was as effective as walking for 30 minutes continuously with respect to reducing systolic blood pressure and postprandial lipaemia.[39] Physical activity improves body composition; however, the most appropriate exercise regimen to achieve this requires clarification.

Mental benefits

In addition to physical benefits, exercise is a recognized strategy for stress reduction and relaxation. Exercise elevates mood, and improves cognition and self-concept. Regular exercise improves mood and helps relieve depression.[40] Brain-derived neurotrophic factors that enhance neurogenesis and influence mood are increased by exercise. Exercise increases circulating β-endorphins and binds stress hormones such as adrenaline, neutralizing their psychological impact. Beta-endorphins produced by acute exercise elevate mood, reduce the pain threshold and enhance neurogenesis.[40] Aerobic exercise expending 17.5 kcal/kg/week is consistent with public health recommendations and is an effective treatment for mild depression.[41]

A prospective study of predominantly white, community-dwelling women over 64 years of age found that women with higher levels of baseline physical activity were less prone to cognitive decline.[42] A randomized, controlled trial in subjects over 50 years of age with subjective memory impairment found that a 6-month physical activity programme modestly improved cognition.[43] The physical activity programme involved three 50-minute sessions of moderate physical activity per week for 6 months.

Exercise risks

Both increased physical activity and fitness decrease all-cause mortality rates; however, research is needed to clarify the contributions of various components of exercise, i.e. intensity, duration, and frequency, to the various dimensions of wellness. Nonetheless, it is recognized that regular physical activity helps prevent cardiovascular disease, hypertension, type 2 diabetes, obesity, and osteoporosis and may also decrease all-cause morbidity and lengthen lifespan. The U.S. Preventive Services Task Force (USPSTF) concluded there was insufficient evidence to recommend for or against routine behavioural counselling in primary care settings to promote physical activity.[44] One reason for this was concerns about adverse effects.

Physical activity is not risk-free and it is unclear which exercise variables are most likely to decrease injuries related to physical activity. Although potential harms of physical activity counselling have not been well defined or studied, the potential for exercise to cause oxidative stress, cardiovascular events, and muscle and fall-related injuries cannot be ignored. In order to maximize the benefits and minimize associated risks, research is needed to determine how exercise regimens should be tailored to meet individual wellness objectives. **Handout 12.3** provides information on how to reduce cardiovascular risk by appropriately monitoring exercise intensity and **Handout 12.4** provides guidelines for limiting other risks associated with exercise.

Oxidative stress

Exercise increases metabolism, and metabolism inevitably releases free radicals. Free radicals attach to various cellular constituents, damage cellular processes and hasten cell death. Free radical damage can be minimized by reducing the production of free radicals or by neutralizing free radicals once they have been formed. Lifestyle choices that reduce metabolism reduce free radical production. This may be achieved by a sedentary lifestyle and a low-energy diet. Free radicals can be quenched by a plant-based diet rich in antioxidants or by selective dietary supplements. A randomized, double-blind, placebo-controlled study has also shown that oral vitamin C supplementation in 1-g doses provides effective prophylaxis against exercise-induced free radical-mediated lipid peroxidation in human diabetic blood.[45] A study of 21 male volunteers suggests that vitamin E may be protective against the exercise-induced oxidative injury.[46] Short-term 30-day supplementation with 800 mg vitamin E each day has no adverse effect on healthy older adults.[47]

While exercise increases metabolism, regular exercise has been shown to enhance antioxidant capacity in adolescent athletes.[48] The enhanced antioxidant capacity in trained adolescent athletes was independent of their dietary antioxidant intake!

Despite these protective compensatory measures, it is desirable that an accurate dose–response relationship for exercise be determined. Exercise intensity appears important for cardiovascular health. Brisk walking for 20 minutes on 3 days of the week does not appear to alter cardiovascular disease risk factors in previously sedentary adults;[49] however vigorous exercise for a similar period decreased the risk of death by 32%.[9] Clinical studies have shown that severe physical exercise can lead to the generation of more free radicals than the endogenous antioxidant systems can scavenge,

whereas moderate-intensity aerobic exercise improves endothelial function and reduces cardiovascular risk.[2] As moderate-intensity exercise causes less free radical activity and hence less lipid peroxidation and inflammation than high-intensity exercise, identification of minimal effective exercise intensity is desirable.[50] Exercise intensity is not the sole factor influencing beneficial cardiovascular outcomes. Other considerations may facilitate constructing a programme least likely to cause oxidative stress without compromising the cardiovascular benefits. One study reported that people aged 50–65 years walking briskly for 30 minutes on 5 days a week improved their cardiovascular risk profile;[21] another found this regimen modified to 3 days of the week was ineffective.[49] The frequency of undertaking exercise is important. In healthy younger men, higher cardiorespiratory fitness but not leisure-time physical activity predicted a reduced risk of coronary heart disease; for older men, high-intensity leisure-time physical activity and fitness appear to be of similar importance in reducing coronary risk.[51] It appears that physical activity interventions may need to emphasize the amount, intensity, and type of weekly leisure-time physical activity for optimal outcomes.[52]

Musculoskeletal injury

Although data on the potential harms of routine physical activity counselling in primary care settings are limited, one study found the rate of musculoskeletal events to be 30% per year.[53] Another reported regular physical activity to be associated with an injury rate as high as 35 injuries per 100 persons per year.[54] High-impact exercise such as running or aerobic dance may result in shin splints, stress fractures, and tendonitis. On the other hand, low-impact aerobic exercises, correct execution of exercises, adequate warm-up and cool-down periods and an appropriate rate of exercise progression can limit musculoskeletal injuries. Exercise planning ranges from choosing the correct shoe for the intended exercise to selecting the exercise suited to a given individual, e.g., jogging is best avoided in persons more than 10 kg over ideal body weight. Brisk walking is a safe, injury-free form of exercise, especially for older persons. For sedentary individuals, a training intensity of 20% less than the desired target is recommended to minimize the risk of musculoskeletal problems. This programme can be increased to the target level after 2 weeks. Further increments may be considered every 2 or 3 months. It should be noted that previously sedentary persons are particularly vulnerable to exercise-related musculoskeletal injury and that back problems are predictors for back injuries.[55] While inappropriate exercise may cause back injury, people with acute low back pain are advised to stay active rather than to rest in bed.[56] Appropriate physical activity promotes health and the risk of exercise-related musculoskeletal injuries can be minimized by adequate pre-exercise preparation and a suitable exercise regimen.

Heat stroke

The exercise environment is important. Vigorous exercise at or above temperatures of 60°F, 100% humidity, 85°F, 50% humidity, or 88°F, 40% humidity, stresses the body's temperature regulatory mechanisms. Sweating with compensatory divergence of circulation to skin areas can result in reduced work capacity and excessive fluid loss. Maintenance of adequate hydration with a hypotonic liquid containing less than 2.5 g of sugar per 100 mL at 46–55°F is recommended. Because prevention is the key, 390–600 mL of this mixture should be taken 15–20 minutes prior to exercise, with some 90–180 mL being taken every 10–15 minutes during exercise.

Cardiovascular strain

Everybody should exercise regularly. **Handout 12.3** provides information on how aerobic exercise intensity may be monitored. For those over 60 years of age undertaking dynamic exercise, the threshold training effect is 40% of heart rate range. Even people with established clinically stable cardiovascular disease should exercise.[57] Their aim, over time, is to achieve 30 minutes or more of moderate-intensity physical activity on most, if not all, days of the week. For those with advanced cardiovascular disease, less intense and even shorter bouts of activity with more rest periods may suffice. Static exercise produces elevation of both systolic and diastolic blood pressure. In healthy persons, low-intensity static exercises at less than 40% of maximum voluntary contraction are well tolerated and may impart a cardiovascular benefit. Regular low- to moderate-level resistance activity, initially

Table 12.1 Maximum desirable age-related heart rates during sustained exercise

Age (years)	Beats per minute	
	Beginners	Fit individuals
25	140	164
30	136	160
35	132	156
40	128	152
45	124	148
50	119	144
55	115	140
60	111	136
65	107	132

See Target Heart Rate Calculator
http://www.mayoclinic.com/health/target-heart-rate/SM00083

under the supervision of an exercise professional, is also encouraged.[57] With adequate attention to training heart rate and cooling down, exercise has a significant cardiovascular benefit.

Prudent programmes limit risk and maximize the benefits for exercise. To maintain cardiovascular fitness and weight control, aerobic exercise performed on 3–5 days per week for 20 to 60 minutes at an intensity of 55–90% of maximum heart rate and 40–85% of maximum oxygen intake reserve is recommended.[58] A compromised cardiovascular system does not preclude controlled exercise. In fact, pain-free walking time increases in persons with peripheral vascular disease when walking at near-maximal pain for 30 minutes at least three times each week.[59]

Table 12.1 provides exercise guidelines for the acceptable heart rates for various age groups.

Sedentary behaviour: an orange flag

While the nature, duration, intensity and frequency of physical activity to most cost-effectively prevent disease requires clarification, it is apparent that all forms of physical activity are beneficial. Compared with inactive persons, 30–60 minutes of moderate- to vigorous-intensity physical activity daily decreases the risk of breast and colon cancer.[60] Furthermore, evidence is accumulating that prolonged periods of inactivity increase the risk of chronic disease independent of exercise.[61] It has become apparent that a lack of physical activity is a health risk.

A lifestyle conspicuous for its paucity of whole body movement has emerged as a risk factor in its own right. A distinct relationship is emerging between 'too much sitting' and biomarkers of metabolic health predictive of, amongst others, an increased risk of type 2 diabetes and cardiovascular disease.[61] A study of healthy adults who met the public health guideline for physical activity reported television-viewing time was positively associated with a number of metabolic risk variables.[62] Significant, detrimental dose–response associations with television-viewing time were observed with respect to waist circumference, systolic blood pressure, and 2-hour plasma glucose in both sexes, and with fasting plasma glucose, triglycerides, and HDL in women. The associations were stronger in women than in men, with significant gender interactions observed for triglycerides and HDL. The subjects in this study were free of clinically diagnosed diabetes or heart disease and reported at least 2.5 hours a week of moderate- to vigorous-intensity physical activity. There is a dose–response relationship between the sedentary time and health risk – the longer the total sedentary time, the greater the risk. However, if the total sedentary time is broken up, risk is reduced. More interruptions in sedentary time have been found to be beneficially associated with metabolic risk variables independent of total sedentary time, moderate- to vigorous-intensity activity time, and mean intensity of the breaks.[63] These findings suggest that it is not only the amount of sedentary time that is important, but also the manner in which it is accumulated!

Inactivity physiology is a new discipline investigating how best to ameliorate specific risk factors related to metabolic diseases through limiting sitting time and doing non-exercise activity.[64] The first potential tenet of an inactivity physiology paradigm is that sitting more and performing less non-exercise activity enhances the health risk exponentially. Prolonged sitting decreases the opportunities for cumulative energy expenditure resulting from the thousands of intermittent muscular contractions throughout the waking period. The second tenet is that sedentary recreational time and exercise-based

leisure-time physical activity are distinct classes of behaviour, with distinct determinants and independent effects on risk for disease. Exercise capacity (fitness) and energy expenditure (recreational inactivity) are independent predictors of risk. The third, and central, tenet is that some of the specific cellular and molecular processes underlying inactivity physiology are qualitatively different from those used during exercise. In essence this means that signals causing harm during excessive inactivity are not always the same signals boosted to promote health during exercise periods. Sedentary behaviours and non-exercise physical activities are distinct sets of behaviours and not simply the lower pole of a physical activity continuum to structured exercise. Although sitting too much, i.e. poor energy expenditure, and being unfit, i.e. poor exercise capacity, both adversely affect the metabolic risk factors for type 2 diabetes and coronary heart disease, they do so by different cellular processes.

Metabolic evidence of the perils of sitting too much and the possible benefits of at least maintaining low-intensity intermittent non-exercise activity throughout most of the day is mounting. Cohorts of highly sedentary people who fail to maintain daily low-intensity intermittent non-exercise activity increase their rates for coronary artery disease, type 2 diabetes, metabolic syndrome, and obesity. Independent from exercise, sedentary time appears to predict the metabolic syndrome and its components. Emerging evidence suggests that maintaining a high level of daily low-intensity activity may be important independently of moderate–vigorous exercise for certain metabolic risk factors. Studies to identify the potentially unique molecular, physiologic, and clinical effects of inactivity physiology are being carried out. One such study is that of Zderic and Hamilton. They identified physical inactivity as a risk factor for lipoprotein disorders and the metabolic syndrome.[65] The most powerful process known to regulate lipoprotein lipase protein may be initiated by inhibitory signals during physical inactivity, independent of changes in lipoprotein lipase messenger RNA.[66] It appears lipoprotein lipase may be regulated by qualitatively different processes over the physical activity continuum. Physical inactivity strongly suppresses muscle lipoprotein lipase activity. Lipoprotein lipase activity in skeletal muscle is the rate-limiting enzyme for hydrolysis of triglyceride-rich lipoproteins. Animal experiments have shown that lipoprotein lipase in the microvasculature of most oxidative muscles is approximately 90% lower in inactive rodents compared with physically active controls. Furthermore, the light ambulatory contractions responsible for non-exercise activity thermogenesis proved sufficient for mitigating these deleterious effects. Experimentally reducing normal spontaneous standing and ambulatory time has a much greater effect on lipoprotein lipase regulation than adding vigorous exercise training on top of the normal level of non-exercise activity.[64] Low-intensity contractile activity may provide one piece of the puzzle for why inactivity is a risk factor for metabolic diseases and why non-vigorous activity provides marked protection against disorders involving poor lipid metabolism.[67]

A study of non-diabetic subjects found that 2-hour plasma glucose was positively associated with sedentary time and negatively associated with both light-intensity and moderate- to vigorous-intensity activity time.[68] As light-intensity physical activity is beneficially associated with blood glucose, substituting light-intensity activity for television viewing or other sedentary activities may be a practical and achievable preventive strategy to reduce the risk of type 2 diabetes and cardiovascular disease. A study on overweight individuals at risk of diabetes found total body movement was significantly and independently associated with fasting triglycerides, insulin, HDL and clustered metabolic risk.[69] Clustered metabolic risk comprises body composition, blood pressure, fasting triglycerides, HDL, glucose, and insulin. Studies have shown that physical inactivity over a 24-hour period may induce negative effects on relatively fast-acting cellular processes in skeletal muscles, or other tissues, that regulate risk factors like plasma triglycerides and HDL.[64] One day of inactivity produces a several-fold greater change in lipoprotein lipase activity than the exercise training response. In theory, this may be in part because non-exercise activity thermogenesis is generally a much greater component of total energy expenditure than is exercise.[64] There is a wide range in the energy demand of non-exercise activity thermogenesis and the sum of thousands of daily muscular contractions during non-exercise activity require more energy than a single episode of continuous exercise. On the other hand, any type of brief, yet frequent, muscular contraction throughout the day may be needed to short-circuit unhealthy molecular signals causing metabolic diseases.[64] In any event, total body movement appears to be associated with intermediary phenotypic risk factors for cardiovascular and metabolic diseases independent of aerobic fitness and obesity.[69]

Independent of time spent in moderate- to vigorous-intensity activity, sedentary time, light-intensity time and average activity intensity have been found to be significantly associated with waist circumference and clustered metabolic risk.[70] It is important for metabolic health to both decrease sedentary time and increase time spent in physical activity. Exercise capacity/fitness and energy expenditure/recreational inactivity are independent predictors of risk and taken together are stronger predictors of all-cause mortality than smoking, hypertension, obesity and diabetes.

The importance of avoiding prolonged uninterrupted periods of sedentary, primarily sitting, time is increasingly evident and new public health recommendations regarding reducing and breaking up sedentary time deserve consideration.[63] There is a case for sedentary behaviour health guidelines for adults to be provided concurrently with public health guidelines on physical activity.

The physical activity road towards health

Despite the proven benefits of physical activity, the majority of persons in the US, England and Australia fail to meet their country's physical activities guidelines.[71–73] Adequate physical activity can provide substantial health benefits.[2]

At the fitness pole of physical activity, the minimum recommendation is some 20–60 minutes of moderate- to high-intensity exercise at 60–90% of maximum heart rate performed three or more times per week. When the aim is to involve a large muscle mass and minimize the ratio between cardiac and total body effort, suitable activities include swimming, cycling, jogging, walking, water aerobics, and dancing. Optimal conditioning, without undue risk of injury, is achieved by three to five exercise sessions per week. Once fit, two sessions per week may suffice. Physically fit individuals have a slower heart rate and show less increase in pulse rate in response to submaximal workloads than do their unfit contemporaries. Fit individuals have enhanced physical work capacity and can do more work and work for longer periods with less fatigue than unfit persons.

Exercise intensity is a determinant of physiological response and safety; while vigorous exercise achieves greater benefits, it also carries higher risks of orthopaedic injury or triggering a heart attack.

In most cases there is no need to perform exercise stress testing for moderate-intensity aerobic exercise such as walking at 3–3.5 mph, or cycling at 5–9 mph. However, exercise stress testing is recommended before undertaking vigorous exercise. Vigorous exercise causes fatigue within 20 minutes, involves over 75% of maximum heart rate, or exertion is perceived as over 5 on a scale of 0–10. Exercise stress testing prior to vigorous exercise is recommended for apparently healthy men over 35 or 40 years of age, for women over 45 or 50 years of age, and for anyone with a cardiovascular risk factor or symptoms regardless of age.

Physiological, epidemiological, and clinical evidence points to the need for every adult to accumulate 30 minutes or more of moderate-intensity physical activity on most, preferably all, days of the week.[74,75] This less demanding schedule of 30 minutes or more of moderate-intensity physical activity expending about 840 kJ (200 kcal) per day appears to achieve most of the exercise-related health benefits. Moderate-intensity exercise may be undertaken in one burst or distributed throughout the day. Moderate exercise utilizes 4–7 kcal per minute. Activities which meet this level of activity include brisk walking (3–4 mph), cycling at 10 mph, racket sports, general home cleaning, house painting, or lawn mowing with a power mower. With advances in inactivity physiology, an added dimension to physical activity recommendations demands consideration. This merely requires frequently interrupting sedentary behaviour with body movements. Health benefit is achieved by increasing thermogenesis with low-intensity activities. The type of exercises chosen and the nature of an exercise schedule are influenced by the desired health benefit. See **Handout 12.5**.

Fitness and recreational physical activity independently promote health. Physical activity goals can be met in formal exercise classes or independently. Older adults who participated in an existing best-practice multiple-component physical activity programme in the US benefited with regard to self-efficacy for exercise adherence, increased upper- and lower-body strength and exercise participation.[76] In fact, it has been suggested that providing twice-weekly exercise classes would achieve a substantial saving to the health bill.[77] While exercise classes may enhance motivation, especially when accompanied by written goal-oriented exercise prescription, individuals can use goal setting, self-monitoring of progress, and self-reinforcement to achieve satisfactory outcomes. See **Handouts 12.6**

and **12.7**. In both instances, components of personal fitness include the elements of aerobic fitness, anaerobic fitness and flexibility.

Aerobic fitness is composed of cardiovascular and respiratory fitness and is best acquired through dynamic exercise involving rhythmic contraction and relaxation of muscle groups. More systemic benefits are derived from isotonic or rhythmic than static exercise programmes. See **Handout 12.6** for guidelines for creating a safe self-care aerobic exercise programme.

Anaerobic fitness comprises muscle strength, power, and endurance. It is best acquired through static exercises involving continuous contraction of a muscle group. Static exercises may be:

- isometric. Muscles are contracted against resistance with no visible motion, e.g. tightening and holding one's abdominal muscles. Isometric exercises carry a risk of more extreme elevations in blood pressure than isotonic exercises
- isotonic. This involves movement of a weight through a specific range of motion, e.g. push-ups, weightlifting
- isokinetic. A machine facilitates movement of a part of the body against a constant resistance at a fixed speed setting.

Strength activities require effort against resistance. Light resistance and increased repetitions are associated with increased strength and toning in the absence of significant muscle building. Initially, one or two sets, with 6–12 repetitions in each set, performed three times per week are recommended. Flexibility comprises activities that extend and maintain the joint range of motion. Stretching movements to the point of tightness, not pain, should be held (static stretch) for 30–45 seconds. Flexibility is joint-specific. Joints should be moved through their range of motion. Neck stretches can for example be performed by slowly and deliberately leaning one's head to the front, back, left and right and then turning the head left and right. Joint flexibility is best maintained through performing static exercises each day.

Training is a form of adaptation to the repeated stimulation of exercise. A safe and effective training programme is one that progressively but moderately overloads the body and permits adequate time for adaptation to each level of stimulation. Progressive increments in fitness require ongoing adaptation of the proposed exercise programme; maintenance of a particular level of fitness requires adherence to the appropriate training programme. Reversion to a sedentary lifestyle is accompanied by a concomitant loss of fitness.

In perspective

Physical activity provides substantial health benefits. Aerobic fitness, strength training and physical activity are three discrete dimensions promoting wellness. In addition to weight-bearing exercises and physical activity leading to cardiorespiratory fitness, consideration is now also being given to avoiding prolonged periods of immobility. Diverse metabolic processes are modulated depending on the intensity and frequency of physical activity. Active fit people enjoy a health advantage over sedentary fit people. Unfit active people are at greater health risk than fit active people. Inactivity physiology has added a new dimension to physical activity considerations.

While further research is required to determine the most cost-effective physical activity regimens, it is apparent that some benefits are not contingent on vigorous activity. Research suggests taking 10,000 steps a day provides a desirable level of physical activity for health.[78] However, this is not normally achievable through routine daily activities. For many, there is a daily deficit of approximately 4000 steps (most from 3000 to 6000 steps), which must be gained from other more rigorous activities. Pedometers are available for measuring activity levels.[79] Observational studies suggest that pedometer users significantly increased their physical activity by 2183 steps per day or 26.9% over baseline.[80] When data from all studies were combined, pedometer users significantly decreased their body mass index by 0.38 and their systolic blood pressure by 3.8 mmHg. Thirty minutes or more of at least moderate-intensity daily physical activity translates to 3000–4000 steps at an intensity of at least 100 steps a minute accumulated in at least 10-minute bouts.[81] To meet these minimal requirements may well require personal commitment that goes beyond everyday work/leisure activity.

References

1. Exercise requirements. http://www. aihw.gov.au/publications/phe/ ihrftav/ihrftav-01.pdf; Accessed 14.12.08.
2. Ignarro LJ, Balestrieri ML, Napoli C. Nutrition, physical activity, and cardiovascular disease: an update. *Cardiovasc Res.* 2007;73:326–340.
3. Sarris J. Depression and exercise. ACSM & AHA Joint Position Statement on exercise to maintain health. *J Comp Med.* 2008;7:50.
4. CDC Report suggests many US adults fall short of guidelines. http://www.rwjf.org/publichealth/ digest.jsp?id=9109; Accessed 14.12.08.
5. Active People Survey. http://wwww.sportengland.org/ index/get_resources /research/ active_people/active_people_ survey_headline_results.htm; Accessed 14.12.08.
6. Australian Bureau of Statistics. http://www.abs.gov.au/ausstats /abs@.nsf/Products/ 0EA5BD9E1A15E374CA 2574D600173D4B?

opendocument; Accessed 14.12.08.
7. Bowen DJ, Fesinmeyer MD, Yasui Y, et al. Randomized trial of physical activity in sedentary middle aged women: effects on quality of life. *Int J Behav Nutr Phys Act.* 2006;3(1):34.
8. Crespo CJ, Palmieri MR, Perdomo RP, et al. The relationship of physical activity and body weight with all-cause mortality: results from the Puerto Rico Heart Health Program. *Ann Epidemiol.* 2002;12 (8):543–552.
9. Leitzmann MF, Park Y, Blair A, et al. Physical activity recommendations and decreased risk of mortality. *Arch Intern Med.* 2007;167(22):2453–2460.
10. Stevens J, Cai J, Evenson KR, Thomas R. Fitness and fatness as predictors of mortality from all causes and from cardiovascular disease in men and women in the lipid research clinics study. *Am J Epidemiol.* 2002;156(9):832–841.
11. Pedersen BK, Saltin B. Evidence for prescribing exercise as therapy in

chronic disease. *Scand J Med Sci Sports.* 2006;16(suppl 1):3–63.
12. Hu G, Tuomilehto J, Silventoinen K, Barengo NC, Peltonen M, Jousilahti P. The effects of physical activity and body mass index on cardiovascular, cancer and all-cause mortality among 47 212 middle-aged Finnish men and women. *Int J Obes (Lond).* 2005;29(8):894–902.
13. Borer KT. Physical activity in the prevention and amelioration of osteoporosis in women: interaction of mechanical, hormonal and dietary factors. *Sports Med.* 2005;35 (9):779–830.
14. Lloyd T, Petit MA, Lin HM, Beck TJ. Lifestyle factors and the development of bone mass and bone strength in young women. *J Pediatr.* 2004;144(6):776–782.
15. Swanenburg J, de Bruin ED, Stauffacher M, Mulder T, Uebelhart D. Effects of exercise and nutrition on postural balance and risk of falling in elderly people with decreased bone mineral density: randomized controlled trial pilot

study. *Clin Rehabil.* 2007;21 (6):523–534.

16. Kemmler W, Lauber D, Weineck J, Hensen J, Kalender W, Engelke K. Benefits of 2 years of intense exercise on bone density, physical fitness, and blood lipids in early postmenopausal osteopenic women: results of the Erlangen Fitness Osteoporosis Prevention Study (EFOPS). *Arch Intern Med.* 2004;164(10):1084–1091.

17. Durstine JL, Grandjean PW, Davis PG, Ferguson MA, Alderson NL, DuBose KD. Blood lipid and lipoprotein adaptations to exercise: a quantitative analysis. *Sports Med.* 2001;31 (15):1033–1062.

18. Kraus WE, Houmard JA, Duscha BD, et al. Effects of the amount and intensity of exercise on plasma lipoproteins. *N Engl J Med.* 2002;347(19):1483–1492.

19. Woolf-May K, Kearney EM, Owen A, Jones DW, Davison RC, Bird SR. The efficacy of accumulated short bouts versus single daily bouts of brisk walking in improving aerobic fitness and blood lipid profiles. *Health Educ Res.* 1999;14(6):803–815.

20. Kokkinos PF, Holland JC, Narayan P, Colleran JA, Dotson CO, Papademetriou V. Miles run per week and high-density lipoprotein cholesterol levels in healthy, middle-aged men. A dose-response relationship. *Arch Intern Med.* 1995;155(4):415–420.

21. Tully MA, Cupples ME, Chan WS, McGlade K, Young IS. Brisk walking, fitness, and cardiovascular risk: a randomized controlled trial in primary care. *Prev Med.* 2005;41 (2):622–628.

22. Cleroux J, Feldman RD, Petrella RJ. Lifestyle modifications to prevent and control hypertension. 4. Recommendations on physical exercise training. Canadian Hypertension Society, Canadian Coalition for High Blood Pressure Prevention and Control, Laboratory Centre for Disease Control at Health Canada, Heart and Stroke Foundation of Canada. *CMAJ.* 1999;160(9 suppl):S21–S28.

23. Ishikawa-Takata K, Ohta T, Tanaka H. How much exercise is required to reduce blood pressure in essential hypertensives: a dose–response study. *Am J Hypertens.* 2003;16(8):629–633.

24. Sugawara J, Inoue H, Hayashi K, Yokoi T, Kono I. Effect of low-intensity aerobic exercise training on arterial compliance in postmenopausal women. *Hypertens Res.* 2004;27(12):897–901.

25. Stewart KJ, Bacher AC, Turner KL, et al. Effect of exercise on blood pressure in older persons: a randomized controlled trial. *Arch Intern Med.* 2005;165(7):756–762.

26. Lee M, Skerrett PJ. Physical activity and all-cause mortality: what is the dose-response relation? *Med Sci Sports Exerc.* 2001;33(6 suppl): S459–S471.

27. Irwin ML, Yasui Y, Ulrich CM, et al. Effect of exercise on total and intra-abdominal body fat in postmenopausal women: a randomized controlled trial. *JAMA.* 2003;289(3):323–330.

28. Ross R, Janssen I, Dawson J, et al. Exercise-induced reduction in obesity and insulin resistance in women: a randomized controlled trial. *Obes Res.* 2004;12 (5):789–798.

29. Mayo MJ, Grantham JR, Balasekaran G. Exercise-induced weight loss preferentially reduces abdominal fat. *Med Sci Sports Exerc.* 2003;35(2):207–213.

30. Després JP, Lemieux I, Bergeron J, et al. Abdominal obesity and the metabolic syndrome: contribution to global cardiometabolic risk. *Arterioscler Thromb Vasc Biol.* 2008;28(6):1039–1049.

31. Oda E. The metabolic syndrome as a concept of adipose tissue disease. *Hypertens Res.* 2008;31 (7):1283–1291.

32. Després JP. Cardiovascular disease under the influence of excess visceral fat. *Crit Pathw Cardiol.* 2007;6(2):51–59.

33. Wijndaele K, Duvigneaud N, Matton L, et al. Sedentary behaviour, physical activity and a continuous metabolic syndrome risk score in adults. *Eur J Clin Nutr.* 2009;63(3):421–429.

34. Laaksonen DE, Lakka HM, Salonen JT, Niskanen LK, Rauramaa R, Lakka TA. Low levels of leisure-time physical activity and cardiorespiratory fitness predict development of the metabolic syndrome. *Diabetes Care.* 2002;25 (9):1612–1618.

35. Leung FP, Yung LM, Laher I, Yao X, Chen ZY, Huang Y. Exercise, vascular wall and cardiovascular diseases: an update (part 1). *Sports Med.* 2008;38(12):1009–1024.

36. Kohut ML, McCann DA, Russell DW, et al. Aerobic exercise, but not flexibility/resistance exercise, reduces serum IL-18, CRP, and IL-6 independent of beta-blockers, BMI, and psychosocial factors in older adults. *Brain Behav Immun.* 2006;20(3):201–209.

37. Weiss EP, Arif H, Villareal DT, et al. Endothelial function after high-sugar-food ingestion improves with endurance exercise performed on the previous day. *Am J Clin Nutr.* 2008;88(1):51–57.

38. Altena TS, Michaelson JL, Ball SD, Thomas TR. Single sessions of intermittent and continuous exercise and postprandial lipemia. *Med Sci Sports Exerc.* 2004;36 (8):1364–1371.

39. Miyashita M, Burns SF, Stensel DJ. Accumulating short bouts of brisk walking reduces postprandial plasma triacylglycerol concentrations and resting blood pressure in healthy young men. *Am J Clin Nutr.* 2008;88(5):1225–1231.

40. Sarris J. Depression and exercise. *J Comp Med.* 2008;7:48–62.

41. Dunn AL, Trivedi MH, Kampert JB, Clark CG, Chambliss HO. Exercise treatment for depression: efficacy and dose response. *Am J Prev Med.* 2005;28(1):1–8.

42. Yaffe K, Barnes D, Nevitt M, Lui LY, Covinsky K. A prospective study of physical activity and cognitive decline in elderly women: women who walk. *Arch Intern Med.* 2001;161(14):1703–1708.

43. Lautenschlager NT, Cox KL, Flicker L, et al. Effect of physical activity on cognitive function in older adults at risk for Alzheimer disease: a randomized trial. *JAMA.* 2008;300(9):1027–1037.

44. U.S. Preventive Services Task Force. Behavioral counseling in primary care to promote physical activity: recommendation and rationale. *Ann Intern Med.* 2002;137 (3):205–207.

45. Davison GW, Ashton T, George L, et al. Molecular detection of exercise-induced free radicals following ascorbate prophylaxis in type 1 diabetes mellitus: a randomised controlled trial. *Diabetologia.* 2008;51(11):2049–2059.

46. Meydani M, Evans WJ, Handelman G, et al. Protective effect of vitamin E on exercise-induced oxidative damage in young and older adults. *Am J Physiol.* 1999;264(5 Pt 2):R992–R998.

47. Meydani M. Vitamin E requirement in relation to dietary fish oil and oxidative stress in elderly. *EXS.* 1992;62:411–418.

48. Carlsohn A, Rohn S, Bittmann F, et al. Exercise increases the plasma antioxidant capacity of adolescent athletes. *Ann Nutr Metab.* 2008;53(2):96–103.

49. Murtagh EM, Boreham CA, Nevill A, Hare LG, Murphy MH. The effects of 60 minutes of brisk walking per week, accumulated in two different patterns, on cardiovascular risk. *Prev Med.* 2005;41(1):92–97.

50. Seifi-Skishahr F, Siahkohian M, Nakhostin-Roohi B. Influence of aerobic exercise at high and moderate intensities on lipid peroxidation in untrained men. *J Sports Med Phys Fitness.* 2008;48(4):515–521.

51. Talbot LA, Morrell CH, Metter EJ, Fleg JL. Comparison of cardiorespiratory fitness versus leisure time physical activity as predictors of coronary events in men aged < or = 65 years and > 65 years. *Am J Cardiol.* 2002;89(10):1187–1192.

52. Malmberg J, Miilunpalo S, Pasanen M, Vuori I, Oja P. Characteristics of leisure time physical activity associated with risk of decline in perceived health. Carlsohn – a 10-year follow-up of middle-aged and elderly men and women. *Prev Med.* 2005;41(1):141–150.

53. Writing Group for the Activity Counseling Trial Research Group. Effects of physical activity counseling in primary care: the Activity Counseling Trial: a randomized controlled trial. *JAMA.* 2001;286:677–687.

54. Eaton CB. Relation of physical activity and cardiovascular fitness to coronary heart disease, Part II: Cardiovascular fitness and the safety and efficacy of physical activity prescription. *J Am Board Fam Pract.* 1992;5(2):157–165.

55. Segwick AW, Smith DS, Davies MJ. Musculoskeletal status of men and women who entered a fitness programme. *Med J Aust.* 1988;148:285–291.

56. Hagen KB, Jamtvedt G, Hilde G, Winnem MF. The updated Cochrane review of bed rest for low back pain and sciatica. *Spine.* 2005;30(5):542–546.

57. Briffa TG, Maiorana A, Sheerin NJ, et al. Physical activity for people with cardiovascular disease: recommendations of the National Heart Foundation of Australia. *Med J Aust.* 2006;184(2):71–75.

58. Morey SS. ACSM revises guidelines for exercise to maintain fitness. *Am Fam Physician.* 1999;59:473.

59. Gardner AW, Poehlman ET. Exercise rehabilitation programs for the treatment of claudication pain. A meta-analysis. *JAMA.* 1995;274(12):975–980.

60. Lee IM. Physical activity and cancer prevention – data from epidemiologic studies. *Med Sci Sports Exerc.* 2003;35(11):1823–1827.

61. Owen N, Bauman A, Brown W. Too much sitting: a novel and important predictor of chronic disease risk? *Br J Sports Med.* 2009;43(2):81–83.

62. Healy GN, Dunstan DW, Salmon J, Shaw JE, Zimmet PZ, Owen N. Television time and continuous metabolic risk in physically active adults. *Med Sci Sports Exerc.* 2008;40(4):639–645.

63. Healy GN, Dunstan DW, Salmon J, et al. Breaks in sedentary time: beneficial associations with metabolic risk. *Diabetes Care.* 2008;31(4):661–666.

64. Hamilton MT, Hamilton DG, Zderic TW. Role of low energy expenditure and sitting in obesity, metabolic syndrome, type 2 diabetes, and cardiovascular disease. *Diabetes.* 2007;56(11):2655–2667.

65. Zderic TW, Hamilton MT. Physical inactivity amplifies the sensitivity of skeletal muscle to the lipid-induced downregulation of lipoprotein lipase activity. *J Appl Physiol.* 2006;100(1):249–257.

66. Hamilton MT, Hamilton DG, Zderic TW. Exercise physiology versus inactivity physiology: an essential concept for understanding lipoprotein lipase regulation. *Exerc Sport Sci Rev.* 2004;32(4):161–166.

67. Bey L, Hamilton MT. Suppression of skeletal muscle lipoprotein lipase activity during physical inactivity: a molecular reason to maintain daily low-intensity activity. *J Physiol.* 2003;551(Pt 2):673–682.

68. Healy GN, Dunstan DW, Salmon J, et al. Objectively measured light-intensity physical activity is independently associated with 2-h plasma glucose. *Diabetes Care.* 2007;30(6):1384–1389.

69. Ekelund U, Griffin SJ, Wareham NJ. Physical activity and metabolic risk in individuals with a family history of type 2 diabetes. *Diabetes Care.* 2007;30(2):337–342.

70. Healy GN, Wijndaele K, Dunstan DW, et al. Objectively measured sedentary time, physical activity, and metabolic risk: the Australian Diabetes, Obesity and Lifestyle Study (AusDiab). *Diabetes Care.* 2008;31(2):369–371.

71. Prevalence of physical activity including lifestyle activities amongst adults – United States, 2000–2001. http://www.cdc.gov/mmwr/preview/mmwrhtml/mm5232a2.htm; Accessed 17.12.08.

72. Percentage meeting physical activity guidelines (England). http://www.heartstats.org/temp/Figsp6.7spweb08.xls; Accessed 17.12.08.

73. *Physical activity in Australia: a snapshot 2004–2005.* http://www.abs.gov.au/AUSSTATS/abs@.nsf/ProductsbyCatalogue/71AB5A496A0B30CACA25724A00108DB6?OpenDocument; Accessed 17.12.08.

74. Consensus Statement from the National Institutes of Health. Physical activity and cardiovascular health. *JAMA.* 1996;276:241–246.

75. Pate RR, Pratt M, Blair SN, et al. Physical activity and public health. *JAMA.* 1995;273(5):402–407.

76. Hughes SL, Seymour RB, Campbell RT, Whitelaw N, Bazzarre T. Best-practice physical activity programs for older adults: findings from the national impact study. *Am J Public Health*. 2009;99 (2):362–368.

77. Munro J, Brazier J, Davey R, Nicholl J. Physical activity for the over-65s: could it be a cost-effective exercise for the NHS? *J Public Health Med*. 1997;19(4):397–402.

78. Choi BC, Pak AW, Choi JC, Choi EC. Daily step goal of 10,000 steps: a literature review. *Clin Invest Med*. 2007;30(3): E146–E151.

79. Rowland K, Schumann SA. Have pedometer, will travel. *J Fam Pract*. 2008;57(2):90–93. Paper available at http://www.jfponline. com/Pages.asp?AID=5928;.

80. Bravata DM, Smith-Spangler C, Sundaram V, et al. Using pedometers to increase physical activity and improve health: a systematic review. *JAMA*. 2007;298 (19):2296–2304.

81. Tudor-Locke C, Hatano Y, Pangrazi RP, Kang M. Revisiting "how many steps are enough?" *Med Sci Sports Exerc*. 2008;40(7 suppl): S537–S543.

Sexual health

Sexual health: an overview

The more traditional notion of sexual health as the absence of sexually transmitted diseases and unwanted pregnancy is being superseded by a more comprehensive approach. Sexual health, consistent with the perspective of the World Health Organization, is largely regarded as:

- a capacity to enjoy and control sexual and reproductive behaviour in accordance with a social and personal ethic
- freedom from psychological factors such as fear, shame, guilt and false beliefs inhibiting sexual response and impairing sexual relationships
- freedom from organic disease, disorders and deficiencies that impair sexual and reproductive functions.

While sexual activity may be both pleasurable and healthy, unsafe sex contributed up to 15% of the total global disease burden in 1990.[1] More than half of American women will have had an unintentional pregnancy by the time they reach the age of 45.[2] The U.S. Preventive Services Task Force (USPSTF) believes: 'All adolescent and adult patients should be advised about the risk factors for human immunodeficiency virus (HIV) infection and other sexually transmitted diseases (STIs) and counselled appropriately about effective measures to reduce the risk of infection.'[3] Sex education needs to address a range of barriers ranging from poor information to gender inequalities; cultural expectations to power distribution.[4] Safe-sex issues at both the level of contraception and sexually transmitted diseases need to be addressed. Gender-specific topics such as breast, cervical, prostate and testicular cancer are also pertinent concerns.

The physiology of sex

Sexual activity is undertaken to experience erotic pleasure, relieve physical tension, relax and induce sleep and to create intimacy and enhance bonding. Sex in these terms is a holistic experience involving mind, body and emotions. Sexual interaction results in an erotic state and passes through the phases of sexual interest, desire, decision and participation. Biologically, sexual interest is strongly influenced by androgen levels. Sexual desire and the motivation to engage in a sexual experience are then modified by a number of other physical and psychological factors. Sexual arousal involves congestion of the pelvis resulting in penile erection in males and vaginal lubrication and clitoral swelling in females. Arousal may be initiated or enhanced by various means including petting, manual genital or breast massage, French kissing, erotic conversation or video viewing. The sexual response cycle progresses from the initial phase of excitement during which erection, vaginal lubrication and a sexual flush develop, to a second phase in which the physiological response plateaus, although subjective feelings of sexual arousal may increase. During phase 3, the tension build-up in the previous two phases is released in an orgasm, which in men is usually accompanied by ejaculation. Orgasm is characterized by rhythmic contractions of the pelvic muscles, tightening of the muscles of the face and extremities, and feelings of intense pleasure. The final phase is one of resolution during which the body returns to its physiological baseline state. There is considerable variation in the sexual responses of individuals.

Contraception

Successful contraception has heralded development of permissive attitudes to women's premarital sexual behaviour and women are experimenting with sex earlier in life, living with partners outside marriage and experimenting with a wider variety of sexual techniques. Among women 'at risk' of pregnancy (16 to 50 years of age) in the UK, 88% used at least one method of contraception in 2007/8.[5] There are a variety of methods that may be used to prevent conception following coitus.[6] Advances in contraceptive technology have made birth control more effective, convenient, and safe. **Handout 13.1** ranks pregnancy risk according to the contraception method used. Periodic counselling is recommended for all persons at risk of unintended pregnancy.

Methods used by males include:

- Coitus interruptus. This method requires that the penis is withdrawn from the vagina before ejaculation. It is highly unreliable.
- The condom. A sheath prevents ejaculation into the vagina. When properly used, condoms are fairly reliable at preventing pregnancy and have the added benefit of protecting against sexually transmitted disease. Condoms are traditionally made of rubber or latex. Oil-based lubricants and vaginal preparations containing mineral or vegetable oil may compromise the integrity of latex condoms.[7] Tougher and thinner polyurethane sheaths that are less allergenic and not affected by oil-based lubricants are also available.[8] The male condom is the second most popular method of contraception and is used by one in four couples.[5] See **Handout 13.2**.
- Vasectomy. This simple operation involves ligation of the vas deferens, thereby interrupting the sperm's pathway from the testis to the urethra. The ejaculate is devoid of sperm after some 10 ejaculations following surgery. In some cases, the operation is reversible. This is the most effective male method of contraception. By 2005, almost 20% of males under the age of 70 years in the UK had had a vasectomy.[9]
- Male injection. A 3-monthly injection of a combination of testosterone and progesterone provides effective contraception.[8]

Ranked in order of effectiveness, contraceptive methods used by women include:

- Oral contraception. This remains the most popular method of contraception.[5] A variety of oral contraception options are available.[10] Various combinations of oestrogen and progesterone in the 'pill' suppress ovulation, make the uterine lining unsuitable for implantation of a fertilized ovum, and alter the cervical mucus so that it becomes thick and hostile to sperm. On a monophasic pill regimen, active pills with a standard dose of oestrogen and progestogen are taken for 21 days followed by 7 pill-free days. On the triphasic pill regimen, pills taken at the beginning of the cycle contain low-dose oestrogen, the level of which increases towards mid-cycle to prevent breakthrough bleeding. The progestogen dose starts very low and increases to a level slightly below that in the standard monophasic pill. Overall, this approach reduces the total progestogen dose. The biphasic pill regimen offers a slightly higher oestrogen dose throughout the 21-day cycle with low progestogen in the first half and increasing progestogen in the second half of the cycle. With combined oral contraception, it is unsafe to extend the 7 pill-free days. If a pill is missed for 12 hours or less, the missed pill is immediately taken and further pills are taken as usual. If more than 12 hours have elapsed since a pill should have been taken, one pill is taken immediately, earlier missed pills are discarded. The rest of the pills in the pack are taken as usual. Another method of birth control should be used for the next 7 days. If intercourse has occurred during the last 7 days and the patient is late in starting the 'active pill' in a new pack or has missed any of the first three 'active' pills in the pack, emergency contraception may be needed. If the patient is more than 12 hours late taking her pill and there are more than seven active hormone pills left in a packet, the pills from the pack should be taken as usual. If there are less than seven active pills left, the 7-day 'pill-free break' is skipped and the active pills in a new pack are started.

Side effects attributable to oestrogen include nausea, dizziness, irritability, cyclical weight gain, bloating, mastalgia and increased vaginal discharge. Side effects attributable to progestogens include vaginal dryness, acne, hirsutism, occasionally sustained weight gain, depression, lassitude and loss of libido. Side effects can be minimized by modifying the combination to each woman's needs.[11] New formulations are being developed that offer effective contraception, acceptable cycle control, and a good tolerability profile.[12]

A progestogen-only pill that contains about 20% of the progestogen of the other pills and no oestrogen is also available. It is taken every day, not cyclically. These pills are a useful option for women who are sensitive to oestrogen and develop nausea on the other combinations.[10] Injections of progesterone and subdermal progestin implants are also available.

Misperceptions about the safety of oral contraceptives and a relative lack of information concerning their numerous non-contraceptive benefits may limit their use.[13] Most concerns regarding oral contraceptive use expressed by Finnish women surveyed related to possible cardiovascular effects, cancer, infertility, mood changes and weight gain.[14] The probability of a patient experiencing a cardiovascular event while taking a low-dose oral contraceptive is very low.[15] In most instances, the non-contraceptive benefits of oral contraceptives outweigh the potential cardiovascular risks. Recent meta-analyses indicate that there is a reduction in the risk of endometrial and ovarian cancer; however, a small increase in the risk for cervical and breast cancer is possible.[15] The risk of breast cancer with oral contraceptive use is equivalent to that in a nulliparous woman over 26 years of age. On the other hand, women who drink have a 40–100% greater risk of breast cancer than teetotallers do. Smoking, hypertension, obesity, and diabetes are also risk factors that must be taken into account by users of oral contraception.

When taken correctly, about 0.5% of sexually active women become pregnant while taking the pill. The risk of pregnancy is increased when women forget to take their hormonally active pills at the beginning or the end of their active pill cycle. Perimenopausal women should be aware that hormone replacement therapy does not offer protection against pregnancy. Certain drugs, e.g. antacids, may impair the bioavailability of oral contraceptives. In addition to a highly effective, reversible method of contraception, possible benefits of oral contraception include a reduction in menstrual flow, dysmenorrhoea and premenstrual tension, a decreased risk of anaemia and amelioration of endometriosis symptoms, fewer ectopic pregnancies, a possible increase in bone density, and possible protection against pelvic inflammatory disease.[15,16]

The decision to use oral contraception should ultimately be made by a fully informed patient.

- Intrauterine device (IUD). The presence of a spiral or coiled device in the uterine cavity substantially reduces the risk of pregnancy following sexual intercourse. Reports of septic abortions and pelvic inflammatory disease have reduced the popularity of this method. However, provided rigid patient-selection guidelines and strict aseptic insertion techniques are used, the IUD can provide safe, long-term, cost-effective, and highly efficacious contraception.[17,18] Despite the longstanding practice of inserting IUDs only for parous women in monogamous relationships, evidence suggests that they can be safely used by both nulliparous and non-monogamous women.[4] IUDs can be inserted mid-cycle. A Finnish survey found that infections, effects on menstruation and ectopic pregnancy were the concerns women most frequently mentioned regarding the use of IUDs.[14] Progesterone-releasing IUDs are now on the market.

- Barrier methods. A vaginal diaphragm can be inserted into the vagina to act as a barrier preventing sperm reaching the cervix. It must be left in place at least 6 hours after intercourse. Fresh spermicide should be applied if intercourse is repeated within 6 hours. A vaginal sponge and cervical cap are other barrier method options. Less than 1% of women in the UK in 2004/5 used the female condom or spermicides.[9] The male condom is more effective, especially when used in conjunction with a spermicide.

- Spermicides. Creams, gels, pessaries or aerosols may be used to deposit spermicidal agents near the cervix prior to intercourse. These are most effective when used in conjunction with other methods. A survey found that one in five physicians who did not wish to become pregnant used more than one type of contraceptive and the most frequently used combination was spermicide with a barrier method.[19] This survey found that these professionals were more likely to use intrauterine devices, diaphragms, or condoms, and less likely to use female or male sterilization than were other women.

- The rhythm method. This involves abstaining from intercourse around the time of ovulation. As sperm may survive for 3 days and ovulation may vary over 48 hours or more in even a regular menstrual period, avoidance of intercourse is recommended between days 9 and 18 of a 28-day cycle. By monitoring her menstrual cycle and taking her early morning temperature, a woman can assess the time of her ovulation. A slight drop in temperature followed by a rise indicates ovulation. Ovulation needs to be monitored over a number of cycles to establish a relatively reliable baseline. This method is unreliable.

Contraception preferences and costs

The type of contraception preferred varies with age. In the UK in 2007/08, single women and those under the age of 30 years were more likely than older women to use the pill or male condom; older women were more likely to rely on their partner's vasectomy or sterilization.[5] Six per cent of UK women under 50 had been sterilized in 2007/08.[5] Recommendations based on good-quality patient-oriented evidence suggests oral contraception should be considered for women who would prefer less frequent menstrual periods; an intrauterine device may be appropriate for women with prior pelvic inflammatory disease, ectopic pregnancy, or

an abnormal Papanicolaou (Pap) smear result, and for many adolescents.[20]

Of unintended pregnancies that occur each year in the US, 52% are to women who used no contraceptive method during the month in which they became pregnant; 43% are to women who used a contraceptive method either inconsistently or incorrectly; and only 5% of unintended pregnancies can be attributed to women in whom the method failed despite correct usage.[21] The direct medical costs of these unintended pregnancies totalled US$5 billion.[22] Contraceptive use saves nearly US$19 billion in direct medical costs each year. Despite the availability of highly effective reversible contraceptive methods, some 49% of the 6.4 million pregnancies each year in the US are unintended.[22]

Emergency contraception

The median age of first intercourse in the US is 17.4 years for females and 17.7 years for males.[23] Furthermore, many sexually active teens either use ineffective methods or do not use contraception – 26% of females aged 15–19 years did not use any method of contraception the first time they had sex and only 28% of females report using condoms every time they had sex in a year.[23] One solution to any suspected unintended pregnancy is emergency contraception.

There are generally two options for emergency contraception: hormonal intervention or insertion of an IUD. In the UK in 2007/08, 91% of women surveyed had heard of the 'morning after pill' and 49% were aware this form of emergency contraception remained effective up to 72 hours after intercourse; however, only one in three were aware of the emergency IUD and fewer than 1 in 10 realized that once inserted this method offered protection for up to 5 days after sex.[5] A major advantage of the hormonal option is that it no longer requires physician intervention in all cases. Between December 2000 and September 2003, various Canadian provinces granted emergency contraception prescriptive authority to pharmacists, and in April 2005, Health Canada granted levonorgestrel non-prescription, behind-the-pharmacy-counter status with no age restriction.[24] Unlike Canada, in the US, Plan B® Emergency Contraception, although available over the counter for women aged 18 and older – as approved by the Food and Drug Administration

(FDA) in August 2006 – requires women younger than age 18 to have a prescription. Plan B[®], the sole dedicated product for emergency contraception on the US market, is progestin only (levonorgestrel) and lacks the risks related to contraceptives containing oestrogen.[25] This emergency contraceptive meets FDA criteria: it is non-toxic, does not cause birth defects, poses no danger of overdose or addiction, and involves no drug interactions or contraindications. Levonorgestrel-only or Plan B[®] Emergency Contraception is 89% effective when used correctly within 72 hours after unprotected sex. It reduces the risk of pregnancy, following a single act of mid-cycle unprotected sexual intercourse, from around 8% to 1.1%.[26] Each 12-hour delay in starting emergency contraceptive treatment halves the efficacy of this approach. Levonorgestrel may interfere with the process of ovulation, fertilization or implantation, depending on the cycle day of unprotected sex and the day on which treatment is initiated. Contraindications to the use of this emergency contraceptive are undiagnosed vaginal bleeding and known allergy to any ingredient.[26] If this emergency contraceptive is used in an existing pregnancy, the pregnancy is not terminated and the fetus is unharmed.[26] The side effects of levonorgestrel are well-characterized, mild to moderate, and self-resolving. Common side effects include nausea, vomiting, dizziness, fatigue, headache, breast tenderness, lower abdominal pain and menstrual irregularities. Levonorgestrel has a significantly lower incidence of side effects compared with combination-method emergency contraceptives.

Emergency contraception should be considered a back-up method for occasional rather than regular use and is intended to be used shortly after sex but before pregnancy has become established. The cost of an unintended pregnancy in women of all ages is estimated as $3795 in a managed-care setting and $1680 in a publicly funded programme; depending on the regimen of emergency contraception used, how it is dispensed, and the health care setting, emergency contraception could save public and managed-care health services between $19 and $498 per year per woman.[26] In addition, modelling suggests obtaining emergency contraception directly from a pharmacy, rather than from a physician or clinic, would save $48 to $158.[26] It should be noted that fears that expanded access to emergency contraception would be associated with increased sexual risk-taking behaviour, or less consistent use of traditional birth control methods, appear groundless.[27]

When contraception fails: preparing for parenthood

In the event of a continuing pregnancy, the following screening procedures are recommended:[3]

* blood typing and antibody screening for all women at their first prenatal visit. Repeat antibody screening is recommended for unsensitized D(Rh)-negative women

* blood pressure measurement to screen for pre-eclampsia at the first prenatal visit and periodically throughout pregnancy

* amniocentesis or chorionic villus sampling for chromosomes studies should be offered to women at high risk of Down syndrome

* maternal serum α-fetoprotein measurement for neural tube defects for all pregnant women who have adequate follow-up services. Folate, in view of its importance in DNA replication, may be important in preventing diverse congenital defects including neural tube defects, cleft palate and cleft lip. Multivitamins with a folic acid content of at least 0.4 mg should be taken daily 1 or more months before conception and continued until the end of the third trimester to reduce the risk of neural tube defects in all women who are planning or capable of pregnancy. In women who have previously had a pregnancy affected by a neural tube defect, the dose of folic acid supplementation should be increased to 1–4 mg/day. The time when folate deficiency may have greatest clinical effect is around 28 days after conception.

All pregnant women should be screened for hepatitis B, HIV, and syphilis; pregnant women at increased risk should be also screened for chlamydial infection and gonorrhoea.

Routine ultrasound examination of the fetus in the third trimester is not recommended. There is insufficient evidence to recommend for or against routine ultrasound screening in the second trimester in low-risk pregnant women. Routine electronic fetal monitoring for low-risk women in labour is also not recommended.

Maternal nutrition is important for the mother and child. Both conception and development of the fetus and neonate is influenced by maternal nutrition during:

* the periconceptional period. Adequate folate is important to prevent congenital defects. See **Handout 9.10**

- pregnancy. The prenatal period is critical for future health and functioning of mother and child. It can be disturbed by undernutrition, a mismatch between prenatal 'programming' by undernutrition and postnatal overconsumption, or by overconsumption/overweight.[28] Intrauterine undernutrition appears to predispose some individuals to insulin resistance and the metabolic syndrome in later life.[29] Low birth weight infants at greatest risk of future cardiovascular diseases, hypertension, dyslipidaemia and type 2 diabetes are those who experience rapid postnatal growth. Healthy in utero programming may be achieved by individual maternal assessment and follow-up coupled with multinutrient supplementation – including iron, zinc, iodine, choline, and long-chain polyunsaturated fatty acids.[28] A case–control study of mothers without anaemia delivering a singleton infant of less than 2500 g showed supplementation with 80 mg ferrous sulphate appeared to lower the risk of low birth weight infants.[30] Docosahexaenoic acid (DHA), an important component of neural and retinal membranes, rapidly accumulates in the brain during gestation and the postnatal period.[31] Positive associations have been shown between the offspring's visual and cognitive development and maternal intake of fish, seafood and omega-3 fatty acids during pregnancy and/or lactation. Maternal DHA intake appears to prolong gestation and reduce the risk of preterm delivery both in low-risk and in high-risk pregnancies. It is recommended that women of reproductive age should achieve an average dietary DHA intake of at least 200 mg/day. However, the minimal threshold for maternal fish intake during pregnancy to achieve beneficial developmental and behavioural outcomes appears to be more than two fish meals, totalling at least 340 g, per week.[32]

In contrast to the benefits of nutritional perspicacity, alcohol and nicotine impair fetal growth. Smoking impairs fetal nutrition as nicotine compromises placental perfusion and carbon monoxide diminishes oxygenation. The impact of alcohol is even more devastating. MicroRNAs (miRNAs) are a class of 18–25 nucleotides long, endogenous, non-coding RNA molecules that post-transcriptionally regulate protein-coding mRNA. MicroRNAs mediate gene silencing by binding to specific target sites within mRNA either to block translation or to bring about degradation of transcripts. These effects can be subtle and in a number of instances result in 'fine-tuning' of gene expression.[33] Animal studies suggest that ethanol treatment affects miRNAs, induces fetal teratogenesis in mice and causes mental retardation in their offspring, both lowering locomotor activity and impairing task acquisition,[34] Normal miRNAs may be required to maintain neuronal integrity.[33] **Handout 9.11** provides some dietary self-care guidelines.

- lactation. There are advantages to breastfeeding for both mother and offspring. In addition to bonding, breast milk concentrates vitamin C, calcium, various B vitamins, vitamin A and carotene. It is also an important source of omega-3 fatty acids. Breast milk is a good source of nutrition for neonates, nonetheless, it should be remembered that alcohol and certain drugs may be secreted in breast milk. See **Handout 9.13**.

Nutrition is also important for the mother. Weight gain during pregnancy should be between 9 and 13 kg. Pregnancy requires an additional 334,880 kJ (80,000 kcal). After the first month, this amounts to 1255 kJ (300 kcal) per day. As dietary restriction during the second half of pregnancy results in a lower than average birth weight infant, mothers should ingest an additional 600 kJ per day during the second and third trimesters of pregnancy. Any increased energy consumption during pregnancy should be directed at foods rich in those nutrients for which there is increased demand, e.g. dairy products rich in calcium, dietary sources of iron. Exclusive breast-feeding for 6 months facilitates postpartum loss of approximately 12 kg of gestational weight gain.[35]

The most prevalent minor complaints of pregnancy, viz. heartburn, constipation and nausea, may be modified by nutritional means. Constipation may by minimized by eating a diet rich in whole grains, fruit, vegetables, nuts and other fibre-rich foods; heartburn by eating small meals more frequently. See **Handout 9.12**.

Sexually transmitted infections (STIs)

In addition to unwanted pregnancy, sexually transmitted infection may be another consequence of unsafe sex. Despite sex education in schools and colleges, the rate of STI between 1996 and 1997 increased in the UK, particularly amongst teenagers.[36]

American teenagers are also at risk. In the US, 53% of high-school students sampled in 1993 reported sexual intercourse; only 52% of these had used a condom at last intercourse.[36] The Centers for Disease Control and Prevention (CDC) estimates that 19 million new infections occur annually in the US, almost one half of which occur in persons 15 to 24 years of age.[37] All adolescent and adult patients should be advised about risk factors for STIs and counselled appropriately about effective measures to reduce the risk of infection.

Orange flags for STIs

Since 2000, the USPSTF has issued eight clinical recommendation statements on screening for sexually transmitted infections.[38] However, routine screening for STIs is not considered necessary in non-pregnant women and men who are not at increased risk. Intervention is particularly targeted at persons with high-risk sexual behaviours.[39] **Handout 13.3** provides a self-screen for risky sexual behaviour. Counselling should be tailored to the individual. In men who have sex with men, it is important to focus on high-risk sexual behaviour and not on sexual orientation. Assessment of risk is based on a careful sexual and drug-use history. The local STI epidemiology should be taken into consideration.

Essential sexual history questions when females present complaining of a vaginal discharge or males complain of urethritis are:

- Are you sexually active?
- How many partners of the opposite sex have you had in the past 3 months and 12 months?
- How many partners of the same sex have you had in the past 3 months and 12 months?
- How many sexual partners have you had in your lifetime?
- Describe your condom use in the last 3 months.

Sexual history includes questions about number of current and past sexual partners, current and previous sexual practices, e.g. anal sex, current and previous illicit drug use, history of prior STI, and the use of condoms or other barrier protection. Females also need to be able to distinguish a normal from an abnormal vaginal discharge. A normal vaginal discharge is a characteristically whitish mucoid discharge accompanied by a vaginal wall transudate which varies from increased moisture during ovulation and premenstrually to thick and mucousy at ovulation.

Handout 13.4 ranks the safety of various sexual behaviours and **Handout 13.5** provides guidelines for practising safe sex. Patients at risk of STIs should receive information on their risk and be advised about measures to reduce their risk. **Handout 13.6** alerts patients to findings suggestive of an STI and indicates the need for professional advice.

Risk reduction

In addition to avoiding exposure due to high-risk behaviours, certain contraceptive methods protect against STIs. High-risk sexual behaviours that should be avoided include having multiple current partners, having a new partner, using condoms inconsistently, having sex while under the influence of alcohol or drugs, and having sex in exchange for money or drugs.[39] Contraceptive measures that offer a degree of protection are spermicides and female barrier methods, e.g. the diaphragm or cervical cap. These reduce the risk of bacterial or chlamydial infection, but are unlikely to be effective against viral transmission. Condoms are the most effective barrier form of STI protection. The degree of risk is enormously reduced by *appropriate* condom use.

Male condoms are made of latex (rubber), polyurethane, or of natural membrane made of sheep intestine. Natural skin condoms are not as effective as latex condoms as they have pores large enough for viruses, but not sperm, to penetrate. Only latex condoms labelled for protection against STIs should be used for disease protection. If one of the partners is allergic to latex, a polyurethane condom can be used. For condoms to be effective, they must be used correctly. **Handout 13.2** provides a checklist for appropriate and safe condom use. Latex condoms are the only form of contraception shown to be highly effective in protecting against the transmission of HIV and other STIs; but their effectiveness is greatly influenced by the way they are stored and used. Despite being effective, condoms are not routinely used; a 1999–2001 UK study found that 38% of men and 48% of women who had had one or more sexual partner in the previous 4 weeks had not used a condom at all.[40] Fortuitously, condoms are the contraceptive method preferred by teenagers.

STIs

The USPSTF recommends that women at increased risk of infection be screened for chlamydia and gonorrhoea and that all sexually active women younger than 25 years be considered at increased risk of these STIs.[38] Compared with older women, younger women are at increased risk of gonorrhoea and chlamydial infection because they may have more new sex partners and because of the relative immaturity of their immune systems and the columnar epithelium lining the adolescent exocervix. In view of the benefits (improved fertility, pregnancy outcomes, and infection transmission) versus the harms (anxiety, relationship problems, and unnecessary treatment of false-positive results) of chlamydial screening, the USPSTF additionally recommends screening for chlamydial infection in older pregnant women who are at increased risk.[41] An estimated 2.8 million new chlamydial infections occur in the US annually.[39]

In view of the ability of asymptomatic carriers to reinfect their partners and spread particular organisms, it is essential that partners of any individual diagnosed with an STI be contacted and treated. As STIs are not always symptomatic, awareness of risky behaviour should act as an orange flag. Asymptomatic persons under 25 years of age who inconsistently use a barrier contraceptive, have changed their sexual partners in the last 6 months, and/or have had contact or infection with another sexually transmitted disease are at particular risk of infection and may be asymptomatic carriers. Male partners asymptomatically house *Trichomonas vaginalis* in their seminal vesicles; their female partners present with a recurrent frothy greenish discharge with dysuria. In contrast, both chlamydial and gonococcal infections are symptomatic in males, and females are asymptomatic carriers. Males present with urethritis. They complain of dysuria and, in the case of gonorrhoea, a urethral discharge is present. As these conditions are symptomatic in males, routine male screening for chlamydia and gonorrhoea is not indicated. In contrast, all individuals at increased risk should be screened for syphilis.[38] While men with primary syphilis may be diagnosed by the presence of a penile chancre, in women the chancre is often hidden.

Self-screening for sexually transmitted disease is advisable for all persons who have had unprotected sex. By recognizing the early signs and symptoms of infection, females may for example avoid pelvic inflammatory disease with distortion of the genital tract and subsequent tubal pregnancies or infertility. Red flags indicating the need for professional evaluation are listed in **Handout 13.6** and common findings associated with many of the prevalent STIs are provided in **Handout 13.7**. Each of the prevalent STIs has its own characteristics.

Viral causes of STIs are difficult to treat. Nonetheless, the USPSTF recommended that all individuals at increased risk should be screened for HIV, while the CDC in 2006 recommended that all persons 13 to 64 years of age be screened for HIV, regardless of risk status.[38,41] Persons whose lifestyle choices increase their risk of exposure to HIV should be tested to reduce the likelihood of their being a source of community infection.

However, even when at-risk individuals submit to laboratory testing, inherent limitations of laboratory-based testing can lead to the failure to identify infected individuals. Limitations include the window between infection and the generation of detectable antibodies and the limited sensitivities of certain antibody tests. The turnaround time of laboratory-based testing further delays patients obtaining test results. Point-of-care or rapid testing attempts to overcome this latter problem. Rapid tests are easy to perform and can give conclusive results within minutes. The OraQuick HIV-1/2 Test, a qualitative immunochromatographic test for the detection of antibodies to HIV-1 and HIV-2, was compared with a conventional enzyme immunoassay (EIA)/Western blot (WB) and found to have 100% sensitivity and specificity.[42] A later UK study largely confirmed these results, reporting OraQuick's sensitivity to be 93.64%, later corrected to 100%; specificity, 99.87%; positive predictive value, 97.78%; and negative predictive value, 99.61%.[43] Of the four current FDA-cleared rapid tests for HIV-specific antibodies, all were found to detect IgG antibodies but only the Uni-Gold Recombigen test was capable of potentially also detecting IgM.[44] As IgM antibodies are the initial antibody response mounted, this test offers a more sensitive option for early detection of infection.

While failure to detect infectious individuals hampers efforts to limit spread of the disease, the psychological cost of false positives is of concern. In fact, even though the incidence of false-positive results is less than 0.005% using combined enzyme immunoassay screening tests and the confirmatory Western blot test, routine screening of a population of 100,000 will result in five non-infected persons being incorrectly diagnosed. The psychological cost of a false-positive test in a low-risk person is deemed to outweigh any possible benefit derived from screening the general population.

Handout 13.8 provides a quiz for patients to check the accuracy of their perceptions regarding acquired immunodeficiency syndrome (AIDS) and spread of this virus. AIDS is the end stage of chronic infection with HIV. There is no effective means of killing the virus once it has infected the host's cells – drugs have difficulty discriminating between viral and host nucleic acids; neither is there currently a means of killing the virus before it infects the host's cells. No vaccine is yet available. End-stage AIDS is fatal usually because the patient cannot overcome intercurrent infections. The immune system of the AIDS patient is so devastated by the AIDS virus that organisms incapable of causing significant infections in healthy people kill AIDS patients. The AIDS virus creates an environment in which opportunistic infections are prevalent. Although drugs capable of impairing the proliferation of these opportunists are available, the host's immune system is incapable of utilizing this assistance to eliminate the infecting organisms. Some individuals appear to have some natural resistance to infection.

One of the most common viral STIs is genital herpes. There are approximately 1.6 million new genital herpes infections annually in the US.[37] In some populations it is thought that at least 20% are infected even though only one-quarter of these have a clinical history. Recurrence of genital herpes due to herpes simplex virus type 1 (HSV-1) occurs an average of once each year; persons with HSV-2 average four recurrences annually. Recurrences affect half of the individuals infected; this may increase to 80% in HSV-2 infection. The annual risk of transmission of genital herpes from an infected partner in a heterosexual couple is 10%. Viral shedding and transmission occur in the absence of genital lesions. See **Handout 13.7**.

Female problems

Sexual activity, in addition to increasing the likelihood of pregnancy and possible exposure to genital infection, may increase the risk of certain genital cancers in females.[45] Cervical cancer is a case in point.

Cervical cancer

All sexually active women between the ages of 18 and 70 are advised to have regular Pap smears. Cervical dysplasia, which may precede pre-invasive neoplastic changes in the cervix, is usually detected on a routine Pap smear. In the UK, a comprehensive cervical screening programme based on cervical cytology is considered to have prevented an epidemic of cervical cancer and projected to have reduced mortality by up to 80%.[46]

A protocol to reduce the risk of cervical dysplasia suggests avoiding:

- first intercourse at an early age
- multiple sexual partners
- HSV-2 exposure
- human papillomavirus (HPV). Persons with condylomata acuminata on the genitalia or a sexually transmitted infection such as herpes, chlamydia or gonorrhoea may also be infected with HPV
- smoking. Smoking doubles or triples the risk of cervical dysplasia. Smoking appears to induce an impaired antibody response to HPV types 16 and 18 in infected women under the age of 30 years[47]
- a high-fat diet. Diets that may reduce the risk of cervical cancer are low in fat and rich in fruit and vegetables.[48] Folic acid, 5 mg twice a day, may also be beneficial.

While abstinence offers good protection, this can scarcely be considered a viable option. In addition to condom use, which offers some protection, vaccination has now become a consideration.[48] Highest prevalence rates for HPV infection are seen following the onset of sexual activity; consequently, vaccination prior to sexual debut is needed. Since 20% of adolescents are sexually active at the age of 14 years, vaccination at the age of 10–12 years has been proposed. Antibody titres following vaccination in girls 12–16 years of age have been shown to be significantly higher than in older women. Two vaccines based on the L1 capsid protein of HPV types 16 and 18 have demonstrated almost 100% efficiency in preventing persistent infection and related HPV pre-malignancy with these viruses in late-stage trials. HPV vaccination in adolescence with continued cervical screening could ultimately lead to a 76% lifetime reduction in cervical cancer deaths after many years and a 50% reduction in cervical screening abnormalities if high coverage of vaccination was achieved.

See Chapter 25 for further information on female cancer.

Premenstrual tension/premenstrual dysphoric disorder

Over 50% of woman experience psychological, physical and/or vegetative symptoms over the course of their menstrual cycle.[49] Symptoms progressively increase in severity, rising to a peak in the 5 days prior to onset of menses. Psychological symptoms predominate and include anger/irritability, anxiety/tension, and mood symptoms. Physical symptoms range from breast tenderness and bloating to increased headache or other pains. Vegetative symptoms such as overeating and oversleeping are reported. Premenstrual tension (PMS), the milder version of this condition, is often self-managed with a variety of lifestyle interventions. Dietary changes include eating more frequent high complex carbohydrate meals and reducing consumption of salt, coffee, chocolate, refined sugar and alcohol. **Handout 13.9** provides some unproven dietary suggestions. Aerobic exercise, relaxation therapy and various stress management techniques may be tried.

Premenstrual dysphoric disorder (PMDD), which presents with severe symptoms during the luteal phase of the menstrual cycle, requires drug intervention. It occurs in an estimated 2% to 9% of menstruating women.[50] Women who develop PMDD appear to have an underlying genetic vulnerability involving the central nervous system neurotransmitter systems, most notably the serotonergic system. Serotonergic dysregulation is possibly triggered by cyclic changes in gonadal steroids. Certainly, many of the typical symptoms of PMDD, such as irritability and poor impulse control, depressed mood, and carbohydrate craving, have been linked to serotonergic dysfunction. Changes in gonadal steroids that occur during the luteal phase appear to amplify any underlying serotonin dysregulation. Treatment with serotonin reuptake inhibitors throughout the menstrual cycle is highly effective in some people. However, as 40% of women with PMDD do not respond to selective serotonin reuptake inhibitors, combined oral contraceptives are being investigated due to their ovulation-suppression effects.[51] A screening test for PMDD is available.[50]

Menopause

Menopause is a physiological phenomenon that leaves women in a state of oestrogen deprivation. The nature and intensity of menopausal symptoms varies in different women and is related to oestrogen fluctuation. Menopause characterized by the permanent cessation of menstrual periods occurs naturally in women, usually in their early 50s. In the US, most women experience menopause between 40 and 58 years of age, with a median age of 52 years.[52] In the UK, the mean age for menopause is 50 years and 9 months.[53] Factors associated with earlier menopause include lower body weight, menstrual length, nulliparity, smoking, never-use of oral contraceptives, lower socioeconomic status, and race or ethnicity. Higher body weight is associated with later onset of menopause.

Menopause passes through a number of phases.[52] Perimenopause or the climacteric, which lasts on average 4 years, includes the menopausal transition, i.e. late reproductive stage and entry into postmenopause, and overlaps the first 12 months of postmenopause. The menopausal transition concludes with the final menstrual period and the beginning of postmenopause. It is characterized by an increase in follicle-stimulating hormone and increased variability in cycle length, two skipped menstrual cycles with 60 or more days of amenorrhoea, or both. Postmenopause begins at the time of the final menstrual period, although it is not recognized until after 12 months of amenorrhoea. Many women have few or no symptoms; others need medical treatment. Table 13.1 summarizes the estimated prevalence of symptoms experienced by woman at various stage of their life cycle.[52]

Most menopausal symptoms can be classified as either physical or psychological. Although it is difficult to differentiate between symptoms truly associated with menopause and those due to ageing, hot flushes, night sweats, and vaginal dryness are clearly tied to the menopausal transition, as is irregular vaginal bleeding secondary to erratic ovulation.

Vasomotor symptoms present with hot flushes, night sweats, palpitations, insomnia, dizziness and headaches or migraine. Women with hot flushes are more likely to experience disturbed sleep, depressive symptoms and significant reductions in quality of life. Hot flushes typically last between 6 months and 5 years after natural menopause, but may persist for as long as 15 years.[53] They occur with the pulsatile release of luteinizing hormone and are characterized by sweating on the face, neck and chest, as well as peripheral vasodilatation. Accompanying the acute rise in the skin temperature of several degrees centigrade, there is a transient increase in heart rate. Symptoms usually last for 4–5 minutes. Oestrogen virtually eliminates hot

Table 13.1 Symptom prevalence

	Premenopause	Perimenopause	Postmenopause
Menstrual cycle	Regular frequency and duration	Erratic	Amenorrhoea
Symptom prevalence			
Vasomotor	14–51%	35–50%	30–80%
Sleep disturbance	16–42%	39–47%	35–60%
Vaginal dryness	16–42%	7–39%	17–30%
Urinary symptoms	10–36%	17–39%	15–36%
Mood changes	8–37%	11–21%	8–38%

flushes but its mechanism of action is unknown. Hot flushes disturb sleep.

Oestrogen and progesterone receptors are found throughout the urogenital tract and are sensitive to menopausal hormonal changes.[53] The vaginal epithelium becomes less cellular and thinner. There is progressive loss of vascularity in the vaginal mucosa. The vagina loses elasticity, shortens, narrows and becomes less distensible. Loss of cellular glycogen and decreased lactic acid change the pH of the vagina from a more acidic environment (pH 4/5) in the premenopausal state to a more alkaline environment (pH 6–8) in the postmenopausal state. All of these changes can cause vaginal irritation, dryness, dyspareunia, vulvovaginal itching, dysuria, frequency and urgency, incontinence, decreased libido and increased susceptibility to infection. Symptoms are noticed months to years after menopause and persist for life. Other complaints include emotional lability, dry skin and hair, joint and limb pains and formication. Women experience a sensation of insects such as ants running over the skin. Biological, psychological and social factors all contribute to the symptom picture in menopause.

Low-dose oestrogen (0.3 mg equivalent), either by itself or with progestins, is the most consistently effective therapy for urogenital and vasomotor symptoms, and the associated sleep disturbance.[52,54] Hormone replacement therapy (HRT) is highly effective at alleviating hot flushes, reducing their frequency by 77%.[53] However, oestrogen therapy at doses equivalent to 0.625 mg of conjugated equine oestrogen increases the risk for serious disease events – specifically, stroke, deep venous thrombosis and/or pulmonary embolism, and, when combined with the progestin medroxyprogesterone acetate, coronary events and breast cancer. Meta-analyses of numerous observational studies and the Women's Health Initiative (WHI) trial confirmed an increased risk of ischaemic heart disease, stroke, thromboembolic events and breast cancer after 5 or more years of HRT.[55] Short-term therapy for vasomotor symptoms therefore appeared a viable option. However, it has more recently been suggested that the increased risks for coronary and thromboembolic events start to emerge in the first year of HRT use; risks for stroke start to increase after 2 years of use; and risks for breast cancer start to increase after 3 to 4 years of use.[52] However, as hot flushes and night sweats are amongst the most bothersome symptoms of menopause and do respond to oestrogen, low-dose oestrogen for less than 5 years deserves consideration in severely affected women. Oestrogen should be used only when lifestyle changes such as relaxation techniques, regular physical activity, weight loss and smoking cessation; and nutraceuticals, including soy isoflavones, red clover isoflavones, black cohosh and vitamin E, have failed.[56] Phytoestrogens in soy products bind weakly to oestrogen receptors and do have a pro-oestrogenic effect in postmenopausal women. The increased risk of incident and fatal breast cancer appears to be substantially greater for oestrogen–progestogen combinations than for other types of HRT.[57] Furthermore, newer classes of antidepressants, selective serotonin reuptake inhibitors, and serotonin and noradrenaline (norepinephrine) reuptake inhibitors show some promising early results for the treatment of vasomotor symptoms.

HRT in postmenopausal women, in addition to relieving menopausal symptoms, reduces the risk of an osteoporotic fracture. Especially when combined with exercise, oestrogen aids remodelling of the skeleton and enhances repair of microfractures. HRT may halve the risk of fractures of the spine, wrist and hip for as long as therapy is continued. HRT also lowers lipoprotein(a) levels and reduces total and LDL-cholesterol. Lipoprotein(a) impedes the dissolution of blood clots and LDL-cholesterol predisposes to atheroma. Long-term use of HRT, however, substantially increases other health risks. Thus, HRT is a therapeutic option with risks and benefits (see **Handout 13.10**). Controversy continues and concern persists. The use of HRT is ultimately the patient's decision; patients need to weigh up the evidence and make an informed choice (see **Handout 13.11**). Patients who reject the HRT option may want to consider dietary changes (see **Handout 13.12**).

Dyspareunia

Painful intercourse may be attributable to psychological or medical factors. Dyspareunia may be superficial or deep. Postmenopausal women may experience pain on intercourse due to urogenital atrophy. Young woman may experience superficial dyspareunia due to muscle spasm (vaginismus) attributable to fear of intercourse or its potential consequences.

Vulvar vestibulitis syndrome is believed to be the most common form of premenopausal dyspareunia and is characterized by severe pain upon vestibular touch or attempted vaginal entry, exquisite tenderness to cotton-swab palpation of the vulvar vestibule, and physical findings limited to vulvar erythema. Overall, women with vestibulodynia demonstrate lower levels of sexual desire, arousal, and frequency of intercourse.[58] They are also prone to anxiety, fear of pain, hypervigilance, catastrophizing, and depression. Childhood physical and sexual abuse are potential risk factors for the development of this condition.

Other medical causes of superficial dyspareunia include an episiotomy scar, genital herpes and candida infection.

Deep dyspareunia may be associated with pelvic endometriosis, cervicitis, chronic salpingitis, retroversion of the uterus, an ovarian cyst, a prolapsed ovary, posterior fibroids or cancer of the cervix.

Handout 13.13 provides a self-screen for patients with dyspareunia.

More information on female sexual dysfunction is available on the Internet;[59] as is other general and specific information about women's health.[60]

Male problems

Routine screening for male genital cancers is somewhat disputed, with Cancer Societies favouring more extreme measures. Although routine screening for prostate cancer with digital examination, serum tumour markers such as prostate-specific antigen, or transrectal ultrasound is not recommended by the USPTF,[3] Cancer Societies advise asymptomatic men over the age of 40 years to have a rectal examination for prostatic carcinoma. Extensive information on men's health can be obtained from the Internet.[61]

Testis self-examination

There is insufficient evidence to recommend for or against routine screening of asymptomatic men for testicular cancer either by physician or by self-examination;[3] nonetheless, the testis, like the breast, is a hormonal target organ. Testicular cancer is extremely rare before the age of 20 and after the age of 60 years. It is, however, a common cancer in white males between the ages of 20 and 34 years. The lifetime risk of developing the disease is substantially higher than the risk of dying from the disease. Detection and removal of a cancer localized to the testis results in cure. Furthermore, in most cases, only one testis is affected and orchidectomy does not impair sexual function.

While some authors feel there is insufficient evidence for routine periodic testicular examination,[62] some health authorities suggest annual and others monthly self-palpation.[63] Monthly self-examinations are certainly recommended for men at increased risk of the disease. Men at increased risk of testicular cancer are those with a family history of testicular cancer and/or a personal history of undescended testes. Regular self-examination should be initiated at puberty. The testicles should be examined after a warm bath or shower. **Handout 13.14** outlines the steps in testicular self-examination. For more information, refer to the Internet.[64]

Impotence

Impotence is the inability of a male to achieve an erection of sufficient quality to achieve satisfactory sexual intercourse. Erectile dysfunction affects 1 in

10 males. Impotence may be due to physical or psychological factors. Psychological causes are common and stress is often implicated. Performance anxiety and relationship problems also need to be considered. Patients with psychogenic causes of impotence usually have normal erections at night, in the early morning and during masturbation. Although they have a good erection, they are unable to maintain it. Psychogenic impotence is often sudden in onset and associated with underlying performance anxiety or a relationship problem. Impotence may only be experienced with a particular partner.

Medical causes of impotence include vascular disease, diabetes, injury and drugs. Antihypertensive agents, psychotropic drugs, digoxin, high-dose steroids and hypolipidaemic agents are all recognized causes of impotence.

Handout 13.15 provides a self-screen for patients with impotence and the Internet provides information on erectile dysfunction.[65]

In perspective

Sexual health goes beyond using birth control and avoiding STIs. It is a global construct grounded in a healthy lifestyle.[66]

References

1. Press Release WHO/86 on 16 Nov 1998. http://www.who.int/inf-pr-1998/en/pr98-86.html; Acccessed 20.12.08.
2. Henshaw SK. Unintended pregnancy in the United States. *Fam Plann Perspect*. 30:1998;24–299(46).
3. U.S. Preventive Services Task Force. *Guide to Clinical Preventive Services*. 2nd ed Baltimore: Williams & Wilkins; 1996.
4. Singh R, Frost J, Jordan B, Wells E. Beyond a prescription: strategies for improving contraceptive care. *Contraception*. 2009;71:1–4.
5. Office for National Statistics. Contraception and sexual health 2007/08. http://www.statistics.gov.uk/STATBASE/Product.asp?vlnk=6988p; Accessed 19.12.08.
6. Qureshi M, Attaran M. Review of newer contraceptive agents. *Cleve Clin J Med*. 1999;66(6):358–366.
7. Rosen AD, Rosen T. Study of condom integrity after brief exposure to over-the-counter vaginal preparations. *South Med J*. 1999;92:305–307.
8. Kubba A. Key developments in family planning. *Practitioner*. 1997;241:604–605.
9. Office for National Statistics. *Contraception & sexual behaviour*. http://www.statistics.gov.uk/cci/nugget.asp?id=326; Accessed 19.12.08.
10. Bagshaw S. The combined OC. *Curr Ther*. 1994;35:49–56.
11. Piegsa K. A GP's guide to choosing combined Pills. *Practitioner*. 1999;244:462–472.
12. Archer DF, Maheux R, DelConte A, O'Brien FB. Efficacy and safety of a low-dose monophasic combination oral contraceptive containing 100 µg levonorgestrel and 20 µg ethinyl estradiol (Alesse). *Am J Obstet Gynecol*. 1999;181(5 Pt 2):39–44.
13. Shulman LP. Oral contraception: safety issues re-examined. *Int J Fertil Womens Med*. 1999;44(2):78–82.
14. Sihvo S, Hemminki E, Kosunen E. Contraceptive health risks – women's perceptions. *J Psychosom Obstet Gynaecol*. 1998;19(3):117–125.
15. Burkman R, Schlesselman JJ, Zieman M. Safety concerns and health benefits associated with oral contraception. *Am J Obstet Gynecol*. 2004;190(4 suppl):S5–S22.
16. Tate P. Minimising the risk in contraception. *Practitioner*. 1997;241:571–580.
17. Kimble-Haas SL. The intrauterine device: dispelling the myths. *Nurse Pract*. 1998;23(11):58 63–69, 74.
18. Canavan TP. Appropriate use of the intrauterine device. *Am Fam Physician*. 1998;58(9):2077–2084, 2087–2088.
19. Frank E. Contraceptive use by female physicians in the United States. *Obstet Gynecol*. 1999;94(5 Pt 1):666–671.
20. Casey PM, Pruthi S. The latest contraceptive options: what you must know. *J Fam Pract*. 2008;57(12):797–805.
21. Kost K, Singh S, Vaughan B, Trussell J, Bankole A. Estimates of contraceptive failure from the 2002 National Survey of Family Growth. *Contraception*. 2008;77:10–21.
22. Trussell J, Lalla AM, Doan QV, Reyes E, Pinto L, Gricar J. Cost effectiveness of contraceptives in the United States. *Contraception*. 2009;71:5–14.
23. Abma JC, Martinez GM, Mosher WD, Dawson BS. Teenagers in the United States: sexual activity, contraceptive use, and childbearing, 2002. *Vital Health Stat*. 2004;23:1–48.
24. Leung VW, Soon JA, Levine M. Emergency contraception update: a Canadian perspective. *Clin Pharmacol Ther*. 2008;83(1):177–180.
25. Harper CC, Weiss DC, Speidel JJ, Raine-Bennett T. Over-the-counter access to emergency contraception for teens. *Contraception*. 2008;77(4):230–233.
26. Camp SL, Wilkerson DS, Raine TR. The benefits and risks of over-the-counter availability of levonorgestrel emergency contraception. *Contraception*. 2003;68(5):309–317.
27. Ziebarth A, Hansen KA. Hormonal emergency contraception: a clinical primer. *S D Med*. 2007;60(3):99–101, 103–105.

28. Shapira N. Prenatal nutrition: a critical window of opportunity for mother and child. *Womens Health (Lond Engl)*. 2008;4:639–656.

29. Beltrand J, Lévy-Marchal C. Pathophysiology of insulin resistance in subjects born small for gestational age. *Best Pract Res Clin Endocrinol Metab*. 2008;22 (3):503–515.

30. Palma S, Perez-Iglesias R, Prieto D, Pardo R, Llorca J, Delgado-Rodriguez M. Iron but not folic acid supplementation reduces the risk of low birthweight in pregnant women without anaemia: a case-control study. *J Epidemiol Community Health*. 2008;62(2):120–124.

31. Cetin I, Koletzko B. Long-chain omega-3 fatty acid supply in pregnancy and lactation. *Curr Opin Clin Nutr Metab Care*. 2008;11 (3):297–302.

32. Makrides M. Outcomes for mothers and their babies: do n-3 long-chain polyunsaturated fatty acids and seafoods make a difference? *J Am Diet Assoc*. 2008;108 (10):1622–1626.

33. Saba R, Goodman CD, Huzarewich RL, Robertson C, Booth SA. A miRNA signature of prion induced neurodegeneration. *PLoS ONE*. 2008;3(11):e3652.

34. Wang LL, Zhang Z, Li Q, et al. Ethanol exposure induces differential microRNA and target gene expression and teratogenic effects which can be suppressed by folic acid supplementation. *Hum Reprod*. 2009;24(3):562–579.

35. Baker JL, Gamborg M, Heitmann BL, Lissner L, Sørensen TI, Rasmussen KM. Breastfeeding reduces postpartum weight retention. *Am J Clin Nutr*. 2008;88(6):1543–1551.

36. Hughes G, Simms I, Rogers PA, Swan AV, Catchpole M. New cases seen at genitourinary medicine clinics: England 1997. *Commun Dis Rep CDR Suppl*. 1998;8(7):S1–S11.

37. Weinstock H, Berman S, Cates Jr W. Sexually transmitted diseases among American youth: incidence and prevalence estimates, 2000. *Perspect Sex Reprod Health*. 2004;36(1):6–10.

38. Meyers D, Wolff T, Gregory K, et al. USPSTF. USPSTF recommendations for STI screening.

Am Fam Physician. 2008;77 (6):819–824.

39. USPSTF. *Recommendations for STI screening* http://www.ahrq.gov/clinic/uspstf08/methods/stinfections.htm; Accessed 19.12.08.

40. Data from the National Survey of Sexual Attitudes and Lifestyles 2000. Use of condoms in the previous four weeks: by number of new partners of the opposite sex, 1999–2001: Social Trends 34 http://www.statistics.gov.uk/cci/nscl.asp?id=6314; Accessed 19.12.08.

41. U.S. Preventive Services Task Force. Screening for chlamydial infection: U.S. Preventive Services Task Force recommendation statement. *Ann Intern Med*. 2007;147(2):128–134.

42. Reynolds SJ, Ndongala LM, Luo CC, et al. Evaluation of a rapid test for the detection of antibodies to human immunodeficiency virus type 1 and 2 in the setting of multiple transmitted viral subtypes. *Int J STI AIDS*. 2002;13 (3):171–173.

43. Zelin J, Garrett N, Saunders J, et al. An evaluation of the performance of OraQuick ADVANCE Rapid HIV-1/2 Test in a high-risk population attending genitourinary medicine clinics in East London, UK. *Int J STI AIDS*. 2008;19(10):665–667.

44. Louie B, Wong E, Klausner JD, et al. Assessment of rapid tests for detection of human immunodeficiency virus-specific antibodies in recently infected individuals. *J Clin Microbiol*. 2008;46(4):1494–1497.

45. Growdon WB, Del Carmen M. Human papillomavirus-related gynecologic neoplasms: screening and prevention. *Rev Obstet Gynecol*. 2008;1(4):154–161.

46. Peto J, Gilham C, Fletcher O, Mathews FE. The cervical cancer epidemic that screening prevented in the UK. *Lancet*. 2004;364 (9430):249–256.

47. Simen-Kapeu A, Kataja V, Yliskoski M, et al. Smoking impairs human papillomavirus (HPV) type 16 and 18 capsids antibody response following natural HPV infection. *Scand J Infect Dis*. 2008;40 (9):745–751.

48. Adams M, Jasani B, Fiander A. Human papilloma virus (HPV) prophylactic vaccination: challenges for public health and implications for screening. *Vaccine*. 2007;25 (16):3007–3013.

49. Pearlstein T, Yonkers KA, Fayyad R, Gillespie JA. Pretreatment pattern of symptom expression in premenstrual dysphoric disorder. *J Affect Disord*. 2005;85(3):275–282.

50. Freeman EW, Sondheimer SJ. Premenstrual dysphoric disorder: recognition and treatment. *Prim Care Companion J Clin Psychiatry*. 2003;5(1):30–39.

51. Halbreich U. Selective serotonin reuptake inhibitors and initial oral contraceptives for the treatment of PMDD: effective but not enough. *CNS Spectr*. 2008;13(7):566–572.

52. NIH State-of-the-Science Conference Statement on management of menopause-related symptoms. *NIH Consens State Sci Statements*. 2005;22(1):1–38.

53. Bruce D, Rymer J. Symptoms of the menopause. *Best Pract Res Clin Obstet Gynaecol*. 2009;23 (1):25–32.

54. Bhavnani BR, Strickler RC. Menopausal hormone therapy. *J Obstet Gynaecol Can*. 2005;27 (2):137–162.

55. Nelson HD, Humphrey LL, Nygren P, Teutsch SM, Allan JD. Postmenopausal hormone replacement therapy: scientific review. *JAMA*. 2002;288 (7):872–881.

56. Umland EM. Treatment strategies for reducing the burden of menopause-associated vasomotor symptoms. *J Manag Care Pharm*. 2008;14(3 suppl):14–19.

57. Beral V. Million Women Study Collaborators. Breast cancer and hormone-replacement therapy in the Million Women Study. *Lancet*. 2003;362(9390):1160.

58. Desrochers G, Bergeron S, Landry T, Jodoin M. Do psychosexual factors play a role in the etiology of provoked vestibulodynia? A critical review. *J Sex Marital Ther*. 2008;34 (3):198–226.

59. *Female sexual dysfunction*. http://www.nlm.nih.gov/medlineplus/femalesexualdysfunction.html; Accessed 24.12.08.

60. *Women's health.* http://www.nlm. nih.gov/medlineplus/womenshealth. html; Accessed 24.12.08.

61. *Men's health.* http://www.nlm.nih. gov/medlineplus/menshealth.html; Accessed 23.12.08.

62. Sladden M, Dickinson J. Testicular cancer. how effective is screening? *Aust Fam Physician.* 1993;22:1350–1356.

63. National Cancer Institute, Division of Cancer Prevention and Control. *Annual Report.* Bethesda, MD: NCI; 1992.

64. *Algorithm testicular problems and indications for professional care.* http://familydoctor.org/online/ famdocen/home/tools/symptom/ 539.printerview.html; Accessed 23.12.08.

65. *Impotence.* http://www.nlm.nih. gov/medlineplus/erectiledys function.html; Accessed 21.12.08.

66. *Eat, exercise, sleep and relax your way to better health.* http://www. webmd.com/sex-relationships/ guide/better-sex-strategies; Accessed 05.03.09.

Mental fitness

14

Mental health: an overview

Psychosocial genomics is an emerging field in the area of mind–body medicine. Gene expression, neurogenesis, and wellness form a complex interrelated system which interacts with and adapts to human experiences, behaviour, and consciousness.[1] Mind–body medicine accepts that thoughts trigger physiological events. Thinking or talking about uplifting and upsetting experiences leads to different psychological responses and biological changes. Choosing and practising beneficial thinking strategies enhances mental fitness and promotes general wellbeing.

The ability to cope with distressing life experiences is an important key to mental fitness. Individuals feel more able to cope when they believe they can exert control over a situation. Animal and human studies have confirmed that helplessness or a lack of control is a stressor and causes immunosuppression.[2] Lack of control disturbs the biochemical balance, resulting in increased corticosteroid release, which in turn suppresses production of:

- serotonin. Serotonin regulates mood, relieves pain, and influences release of endorphins

- dopamine. Dopamine is largely responsible for a sense of reward or pleasure
- noradrenaline. Noradrenaline depletion causes depression.

Perceived control: a powerful strategy

A sense of control can be enhanced by improving one's coping skills. **Handout 14.1** identifies strategies for improving coping skills. A sense of increased control can be achieved by:[3]

- gaining information. When informed about a situation, individuals experience an increased sense of control because the situation becomes predictable and is seen as more manageable
- being prepared. When people feel prepared for something, they believe they are better able to control difficult situations. Thorough preparation for an event by using both intellectual and emotional strategies enhances control. When improved problem-solving skills are combined with positive visualization, positive outcomes seem more likely
- placing faith in someone or something we deeply trust. The practitioner is a good source of support; however, dependency can be a problem
- adopting a less pessimistic outlook. Mindset influences clinical outcome. In HIV patients, negative expectations are associated with health decline while the ability to anticipate an active future through 'self-oriented active optimistic coping behaviour' is associated with a positive

outcome.[4] Research suggests the thinking strategy chosen can be brought under cognitive control when an appropriate self-regulatory strategy is implemented[5]

- building a stronger support system. Encouragement mobilizes healing forces. Key components of a good social support system include:[6]
  - being loved and cared for
  - being valued
  - sharing companionship
  - having access to information and guidance
  - physical and material assistance
- learning a new coping skill. The acquisition of new coping skills includes refining information-gathering and information-interpreting skills. Better coping skills result in being better prepared. **Handout 14.2** shows how task-orientated problem-solving skills can be used to enhance coping.

Self-efficacy: self-belief

Efficacy expectancies are the belief that one can successfully execute the behaviour necessary to achieve the desired outcome.[7] The consultation can be used to enhance patients' efficacy expectations. By focusing on the patient's coping skills, the consultation can specifically enhance self-efficacy. Self-efficacy is the belief that performing a chosen behaviour will lead to a desired outcome; that one can successfully perform that behaviour and the intended outcome of a given behaviour is of personal value. Self-efficacy is one of a number of constructs hypothesized to explain phenomena which help an individual stay healthy under various kinds of stress. Similar constructs include Antonovsky's sense of coherence, Kobasa's hardiness and Rosenbaum's learned resourcefulness.[8] Rosenbaum's individual with learned resourcefulness resembles the individual with high efficiency.[9] Learned resourcefulness is the belief that one can effectively deal with 'manageable' levels of stress. It includes personal beliefs, self-control skills and behaviours. Any stressors that disrupt habitual goal-directed behaviour trigger a process of self-regulation consisting of conscious evaluation of the event followed by actions aimed at regulating the disruption. This process includes self-monitoring of maladaptive thoughts, feelings and behaviours; it involves application of problem-solving skills and incorporates emotional regulation and self-control. Learned resourcefulness is the development of mechanisms whereby persons self-regulate internal responses that interfere with the smooth execution of behaviour – it is the development of good coping skills.

Hardy individuals tend to experience life in ways similar to persons rich in learned resourcefulness. Hardiness enables people to modify the effects of stress by transformational coping which includes: reinterpreting the situation, actively imagining new ways of confronting a stressful situation, and considering the effective use of available resources. Personality constructs relevant to hardiness are commitment, control and challenge. Commitment is belief in the truth, importance and value of what one is doing; control is the tendency to believe and act as if one can influence the course of events; and challenge is based upon acceptance of change as normal. Change is also perceived to hold the promise of future opportunity. Hardy people have a number of characteristics in common with persons with a strong sense of coherence.

Persons with a strong sense of coherence (SOC) tend to be more self-efficient, hardy and resourceful than persons with a weak SOC. SOC may be construed as a coping style characterized by an enduring tendency to see one's life as more or less ordered, predictable and manageable.[10] A SOC is composed of the three elements of comprehensibility, manageability and meaningfulness. Comprehensibility is high when the individual perceives that stimuli arising from the external and internal environment are structured, predictable and explicable. Manageability is high when individuals believe they have adequate resources available to manage demands. Meaningfulness is present when challenges being confronted are regarded as worthy of engagement and investment. A person with a strong SOC is less likely, than one with a low SOC, to perceive stressful situations as threatening and anxiety provoking.

Learned resourcefulness, hardiness and a sense of coherence are thought to mitigate stressful events at different phases of the self-control process. Learned resourcefulness is postulated to reduce unhelpful reactions to stressors. In contrast, hardiness and a sense of coherence are thought to influence the initial evaluation of the stressful event. Persons with a low SOC are more likely both to show distress and to appraise and cope with stressful situations in ways less likely to resolve or alleviate their distress.[11]

Learned resourcefulness, hardiness and sense of coherence are conducive to mental fitness. Mental fitness can be enhanced by acquiring improved coping skills. The first phase in coping is to appraise the stressor. If the stressor is perceived as non-threatening, it is not a cause for concern. If the stimulus is potentially threatening, then it is necessary to appraise one's resources. The more control one perceives one has over a situation, the less threatening the stressor. When selecting and implementing a coping strategy, consideration is given both to the nature of the stressor and to available resources. It is beneficial to combine multiple interventions.

Coping

Coping is a life skill. It can be refined using strategies that range from changing perceptions to enhancing coping skills. Perceptions of self, specific stressors and one's general life situation are all subject to change. Creative problem solving is a skill that can be acquired and improved. Transformational coping takes constructive action to change the stressor; regressive coping avoids the stressor. The former is associated with a fundamentally optimistic attitude; the latter with a pessimistic approach. Both coping strategies and illness perceptions have been shown to influence the level of psychological distress amongst allergy sufferers.[12] Coping strategies explained between 12% and 25% while illness perceptions explained between 6% and 26% of the variance on diverse measures of psychological distress. This study concluded that health interventions aimed at increasing a sense of control, using more adaptive coping strategies and changing perception of the condition would prove beneficial. Just as a patient can reduce the impact of a disorder by changing their perceptions of the illness, so can individuals enhance their mental health by modifying unhelpful self-perceptions.

Changing self-perceptions

Changing perceptions is a powerful intervention tool. Optimism, explanatory style, and self-esteem are conducive to mental health. Potential weaknesses in perceptual thinking processes include:

- distorting information. Faulty self-perception and poor self-esteem may result in information being distorted so that it fits with erroneous perceptions. It is possible to change one's self-perception and improve one's self-esteem

- an inadequate conceptual framework. Awareness of different ways of viewing a situation can lead to changes in perception. Perceptual errors often result from failure to discriminate between fact and inference. Tools are available to help one view situations from different viewpoints

- self-reindoctrination. Repetitive self-talk of illogical beliefs sustains defective thinking. Self-talk can be changed.

You can change your outlook by changing your perceptions. Self-perception or self-concept is one's self image. Self-perception is one's self-evaluation and consists of:[13]

- Self-awareness – being aware that one has an impact on others (and vice versa).

- Self-worth and self-love. These inborn capacities include self-forgiveness.

- Self-confidence. Self-confidence is learned. The positive reinforcement of success builds confidence. Confidence is built by:
  - positive visualization/imagery
  - positive self-talk
  - working hard to master challenges.
  Self-confidence reflects how highly one values one's abilities and achievements; self-esteem is how one values oneself.

- Self-esteem. Self-esteem is self-liking or self-acceptance. Self-esteem is an objective and favourable impression of one's self that influences all one's experiences. Esteem is compassion for self and is learned from one's actions. A lack of self-esteem reduces the capacity for satisfaction. Self-esteem is the reputation we acquire with ourselves. It is earned and comes from meeting personal standards. When rewarded internally it enhances self-concept. Self-esteem has two components:
  - self-respect. This is the ability to appreciate one's emotional nature and express feelings when they are felt. Self-respect incorporates a personal sense of worthiness, a sense of being worthy of happiness
  - self-efficacy. This is a basic confidence in one's ability to face life's challenges, a sense of knowing we can succeed insofar as this depends on our own efforts. Self-efficacy generates a sense of control over one's life and is associated with psychological wellbeing.

Self-esteem is due to one's internal representation of oneself – it does not necessarily reflect the reality of how one actually is. While, in the short term, heightening self-esteem may require the discomfort of moving out of one's comfort zone, in the long run, high self-esteem promotes hardiness.

Handout 14.3 provides tips for improving one's self-perception.[14]

Changing perceptions of the world

Expectations, both positive and negative, modify how events are experienced. Nocebo suggestions, in which expectation of pain increase is induced, are capable of producing both hyperalgesic and allodynic responses.[15] Expectations are further modulated by explanatory style. The way people perceive events in their life affects their health.[3] Pessimists assume a problem is stable or never-ending. They suppose it is global, i.e. not an isolated incident, and they internalize the problem, believing that everything is their fault. Pessimists tend to attribute their problems to permanent personal inadequacies that undermine what they do. They tend to blame themselves for bad things that happen and attribute good things to chance. A negative explanatory style harms health and predisposes to unhealthy behavioural choices. The ability to reflect on negative autobiographical experiences without ruminating is critical to mental health. Neural activity in different brain areas is detected when attempts to cope with negative autobiographical memories use emotionally charged cognitive strategies compared with thinking processes that analyse and accept previous experiences.

While depressed individuals may spontaneously engage in the same type of self-focused rumination triggered by emotion-based strategies,[5] cheerful individuals use a positive explanatory style. Optimists' explanatory style is to recognize that problems pass. They localize problems, i.e. they do not permit problems in one area to cloud other aspects of life. They do not inappropriately assume blame and are realistic in their self-beliefs. Optimists are flexible and welcome the need to make life changes. They implement changes in small steps by setting goals that are small enough to be quickly achieved and then reward themselves when they reach their goals. They also seek out optimistic people and actively practice being optimistic!

Handout 14.4 demonstrates how to 'turn lemons into lemonade'. A fundamental requirement is to learn to recognize and appreciate life's joys. The message is, instead of documenting your woes, keep a record of the good things that happen each day. Count your blessings. Become aware of how much you have to be grateful for – the warmth of the sun, the song of the birds, a smile of a friend. Consciously jotting down the little pleasures in life provides a simple strategy to help you to live in and appreciate the moment.

Improving coping skills

Coping may be cognitive, emotional, physical or any combination of these. Problem-focused or active coping may be suitable only for situations that can be changed; emotional or passive coping may be more applicable for those aspects of stressful situations which are unchangeable. Relaxation or coping at a physical level may be equally helpful in either situation.

1. Refining cognitive coping skills

In pain management, active coping strategies in which the individual attempts to function in spite of pain are associated with better adaptive functioning than are passive coping strategies, which tend to result in greater incapacity.[16] Appraising pain as a challenge is predictive of active coping and mastery; appraising pain as a threat predisposes to passive coping, depression and reduced self-esteem.[17] Active coping is facilitated when individuals get problems into perspective. A balanced view is fundamental to good cognitive coping. A balanced view is facilitated when problems are viewed from different perspectives. Edward de Bono's Six Thinking Hats provide a user-friendly approach to seeing situations from different points of view.[18] By deliberately using the thinking hats in sequence, various options for responding to a problem become apparent. By wearing each of the thinking hats, a better appreciation of the nuances of a stressful situation can be explored. By examining a problem from different angles, the six hats enable users to create novel perceptions of old – and new – problems. Figure 14.1 describes the six hats.

In all cases, a balanced view of a situation includes identifying[19]:

- the good, the pluses
- the bad, the minuses
- the possibilities

The **white hat** deals with data and information. When confronted by a situation it is helpful to:

- find out what information is available
- identify what information you would like to have
- ascertain what data are missing
- decide how missing data can be collected

The **red hat** deals with intuition, emotions and feelings. Faulty thinking from overuse of red hat thinking may result in:

- making assumptions about what others think (mind reading)
- taking things personally (wearing the hat regardless of fit)
- taking the blame, assuming responsibility whatever the cause
- mistaking feeling for facts
- name calling/labelling... 'idiot'
- scare mongering... what if?
- wishful thinking... if only

The **black hat** is cautious thinking concerned with assessing risk and critically evaluating the situation. This is the pessimistic perspective. Faulty thinking patterns associated with thinking confined to the black hat includes:

- predicting the worst possible outcome (catastrophizing)
- assuming that what happened on one occasion will always happen (over-generalizing)
- making a mountain out of a molehill (exaggerating – the importance or magnitude of the problem)
- looking on the dark side (overlooking the positive)

The **yellow hat** provides a logical positive view, it represents the optimists view. It identifies benefits and why the notion is feasible.

The **green hat** is for new ideas; it considers the possibility of changing the current situation into something better. The green hat is for creativity.

The **blue hat** overviews the thinking process. It defines and redefines the problem and ensures that the viewpoints identified when wearing each of the other hats is organized into a realistic appraisal of the situation. The blue hat checks that the other hats have been used.

Figure 14.1 • The Six Thinking Hats

- other people's views
- possible consequences.

Handout 14.5 provides a quick guide describing how the thinking hats can be used to solve problems in different situations.

2. Refining emotional coping skills

Emotion has been linked with disease risk. According to a 13-year study involving 2000 individuals, specific emotional factors are more predictive of who will develop cancer or coronary heart disease than is cholesterol, blood pressure or smoking.[20] High anxiety impairs thinking by blocking factual information and reducing awareness of personal thoughts and feelings. Poor thinking skills in turn contribute to anxiety. You can interrupt this cycle by:

- identifying thoughts and recognizing how self-talk influences mood
- changing self-talk. Self-talk influences emotions, thoughts, physiology and behaviour. As self-talk

is self-fulfilling and can be self-regulated, it is important to tune into and optimize self-talk. Self-talk can be uplifting or belittling, blocking personal growth.

Handout 14.6 provides tips for improving emotional coping skills.

3. Controlling physical feedback

In view of the interconnections between mind and body, psychosocial stressors may be expressed as physical tension and awareness of muscle tightness conveys a message of unease to the nervous system. Awareness of muscle tension exacerbates feeling of distress. Reduction of muscle tension can in turn enhance psychological wellbeing. A variety of techniques can be used to reduce muscle tension.

Handout 14.7 lists strategies that can be used to reduce the physical impact of stress. **Handout 14.8** can be used as a self-check to determine if residual tension persists and additional muscle relaxation measures should be included.

Getting professional help

While improving coping skills requires personal application, some individuals may also benefit from professional assistance. **Handout 14.9** provides a brief self-screen to alert persons who need additional assistance with coping. **Handouts 14.10–14.12** can then be used to try to more precisely identify the nature of the problem. Both prolonged exposure to stimuli perceived as stressful and/or persistent use of inappropriate responses to life events lead to a chronic stress response. When body 'tone' is set too high, the capacity of the body to adapt is impaired and organ reserves are depleted. Managing stress is an essential life task in modern society. **Handouts 14.8** and **14.10** provide a self-check for assessing personal stress.

Depression is also a prevalent problem. **Handout 14.11** identifies red flags for depression. In fact, depression is considered a normal accompaniment of ageing. One in five elderly people will, at some stage, suffer some form of depression. Dysthymia is chronic mild depression. Sufferers experience mild depression on most days over 2 or more years. Only one in three depressed people ever seeks help, yet depression is treatable.

It is anticipated that one in ten people will be affected by anxiety in the next year and that one in four people will be affected by anxiety at some point in their life. Anxiety may be self-imposed when people try to meet the expectations of others and/or compare themselves with others rather than their previous self. Anxiety may also be encountered when family or work demands are perceived as excessive. **Handout 14.12** provides a self-screen to detect clinical anxiety.

Anxiety disorders range from generalized anxiety, through panic attacks to phobias. Generalized anxiety presents as a pervading persistent sense of apprehension. In all cases, no realistic anxiety trigger can be identified to explain the attack. Generalized anxiety is a feeling of distress in the absence of an identifiable threat and is characterized by excessive worry about trivial or unrealistic problems. Anxiety is worsened by awareness of and by reacting adversely to physical symptoms. Awareness of and reaction to a dry mouth, pounding heart and rapid respiration may heighten tension and convert feelings of anxiety into panic. Panic attacks are experienced as recurrent, unexpected episodes of intense anxiety. A diagnosis is made when a single attack is followed by 4 weeks during which fear of a second attack is experienced or when four attacks occur in a 4-week period. Panic attacks are episodes of sudden inexplicable terror.

Phobias are inordinate fears of certain objects or situations. This differentiates phobias from generalized anxiety, when anxiety is free-floating and is unrelated to any specific event or situation. Persons with a phobia associate fear with particular situations or objects. Simple phobias include fear of snakes, thunder, spiders or cancer.

Special skills

Modern life requires that individuals learn to cope with, rather than act out, their anger; that they are assertive without being aggressive; and that they manage time effectively and efficiently.

Coping with anger

Negative anger results in hostility. Aggressive impulses are often turned inward and enhance personal stress. Negative anger is self-destructive. Behaviour that changes the environment ultimately reduces stress. Positive anger energizes and results in action. **Handout 14.13** provides tips for handling anger.

Dealing with angry people is another potential source of stress. When dealing with angry people the situation may be defused by listening to what the other person is trying to convey. The characteristics of good listeners are that they:

* stop talking
* focus on the speaker
* notice *how* things are said
* notice what is and what isn't said
* stop for clarity checks.

Poor listening may escalate tense situations. Poor listening behaviour includes:

* faking attention
* interrupting others
* dominating the conversation
* correcting – waiting for factual errors, then pouncing
* criticizing or judging others rather than listening to what is being said.

Being assertive

Assertive people respect their own rights and those of others. Assertiveness is different to aggression, submission and manipulation. People are aggressive because they are scared, it sometimes works and/or they are angry. People are submissive because they are scared, think it is polite and/or do not know how to be assertive.

There are various types of assertion:

- basic assertion: used when expressing beliefs, opinions and sticking up for your rights
- empathic assertion: disagree with someone but acknowledge their right to have an opinion. *'I hear what you are saying but I have a different view'*
- escalating assertion: handle a drawn-out confrontation by escalating your assertiveness to the minimal level required
- confrontation assertion: used when someone says one thing and does another. Stick to the behaviour and don't attack the person
- language assertion: *'When you do A, the effect on me is B and I feel C'*
- persuasive assertion: tact and timing.

Become assertive by preparing yourself mentally with assertive self-talk and a belief in your right and that of others to: be treated with respect, be heard, set your own priorities, ask for what you want, make mistakes, and to say 'no'.

Handout 14.14 provides tips for becoming assertive.

Managing time

Time can be wasted due to unnecessary personal behaviours. Beware of:

- perfectionism. Yesterday's standards may not be realistic in today's world. Challenge old standards. It may be necessary to question whether cleanliness is indeed next to godliness and vacuum the carpet once a fortnight instead of once a week
- confusion. Understand why you are performing a task. Know your goals
- indecision. Decide how best to reach the desired destination
- overload. There may simply be too much to do in the time available. About 80% of all human knowledge has been obtained since the mid-1960s. On average, we expect ourselves to do 30% more in a week than we did 20 years ago
- procrastination. Leaving it for later can mean that the decision to leave it for later is taken repeatedly.

- avoidance. Putting off a task in the hope that it will go away seldom works
- interruptions. Distraction from the task at hand by people in person or on the phone can greatly prolong tasks
- being unable to say 'no'. By saying 'yes' to one task you are really saying 'no' to something else. Make the right choices.

Useful suggestions for efficient time management are found in **Handout 14.15**.[21,22]

Managing cognitive ageing

As many as 1 in 10 people over 65 years have cognitive and functional difficulties; this number escalates to 4 in 10 for those over 85 years of age.[23] A North American study estimated that the risk of dementia doubles every 5 years after the age of 65 years;[24] a UK study estimated that the prevalence of dementia almost doubles every 5 years after the age of 35 years![25] Being mentally active enhances neuronal connections and tasks that stimulate thinking appear to delay cognitive ageing. Brain training packages are available which assess cognitive age and provide mental exercises to slow cognitive decline.[26] In addition to brain exercises, dietary choices may be important.

Adherence to the Mediterranean diet may promote cognitive health.[27] The Mediterranean diet is rich in cereals, wine, fruits, nuts, legumes, whole grains, fish and olive oil. A double-blind, placebo-controlled, randomized trial found that pregnant women who consumed a functional food rich in a long-chain omega-3 fatty acid (DHA) produced infants who at 9 months appeared to have better problem-solving ability.[28] Recognition memory was not enhanced. At the other end of the age spectrum, a 3-year cross-sectional study found that increased intake of long-chain plasma omega-3 fatty acids was associated with less decline in sensorimotor speed and complex speed but not in memory, information-processing speed or word fluency.[29] A double-blind study found omega-3 supplementation improved the cognitive scores for people with mild cognitive impairment.[30] Another study suggested that seafood intake is associated with better cognitive performance in a dose-dependent manner – subjects whose mean daily intake of fish and fish products was at least 10 g/day did better, with the maximum effect observed at an intake of approximately 75 g daily.[31] Benefit was greatest with non-processed lean fish and fatty fish. Another study found a significant positive trend in mental wellbeing associated with the ratio of eicosapentaenoic to arachidonic acid rather than the proportion of omega-3 fatty acids consumed.[32]

Fish is not the only component of the Mediterranean diet associated with cognitive health. Inflammation and oxidative stress play important roles in brain ageing. Inflammatory markers, along with cellular and molecular oxidative damage, increase during normal brain ageing. This increase is accompanied by a decline in cognitive and motor performance in elderly people, even in the absence of neurodegenerative diseases. Research suggests that dietary supplementation with fruit or vegetable extracts can decrease the age-enhanced vulnerability to oxidative stress and inflammation.[33] In elderly subjects, reduced levels of folate and vitamin B12 have also been found to be independently associated with cognitive decline.[34] Vitamin B12 status is suspected to be a modifiable cause of brain atrophy and subsequent cognitive impairment.[35]

Children's cognitive development is also susceptible to dietary intake. A 2-year, longitudinal, randomized, controlled, feeding intervention study involving rural children in Kenya found that dietary intake of various micronutrients was associated with improvement in cognitive function, with iron, zinc, vitamin B12 and riboflavin being significantly associated with improved cognitive test scores.[36] Another study found that children's performance declined throughout the morning but that the decline in accuracy, attention and secondary memory could be significantly reduced following the intake of a breakfast cereal with a low, rather than an high, glycaemic index.[37] The Mediterranean diet is rich in micronutrients and fibre.

The brain is the most cholesterol-rich organ in the body, containing about 25% of total body cholesterol. The major pathway of elimination of excessive brain cholesterol, derived from excessive synthesis or cell death, is the conversion of cholesterol into 24S-hydroxycholesterol. This brain-specific oxysterol passes through the blood–brain barrier into the peripheral blood. The concentration of 24S-hydroxycholesterol declines as dementia progresses. The ratio of 27-hydroxycholesterol, another oxidated product of cholesterol able to cross the blood–brain barrier, to cholesterol is significantly lower in persons with mild cognitive impairment and dementia.

Lower levels of serum total cholesterol may be viewed as a frailty marker, predictive of lower cognitive functioning in older persons.[38] Lower cholesterol is negatively associated with both general cognition and information-processing speed. Another cholesterol moiety has also been linked with cognition. Subjects with low HDL-cholesterol (<40 mg/dL) were found to have a greater odds of short-term verbal memory deficits.[39] This study reported that decreases in HDL cholesterol were associated with declines in memory in middle-aged adults over a 5-year follow-up period. The Mediterranean diet reduces total and LDL cholesterol but increases HDL cholesterol.

In addition to diet, exercise prevents decline in HDL levels. A cohort study found that men with poor physical function who increased physical activity significantly reduced their risk of dementia. During a mean follow-up of 6.1 years, increasing physical activity and function were associated with a decreasing trend in risk of dementia.[40]

While much has yet to be learnt to maximize brain function with increasing age, mental and physical activity and a healthy diet can only enhance the wellbeing of an ageing population.

In perspective

Exercises, relaxation, good nutrition, a sense of humour, good time management and communication skills plus a strong social support network are the ingredients of mental fitness. Good mental health is a challenge and a blessing. It is a challenge worth pursuing given modern lifestyle and a blessing when achieved. **Handout 14.16** provides a protocol for improving mental health.

References

1. Rossi EL. Psychosocial genomics: gene expression, neurogenesis, and human experience in mind-body medicine. *Adv Mind Body Med.* 2002;18(2):22–30.

2. Bolletino RC. Cancer: the roots of mind-body treatment of cancer patients. In: Watkins A, ed. *Mind-Body Medicine.* New York: Churchill Livingstone; 1997:87–111.

3. Hafen BQ, Karren KJ, Frandsen KJ, Smith NL. *Mind/Body Health: The Effect of Attitudes, Emotions, and Relationships.* Needham Heiths, MA: Simon & Schuster; 1996:475.

4. Ironson GH, Woods TE, Antoni MH. HIV disease: psychological well-being, health and immunity. In: Watkins A, ed. *Mind-Body Medicine.* New York: Churchill Livingstone; 1997:113–128.

5. Kross E, Davidson M, Weber J, Ochsner K. Coping with emotions past: the neural bases of regulating affect associated with negative autobiographical memories. *Biol Psychiatry.* 2009;65(5):361–366.

6. Luskin F, Newell K. Mind-body approaches to successful aging. In: Watkins A, ed. *Mind-Body Medicine.* New York: Churchill Livingstone; 1997:251–268.

7. Bandura A. Self-efficacy: towards a unifying theory of behavioral change. *Psychol Rev.* 1977;84:191–215.

8. Orr E, Westman M. Does hardiness moderate stress and how?: a review. In: Rosenbaum M, ed. *Learned Resourcefulness: On Coping Skills, Self-Control and Adaptive Behavior.* New York: Springer; 1990:64–94.

9. Rosenbaum M. The role of learned resourcefulness in the self-control of health behavior. In: Rosenbaum M, ed. *Learned Resourcefulness: On Coping Skills, Self-Control And Adaptive Behavior.* New York: Springer; 1990:3–30.

10. Antonovsky H, Sagy S. The development of a sense of coherence and its impact on stress situations. *J Soc Psychol.* 1986;126(6):213–225.

11. Mc Sherry WC, Holm JE. Sense of coherence: its effects on psychological and physiological processes prior to, during and after a stressful situation. *J Clin Psychol.* 1994;50:476–487.

12. Knibb RC, Horton SL. Can illness perceptions and coping predict psychological distress amongst allergy sufferers. *Br J Health Psychol.* 2008;13(Pt 1):103–119.

13. Cleghorn P. *The Secrets Of Self-Esteem.* Brisbane: Element; 1996.

14. Branden N. *Six Pillars Of Self-Esteem.* New York: Bantam Books; 1994.

15. Colloca L, Sigaudo M, Benedetti F. The role of learning in nocebo and placebo effects. *Pain.* 2008;136(1–2):211–218.

16. Ramírez-Maestre C, Esteve R, López AE. Cognitive appraisal and coping in chronic pain patients. *Eur J Pain.* 2008;12(6):749–756.

17. Dysvik E, Natvig GK, Eikeland OJ, Lindstrøm TC. Coping with chronic pain. *Int J Nurs Stud.* 2005;42(3):297–305.

18. De Bono E. *Six Thinking Hats.* Victoria: Penguin Books; 1990.

19. De Bono E. *Serious Creativity.* London: Harper Collins; 1992.

20. Crawford RJM. Emotional health, cancer and heart disease. *N Z Med J.* 1993;10:87.

21. De Bono E. *Teach Your Child How to Think.* London: Penguin Books; 1993.

22. Butler G, Hope T. *Managing Your Mind: The Mental Fitness Guide.* New York: Oxford University Press; 1995.

23. Lechky O. Diagnosing dementia. *Canadian Medical Association Leadership Series: Elder Care.* 2005;4:25–28.

24. Frenette G, Beauchemin JP. Sad but true: your father has dementia. An approach to announcing the diagnosis. *Can Fam Physician.* 2003;49:1296–1301.

25. Harvey RJ, Skelton-Robinson M, Rossor MN. The prevalence and causes of dementia in people under the age of 65 years. *J Neurol Neurosurg Psychiatry.* 2003;74:1206–1209.

26. *Brain Taining.* <http://en.wikipedia.org/wiki/Brain_Age>; Accessed 28.12.08.

27. Scarmeas N, Luchsinger JA, Mayeux Y, Stern Y. Mediterranean diet and Alzheimer disease mortality. *Neurology.* 2007;69(11):1084–1093.

28. Judge MP, Harel O, Lammi-Keefe CJ. Maternal consumption of a docosahexaenoic acid-containing functional food during pregnancy: benefit for infant performance on problem-solving but not on recognition memory tasks at age 9 mo. *Am J Clin Nutr.* 2007;85(6):1572–1577.

29. Dullemeijer C, Durga J, Brouwer IA, et al. n 3 fatty acid proportions in plasma and cognitive performance in older adults. *Am J Clin Nutr.* 2007;86(5):1479–1485.

30. Chiu CC, Su KP, Cheng TC, et al. The effects of omega-3 fatty acids monotherapy in Alzheimer's disease and mild cognitive impairment: a preliminary randomized double-blind placebo-controlled study. *Prog Neuropsychopharmacol Biol Psychiatry.* 2008;32:1538–1544.

31. Nurk E, Drevon CA, Refsum H, et al. Cognitive performance among the elderly and dietary fish intake: the Hordaland Health Study. *Am J Clin Nutr.* 2007;86(5):1470–1478.

32. Crowe FL, Skeaff CM, Green TJ, Gray AR. Serum phospholipid n 3 long-chain polyunsaturated fatty acids and physical and mental health in a population-based survey of New Zealand adolescents and adults. *Am J Clin Nutr.* 2007;86(5):1278–1285.

33. Lau FC, Shukitt-Hale B, Joseph JA. Nutritional intervention in brain aging: reducing the effects of inflammation and oxidative stress. *Subcell Biochem.* 2007;42:299–318.

34. Koike T, Kuzuya M, Kanda S, et al. Raised homocysteine and low folate and vitamin B-12 concentrations predict cognitive decline in community-dwelling older Japanese adults. *Clin Nutr.* 2008;27(6):865–871.

35. Vogiatzoglou A, Refsum H, Johnston C, et al. Vitamin B12 status and rate of brain volume loss in community-dwelling elderly. *Neurology.* 2008;71(11):826–832.

36. Gewa CA, Weiss RE, Bwibo NO, et al. Dietary micronutrients are associated with higher cognitive function gains among primary school children in rural Kenya. *Br J Nutr.* 2009;101(9):1378–1387.

37. Ingwersen J, Defeyter MA, Kennedy KA, Wesnes KA, Scholey AB. A low glycaemic index breakfast cereal preferentially prevents children's cognitive performance from declining throughout the morning. *Appetite.* 2007;49(1):240–244.

38. van den Kommer TN, Dik MG, Comijs HC, et al. Total cholesterol and oxysterols: early markers for cognitive decline in elderly? *Neurobiol Aging.* 2009;30 (4):534–545.

39. Singh-Manoux A, Gimeno D, Kivimaki E, Brunner E, Marmot HDL, Low HDL. cholesterol is a risk factor for deficit and decline in memory in midlife. The Whitehall II Study. *Arterioscler Thromb Vasc Biol.* 2008;28:1556–1562.

40. Taaffe DR, Irie F, Masaki KH, et al. Physical activity, physical function, and incident dementia in elderly men: the Honolulu-Asia Aging Study. *J Gerontol A Biol Sci Med Sci.* 2008;63(5):529–535.

PART 3

Orange flags: alerts for risky choices

Points to Ponder !

- Unhealthy habits are the currency of ill health – they raise orange flags warning of health hazards ahead.
- Logic alone fails to change bad habits – a change of heart is needed.

We live in an environment that offers great opportunities and substantial risks. Individuals can avoid or limit exposure to health hazards, yet a US physicians' survey found that only 1 in 10 patients reported a lifestyle free of four common risky choices.[1] Risky behaviours associated with cardiovascular disease or cancer, the two diseases responsible for 59% of American deaths, are present during adolescence.[2] The physicians' survey reported 2 in 3 patients physically inactive, 1 in 2 overweight, 1 in 5 smoked cigarettes and almost 1 in 10 abused alcohol. One-third of participants reported one of these risky behaviours; 2 in 5 had indulged in two. Smoking and obesity, in combination with physical inactivity, are the top behavioural causes of premature death in the US.[3] Risky choices in adolescents persist into adulthood. During the 2007 calendar year, the national Youth Risk Behavior Surveillance reported more than 1 in 10 high school

students were obese. During the 30 days before the survey, 1 in 5 had smoked cigarettes and almost 1 in 3 had ridden in a car or other vehicle driven by someone who had been drinking alcohol.[2] In addition, 3 in 4 high school students had drunk alcohol, and almost 1 in 20 had used methamphetamines.[2] Similarly, 4 of the top 10 risky choices made by Australians in 2006 were being overweight, smoking tobacco, abusing alcohol and using illicit drugs.[4] As risky behaviours among youth are strongly linked to unhealthy habits in adulthood, orange flags suggesting risky lifestyle choices are best detected early.

Positive messages appear more effective in achieving change than negative health communications. Efforts to persuade people to change negative behaviours are likely to be more successful if linked to health gains rather than disease risk. The Behaviour Image Model suggests that health-promoting behaviours are best framed as leading to greater health/personal development (i.e. gains), while risky behaviours can be described as interfering with health enhancement and personal growth.[5] Risky behaviours are more likely to be avoided when messages are framed in terms of the health benefits achieved by change. The behaviour image model is based on Prospect Theory, which states that information presented in terms of either positive gains (benefits) or negative losses (costs) influences behavioural decisions differentially. The underlying assumption of Prospect Theory is that people are risk seeking when they consider losses, but risk averse when they consider gains. Generally speaking, gain-framed messages are thought to be more effective for influencing decisions regarding behaviours with low-risk and certain outcomes. Gain-framed messages are well suited to health-promoting and disease-prevention behaviours. The behaviour image model furthermore uses an image appeal linking a target health behaviour, e.g. safe alcohol use, with a socially responsible behaviour, e.g. fewer roads accidents.

When attempting to change behaviours, the focus is to change behaviours rather than to convey facts and principles. The desired behaviour, its rationale and the language in which it is conveyed must match the patient's experience, reasoning and learning style. New information is learnt by adding it to what is already known. Behaviours are most likely to be changed when the individual's personal interests and values are reflected in the goal.

The decision to undertake risky behaviour is influenced by:[6]

- the personal estimate of the likelihood of being harmed
- the perceived severity of potential consequences
- whether effects are likely to be everyday or catastrophic
- whether the consequences will be immediate or delayed
- whether the risk is natural or contrived, i.e. manmade
- whether the event or risky behaviour is familiar or unfamiliar
- whether exposure is voluntary or imposed.

The decision to break a bad habit moves through a number of phases. Behaviour change has been described as passing through the phases of pre-contemplation, contemplation, action, maintenance and relapse.[7] In phase I, the pre-contemplation phase, individuals intend to continue with their unhealthy behaviour patterns. At this stage, however, the health professional can plant the idea that the behaviour is a problem. In phase II, the contemplation phase, individuals weigh up the pros and cons of continuing with an unhealthy behaviour pattern. At this stage, the practitioner can provide factual information and motivate the patient to change. During this phase, the individual can be assisted to recognize how the

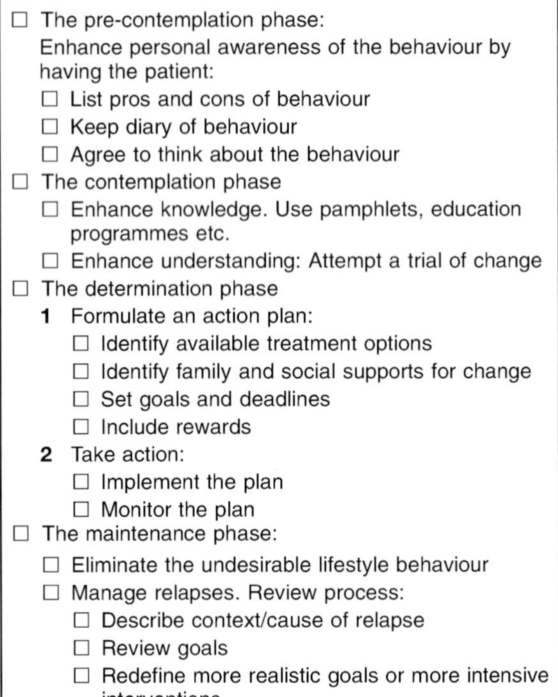

Figure P3.1 • The phases of change.

negative effects of the habit outweigh any benefits (see Figure P3.1). Important considerations include:[8]

- Deciding to change. When the advantages of changing are seen to outweigh the disadvantages of continuing, then change becomes a consideration. Weighing the risks of continuing a current behaviour against the benefits of change provides strong motivation for persisting with a new behaviour. Awareness of personal risk should not be assumed. A US national telephone survey found smokers underestimated their relative risk compared to non-smokers, believed they had a lower risk of developing lung cancer than the average smoker, and failed to appreciate the dose–response relationship between lung cancer and number of cigarettes smoked.[9]

- Increasing awareness of the habit. As many habits are automatic, a preliminary step towards changing a habit is to become aware of the habit. Preliminary awareness of a potential problem may be raised by asking: 'In the last year, have you ever drank or used drugs, including nicotine, more than you meant to?' and 'Have you felt you wanted or needed to cut down on your drinking or drug use in the last year?' One positive response has around an 81%

Increase awareness of behaviour by recording stimuli leading to that behaviour. Identify what triggers that behaviour and rate the satisfaction associated with that behaviour on each occasion. Use this as a guide to help decide how best to change risky behaviour.

DATE . . . .   DAY . . . .

TIME	BEHAVIOUR TRIGGER	NATURE/CHARACTERISTICS OF THE BEHAVIOUR	OCCASION	SATISFACTION

Figure P3.2 • Self-awareness diary.

sensitivity and specificity for current substance use disorders.[10] A more precise measure is development of a habit diary (see Figure P3.2).

Once motivated, a number of steps need to be taken to achieve and maintain the desired change. In phase III, the action phase, a successful behaviour change strategy is negotiated. Professionals provide support, information and explanation. The options for change are clarified. In phase IV, the maintenance phase, the practitioner provides ongoing support and counselling. In phase V, relapses may occur. Professional intervention varies depending on the current phase. In general, support is maintained and monitoring continued. Whereas the phases of change Figure P3.1 views change from the patient's perspective, Figure P3.3 focuses on the complementary steps the practitioner needs to follow to assist patients to acquire a well-ness-promoting lifestyle.[11] Two vital steps are to:

- Devise strategies for changing the habit. The habit diary can provide useful information and help individuals become aware of early warning cues. Recognizing and avoiding 'danger' periods can help self-control. It is imperative that old habits are replaced with health-promoting alternative behaviours. Replace cigarettes with celery or a carrot rather than chocolate. Replace coffee with water or green tea rather than alcohol. Replace tranquillizers with exercise.

- Monitor progress. Self-monitoring should include constant reminders of the advantages of stopping. The process is one of ongoing reflection. Motivation is maintained by referring to the same cost:benefit analysis that initially acted as a stimulus to embracing change.

All behavioural programmes rely on certain basic elements. These include:[12]

- self monitoring. Behaviour analysis creates awareness of current inappropriate lifestyle choices. Ongoing behavioural self-evaluation provides a record of progress and acts as a source of encouragement or warning.

- controlling stimuli that precede unhealthy behaviours. Stimuli associated with unhealthy choices should be replaced by health-promoting options. Watching television may act as a stimulus to eating chocolate. Risky eating behaviour can be changed by modifying the type of food eaten. For overweight persons, this may be celery, whereas for persons with an ideal or low body weight, nuts may be the preferred replacement snack.

- developing techniques to control the behaviour. Counting mouthfuls, placing eating utensils on the plate between mouthfuls, and swallowing one mouthful before preparing the next are all measures that overweight persons may use to prolong eating without increasing energy intake.

Step 1: Identify bad habits/risky health behaviours
Step 2: Seek motivation to change
☐ Explore general reasons for changing.
☐ List the benefits resulting from performance of each bad habit
☐ List the adverse outcomes resulting from performance of each bad habit
☐ Identify reasons for changing the habit now
Step 3: Describe the unwanted behaviour. Use a diary to record:
☐ when the habit is performed: date and time
☐ why the habit is performed: the cue or stimulus triggering the habit
☐ the satisfaction gained from the habit on each occasion
Step 4: Break the bad habit. Formulate a strategy for changing the habit:
☐ Set attainable goals:
   ☐ specify targets
   ☐ set dates by which the frequency of risky behaviours will be reduced
   ☐ set dates by which the risky behaviours will be eliminated
☐ Develop a strategy for eliminating the habit:
   ☐ omit the behaviour on occasions when it is least 'enjoyed'
   ☐ identify good habits to replace the risky behaviour
   ☐ reward success
☐ Prepare a change schedule:
   ☐ clearly outline each behavioural step to eliminate the bad habit
   ☐ build on current good habits
   ☐ select changes most compatible with the preferred lifestyle
☐ Determine how the new behaviour pattern will be monitored
Step 5: Identify failures and modify the programme to meet achievable interim goals

Figure P3.3 • Steps to changing risky behaviours.

Similarly, counting puffs, placing the cigarette in the ashtray between puffs, and only inhaling on every second puff are all measures that smokers may use to prolong the act of smoking without the associated risk.

• reinforcing prescribed behaviours. Appropriate behaviours should be rewarded.

• cognitive restructuring. Positive monologues are learned to replace negative, discouraging self-statements.

Maximize success by replacing old risky habits with new health-promoting ones. Convert orange flags of hazard to green flags of wellness.

References

1. Coups EJ, Gaba A, Orleans CT. Physician screening for multiple behavioral health risk factors. *Am J Prev Med.* 2004;27 (2 Suppl):34–41.

2. Eaton DK, Kann L, Kinchen S, et al. Centers for Disease Control and Prevention (CDC). Youth risk behavior surveillance—United States, 2007. *MMWR Surveill Summ.* 2008;57(4):1–131.

3. Schroeder SA. Shattuck Lecture. We can do better—improving the health of the American people. *N Engl J Med.* 2007;357 (12):1221–1228.

4. AIHW Australian Health. Number 10; 2006. http://www.AIHW.gov. au/publications/index.CFM/title/ 10321 Accessed 11.12.07.

5. Werch CC. The Behavior-Image Model: a paradigm for integrating prevention and health promotion in brief interventions. *Health Educ Res..* 2007;22(5):677–690.

6. Anonymous. *Risk Analysis: Perception and Management.* London: Royal Society; 1992.

7. Hettema J, Steele J, Miller WR. Motivational interviewing. *Annu Rev Clin Psychol.* 2005;1:91–111.

8. Butler G, Hope T. *Managing Your Mind: The Mental Fitness Guide.* New York: Oxford University Press; 1995.

9. Weinstein ND, Marcus SE, Moser RP. Smokers' unrealistic optimism about their risk. *Tob Control.* 2005;14(1):55–59.

10. Brown RL, Leonard T, Saunders LA, Papasouliotis O. A two-item screening test for alcohol and other drug problems. *J Fam Pract.* 1997;44:151–160.

11. Prochaska JO, DiClement CC. Stages and processes of self-change of smoking. Toward an integrative model of change. *J Consult Psychol.* 1983;51:390–395.

12. Stukard AJ. Behavioural management of obesity. *Med J Aust.* 1985;142:S13–S20.

Substance abuse

- Everybody takes drugs in one form or another.
- Drugs are neither inherently good nor bad; they can help and/or harm – it's a question of how they are used.

An illicit drug is defined as any chemical, not required for maintenance of health, which alters biological function. Many young people use illicit drugs. In 2005, 8.1% of Americans reported using illicit drugs in the past month, this figure rose to 20% amongst 18- to 25-year-olds.[1] The prevalence of drug use increases sharply with age amongst young people: in England, only 8% of 11-year-olds had used drugs in the last year compared with 38% of 15-year-olds.[2] In 2007 in England, 25% of those aged 11 to 15 said they had tried drugs at least once, 17% reported taking drugs in the last year, 10% in the last month.[3] Encouragingly, these proportions have fallen since 2001, when they were 29%, 20% and 10% respectively.[3] In 2004, 38% of Australians aged 14 years and over had used any illicit drug at least once in their lifetime, and 15% had used any illicit drug at least once in the last 12 months.[4] Recent illicit drug use was most prevalent among persons aged between 18 and 29 years in 2004, with almost one in three people (31%) in this age bracket having used at least one illicit drug in the last 12 months.

Tobacco and alcohol are not classified as illicit drugs for adults; however, their use appears to predispose to illicit drug use. Alcohol use often leads to use of tobacco, marijuana, psychedelics and other illicit substances. Smokers are over three times as likely to use another illicit drug as non-smokers.[4] Experimentation with alcohol generally occurs earlier and more widely than with tobacco.[5] Adolescent access to cigarettes, alcohol and marijuana in the home is positively associated with illicit drug use.[6] The earlier the age of first use of any drug, the greater the likelihood of dependence.[7]

Persons who have used an illicit drug, other than marijuana, at least once in their lifetime are almost twice as likely to have been diagnosed with and/or treated for a mental health disorder.[4] Illicit drug use is also associated with an increased risk of hepatitis C, HIV, pneumonia, motor vehicle injury, and violence. Related deaths may be due to homicide, suicide, or accidental overdose. Accidental opioid overdose led to 31.5 deaths per million persons in 2003.[4] Furthermore, in Australia, opioid overdose deaths tend to occur at earlier ages in successive birth cohorts.[8] The social and economic cost of illicit drug use is high. Over a decade ago, a British study found that the total costs accumulated during 1 year by 1075 drug users amounted to over £12 million; the major cost was attributable to self-reported criminal behaviour.[9] Despite the undesirable repercussions of drug use, there is insufficient evidence to recommend for or against routine screening for drug abuse using standardized questionnaires or biological assays.[10]

Definitions and terminology

Drug abuse is defined as a maladaptive pattern of use. By definition, drug abuse is recurrent use of a substance within a 12-month period that has resulted in at least one of the following:

- failure to fulfil occupational or social obligations due to substance abuse
- use in physically hazardous situations
- use leading to legal problems
- continued use despite persistent social or interpersonal problems.

The five stages of substance abuse, often initiated in adolescence, have been described as:[11]

1. The potential for abuse. Circumstances such as peer and family drug use may predispose to experimentation.
2. Drug experimentation. It is during this stage that the individual discovers the drug 'high'. At this stage no adverse effects are detected.
3. Routine drug use. With routine use, adverse behavioural changes emerge, e.g. lying, mood swings, stealing.
4. Preoccupation with the drug. As dependency increases, stronger substances are sought. Larger doses are required to achieve the drug high. Risks are taken to get drugs. Lifestyle disruption is noted.
5. Burnout. Behavioural aberration finally becomes pronounced. Depression, self-disgust, withdrawal and suicide risk are common.

Drug abuse has acquired its own terminology. Hazardous use of a substance implies that the quantity and/or pattern of use places the user at risk of adverse consequences. Harmful use indicates there is evidence that use of the substance is having adverse physical and/or psychological consequences. The effects of drug use depend on the type of drug, the amount taken and, particularly with respect to illegal drugs, the quality and purity of the drug.

Dependence is a harmful manifestation of abuse. It is defined as a maladaptive pattern of recurrent use that has resulted, within a 12-month period, in at least three of the following:

- tolerance. A diminished effect follows continued use. Increased amounts are required to achieve the desired 'high'
- withdrawal symptoms. A dependent person presents with a characteristic syndrome when the drug is withheld. Dependent persons actively seek to relieve or avoid withdrawal symptoms by taking the substance
- impaired control. Larger amounts of the substance are taken over a longer period than initially intended

- preoccupation. Drug dependence results in preoccupation with the acquisition or use of the substance
- difficulty quitting. Dependence implies a persistent desire for the substance and hence attempts to quit are often difficult.
- sustained social, occupational or recreational disability
- continued use, despite adverse consequences.

Addiction is a behavioural pattern characterized by an overwhelming compulsion to obtain and use the drug. Tolerance and withdrawal are encountered in, but not synonymous with, addiction. Rat models used to explore the course of addiction found that forced intake led to tolerance and withdrawal, i.e. physical dependence, but not addiction.[12] When the drug was withdrawn, hyperreactivity developed, but retesting, by making the drug freely available in a bitter mixture, did not result in drug intake. In contrast, free intake over 47 weeks resulted in addiction. After 6 months of drug deprivation, retesting with the drug freely available in a bitter mixture found that rats selected the bitter drug-rich water in preference to fresh water.[12] In addicted humans, both a physical and psychological need for the drug results in continued use despite adverse consequences. In an experimental study it was found that although as the price of heroin increased, purchases decreased, reductions in heroin purchases were proportionally less than price increases.[13] The authors suggested that demand for heroin is inelastic. The demand for marijuana, alcohol and valium purchases did not vary with income in this study.

A physiological explanation for abuse

Intranasal absorption, inhalation and intravenous drug administration are highly efficacious routes for the delivery of drugs. Delivery of inhaled (smoked) drug to the brain is largely equivalent to intravenous drug injection, as the peak blood concentrations and time lapse between exposure and experiencing the effects of the drug are similar with both routes.[14]

The desire to use drugs and the process of addiction result from the effect the drug has on brain function. Drugs of abuse probably produce their rewarding effects by acting on a common brain reward circuit, the extended amygdala. The extended amygdala involves the mesolimbic dopamine system and specific subregions of the basal forebrain. Psychostimulants, opiates, ethanol, cannabinoids and nicotine all increase dopamine transmission in limbic regions of the brain through interactions with a variety of transporters, ionotropic receptors and metabotropic receptors.[15] Behavioural pharmacological experiments indicate that increased dopamine transmission is both necessary and sufficient to promote psychostimulant reinforcement. Although increasing mesolimbic dopamine transmission plays an important role in the reinforcing effects of opiates, ethanol, cannabinoids and nicotine, there are also dopamine-independent processes that contribute significantly to the reinforcing effects of these compounds.[15] Recent evidence confirms the importance of dopamine-independent mechanisms in reward-related behaviours.[16] The cannabinoid, opioid, nociceptin, corticotropin-releasing factor and hypocretin systems are all potential candidates. Although drugs of abuse possess diverse neuropharmacological profiles, activation of the mesocorticolimbic system, particularly the ventral tegmental area, nucleus accumbens, amygdala and prefrontal cortex via dopaminergic and glutamatergic pathways, constitutes a common pathway by which various drugs of abuse mediate their acute reinforcing effects.[17] Long-term neuroadaptations in this circuitry probably underlie the transition to drug dependence and cycles of relapse. Progressively greater drug-induced motor responses lead to behavioural sensitization. Environmental cues are believed to play a role in drug addiction by increasing brain reward function through lowering intracranial self-stimulation thresholds. Repeated and prolonged drug abuse leads to compulsive use at the behavioural level and a progressive dysregulation of brain reward circuitry and recruitment of brain stress systems such as corticotropin-releasing factor at the molecular level. The molecular mechanisms of signal transduction in these systems are a likely target for residual changes as they convey allostatic changes in reward set points.[18] This leads to vulnerability to relapse. Drug addiction is a chronic relapsing disorder characterized by persistent drug-seeking and drug-taking behaviours.

A problem in search of a solution

Health authorities suggest that measures to control supply are failing and that new initiatives should be directed at changing the demand for drugs. Early recognition of substance abuse by health professionals, abusers and/or the family provides a potentially important strategy for damage limitation. The earlier the problem is identified and acknowledged, the sooner help can be sought. An affirmative response to a simple question such as 'In the last year have you used drugs more than you meant to?' or 'Have you felt you wanted or needed to cut down on your drinking or drug use in the last year?' has around an 81% sensitivity and specificity for a current substance use disorder.[19] Drugs of concern include: marijuana or its derivatives, amphetamines or its variants, barbiturates or other sedatives, tranquillizers, heroin, various forms of cocaine or any of the opiates, and psychedelics. A personal decision either to take a drug of dependence or to exceed a prescribed dose on a number of occasions (possibly more than five) is cause for concern.

When undertaking drug screening, it is important to evaluate the decision to use a drug and to ascertain the presence of tolerance and whether adverse psycho-emotional effects are experienced as a result of taking the drug.

The nature of the drug influences the propensity towards tolerance and withdrawal symptoms. One study found that the proportion of dependent individuals who denied tolerance or withdrawal ranged from 30% for marijuana to 4% for opiates.[20] Most mood-altering drugs increase brain dopamine levels and higher steady states are established with chronic use of such drugs. Resistance to acknowledging a drug problem is marked and a checklist may be needed to enhance self-awareness. **Handout 15.1** provides a self-screen for a drug problem. **Handout 15.2** provides a list of red flags that may serve as a warning of a potential drug problem in others. As many of the signs of drug abuse, such as sudden changes in mood, difficulty in getting along with others, irritability, and depression, may be due to other causes, only direct observation of drug use is confirmatory. As the use and abuse of most legal and illicit psychoactive drugs have been shown to be substantially heritable, family drug abuse may serve as a warning to other family members.

Substances of abuse

Illicit use of drugs accounted for 17,000 deaths in the US in 2000.[21] However, socially approved recreational drugs were responsible for an even greater number of deaths. The leading causes of death in 2000 were tobacco (435,000 deaths; 18.1% of total

US deaths), poor diet and physical inactivity (365,000 deaths; 15.2%), and alcohol consumption (85,000 deaths; 3.5%).[21]

Socially acceptable substances used in excess or medications used inappropriately can become substances of abuse.

Coffee

Caffeine is by far the most commonly consumed of all psychoactive substances. Most people drink caffeine in coffee, tea or cola drinks, or eat it in chocolate. Over 400 billion cups of coffee are consumed annually worldwide and 75% of caffeine consumed in the US is in the form of coffee.[22] Some 24.2 gallons of coffee were consumed per person in the US in 2005.[23] The caffeine content of coffee in a 150-mL cup varies from 80–350 mg in brewed coffee to 60–100 mg in instant coffee or 2–4 mg in decaffeinated coffee. Brewed tea contains 8–90 mg of caffeine while cocoa or hot chocolate contain 10–70 mg per cup. A 200-g chocolate bar contains 20–60 mg. Caffeine content in milk chocolate is estimated to be about half that in dark chocolate.

In addition to coffee drinking being a social custom, there appears to be a genetic predisposition to caffeine consumption. The resemblance and differences between mono- and dizygotic twin pairs for total caffeine consumption, heavy caffeine use, caffeine intoxication, caffeine tolerance, and caffeine withdrawal suggested that between 35% and 77% of coffee consumption is genetically determined.[24] Caffeine is an adenosine receptor antagonist and a recognized ergogenic, i.e. it enhances physical performance. Although well tolerated in low doses, excess caffeine consumption is not without its hazards. In moderate doses caffeine is used to stimulate thinking, stay awake, suppress appetite, improve alertness and quicken reaction time. However, a double-blind study found no evidence to support the notion that caffeine improves performance, either in the context of acute or habitual use.[25] On the contrary, performance was found to be significantly impaired when caffeine was withdrawn abruptly following habitual use. Participants reported feeling more alert and less tired following acute ingestion of caffeine, but feeling less alert in conjunction with chronic exposure to the drug. Caffeine has been found to fragment sleep, causing sleep disruption especially in the latter part of the night.[26] The half-life of caffeine is 3–7 hours.

In higher doses caffeine may raise blood pressure. Meta-analysis of 11 trials found that subjects having a median dose of coffee of five cups/day had increased systolic and diastolic blood pressure levels.[27] The effect of coffee drinking on blood pressure was greatest among younger participants. Another study found that caffeine (3.3 mg/kg or 260 mg) raised both systolic and diastolic blood pressure into the hypertensive range in 19% of those with high-normal blood pressure, 15% of those with stage 1 hypertension and 89% of diagnosed hypertensive patients.[28] Caffeine appears to carry an increased risk of persistent atrial fibrillation[29] and a modest risk of chronic daily headache onset, regardless of headache type.[30] It is also worth noting that compared with coffee nondrinkers, people who consumed >200 mL coffee daily had raised inflammatory markers, including increased levels of at least 50% in interleukin 6 (IL-6) and 30% in C-reactive protein (CRP).[31] Caffeine consumption throughout pregnancy, moreover, is associated with a risk of fetal growth restriction, particularly in women with a fast caffeine clearance rate.[32] It has been suggested that pregnant women limit their caffeine intake to 200 mg a day. On the other hand, coffee consumption appears to lower the risk of dying from ischaemic heart disease or, in older subjects without moderate or severe hypertension, of developing heart valve disease.[33] These beneficial effects, however, may not be attributable to caffeine. A lower risk of coronary heart disease among moderate coffee drinkers might be due to antioxidants found in coffee.[34] Similarly, the reduced risk of diabetes type 2 in coffee drinkers is probably not due to caffeine, as the inverse association between coffee and type 2 diabetes mellitus in a cohort of postmenopausal women was particularly strong with decaffeinated coffee.[35]

Sudden cessation of caffeine produces withdrawal symptoms. Caffeine, in doses that reflect many people's daily consumption levels, leads to release of dopamine in the prefrontal cortex. This phenomenon is consistent with caffeine's reinforcing properties. Abstinence from 100 mg daily can produce symptoms! Withdrawal effects are reported in people drinking one to three cups of coffee daily or two cups of tea daily or three cans of caffeinated soft drink daily.[36] Symptoms present 12–24 hours after abstinence, peak in intensity at 20–51 hours and may persist for 2–9 days. There is a direct dose relationship with both the incidence and severity of symptoms. Caffeine-withdrawal syndrome is characterized by headache in 50% of people. Clinically significant distress or functional impairment is encountered in 13% of persons.

Symptoms range from fatigue and drowsiness, to having difficulty concentrating, being irritable, to experiencing flu-like symptoms, muscle stiffness and nausea. A toxic overdose of caffeine occurs when over 7 mg/kg of caffeine is ingested daily. Symptoms of caffeinism include anxiety, tension, headaches, insomnia, irritability, anorexia and dizziness. Flushing and arrhythmias as well as epigastric pain, diarrhoea and vomiting have been described.

Caffeine fulfils some of the criteria for drug dependence. It shares with amphetamines and cocaine a certain specificity of action on the cerebral dopaminergic system, but does not act on the dopaminergic structures related to reward, motivation and addiction.[35] When compared with nicotine and alcohol, there seems to be no significant differences in the psychosocial manifestations of the difficulty in abstaining from caffeine.[36] However, there appears to be very little health risk when caffeine intake is limited to an amount equivalent to two cups of coffee daily. Indeed, one study found that consumption of caffeine was associated with a reduced risk of depression and may even benefit cognitive functioning in a non-working population.[37] In fact, caffeine consumption exhibits a U-shaped mortality curve. Moderate caffeine consumers, 100–399 mg/day, have a significantly reduced risk of death.[38] Caffeine is used, in combination with other drugs, to treat migraine, and also as a mild stimulant. Its metabolites paraxanthine, theobromine, and theophylline relieve mild bronchospasm.

Handout 15.3 provides a protocol for managing caffeine consumption.

Nicotine *(fag, coffin nail)*

Tobacco kills nearly 500,000 Americans each year and one in six deaths are smoking related.[39] Nicotine is the primary reason cigarettes are addictive. Nicotine may be inhaled in cigarette smoke or snuff or it may be absorbed from the buccal mucosa in the form of chewing tobacco. It occurs naturally in the tobacco plant. Each cigarette contains 1–2 mg of nicotine. Nicotine levels peak in the brain within 10 seconds of inhalation. On reaching the brain, nicotine releases dopamine. Smokers report mood improvement after smoking. Nicotine has a biphasic effect. The initial stimulatory effect of nicotine is due to adrenaline release, which increases blood glucose, heart rate and blood pressure. The calming effect is probably due to dissipation of nicotine

levels. Although smokers perform better in some tasks requiring sustained concentration following nicotine intake, nicotine does not improve general learning. Usually taken for relaxation, nicotine causes psychological and possibly physical dependence. Its potential to cause dependence has resulted in nicotine replacement being used as a quitting aid.[40]

In large quantities nicotine is extremely toxic. In excessive amounts it causes anorexia. In fact, smokers tend to weigh less than non-smokers and gain an average of 2.3 kg when they quit smoking.[41] New smokers may experience the unpleasant toxic effects of nicotine, but soon develop a tolerance following chronic tobacco use. Nicotine is highly addictive and the level of daily nicotine exposure required to establish and sustain addiction is estimated to be 5 mg per day.[42] Smoking as few as four cigarettes daily can lead to addiction! Over one in three young people who 'experiment' end up being addicted by the time they are 20.[43] Cigarette smokers become physically and psychologically dependent and suffer withdrawal symptoms, including changes in body temperature, heart rate, digestion, muscle tone, and appetite. Psychological symptoms include irritability, anxiety, sleep disturbances, nervousness, headaches, fatigue, and nausea. Symptoms are experienced within 2 hours of last nicotine exposure, peak at 24–48 hours, and gradually decline in intensity over 2 weeks. Tobacco craving can last days, weeks, months, years, or an entire lifetime. An additional caution for smokers is that nicotine interacts with and affects the action of theophylline (a bronchodilator), insulin and high-dose oestrogen oral contraceptives.

Handout 15.4 provides a self-screen to detect evidence of nicotine withdrawal following smoking cessation. Chapter 16 considers smoking as a risky choice.

Marijuana *(cannabis, pot, grass, joint, reefer, locoweed, sticks, giggle smoke, griffo, mohasky, jive)*

Marijuana is the most frequently used illicit drug worldwide. In 2000/2001 the estimated annual prevalence of marijuana use was around 3.9% of the global population aged 15 years or over.[44] In 2005 in the US 74.2% of the 19.7 million illicit drug users used marijuana, with around 6000 first-time users trying the drug each day.[45] A survey found that 40.2% of high school students had tried marijuana during their lifetime, and 22.4% of students had used marijuana at least once during the 30 days prior to the study.[46] Marijuana is a particularly popular drug amongst young people. In England in 2007 marijuana was used by 13% of those aged 11 to 15, and in 2002/03 in England and Wales it was the most frequently reported illicit drug, used by 26% of 16- to 24-year-olds.[2] In Australia in 2004 one in three persons had used marijuana at least once in their lifetime and 11% of the population had used it in the previous 12 months.[4] Marijuana accounted for 72% of illicit drug arrests in 2003–04 in that country.

Marijuana, a coarse tobacco-like mixture, and hashish, a resin, come from the dried leaves and flowers of the hemp plant, *Cannabis sativa*. *Cannabis sativa* contains over 400 compounds and a total of 66 cannabinoids. One of the major cannabinoids is tetrahydrocannabinol (THC). Marijuana is usually smoked in water pipes (bongs) or in hand-rolled cigarettes (joints). When smoked it has a sweetish odour. Hash is usually mixed with tobacco and smoked. The concentration of THC is higher and more potent in hash than in the leaf and flower heads. Experience with cultivation has resulted in marijuana in the 1990s being about 20 times more potent than that in the 1960s. A cannabis hybrid, 'skunk', has a THC content of up to 30%, over sixfold stronger than standard marijuana. Marijuana and hashish can also be cooked in foods and eaten.

THC affects the central nervous system and has well-documented behavioural and cardiovascular effects. Symptoms of dependence and withdrawal have been reported at high doses (210 mg/day) but dependence has also been shown to develop following exposure to daily doses of THC between 80 and 120 mg.[47] These levels more closely approximate levels attained by smoking marijuana. When smoked, the effects of THC are experienced within minutes and last 1–3 hours; cardiovascular side effects peaking in 20 minutes.[48] This drug is usually taken for relaxation, its mood-enhancing effects, and its ability to alter consciousness.[49] These psychoactive effects last 4–6 hours and may include impaired coordination, mood and perception. As marijuana is fat-soluble, its effects persist for longer than alcohol, which is water-soluble.

Tasks most impaired by marijuana are those requiring short-term memory, sustained or divided attention, complex decision-making, and reaction time.[50] Chronic build-up of cannabinoids over a number of years progressively impairs concentration and the ability to filter out irrelevant information. Increased frequency of use delays the speed of information processing. Meta-analysis of 15 studies of the residual effects of recreational marijuana use on neurocognitive ability found a modest, long-term reduction in learning and memory but no long-term effects on reaction time, attention, language, reasoning ability, or perceptual or motor skills.[51] Other side effects are hypertension and tachycardia. When cannabis users were asked to rate the effects of their own cannabis use as positive, neutral, or negative, they gave overwhelmingly negative ratings of the effects that cannabis had had on their social life (70%), their physical health (81%), their mental health (60%), their cognition (91%), their memory (91%), and their career (79%).[52] The most commonly cited negative aspects of use volunteered were cost, negative psychological effects and legal status.[49] **Handout 15.5** provides a self-screen for the effects of marijuana. Telltale signs include dilated pupils and erratic behaviour.

Abstinence following daily marijuana use is often characterized by a time-dependent constellation of clinically significant symptoms that include anxiety, depression, irritability, marijuana craving, decreased food intake, and less and poorer quality sleep.[52] Withdrawal in humans has been reported to occur for the first 14 days after cessation of marijuana use. The previously mentioned placebo-controlled study reported that abstinence from THC increased ratings of 'Anxious', 'Depressed' and 'Irritable', decreased the reported quantity and quality of sleep, and decreased food intake by 20–30% compared with baseline.[47] Symptoms can be alleviated by the resumption of marijuana smoking. Alleviation of abstinence symptoms may be an important factor in the maintenance of daily marijuana use.[47] Daily use carries a high risk of dependence; however, behavioural therapies are efficacious for facilitating abstinence from marijuana.

In 1996, California legalized the 'compassionate use' of marijuana.[52] The cannabinoid system is a major medication target area to treat marijuana withdrawal and dependence along with a variety of other conditions.[53]

THC derivatives offer an avenue for stimulating the appetite of cancer patients and counteracting nausea associated with cancer chemotherapy.[54] Despite the potential for their medicinal use, THC derivatives are seldom used. Although 30% of oncologists surveyed favoured rescheduling, they estimated writing less than one prescription per month for marijuana cigarettes.[55] Nonetheless, marijuana is an effective antiemetic – its therapeutic effect is experienced 30–60 minutes after exposure and peaks in 2–4 hours.[56] In a placebo-controlled trial of healthy marijuana smokers, THC increased food intake by 35–45% and tolerance did not develop to this effect.[47] One function of the endocannabinoid system may be to maintain a steady state. Therapeutic use of botanical cannabis or synthetic molecules as agonists or antagonists holds promise and may be of value in the treatment of certain types of pain, spasticity, eating disorders, inflammation, and possibly blood pressure control.[57] Even multiple sclerosis, neurodegenerative disorders, epilepsy, glaucoma, and schizophrenia are being treated or have the potential to be treated by cannabinoid agonists/antagonists/cannabinoid-related compounds.[58] It should however be noted that delivery of THC by smoking a cannabis cigarette is problematic. Compared with tobacco, smoking cannabis increases carboxyhaemoglobin concentrations by a factor of 5 and tar inhalation and retention by a factor of 4. Pulmonary defences are impaired. Deep inhalation and breath-holding techniques increase respiratory damage.[59]

The effects of cannabis depend on the amount taken, the user's expectations, the psycho-emotional state in which the drug is taken and the way in which the drug is taken. Small amounts can produce a feeling of wellbeing and a tendency to talk and laugh. Users experience distortion of time and space. Impaired coordination and reduced concentration can have disastrous outcomes. An experiment on pilots, using a computerized flight simulator, showed their ability to land a plane was still impaired 24 hours after smoking a single marijuana joint.[60] The pilots reported no awareness of impaired performance. Such risk is not confined to air travel. A roadside study of reckless drivers found that 45% tested positive for marijuana.[61] The effects of THC on psychomotor performance and driving skills are dose related. Drivers with blood THC concentrations above 3 ng/mL had an increased risk for being judged impaired compared with drivers at lower concentration.[62] A comparison of meta-analyses of experimental studies on the impairment of driving skills by alcohol and marijuana suggested that a THC concentration in the serum of 7–10 ng/mL results in impairment equivalent to that caused by a blood alcohol concentration of 0.05%.[63] As the concentration of THC in blood at the time of driving is probably a great deal higher than at the time of sampling (30–90 minutes later), a 'zero tolerance' legislative approach has been suggested.[64] Certainly it appears that for young people the risks of driving under the influence of cannabis may now be greater than the risks of driving under the influence of alcohol.[65] Furthermore, as response time slows down and motor control worsens with increasing THC doses, the increase in the average THC content of some cannabis cigarettes (up to approximately 60 mg per cigarette) is of additional concern.[66]

Polydrug use is common amongst marijuana users, with alcohol and tobacco almost universally used on a regular basis.[49] Statistics suggest that use of marijuana tends to lead to the use of other drugs. In fact, it appears that three in four persons who use marijuana at least 100 times become cocaine users.[67]

Cocaine *(coke, 'C', crack, snow, nose candy, blow, toot, rock, snort, white lady, flake, dust)*

Cocaine is more addictive than alcohol, marijuana or opiates.[68] In 2006 it was reported that 2.8% of persons in the US between the ages of 15 and 64 had used cocaine at least once in the previous year; the figure for England and Wales was 2.4%, and for Australia was 1.2%.[69] In Australia, cocaine ranks as the fifth most likely cause of a drug-related death: in 2004, in persons aged 14 years and over, tobacco accounted for 46.4% of drug-related deaths, alcohol for 24.2%, opiates/opioids such as heroin for 13%, ecstasy/designer drugs for 6.5% and cocaine for 4.6%.[70] In the 12 months prior to 2003, 1% of 11- to 15-year-olds in England had used cocaine; among 16- to 24-year-olds in England and Wales, 5% had used cocaine while fewer than 1% had used crack.[2] The physiological and psychoactive effects of cocaine are similar regardless of whether it is in the form of cocaine hydrochloride or crack cocaine (cocaine base). Abuse and propensity for dependence are most likely when cocaine is smoked or injected intravenously compared with intranasal administration. The immediacy, duration, and magnitude of cocaine's effect seem to be important determinants.

Cocaine directly affects the central nervous system, reducing cerebral blood flow, especially to the frontal lobes. This persists for 10 days after drug withdrawal. A 1–3-mg dose of cocaine produces stimulation by releasing noradrenaline. Euphoria is followed within 30–60 minutes by a 'let down' of depression and dullness. Cocaine may be sniffed through the nose ('snorted') or injected. When converted into freebase, cocaine can be sold as cocaine crystals or in solvent form that is heated and the vapour inhaled. Crack is a cocaine freebase preparation made by adding baking soda to a solution of cocaine hydrochloride and then heating the mixture. Freebasing cocaine results in an intense rush within 10–15 seconds after inhalation. Euphoria lasts 10 to 20 minutes before the let down and craving for another dose.[48] Freebase cocaine increases cerebral dopamine release. Tolerance develops and withdrawal symptoms range from deep depression and suicidal feelings to nausea, vomiting, shaking fits, fatigue, irritability and muscle pain. Addiction takes place faster than with any other drug and marked tolerance develops rapidly. Crack is associated with an alarming increase in crime and violence.

The effects of cocaine will vary from person to person. They will depend on: how much cocaine is taken; the way in which cocaine is taken; the person's size, weight and health; the person's experience with cocaine over a period of time; whether it is taken on its own or in combination with other drugs; and whether the person is alone or with others. Immediate effects occur rapidly after a single dose and can last from a few minutes to several hours. They include:

- anorexia
- tachycardia
- agitation
- sexual arousal
- increased body temperature
- dilated pupils
- increased alertness, energy and euphoria
- inability to judge risks
- unpredictable and aggressive behaviour.

Chronic users may lose touch with reality and withdraw from friends, family, sports, hobbies, and other activities.

About 10 mg, one-tenth of the dose users commonly inhale, has been known to kill individuals who have a particularly strong reaction to cocaine. Convulsions may occur. Other users merely become violent, erratic, or paranoid. Cocaine psychosis may result from one or more high doses over a period of time. Symptoms include hearing voices, delusions, suspicion and fear of persecution. Users may experience tactile hallucinations and report a sensation of imaginary insects crawling over the skin. Cocaine increases blood pressure, and cardiac and respiratory rates. Users are at increased risk of heart attacks, strokes, and respiratory failure. Smoking freebase cocaine can cause breathing difficulties, a chronic cough and lung damage. Snorting cocaine can lead to nosebleeds, sinusitis and tearing of the nasal wall. Chronic nasal use results in membrane damage, and perforation of the nasal septum may occur. Injecting cocaine with used or dirty needles increases the risk of AIDS, hepatitis and skin abscesses.

Handout 15.6 provides a self-screen to detect the short- and long-term effects of cocaine use.

Amphetamines *(pep pills, speed, hearts, ups, crystal, footballs, gooey, bennies, black beauties, copilots, crystal, dexies, eye openers, lid poppers, meth, uppers, wake-ups, buzz, whiz, amphet, sulph)*

Street combinations:

goofballs (amphetamines and barbiturates)
speedballs (methamphetamine, cocaine and heroin)
zoom (cocaine, heroin and amphetamines)
ecstasy (mainly MDMA [3,4 methylenedioxymethamphetamine])

Like cocaine, amphetamine and its derivatives are popular stimulants.[48] The main pharmacological difference is that the effect of amphetamines lasts three to five times longer than that of cocaine. Both drugs stimulate the sympathetic nervous system and initially increase neural pathway activity by inhibiting reuptake of neurotransmitters. Moderate doses produce euphoria, a sense of elation and heightened arousal. Evidence of stimulant overdose includes agitation, hallucinations, fever and convulsions.

Amphetamines and the amphetamine derivative ecstasy are now among the most available drugs for youth. In the year leading up to 2003, among 16- to 24-year-olds in England and Wales, 5% had used ecstasy and 4% had used amphetamines.[2] In 2004, 7% of 12–24-year-old Australians had used ecstasy and/or amphetamines in the last 12 months and in 20–24-year-old group 13% had used ecstasy and 11% amphetamines.[4] In that year 12% of arrests related to amphetamine-type stimulants. Amphetamines are a popular stimulant amongst long-haul truck drivers.

Amphetamines produce euphoria, increase energy, are relatively inexpensive to purchase and have the reputation of being fairly safe. Amphetamines may be injected, sniffed, mixed with cannabis or tobacco and smoked, or smoked straight off tin foil. The powder form is commonly taken orally. It can be dissolved in a drink, licked off a finger, or the powder can be rubbed into the gums. The effects depend on: the amount taken; the person's experience with the drug; their expectations; their current mood; the quality/purity of the drug; and the mode of drug administration. Small doses reduce appetite and produce feelings of wellbeing, self-confidence, increased energy and alertness. The increased alertness results in insomnia, increased resistance to fatigue, and boredom. State-dependent learning is improved. However, as information is best recalled when the person is in a similar drug-induced state, some aspects of the learner's ability may actually be impaired. Adverse effects are confused thinking, extreme restlessness, and irritability. Dilated pupils are common. Psychological dependence develops quickly in most regular users and chronic high-dose users become physically dependent. Extreme fatigue, followed by prolonged but disturbed sleep, occurs on withdrawal. Agitation, irritability, apathy, depression, disorientation and feelings of being unable to cope are also described. Chronic dependence produces impairment of the frontal cortex and methamphetamine psychosis may result in persistent central noradrenergic dysregulation after acute psychotic symptoms have resolved.[71]

Medicinal uses for amphetamines include: narcolepsy (uncontrolled episodes of sleep); attention deficit disorder; sedation caused by drugs prescribed for epilepsy; Parkinson's disease; abnormally low blood pressure associated with anaesthesia; obesity due to improper diet; and depression. Prolonged use can precipitate other health problems, including malnutrition due to anorexia and sometimes diarrhoea, poor resistance to infection, hypertension and emotional disturbances.

MDMA (3,4-methylenedioxymethamphetamine) is a semisynthetic, amphetamine-type psychoactive drug and the major constituent of the 'rave' drug ecstasy.[72] The rapidly increasing use of methamphetamine in the West over the last decade is raising safety concerns.[73] Ecstasy has an energizing effect, producing feelings of euphoria and emotional warmth while distorting tactile experiences and time perception. Repeated exposure to ecstasy produces a persistent decrease in serotonergic activity.[74] Serotonin plays an important role in regulating mood, aggression, sexual activity, sleep, and sensitivity to pain. Serotonin modulates learning and memory. It appears that ecstasy may be responsible for memory deficits in recreational users. The extent of memory impairment correlates with the degree of exposure to ecstasy; higher exposure leads to greater impairment in immediate verbal memory and delayed visual memory.[75] Verbal and visual memory impairment persist with abstinence. While tolerance to ecstasy's positive effects develops rapidly with continued use, the impact of negative effects increase on continued use.[76] This finding suggests that ecstasy would not lend itself to regular and frequent use and has led some to believe it is safe. Nonetheless, nearly 75% of the respondents in a survey associated ecstasy with at least some risk; 24% considered its use dangerous or very dangerous.[77] Ecstasy admissions to emergency departments tend to be due to overdose and unexpected reactions.[78]

Handout 15.7 lists some of the dose-related responses to amphetamines.

Hallucinogens

The US Office of National Drug Control Policy categorizes ecstasy as a manmade hallucinogen.[79] Other manmade hallucinogens are lysergic acid diethylamide (LSD), phencyclidine (PCP) and ketamine; psilocybin mushrooms and the herb *Salvia divinorum* are natural hallucinogens. Hallucinogens or 'psychedelic' drugs distort perceptions. They work directly on the brain and affect all the senses, producing illusions or hallucinations. In addition to visual and auditory hallucinations, these drugs induce feelings of detachment from one's environment and oneself, and distortions in time and perception. The effects of hallucinogens can last for 12 hours. These mind-altering substances are taken to increase insight and enhance energy. They can produce mood swings, and elevate body temperature and blood pressure. A catatonic syndrome characterized by lethargy, disorientation, meaningless repetitive movements, and behaviour similar to schizophrenic psychosis, however, may be precipitated.

PCP (phencyclidine) *(angel dust, clicker, crystal, dummy dust, killer, weed, mint weed, super grass, horse, hog, sherms)*

This manmade hallucinogen may be the most destructive drug known. It is highly unpredictable. It may be taken orally, smoked, injected or snorted.

Adverse effects include slurred speech, blurred vision, confusion, agitation, anxiety, impaired memory and perception, convulsions, hypertension, and death from overdose. In 2006, the National Survey on Drug Use and Health (NSDUH) found 2.7% of persons aged 12 or older surveyed had used PCP in their lifetime.[79]

LSD (lysergic acid diethylamide) *(acid, big D, sunshine, blue dragon, sugar cubes, blotters, barrels, windowpanes, purple haze)*

LSD is less potent than PCP but is nonetheless a dangerous drug. It is highly water-soluble and can be absorbed through the skin. It is usually taken as a drop on 'blotting' paper. Effects are felt within 30–90 minutes and last up to 16 hours. Adverse effects include mood swings, breaks from reality and emotional breakdown. Flashbacks occur for up to 6 months. LSD causes dependency but has no withdrawal symptoms. In 2006, the NSDUH found 9.5% of persons aged 12 or older surveyed had used LSD in their lifetime.[79]

Mescaline and psilocybin *(buttons, cactus, magic mushrooms, mesa)*

Like LSD, mescaline causes hallucinations, illusions, mood swings, breaks from reality and emotional breakdown.

Ketamine

This drug is used medicinally to produce dissociative anaesthesia. It produces profound analgesia. It is particularly useful for invasive diagnostic procedures such as sigmoidoscopy.

Handout 15.8 lists some of the physical and psychological risks associated with the use of hallucinogens.

Inhalants *(gas, glue, laughing gas, liquid paper, sniff, whippets)*

Inhalants refer to substances that are sniffed or huffed to give the user an immediate high. They include a diverse group of chemicals found in consumer products such as aerosols, cleaning solvents and glues. The five substances most frequently used as inhalants are gasoline (by 57.4%), Freon (40.45%), butane lighter fluid (38.3%), glue (29.8%), and nitrous oxide (23.4%).[80] Abused solvent-based glues include those commonly used for gluing laminates, vinyl floor tiles, wood and plastic. Adolescents tend to abuse different products at different ages.[81] Among new users aged 12–15, the most commonly abused inhalants were glue, shoe polish, spray paints, gasoline, and lighter fluid. Among new users aged 16 or 17, the most commonly abused products were nitrous oxide or whippets. Nitrites are the class of inhalants most commonly abused by adults.

Inhalants can be 'sniffed' directly from the container; from a plastic bag placed over the user's mouth and nose; or from the fume-filled air in a confined space; or by placing a soaked rag in the mouth ('huffing').

Use of inhalants may result in slurred speech, poor coordination, euphoria, lightheadedness, hallucinations, and delusions. Outcomes differ depending on the chemicals involved. Hypoxia leading to brain damage and death may result from asphyxia, suffocation, choking on vomit, or cardiac arrest. Single use of inhalants may also cause visual hallucinations, severe mood swings, and numbness and tingling of the extremities. Early clues to inhalant sniffers may be the smell of glue or other solvents on their breath. Judging by children incarcerated in a juvenile detention facility, inhalant abuse is associated with the later use of other substances of abuse.[82]

Handout 15.9 provides information on the risks associated with the use of inhalants.

Opiates

Opiates are derived from the opium poppy. Morphine is the major psychoactive substance. Both morphine and codeine are used in pain relief. Narcotic users have pinpoint pupils. A narcotic overdose should be suspected in users with cold, clammy skin; slow, shallow respiration; convulsions; and coma.

Handout 15.10 lists some of the adverse consequences of opiate use.

Codeine *(schoolboy)*

Codeine causes moderate physical and psychological dependence. A study comparing dependent and nondependent users found that dependent subjects reported problems with other drugs more often than did nondependent users (alcohol, 57% vs. 26%; cannabis, 23% vs. 5%; sedative/hypnotics, 33% vs. 12%; and heroin, 11% vs. 2%, respectively).[83] Dependent subjects are most likely to use codeine for pleasurable effects, to relax, or to prevent withdrawal symptoms. They find codeine less effective for treating pain than nondependent subjects.

Codeine is sometimes used in mixtures to suppress a cough or reduce diarrhoea. Taken in excess, it causes confusion, poor coordination, and itching.

Heroin *('H', smack, junk, stuff, scag, brown sugar)*

Heroin is derived from morphine. In the 12 months prior to 2003, approximately 1.3% of Americans had ever used heroin;[84] in England and Wales fewer than 1% of 16- to 24-year-olds had used heroin.[2] Most users stop by the age of 40 and the majority are employed.[84] Nonetheless, the potential for physical and psychological dependence on heroin is high. A survey found respondents believed heroin to be the most dangerous drug in terms of both absolute and relative risk compared with other substances.[78] Death from an overdose, AIDS, and serum hepatitis are real risks of heroin use. Telltale signs of use are hypodermic syringes and needle marks. Heroin injectors are more likely than heroin 'chasers' to be deeply involved in a heroin-using culture and to be using heroin daily.[85]

Prevention is better than cure. Before embarking on an illicit drug, adventurers would be well advised to consider the risks. See **Handout 15.11**.

Drugs in sport

Athletes may use drugs to enhance their performance. 'Doping' not only is cheating but also poses a grave threat to an athlete's health and safety. The World Anti-Doping Agency has developed a World Anti-Doping Code which sets out the procedural ground rules.[86] Substances banned in Olympic sports include anabolic agents, narcotics, and growth hormones, as well as stimulants and illicit drugs such as cocaine and marijuana. Athletes are randomly drug tested. Medications which athletes need to avoid include:

- Sympathomimetic amines. Drugs such as adrenaline (epinephrine) increase alertness and improve endurance. They are commonly found in over-the-counter cold and flu medications. Asthma medications such as Ventolin have a similar effect.
- Narcotic analgesics. Used to relieve pain, these drugs are psychostimulants. Codeine may be combined with other analgesics or in cough mixtures sold over the counter.
- Anabolic steroids. These synthetic derivatives of testosterone enhance performance and increase muscle bulk, enhancing strength and stamina. Adverse effects from misuse include: high blood pressure; heart, liver and kidney problems; mood swings; and, in females, male secondary sexual

characteristics. Tolerance develops with continued use. Corticosteroids, drugs used to reduce inflammation, are also banned.

- Human growth hormone. This anabolic hormone promotes physical development, stimulating collagen synthesis, increasing muscle bulk and boosting energy release from fat.
- Blood doping. Infusion of red cells just prior to an event increases the oxygen-carrying capacity of the blood. Erythropoietin, the hormone responsible for stimulating red cell production, is also banned.

Medications

Drug-related morbidity and mortality are common and are not confined to illicit drug taking. Overall, the cost of medication-related morbidity and mortality in the US exceeded $177.4 billion in 2000.[87] In ambulatory settings, the mean cost for a treatment failure was $977; for a new medical problem, the mean cost was $1105, and the cost of a treatment failure resulting in a new medical problem was $1488. Hospital admissions accounted for nearly 70% and long-term-care admissions 18% of total costs. Since 1995, the costs associated with drug-related problems have more than doubled. The most common types of medication-induced disorders are dose-dependent, predictable and preventable. Drug reactions may result from an exaggeration of the normal pharmacological effects of a drug, by excess intake of the drug or by a drug–drug, drug–disease or drug–food interaction. The two most common drug–disease interactions in older adults are first-generation calcium channel blockers used in patients with congestive heart failure and aspirin used in patients with peptic ulcer disease (both, 3.7%).[88] Other drugs causing problems due to interactions are antihistamines and tranquillizers.

Antihistamines are used to treat certain allergies, e.g. hayfever, to dry secretions in the common cold, to sedate and to prevent motion sickness. Excess sedation results if used in combination with alcohol or benzodiazepines. Benzodiazepines are minor tranquillizers. They are depressants slowing down physical, mental and emotional responses. The most common benzodiazepine tranquillizers are Valium, Serepax and Mogadon. Minor tranquillizers are usually prescribed for anxiety or sleep problems.

When prescribing drugs, patients are cautioned about drug–drug and drug–nutrient interactions.

Screening for abuse

Two questions have emerged as invaluable for briefly screening individuals for substance abuse.[89] A positive response to 'In the last year, have you ever drunk or used drugs more than you meant to?' has a sensitivity of over 70% and a specificity of over 80%. This is an excellent screening question. To reduce the risk of a false positive, a second question, 'Have you felt you wanted or needed to cut down on your drinking or drug use in the last year?', is useful. This question, while having a sensitivity of just over 56%, has a specificity of over 91%. This two-item conjoint screen has been shown to be particularly sensitive to polysubstance use disorders. Respondents who gave 0, 1, and 2 positive responses had a 7.3%, 36.5%, and 72.4% chance of a current substance use disorder, respectively; likelihood ratios were 0.27, 1.93, and 8.77.

Other questions with lower sensitivity and therefore less useful as screening tools are:

- In the last year, have you drunk or used nonprescription drugs to deal with your feelings, stress, or frustration?
- In the last year, how many times have you not remembered things that happened while you were drinking or using drugs?
- As a result of your drinking or drug use, did anything happen in the last year that you wish didn't happen?

These last two questions have a specificity in excess of 92%.

Screening for drug abuse using the two-item conjoint screening method provides health professionals with a useful tool for the brief clinical interview. See **Handout 15.11**.

In perspective

Drug dependence is a physical and psychological phenomenon. While some individuals may have a genetic predisposition to dependence, currently it is not possible confidently to predict who is at increased risk. Prevention is the best approach. It is easier to avoid drug abuse than to recover from drug addiction.

References

1. National Centre for Health Statistics. *Health, United States, 2007. With Chartbook on Trends in the Health of Americans*. Hyattsville, MD: US Department of Health and Human Services; 2007.

2. *Statistics on young people and drug misuse: England, 2003*. Last modified date: 8 February. http://www.dh.gov.uk/en/Publicationsandstatistics/Statistics/StatisticalWorkAreas/Statisticalpublichealth/DH_4087896; Accessed 05.01.09.

3. *NHS: The Information Centre. Drug use, smoking and drinking among young people in England 2007*. http://www.ic.nhs.uk/statistics-and-data-collections/health-and-lifestyles-related-surveys/smoking-drinking-and-drug-use-among-young-people-in-england; Accessed 05.01.09.

4. Australian Institute of Health and Welfare. *Statistics on Drug Use in Australia 2004*. Drug Statistics Series No. 15. AIHW Cat. No. PHE 62 Canberra: AIHW; 2005.

5. Hill DJ, White VM, Williams RM, Gardner GJ. Tobacco and alcohol use among Australian secondary school students in 1990. *Med J Aust.* 1993,158:228–234.

6. Resnick MD, Bearman PS, Blum R, et al. Protecting adolescents from harm. *JAMA.* 1997;278:823–832.

7. Robins LN, Przybeck TR. Age of onset of use: a predictor in drug and other disorders. In: Battjes RJ, ed. *Etiology of Drug Abuse: Actions for Prevention*. Washington, DC: USA Printing Office; 1985.

8. Hall WD, Degenhardt LJ, Lynskey MT. Opioid overdose mortality in Australia, 1964–1997: birth cohort trends. *Med J Aust.* 1999;171:34–37.

9. Healey A, Knapp M, Astin J, et al. Economic burden of drug dependency. Social costs incurred by drug users at intake to the National Treatment Outcome Research Study. *Br J Psychiatry.* 1998;173:160–165.

10. U.S. Preventive Services Task Force. *Guide to Clinical Preventive Services*. 2nd ed. Baltimore: Williams & Wilkins; 1996:583.

11. Comerci GD, Fuller PG, Morrison SF. Cigarettes, drugs, alcohol and teens. *Patient Care.* 1997;31:57–84.

12. Heyne A, Wolffgramm J. The development of addiction to d-amphetamine in an animal model: same principles as for alcohol and opiate. *Psychopharmacology.* 1998;140(4):510–518.

13. Petry NM, Bickel WK. Polydrug abuse in heroin addicts: a behavioral economic analysis. *Addiction.* 1998;93(3):321–335.

14. Cone EJ. Recent discoveries in pharmacokinetics of drugs of abuse. *Toxicol Lett.* 1998;102:97–101.

15. Pierce RC, Kumaresan V. The mesolimbic dopamine system: the final common pathway for the reinforcing effect of drugs of abuse?

Neurosci Biobehav Rev. 2006;30 (2):215–238.

16. Boutrel B. A neuropeptide-centric view of psychostimulant addiction. *Br J Pharmacol.* 2008;154 (2):343–357.

17. Feltenstein MW, See RE. *The neurocircuitry of addiction: an overview. Br J Pharmacol.* 2008;154 (2):261–274.

18. Leshner AI, Koob GF. Drugs of abuse and the brain. *Proc Assoc Am Physicians.* 1999;111(2):99–108.

19. Brown RL, Leonard T, Saunders LA, Papasouliotis O. A two-item screening test for alcohol and other drug problems. *J Fam Pract.* 1997;44:151–160.

20. Schuckit MA, Daeppen JB, Danko GP, et al. Clinical implications for four drugs of the DSM-IV distinction between substance dependence with and without a physiological component. *Am J Psychiatry.* 1999;156 (1):41–49.

21. Mokdad AH, Marks JS, Stroup DF, Gerberding JL. Actual causes of death in the United States, 2000. *JAMA.* 2004;291(10):1238–1245.

22. http://www.top100espresso.com/ coffee_consumption_statistics_ report.html; Accessed 05.01.09.

23. http://www.ers.usda.gov/ AmberWaves/June07/Findings/ Coffee2.htm; Accessed 05.01.09.

24. Kendler KS, Prescott CA. Caffeine intake, tolerance, and withdrawal in women: a population-based twin study. *Am J Psychiatry.* 1999;156:223–228.

25. James JE. Acute and chronic effects of caffeine on performance, mood, headache, and sleep. *Neuropsychobiology.* 1998;38 (1):32–41.

26. National Centre on Sleep Disorders Research Working Group. Recognizing problem sleepiness in your patients. *Am Fam Physician.* 1999;59:937–944.

27. Jee SH, He J, Whelton PK, Suh I, Klag MJ. The effect of chronic coffee drinking on blood pressure: a meta-analysis of controlled clinical trials. *Hypertension.* 1999;33 (2):647–652.

28. Hartley TR, Sung BH, Pincomb GA, Whitsett TL, Wilson MF, Lovallo WR. Hypertension risk status and effect of caffeine on blood pressure. *Hypertension.* 2000;36(1):137–141.

29. Mattioli AV, Bonatti S, Zennaro M, et al. Effect of coffee consumption, lifestyle and acute life stress in the development of acute lone atrial fibrillation. *J Cardiovasc Med (Hagerstown).* 2008;9(8):794–798.

30. Scher AI, Stewart WF, Lipton RB. Caffeine as a risk factor for chronic daily headache: a population-based study. *Neurology.* 2004;63 (11):2022–2027.

31. Zampelas A, Panagiotakos DB, Pitsavos C, Chrysohoou C, Stefanadis C. Associations between coffee consumption and inflammatory markers in healthy persons: the ATTICA study. *Am J Clin Nutr.* 2004;80(4):862–867.

32. CARE Study Group. Maternal caffeine intake during pregnancy and risk of fetal growth restriction: a large prospective observational study. *BMJ.* 2008;337:a2332.

33. Greenberg JA, Chow G, Ziegelstein RC. Caffeinated coffee consumption, cardiovascular disease, and heart valve disease in the elderly (from the Framingham Study). *Am J Cardiol.* 2008;102 (11):1502–1508.

34. Cornelis MC, El-Sohemy A. Coffee, caffeine, and coronary heart disease. *Curr Opin Clin Nutr Metab Care.* 2007;10(6):745–751.

35. Pereira MA, Parker ED, Folsom AR. Coffee consumption and risk of type 2 diabetes mellitus: an 11-year prospective study of 28 812 postmenopausal women. *Arch Intern Med.* 2006;166 (12):1311–1316.

36. Juliano LM, Griffiths RR. A critical review of caffeine withdrawal: empirical validation of symptoms and signs, incidence, severity, and associated features. *Psychopharmacology (Berl).* 2004;176(1):1–29.

35. Nehlig A. Are we dependent upon coffee and caffeine? A review on human and animal data. *Neurosci Biobehav Rev.* 1999;23(4):563–576.

36. Miyata H, Hironaka N, Takada K, Miyasato K, Nakamura K, Yanagita T. Psychosocial withdrawal characteristics of nicotine compared with alcohol and caffeine. *Ann N Y Acad Sci.* 2008;1139:458–465.

37. Smith AP. Caffeine, cognitive failures and health in a non-working community sample. *Hum Psychopharmacol.* 2009;24 (1):29–34.

38. Paganini-Hill A, Kawas CH, Corrada MM. Non-alcoholic beverage and caffeine consumption and mortality: the Leisure World Cohort Study. *Prev Med.* 2007;44 (4):305–310.

39. *National Institute on Drug Abuse Research Report.* http://www.nida. nih.gov/ResearchReports/Nicotine/ Nicotine.html; Accessed 06.01.09.

40. Balfour D, Benowitz N, Fagerstrom K, Kunze M, Keil U. Diagnosis and treatment of nicotine dependence with emphasis on nicotine replacement therapy. A status report. *Eur Heart J.* 2000;21 (6):438–445.

41. Kawachi I, Troisi RJ, Rotnitzky AG, Coakley EH, Colditz GA. Can physical activity minimize weight gain in women after smoking cessation? *Am J Public Health.* 1996;86(7):999–1004.

42. Benowitz NL, Henningfield JE. Establishing a nicotine threshold for addiction. *N Engl J Med.* 1994;331:123–125.

43. Russell MAH. The nicotine addiction trap: a 40-year sentence for four cigarettes. *Br J Addict.* 1990;85:293–300.

44. United Nations Office on Drugs and Crime. *Global illicit drug trends— 2003.* Vienna, Austria: United Nations International Drug Control Programme Research Section; 2003.

45. Substance Abuse and Mental Health Services Administration, Office of Applied Studies. *Results from the 2005 National Survey on Drug Use and Health: national findings.* NSDUH Series H-30. DHHS Publication No. SMA 06-4194 Rockville, MD: US Department of Health and Human Services; 2006.

46. Centers for Disease Control and Prevention. Surveillance summaries. *Morb Mortal Wkly Rep.* 2004;53 (No. SS-2).

47. Haney M, Ward AS, Comer SD, Foltin RW, Fischman MW. Abstinence symptoms following oral THC administration to humans. *Psychopharmacology.* 1999;141 (4):385–394.

48. Johnson MC, Heriza TJ, St Dennis C. How to spot illicit drug abuse in your patients. *Postgrad Med.* 1999;106:199–218.

49. Swift W, Hall W, Copeland J. Characteristics of long-term cannabis users in Sydney, Australia. *Eur Addict Res.* 1998;4(4):190–197.

50. Kalant H. Adverse effects of cannabis on health: an update of the literature since 1996. *Prog Neuropsychopharmacol Biol Psychiatry.* 2004;28:849–863.

51. Grant I, Gonzalez R, Carey CL, et al. Non-acute (residual) neurocognitive effects of cannabis use: a meta-analytic study. *J Int Neuropsychol Soc.* 2003;9(5):679–689.

52. Elkashef A, Vocci F, Huestis M, et al. Marijuana neurobiology and treatment. *Subst Abus.* 2008;29(3):17–29.

53. Hanuš LO. Pharmacological and therapeutic secrets of plant and brain (endo)cannabinoids. *Med Res Rev.* 2009;29(2):213–271.

54. Voth EA, Schwartz RH. Medicinal applications of delta-9-tetrahydrocannabinol and marijuana. *Ann Intern Med.* 1997;126(10):791–798.

55. Schwartz RH, Voth EA, Sheridan MJ. Marijuana to prevent nausea and vomiting in cancer patients: a survey of clinical oncologists. *South Med J.* 1997;90(2):167–172.

56. Capaldini L, Tashkin D, Vilensky W. Does marijuana have a place in medicine? *Patient Care.* 1998;32:41–53.

57. Grant I, Cahn BR. Cannabis and endocannabinoid modulators: therapeutic promises and challenges. *Clin Neurosci Res.* 2005;5(2–4):185–199.

58. Kogan NM, Mechoulam R. Cannabinoids in health and disease. *Dialogues Clin Neurosci.* 2007;9(4):413–430.

59. Hall W. The health risks of cannabis. *Aust Fam Phys.* 1995;24:1237–1239.

60. Leirer VO, Yesavage JA, Morrow DG. Marijuana carry-over effects on aircraft pilot performance. *Aviat Space Environ Med.* 1991;62(3):221–227.

61. Brookoff D, Cook CS, Williams C, Mann CS. Testing reckless drivers for cocaine and marijuana. *N Engl J Med.* 1994;331(8):518–522.

62. Khiabani HZ, Bramness JG, Bjørneboe A, Mørland J. Relationship between THC concentration in blood and impairment in apprehended drivers. *Traffic Inj Prev.* 2006;7(2):111–116.

63. Grotenhermen F, Leson G, Berghaus G, et al. Developing limits for driving under cannabis. *Addiction.* 2007;102(12):1910–1917.

64. Jones AW, Holmgren A, Kugelberg FC. Driving under the influence of cannabis: a 10-year study of age and gender differences in the concentrations of tetrahydrocannabinol in blood. *Addiction.* 2008;103(3):452–461.

65. Fergusson DM, Horwood LJ, Boden JM. Is driving under the influence of cannabis becoming a greater risk to driver safety than drink driving? Findings from a longitudinal study. *Accid Anal Prev.* 2008;40(4):1345–1350.

66. Hunault CC, Mensinga TT, Böcker KB, et al. Cognitive and psychomotor effects in males after smoking a combination of tobacco and cannabis containing up to 69 mg delta-9-tetrahydrocannabinol (THC). *Psychopharmacology (Berl).* 2009;204(1):85–94.

67. Kleber HD. Cocaine abuse: historical, epidemiological and psychological perspectives. *J Clin Psych.* 1988;49(2 suppl):3–6.

68. Bierut LJ, Strickland JR, Thompson JR, Afful SE, Cottler LB. Drug use and dependence in cocaine dependent subjects, community-based individuals, and their siblings. *Drug Alcohol Depend.* 2008;95(1–2):14–22.

69. *World Drug Report 2006 figures.* http://en.wikipedia.org/wiki/List_of_countries_by_prevalence_of_cocaine_use#cite_note-wdr_2006-0; Accessed 06.01.09.

70. *National Drug Strategy household survey.* http://www.aihw.gov.au/publications/index.cfm/title/10190 Accessed; 06.01.09.

71. Iwanami A, Kuroki N, Iritani S, Isono H, Okajima Y, Kamijima K. Event-related potential in chronic methamphetamine dependence. *J Nerv Ment Dis.* 1998;186(12):746–751.

72. Hegadoren KM, Baker GB, Bourin M. 3,4-Methylenedioxy analogues of amphetamine: defining the risks to humans. *Neurosci Biobehav Rev.* 1999;23(4):539–553.

73. Albertson TE, Derlet RW, Van Hoozen BE. Methamphetamine and the expanding complications of amphetamines. *West J Med.* 1999;170(4):214–219.

74. Morgan MJ. Memory deficits associated with recreational use of "ecstasy" (MDMA). *Psychopharmacology.* 1999;141(1):30–36.

75. Bolla KI, McCann UD, Ricaurte GA. Memory impairment in abstinent MDMA ("Ecstasy") users. *Neurology.* 1998;51(6):1532–1537.

76. Elk C. MDMA (Ecstacy): useful information for health professionals involved in drug education programs. *J Drug Educ.* 1996;26(4):349–356.

77. Gamma A, Jerome L, Liechti ME, Sumnall HR. Is ecstasy perceived to be safe? A critical survey. *Drug Alcohol Depend.* 2005;77(2):185–193.

78. Landry MJ. MDMA: a review of epidemiologic data. *J Psychoactive Drugs.* 2002;34(2):163–169.

79. *NSDUH Report: Use of Specific Hallucinogens.* http://www.whitehousedrugpolicy.gov/DrugFact/hallucinogens/index.html; Accessed 06.01.09.

80. McGarvey EL, Clavet GJ, Mason W, Waite D. Adolescent inhalant abuse: environments of use. *Am J Drug Alcohol Abuse.* 1999;25(4):731–741.

81. National Institutes of Health. Infofacts http://www.nida.nih.gov/Infofacts/Inhalants.html; Accessed 06.01.09.

82. Young SJ, Longstaffe S, Tenenbein M. Inhalant abuse and the abuse of other drugs. *Am J Drug Alcohol Abuse.* 1999;25(2):371–375.

83. Sproule BA, Busto UE, Somer G, Romach MK, Sellers EM. Characteristics of dependent and nondependent regular users of

codeine. *J Clin Psychopharmacol.* 1999;19(4):367–372.

84. Heroin use USA http://www. alcohol-and-drug-guide.com/heroin-use-usa.html; Accessed 06.01.08.

85. Strang J, Griffiths P, Powis B, Gossop M. Heroin chasers and heroin injectors: differences observed in a community sample in London, UK. *Am J Addict.* 1999;8(2):148–160.

86. *Drugs and Sport* http://www. whitehousedrugpolicy.gov/ PREVENT/sports/index.html; Accessed 06.01.09.

87. Ernst FR, Grizzle AJ. Drug-related morbidity and mortality: updating the cost-of-illness model. *J Am Pharm Assoc (Wash).* 2001;41 (2):192–199.

88. Lindblad CI, Hanlon JT, Gross CR, et al. Clinically important drug-disease interactions and their prevalence in older adults. *Clin Ther.* 2006;28(8):1133–1143.

89. Brown RL, Leonard T, Saunders LA, Papasouliotis O. A two-item conjoint screen for alcohol and other drug problems. *J Am Board Fam Pract.* 2001;14(2): 95–106.

Smoking

Smoking: a health risk

Tobacco contributed 2.6% of the total global disease burden in 1990 and 'by 2020, tobacco is expected to kill more people than any single disease, surpassing even the HIV epidemic'.[1] In the UK, one in five of all deaths were caused by smoking in 1995,[2] while 435,000 Americans died up to 15 years prematurely in 2005 due to this habit.[3] Fortunately, the prevalence of smoking in the US, England and Australia is declining.[2–4] Nonetheless, in 2005, 23% of men and 18% of women in the US were still smoking,[3] as were 24% of men and 21% of women in England in 2006.[2] In Australia, 17% of the population aged 14 years and over were daily smokers, with the highest smoking rates recorded in the 20–29 year age group.[4] A survey of high school students in the US during 2007 found 20% had smoked cigarettes during the 30 days before the survey.[5] The prevalence of cigarette use among adolescents is second only to alcohol consumption, with 58.4% of high school students in the US having tried cigarettes; 9.7% smoke on at least 20 out of 30 days.[6] In 2007, in England, 33% of pupils had tried smoking and pupils classified as regular smokers smoked an average of 44.1 cigarettes weekly.[7]

Smoking is implicated in 30% of all cancer deaths and in 87% of deaths attributed to lung cancer. Smoking is also causally linked to 82% of deaths from chronic obstructive airways disease, 21% of deaths from coronary artery disease and 18% of stroke deaths. About half of all regular cigarette smokers will ultimately die of a smoking-related disease and 40% of people who smoke 20 or more cigarettes a day will die before the age of 65 years. A US national telephone survey found that smokers underestimated the health hazard presented by smoking.[8] Smokers perceived that their risk of lung cancer and of cancer in general barely increases with the number of cigarettes smoked daily; more than half surveyed felt exercise neutralized most of the effects of smoking![8] Fewer women give up tobacco than alcohol during pregnancy.[4] Smoking during pregnancy restrains fetal growth and induces neuroendocrine dysfunction through placental vascular effects and possibly also via altered leptin metabolism.[9] A longitudinal study suggests maternal smoking in pregnancy is associated with an increased rise in total cholesterol levels and a tendency towards an adverse lipoprotein profile in offspring.[10] Prenatal nicotine exposure produces cognitive and behavioural impairment in children and appears to increase the likelihood of subsequent tobacco use.[11] Prenatal and postnatal nicotine exposure may cause the upregulation of nicotine receptors in the brain.

Passive smoking also carries considerable risk. Sidestream smoke has higher concentrations of carbon monoxide, nicotine, carcinogens, and formaldehyde (which inhibits respiratory cilia) than the mainstream smoke inhaled by the smoker. There is some evidence to suggest that secondhand smoke exposure may yield nicotine levels similar to those obtained through active smoking![11] A non-smoker sharing an office with a smoker could potentially inhale the equivalent of five cigarettes a day in respiratory suspended particles. Passive smoking recently has been accepted as a major risk for coronary artery disease, stroke, and cancers.[12] Exposure to 30 minutes of secondhand smoke affects coronary flow velocity reserve in non-smokers, indicating endothelial dysfunction in coronary circulation.[13] The relative risk of lung cancer in a two-packet-a-day smoker is 20 times that of the non-smoker;[14] it is about 20% greater in a never-smoking spouse of a smoker.[15] A non-smoker increases their lung cancer risk by 30% by marrying a smoker. In addition to lung cancer, passive smoking is a risk factor for recurrent sore eyes, headaches, premature ventricular contractions, asthma attacks and respiratory problems in infancy or early childhood.[16] Exposure to tobacco smoke is widespread, with 60% of the US population being exposed to secondhand smoke.[17]

The excess morbidity and mortality associated with smoking is greater in cigarette than pipe and cigar smokers. The constituents of burning tobacco that appear to be implicated in the pathogenesis of tobacco-related disorders are tar and hydrocarbons, nicotine and carbon monoxide.

Tar and hydrocarbons

The potential toxicity of airborne particles appears related to both the size and composition of the particle itself, as well as the gaseous or liquid-phase pollutants – that coexist with the particles. Particles with a diameter of 1–10 μm in diameter penetrate and remain in the lower respiratory tract. These particles may exert a direct toxic effect or may passively carry biologically active hydrocarbons or inorganic metals in a thin film of absorbed material. Certain ring and straight chain hydrocarbons can be oxidized to form compounds such as aldehydes. These, like other oxidants, irritate mucous membrane and conjunctiva. In addition to accelerating the production of ozone, certain hydrocarbons are known to be carcinogenic. Adsorption of polycyclic aromatic hydrocarbons onto the surface of particulate matter may transfer carcinogenic substances into the lower respiratory tract. Smoking in the workplace can enhance the risk of carcinogenesis on exposure to industrial chemicals, including asbestos, arsenic, nickel, chromates, and ionizing radiation.

Smoking is considered an additive factor in lead toxicity.

Tar, hydrocarbons, and particulate matter, when regularly inhaled, can lead to

- persistent bronchial irritation. Manifest early as the 'smoker's cough', persistent irritation presents at a later stage as chronic bronchitis
- alveolar damage. Progressive dyspnoea is later accompanied by the increased anteroposterior chest diameter characteristic of emphysema. Cor pulmonale, right heart failure attributable to lung disease, is a relatively late complication
- neoplastic change. Cancer may be initiated and/or promoted by compounds in cigarette smoke. Bronchogenic carcinoma may result from inhaled carcinogens and bladder cancer may result from increased urinary excretion of free radicals. Mucosal damage attributable to free radicals may be minimized by antioxidants. A double-blind, placebo-controlled trial found that plasma ascorbic acid was depleted by smoking and restored by moderate supplementation or 272 mg of vitamin C daily.[18] This exceeds the RDA for vitamin C some sixfold.

Carbon monoxide

Carbon monoxide is produced by incomplete combustion of hydrocarbons. It competes successfully with oxygen for combination with haemoglobin. Smokers who inhale frequently have blood carboxyhaemoglobin levels double that of urban non-smokers. A number of studies have found carboxyhaemoglobin levels in smokers to be around 5%. At this level, neurological effects include restlessness, irritability, impaired concentration, and delayed reaction time. The long-term effects of excessive exposure to carbon monoxide include structural changes in the myocardium and arterial walls. Increased carboxyhaemoglobin is one good reason for not smoking during pregnancy. Nicotine is another.

Nicotine

Tar particles and hydrocarbons are responsible for lung damage, carboxyhaemoglobin impairs tissue oxygenation, but it is nicotine that induces physical and psychological dependence. Inhaled nicotine rapidly reaches the central nervous system, providing rapid gratification and strong behavioural reinforcement. The clinical effects of nicotine include:

- psychic satisfaction. Cigarette smoke is more acidic and inhalation enhances nicotine absorption. Cigar smoke is more alkaline; adequate absorption is achieved through the buccal mucosa. Cigarette smokers inhale; cigar smokers do not. However, cigarette smokers switching to cigars do not change their smoking patterns and as they continue to inhale they retain the enhanced morbidity risk of cigarette smoking
- release of catecholamines. Secondary effects of smoking include free fatty acid mobilization and elevated blood triglyceride levels; tachycardia and hypertension; increased platelet adhesiveness and aggregation with resultant promotion of blood coagulation; and a reduced appetite due to slow stomach emptying and increased duodenal reflux.

Addictive characteristics encountered in nicotine use include:[19–21]

- a psychoactive effect of euphoria, stimulation, or relaxation. Nicotine improves the performance of repetitive tasks, attention, problem solving, and learning
- compulsive use. Awareness of its deleterious effects does not automatically lead to smoking cessation
- regular use. Deprivation increases the desire to use the drug
- the paired stimulus–response of inhalation. Nicotine affects the central nervous system within 7 seconds of inhalation – this provides powerful reinforcement of the habit
- the development of nicotine tolerance. Smokers adapt to the subjective effects and tachycardia of nicotine inhalation within 24 hours. Persons with persistently high nicotine blood levels report tolerance to the pallor, nausea, and vomiting of nicotine toxicity
- physical dependence and a withdrawal syndrome. Symptoms are usually most severe 48–96 hours after the last cigarette. Irritability, restlessness, inability to concentrate, sleep disturbance, weight gain, constipation or diarrhoea, and nicotine craving are recognized manifestations of nicotine withdrawal. A second peak of withdrawal symptoms is experienced about 10 days after quitting
- a high relapse rate after smoking cessation.

Persons who are highly dependent on nicotine are those most likely to suffer withdrawal and relapse after smoking cessation. Nicotine dependence is most likely to be high in persons who always inhale, who smoke one or more cigarettes every 30 minutes and who show evidence of a withdrawal syndrome. Analysis of various tobaccos found that mainstream smoke deliveries varied from 0.5 to 1.6 mg for nicotine, 6.8 to 21.6 mg for tar, and 5.9 to 17.4 mg for carbon monoxide per cigarette, with cigarettes from European, American, or African WHO regions tending to have lower smoke deliveries than those from other countries surveyed.[22]

As nicotine is the addictive component of tobacco, sources and modes of delivery of nicotine have been sought that are free of the adverse lung effects of tobacco smoke. Analysis of the nicotine content of 11 popular brands of smokeless tobacco found the nicotine content to be highest in moist snuff, moderate in plug tobacco and lowest in loose-leaf chewing tobacco.[23] The toxicity of smokeless tobacco varies by brand and across countries; however, cigarette smoking does produce more negative health effects and probably has a higher addiction potential with more severe withdrawal. While smokeless tobacco reduces the risk of lung diseases, it remains a significant cause of oral pathology, is toxic for the fetus and may increase the risk for cardiovascular disease.[23] All tobacco use increases heart rate and blood pressure, but products with lower nicotine content evoke smaller cardiovascular responses. Overall, 11% of the general population in the US have 'ever tried' chewing tobacco, snuff, or other smokeless tobacco.[24] Converting to smokeless tobacco is a poor alternative to quitting. However, quitting is difficult.

In the US in 2005, of the 44.5 million smokers, 70% claimed they would like to quit,[3] and in 2007 in the UK, 73% of current smokers said they would like to give up smoking.[25] Globally, premature tobacco-attributable deaths are projected to rise from 5.4 million in 2004 to 8.3 million in 2030, yet two out of three countries have no, or a minimal, tobacco control policy.[26] Even in countries with tobacco control policies, the social and economic costs are substantial. In the US during 2000–2004, smoking resulted in an estimated annual average of 269,655 deaths among males and 173,940 deaths among females.[27] The total economic burden of smoking in the US is approximately $193 billion per year; investments in comprehensive, state-based tobacco prevention and control programmes in fiscal year 2007 totalled $595 million – approximately 325-times less than the smoking-attributable costs.[27]

Increasing the baseline quit rate from the current 2.5% of smokers to 10% would prevent 1,170,000 premature deaths in the US![3]

Smoking and disease

Tobacco use is the leading preventable cause of death in the US, where more deaths are caused each year by tobacco use than by all deaths from human immunodeficiency virus, illegal drug use, alcohol use, motor vehicle injuries, suicides, and murders combined.[28] The major impact of smoking is on the respiratory and cardiovascular systems. The three leading specific causes of smoking-attributable death were lung cancer, ischaemic heart disease and chronic obstructive pulmonary disease. An estimated 49,400 lung cancer and heart disease deaths annually were attributable to exposure to secondhand smoke.[27]

The cardiovascular system

Smoking was responsible for 126,005 deaths from ischaemic heart disease annually in the US in 2000–2004; in adults 35 years of age and older, 32.6% of smoking-attributable deaths were caused by cardiovascular diseases.[27] Cigarette smoking doubles or trebles the risk of dying from a heart attack;[28] in women more so than in men.

Nicotine adversely affects lipids, blood coagulation and vascular stability. The event that precipitates a heart attack or ischaemic stroke is usually either arterial spasm or a thrombus. Secondhand smoke also increases the risk of coronary heart disease. Platelet and endothelial function, arterial stiffness, atherosclerosis, oxidative stress, inflammation, heart rate variability and energy metabolism are exquisitely sensitive to the toxins in secondhand smoke. The effects of brief passive smoking are often nearly as large as chronic active smoking! Passive smokers have disproportionately high levels of fibrinogen and homocysteine, two biomarkers of cardiovascular disease risk.[29] Tobacco smoke increases the risk both of atheroma formation and coagulation.

Giving up smoking can halve the risk of dying in 5–10 years. Women who stop smoking reduce their excess risk of coronary heart disease by 25–33% within 2 years and approximate the risk of those who have never smoked in 10 to 14 years.[30] This pattern of reduced excess risk also applies to stroke and is consistent regardless of the number of cigarettes smoked, the age of starting or the presence of other risk factors for stroke.[31]

Lung disease

Smoking was responsible for 128,922 deaths from lung cancer annually in the US in 2000–2004, and in adults 35 years of age and older, 41% of smoking-attributable deaths were caused by cancer and 26.3% by respiratory diseases.[27]

Obstructive airway disease

Smoking impairs normal respiratory function. Cigarette smoking increases the risk of dying from chronic obstructive lung disease by a factor of 10; in fact, some 90% of all deaths from chronic obstructive lung diseases are attributable to cigarette smoking.[28] Chronic obstructive airways disease is a syndrome of progressive airflow limitation characterized by an abnormal inflammatory reaction. The condition is the result both of an environmental insult and of a host reaction which is likely to be genetically predetermined. Chronic tobacco smoking and indoor air pollution are major causes. Smoking is responsible for more cases of obstructive airways disease than dusty occupational environments. However, only a fraction of smokers develop clinically relevant obstructive airways disease.[32] Changes associated with obstructive lung disease may be detected early using spirometry. Figure 16.1 provides information on normal lung capacity. Other normal parameters of respiratory function are listed in Table 16.1.

A prolonged expiration suggests the need to assess ventilatory capacity using spirometry. Noninvasive spirometric lung function tests can measure the ventilatory capacity of the lung. Normal indices are as follows:

- TLC (5800 mL) = VC (4600 mL) + RV (1200 mL), where TLC is total lung capacity, VC is vital capacity, and RV is residual volume.
- VC (4600 mL) = IC (3500 mL) + ERV (1100 mL), where IC is inspiratory capacity and ERV is expiratory residual volume.
- IC (3500 mL) = TV (500 mL) + IRV (3000 mL), where TV is tidal volume and IRV is inspiratory residual volume.
- TLC (5800) = IC (3500 mL) + FRC (2300 mL), where FRC is the functional residual capacity.

The disease is initially asymptomatic, becoming symptomatic once the forced expiratory volume in one second (FEV1) falls below 70% of the predicted

Normal indices on non-invasive spirometric lung function testing of an adult are of the order of:
total lung capacity (TLC) = 5800 mL
vital capacity = 4600 mL
residual volume (RV) = 1200 mL
inspiratory capacity (IC) = 3500 mL
expiratory residual volume (ERV) = 1100 mL
tidal volume (TV) = 500 mL
inspiratory residual volume (IRV) = 3000 mL
functional residual volume (FRV) = 2300 mL
forced expiratory volume in 1 second (FEV1) = 3700 mL
forced vital capacity (FVC) = 4600 mL

The relationship between these parameters is expressed as:
TLC (5800 mL) = VC (4600 mL) + RV (1200 mL)
VC (4600 mL) = IC (3500 mL) + ERV (1100 mL)
IC (3500 mL) = TV (500 mL) + IRV (3000 mL)
TLC (5800) = IC (3500 mL) + FRC (2300 mL)
FEV1/FVC = 80%

Feather I. Spirometry; a practical guide for GPs. Modern Medicine of Australia March 1996, 103–110.

Figure 16.1 • Spirometric assessment of ventilatory capacity.

Table 16.1 Parameters of adult respiratory health

Respiration	Wellness	Dysfunction
Rate	16–20/min*	>20/min
Rhythm	Regular	Irregular
Respiratory:pulse rate ratio	1:4[†]	> or <1:4
A-P:transverse diameter	1:2 to 5:7	<1:2 or >5:7
Respiratory expansion	Symmetrical	Asymmetrical
Diaphragmatic excursion	3–5 cm	<3 cm
Palpation	Trachea central	Tracheal deviation
Percussion note	Resonant	Dull or hyperresonant
Auscultation	*Breath sounds:*	*Breath sounds:*
Lung periphery	Vesicular breath sounds	Bronchial breathing
1st/2nd interspace at sternal border	Bronchovesicular	Bronchial
Between the scapulae	Bronchovesicular	Bronchial
	Adventitious sounds:	*Adventitious sounds:*
Lung fields	Absent	Detected
Spirometry (see Figure 16.1)	Within normal parameters	Altered parameters

*<40/min in 1–5-year-olds, <30/min in 6–8-year-olds.
[†]1:3 in children.

value. In smokers, the early stages of lung damage include increased total lung capacity due to an increased functional residual volume and decreased vital capacity. Vital capacity is best detected by a prolonged forced expiration. In the absence of lung damage, it is possible to exhale 75% of one's vital capacity in one second and almost all of the vital capacity in 3 seconds. A prolonged FEV1 is a useful measure of airways obstruction; when this is impaired and fails to improve after administration of bronchodilators, then structural change is likely. The alternative approach is to measure maximum voluntary ventilation (MVV). In healthy people, about half of the vital capacity can be breathed with each breath at a respiratory rate of 40–70 breaths per minute; this is reduced in chronic obstructive airways disease. Dyspnoea and the degree of airflow limitation are the most troubling subjective variables.[33]

Cancer

Smoking accounts for about a third of all cancers in the US. While 90% of deaths from lung cancer are estimated to be due to smoking, smokers are also at increased risk of bladder, renal, oral, oesophageal, stomach, pancreatic and breast cancer. Tobacco use is believed to be the main cause of 90% of all male and 79% of all female lung cancers.[34] In fact, it has been suggested: 'There is no cancer epidemic except for cancer of the lung due to smoking.'[35] By 2025, one-third of all adult deaths are expected to be related to cigarette smoking and, compared with non-smokers, the risk of lung cancer is estimated to be 20–40 times higher in lifelong smokers.[34] Current smokers have a far greater risk of lung cancer than those who have stopped smoking or have never smoked. Compared to never-smokers, the risk of dying from lung cancer is more than 22 times higher among male and about 12 times higher in female smokers.[28]

Tobacco smoke not only delivers carcinogens, it also has an immunosuppressive effect. Smoking affects innate immunity through structural and functional changes in the respiratory ciliary epithelium, lung surfactant protein, and immune cells such as alveolar macrophages, neutrophils, lymphocytes and natural killer cells.[36] Lung cancer rates increase with exposure to tobacco's carcinogens. More than 50 carcinogens have been identified in tobacco, including polynuclear aromatic hydrocarbons, aromatic amines, and N-nitrosamines.

Since 1950, the makeup of cigarettes and the composition of cigarette smoke have gradually changed. On average, 'tar' and nicotine yields have declined from a high of 38 mg 'tar' and 2.7 mg nicotine to 12 mg and 0.95 mg respectively. Smoking non-filtered cigarettes with tar ratings of 22 mg or over poses the greatest risk of lung cancer.[37] However, low-tar cigarettes do not offer a solution, as lung cancer risk is similar in people who smoke medium-tar, low-tar, or even very-low-tar cigarettes with no more than 7 mg of tar per cigarette.[37] This paradox is explained by smokers of low-yield cigarettes compensating for the low delivery of nicotine by inhaling smoke more deeply and by smoking more intensely. Under these conditions, the peripheral lung is exposed to increased amounts of smoke carcinogens that are suspected to lead to lung adenocarcinoma. Furthermore, the more intense smoking by the consumers of low-yield cigarettes increases N-nitrosamines in the smoke two- or three-fold. A powerful lung carcinogen, 4-(methylnitrosamino)-1-(3-pyridyl)-1-butanone (NNK), is exclusively formed from nicotine! Depending on the yield of the brand chosen, the threshold risk level for lung cancer appears to be 20 pack-years, i.e. smoking an average of one or more packets a day over 20 years. Smoking 25 cigarettes per day increases the risk of lung cancer 30-fold and that of bladder cancer 3-fold.[38] Compared with non-smokers, there is a 40% increased mortality rate among smokers who smoke less than 10 cigarettes daily and a 120% increased mortality rate among smokers who smoke over 40 cigarettes a day.[39] The duration of exposure has emerged as a critical determinant for lung cancer.[39] The earlier a smoking habit is acquired, the greater the potential long-term health hazard. In 2002 in the UK, 10% of children aged 11–15 smoked cigarettes regularly.[40]

Persons who quit reduce their health risk compared with those who continue smoking, but do not revert to a non-smoker's baseline level.[41] Nonetheless, smokers who stop before the age of 35 years may achieve a life-expectancy not significantly different from a non-smoker! Unfortunately, many smokers are in denial. A French national telephone survey reported that 44% of current smokers agreed smoking can cause cancer but only in persons whose daily consumption was higher than their own; an additional 20% considered that the cancer risk became high only for a smoking duration higher than their own.[42] Most smokers surveyed subscribed to misconceptions such as 'smoking is not more dangerous than air pollution' and 'some people smoke their whole life but never get sick'.[42]

Lung cancer is usually asymptomatic until late in the disease and prognosis is influenced by the stage of development of the lesion at the time of diagnosis. Early recognition may be life saving. While exposure to tobacco smoke raises suspicion of future disease, more definitive risk markers are urgently required for early disease diagnosis.[43] Smoking is estimated to trigger some 10 to 20 genetic events that persist for many years after smoking cessation. These genetic alterations may be detected by biopsy, and, more recently, alterations in the DNA extracted from the exhaled breath condensate of smokers looks promising.[44] Detection of an epithelial biomarker that recognizes a heterogeneous nuclear ribonuclear protein expressed by sputum epithelial cells is also possible.[45] This biomarker is particularly useful for the detection of early localized disease.[45] Compared to cytology with its 21% and chest X-ray with its 42% sensitivity, this biomarker with a sensitivity of 74% provides a good initial screening test for lung carcinogenesis. However, definitive diagnosis still requires a more specific test such as cytology with a 100% and chest X-ray with 90% specificity.

Women's health

The three leading smoking-related causes of death in women, ranked in order of importance, are lung cancer, chronic lung disease and heart disease. Ninety percent of all lung cancer deaths in women smokers are attributable to smoking, and by 1987, lung cancer had surpassed breast cancer as the leading cause of cancer-related deaths in women.[46] Smoking is furthermore one of the recognized risk factors for breast cancer. Women have a 1-in-8 lifelong risk for developing breast cancer and a 1-in-28 risk of dying of breast cancer.[47] In addition to cigarette smoke delivering carcinogens, other mechanisms deserve consideration. Smoking alters genetic expression, substantially increasing the likelihood of breast cancer in female carriers of mutations in the ataxia-telangiectasia gene.[48] Smoking also has an anti-oestrogenic effect insofar as it appears related to the early onset of menopause.[49]

Compared with women who never have smoked, postmenopausal smokers have lower bone density and an increased risk for hip fractures.[46] Consistent risk factors for low bone mineral density/bone loss are advancing age, smoking, low weight and weight loss.[50] Current smoking, along with a plethora of other risk markers, is predictive of 5-year hip fracture risk.[51] Postmenopausal bone loss is greater in current smokers than non-smokers. Bone density decrease is accelerated in smokers by an additional 2% for every 10 years after menopause. Compared with non-smokers, in current smokers the relative risk of a hip fracture is similar at age 50, 17% greater at the age of 60 years, 41% higher at 70, 71% at 80, and 108% greater at 90 years.[52] Compared with a non-smoker, the relative risk of a female smoker with a BMI of 25 kg/m^2 suffering a hip fracture is increased 1.5 times.[53] This risk increases to threefold in females with a BMI of 20. For lean females, the association with current smoking is as large as adding 10 years to their age!

Tobacco use among pregnant women is associated with pregnancy complications ranging from placental dysfunction, preterm labor, and premature rupture of membranes to spontaneous abortions and stillbirths.[54] Cigarette smoking increases the risk for infertility, low birth weight, and sudden infant death syndrome.[46] A long-term negative association between maternal smoking during pregnancy and later growth and bone mass of term infants has been noted.[55] Children exposed to mothers who smoke are at increased risk for various conditions ranging from developing otitis media and asthma to learning disorders.[54]

The timing of exposure to tobacco rather than the dose or duration may be critical. It has been suggested that quitting is harder for pregnant women because the physiological adaptations of pregnancy increase the clearance of nicotine, thus lowering nicotine levels and increasing the desire to smoke.[56] An Australian survey reported that 22% of women smoked when they were not pregnant and/or breastfeeding, and 20% continued to smoke during pregnancy and/or while breastfeeding.[4]

There is an additional adverse effect of smoking of particular concern to women. After 10 pack-years, women smokers are twice or three times as likely as non-smokers to develop severe facial wrinkling.[57] In men, similar effects occur after 20 pack-years. In both sexes, the increased risk of wrinkling is equivalent to about 17 months of ageing.

Reduced productivity

Smoking imposes an economic burden on society. Sleepiness is one factor that contributes to the financial cost of employing smokers. Nicotine impairs sleep. Disturbed sleep has deleterious daytime consequences, ranging from sleepiness to dysphoric mood. Nicotine increases vigilance, disrupts sleep and reduces total sleep time.[58] Awakenings provide repetitive bursts of sympathetic nervous system activation, possibly explaining the increased cardiovascular and cerebrovascular morbidity noted. Cigarette smoking is associated with difficulty both initiating and maintaining sleep, while nicotine withdrawal precipitates insomnia. In fact, nicotine replacement therapy induces frequent awakenings and decreases total sleep duration.[58]

Worker sleepiness, resultant industrial accidents and absenteeism all contribute to the adverse impact smoking has on productivity. In 1988, it was estimated that employing a smoker carried an additional cost of $5000 per smoker per year.[59] In 2007, the total economic costs associated with cigarette smoking were estimated at $7.18 per pack of cigarettes sold in the US.[60] In that year, cigarette companies spent more than $45 for every person in the US and more than $290 for each US adult smoker on advertising and promotion.

Quitting

On average, adults who smoke cigarettes die 14 years earlier than non-smokers.[28] However, smokers who quit before the age of 50 halve their risk of dying in the next 15 years.[61] Smokers who quit reduce their risk of smoking-related disorders.[62] Stroke risk decreases to that of a never-smoker within 5 to 15 years of quitting. The risk is halved for cancers of the mouth, throat, and oesophagus after 5 years and for lung cancer after 10 years of abstinence. The risk of dying from chronic obstructive pulmonary disease is reduced. Coronary heart disease risk is halved after 1 year and is nearly the same as someone who never smoked 15 years after quitting.

Quitting is however associated with an increase in weight as compared to those who continue smoking.[63] In quitters there was a significant, positive relationship between number of cigarettes smoked and increase in BMI. Compared to those who continue to smoke, the excess weight gained over a 10-year period following quitting was 4.4 kg for men and 5.0 kg for women.[64] Despite potential weight gain, quitting appears to be the only really satisfactory alternative.

Strategies for quitting

Quitting is difficult. Never starting to smoke is a much preferred option. Quit programmes need to be targeted at all age groups. The urgency of quitting should not be underestimated. Smoking, along with raised serum cholesterol levels, has been implicated in the early coronary atherosclerosis or precursors of atherosclerosis detected in autopsies on children and adolescents.[65] Quit programmes range from mass media campaigns[66] to programmes targeted at families, schools or the workplace.[67] Counselling in primary practice is encouraged. The U.S. Public Health Service recommends that primary care physicians counsel smokers and use the five As (Ask, Advise, Assess, Assist, Arrange) model when treating patients with nicotine addiction.[68] Even 5 minutes' advice on smoking cessation by physicians during an office visit can increase quitting rates;[68] these rates can be most effectively increased when interventions are tailored to patient needs. Behaviour modification has been shown to improve long-term smoking cessation success; indeed, self-help interventions appear to be more effective than standard care.[69] Intervention can be particularly helpful when counselling alerts smokers to self-help interventions tailored to meet their particular needs.

The Transtheoretical Model of behaviour change, conceptualized as involving temporal, dependent and independent dimensions, provides a framework for customizing lifestyle modification.[70,71] The temporal dimension represents the Stages of Change, which categorize readiness to change through a process of five motivational stages.[68] In the pre-contemplation stage, the individual is not planning to quit within the next 6 months; in the contemplation phase, consideration is given to quitting within the next 6 months; in the preparation phase, the person plans to quit within the next 30 days; in the action phase, he or she has quit but for less than 6 months. Once the person has quit for at least 6 months, he or she is considered to be in the maintenance phase. Interventions based on the stages of change model have been shown to enhance motivation and predict cessation. The dependent variable in the Transtheoretical Model encompasses cognitive considerations including decisional balance, the pros and cons of change, and situational temptations. The independent dimension contains variables affecting the processes of change. The processes of change comprise experiential and behavioural dimensions. Experiential processes of change embrace consciousness raising, self-reevaluation, environmental reevaluation, dramatic relief and social liberation; behavioural processes of change include helping relationship, counter conditioning, stimulus control, self-liberation and reinforcement management. By identifying smokers' readiness to change, having smokers analyse the cost:benefits of quitting and evaluating how various strategies may impact on their lifestyle, health professionals can motivate and enable smokers to take increased personal responsibility for their quit programme. When behavioural measures fail, pharmaceutical options are available.

The three first-line medications for smoking cessation are nicotine replacement therapy, varenicline (a partial nicotine receptor agonist) and slow-release bupropion.[72] All three agents approximately double 1-year quit rates when used for 3 months. The first agent to be used in smoking cessation should be nicotine replacement therapy. The aim of nicotine replacement therapy is to ease the transition from cigarette smoking to abstinence by temporarily replacing nicotine to reduce the motivation to smoke and avoid or lessen withdrawal symptoms.[73] Different forms of nicotine replacement therapy include chewing gum, transdermal patches, nasal spray, inhalers and tablets/lozenges. Optimal intervention may be a combination of the patch with gum, inhaler, sublingual tablets or nasal spray. In highly dependent smokers, significant benefit from 4-mg gum compared with 2-mg gum or higher-dose patches has been detected. The 4-mg nicotine gum should be used on persons who smoked 25 or more cigarettes a day. Patients on 2-mg strength should never use more than 30 pieces a day, and those on 4 mg should use no more than 20 pieces a day. Gum should be chewed on a fixed schedule and used when the urge to smoke is experienced. The absorption of nicotine from buccal mucosa is slower than following inhalation. The rapid blood levels of nicotine achieved with smoking are not achieved with gum chewing. Gum should therefore be chewed starting 30 minutes prior to the anticipated peak craving time. The gum should be chewed

briefly and then placed between the gum and upper lip. When the tingling sensation ceases, the procedure of chewing, shaping the gum into a rectangle and placing it under the upper lip should be repeated. Acidic beverages interfere with buccal absorption of nicotine and therefore only water should be consumed 15 minutes before and after gum chewing. Because 10% of individuals become dependent on nicotine gum, prescription of the gum should be limited to a period of 3 months and withdrawal of the gum should be tapered over the last 3 or 4 weeks. Nicotine replacement therapy increases the rate of quitting by 50–70%, regardless of setting.[73]

Nicotine receptor partial agonists appear to help smokers quit by maintaining moderate levels of dopamine to counteract withdrawal symptoms and by reducing smoking satisfaction.[74] More participants quit successfully with varenicline than with bupropion.

Tailoring a quit programme

Handouts are provided to enable health professionals assist smokers develop and implement a tailored behaviour modification based quitting programme.

Handout 16.1 provides a self-screen to help smokers become aware of the nature and impact of their smoking behaviour. **Handout 16.2** helps smokers to ascertain their preparedness to quit, while **Handouts 16.3** and **16.4** may be used to provide an incentive to those who are undecided.

When attempting to stop smoking, it is important to:

- determine the current motivation to change the habit. Why quit now?
- identify any perceived reasons or justifications for becoming a non-smoker. What are the benefits of becoming a non-smoker?
- ascertain and appropriately characterize the 'rationale' underlying the smoking habit. Why do I smoke?

There are two recommended quit methods: either gradual tapering of smoking prior to complete abstinence ('cut down') or abrupt abstinence from cigarettes ('cold turkey'). It has been cautiously suggested that cold turkey should be the recommended strategy for smokers who want to quit on their own.[75] In the gradual-tapering strategy, important aides to quitting include:

1. Keeping a smoker's diary. The simplest home approach is outlined in **Handout 16.5**.
2. Focusing on behavioural change. Various options are outlined in **Handout 16.6**. Combining various approaches is often beneficial.
3. Appreciating the rationale for continuing to smoke. It is helpful when developing a personalized quitting schedule to identify individual reasons for smoking. **Handout 16.7** provides a general self-assessment schedule and **Handout 16.8** focuses on nicotine dependence.

Nicotine dependence is the major barrier to quitting. Persons who smoke within 5 minutes of waking up are likely to be dependent. Smoking within 5 minutes of waking was much more common among those who smoked at least 20 cigarettes daily than amongst those who smoked less often.[25] Nicotine-dependent smokers often do best when quitting abruptly or going cold turkey. They are the group of smokers most likely to need nicotine replacement therapy. While nicotine replacement reduces craving and the adverse effects of tobacco smoke, it does not eliminate all the cardiovascular consequences associated with smoking. Persons who use nicotine replacement when quitting may fail to achieve lower ambulatory blood pressure and reduce their heart rate within 24 hours of their last cigarette.[76] Nonetheless, nicotine replacement avoids lung damage and eliminates exposure to inhaled carcinogens and carbon monoxide. In contrast, nicotine fading, which involves gradually reducing nicotine by changing to brands with less tar and nicotine and smoking fewer cigarettes per day, does not. In fact, it has been found that smokers, when changing to low-nicotine cigarettes, either smoke more cigarettes, or puff and inhale more deeply, to achieve their usual nicotine dose. Persons addicted to nicotine experience the greatest difficulty quitting. **Handout 16.9** provides an approach that links the rationale for smoking with possible intervention options. Persistent use of nicotine replacement should be avoided.

Individualized smoking cessation contracts can be formulated (see **Handout 16.10**). Smoker typology provides helpful hints for selecting the message content most likely to be helpful. The manner in which advice is provided can also have an impact. Health professionals can adapt the delivery of the message depending on the smoker's preferred behaviour style (see Table 5.5). Analysis of the smoker's locus of control (see Table 5.4) can provide a guideline for determining the amount of support required. Persons with an external locus of control may need more collaboration. Personalized contracts have an inherent flexibility that permits maximization of the positive correlation between successful smoking cessation and the frequency and intensity of practitioner contact coupled with the use of multiple intervention modalities.[77] While tailored intervention programmes may be more effective, they are more time consuming. It is therefore important to remember that even simple advice has an, albeit small, effect on cessation rates.[78]

In perspective

It has been suggested that, compared with routine care, providing advice consistently to all smoking patients is more effective than doubling the federal excise tax![79] According to smoking patients, provider advice doubles their chances of quitting – in fact, the probability of quitting by the end of a 12-month reference period increases from 6.9% to 14.7%.[79] In the longer term, routine provider advice is also deemed likely to outperform other tobacco control policies such as banning smoking in private workplaces.[79]

Assuming an unassisted quit rate of 2–3%, even a brief advice intervention can increase quitting by a further 1–3%. In fact, it has been suggested that there is only a small additional benefit of more intensive interventions compared with very brief interventions![77] As the real risk of tobacco use still appears to be poorly appreciated, everybody should perhaps be provided with an awareness handout (see **Handout 16.11**). Health professionals are an invaluable quitting resource!

References

1. Murray CJL, Lopez AD, eds. *The Global Burden Of Disease: Summary*. Published by Harvard School of Public Health on behalf of the WHO & World Bank. Boston: Harvard University Press; 3,28:1996.

2. NHS: The Information Centre. Health Survey for England 2006. http://www.ic.nhs.uk/statistics-and-data-collections/health-and-lifestyles-related-surveys/health-survey-for-england/health-survey-for-england-2006:-cvd-and-risk-factors-adults-obesity-and-risk-factors-children; Accessed 02.01.09.

3. Schroeder SA. Shattuck Lecture. We can do better—improving the health of the American people. *N Engl J Med*. 2007;357 (12):1221–1228.

4. Australian Institute of Health and Welfare. *Statistics on Drug Use in Australia 2004*. Drug Statistics Series No. 15. AIHW Cat. No. PHE 62. Canberra: AIHW; 2005.

5. Eaton DK, Kann L, Kinchen S, et al. Centers for Disease Control and Prevention (CDC). Youth risk behavior surveillance—United States, 2007. *Morb Mortal Wkly Rep Surveill Summ*. 2008;57 (4):1–131.

6. Centers for Disease Control and Prevention. Surveillance summaries. *Morb Mortal Wkly Rep*. 2004;53 (No. SS-2).

7. NHS: The Information Centre. Drug use, smoking and drinking among young people in England 2007. http://www.ic.nhs.uk/statistics-and-data-collections/health-and-lifestyles-related-surveys/smoking-drinking-and-drug-use-among-young-people-in-england; Accessed 06.01.09.

8. Weinstein ND, Marcus SE, Moser RP. Smokers' unrealistic optimism about their risk. *Tob Control*. 2005;14(1):55–59.

9. Kayemba-Kay's S, Geary MP, Pringle J, Rodeck CH, Kingdom JC, Hindmarsh PC. Gender, smoking during pregnancy and gestational age influence cord leptin concentrations in newborn infants. *Eur J Endocrinol*. 2008;159 (3):217–224.

10. Jaddoe VW, de Ridder MA, van den Elzen AP, Hofman A, Uiterwaal CS, Witteman JC. Maternal smoking in pregnancy is associated with cholesterol development in the offspring: a 27-years follow-up study. *Atherosclerosis*. 2008;196 (1):42–48.

11. Fujiwara H. Anti-smoking declaration. *Circ J*. 2003;67(1):1–2.

12. Okoli CT, Kelly T, Hahn EJ. Secondhand smoke and nicotine exposure: a brief review. *Addict Behav*. 2007;32(10):1977–1988.

13. Ahijevych K, Wewers ME. Passive smoking and vascular disease. *J Cardiovasc Nurs*. 2003;18 (1):69–74.

14. Wolpaw DR. Early detection of lung cancer. *Med Clin North Am*. 1996;80:63–82.

15. Cardenas VM, Thun MJ, Austin H, et al. Environmental tobacco smoke and lung cancer mortality in the American Cancer Society's Cancer Prevention Study. II. *Cancer Causes Control*. 1997;8(1):57–64.

16. Magnus P. Passive smoking. *Patient Management*. 1987;11:49–60.

17. Centers for Disease Control and Prevention. Second national report on human exposure to environmental chemicals: Tobacco smoke. NCEH Pub. No. 03-0022. http://www.cdc.gov/exposurereport/2nd/pdf/secondner.pdf;2003. Accessed 1.02.09.

18. Lykkesfeldt J, Christen S, Wallock LM, Chang HH, Jacob RA, Ames BN. Ascorbate is depleted by smoking and repleted by moderate supplementation: a study in male smokers and nonsmokers with matched dietary antioxidant intakes. *Am J Clin Nutr*. 2000;71 (2):530–536.

19. Benowitz NL. Pharmacological aspects of cigarette smoking and nicotine addiction. *N Engl J Med*. 1988;319:1318–1330.

20. Sohn M, Hartley C, Froelicher ES, Benowitz NL. Tobacco use and dependence. *Semin Oncol Nurs*. 2003;19(4):250–260.

21. Milhorn HT. Nicotine dependence. *Am Fam Physician*. 1989;39:214–224.

22. Calafat AM, Polzin GM, Saylor J, Richter P, Ashley DL, Watson CH. Determination of tar, nicotine, and carbon monoxide yields in the mainstream smoke of selected international cigarettes. *Tob Control*. 2004;13(1):45–51.

23. Hatsukami DK, Lemmonds C, Tomar SL. Smokeless tobacco use: harm reduction or induction approach? *Prev Med*. 2004;38 (3):309–317.

24. Tilashalski K, Rodu B, Mayfield C. Assessing the nicotine content of smokeless tobacco products. *J Am Dent Assoc*. 1994;125(5):590–592 594.

25. Lader D. *Omnibus Survey Report No. 36. Smoking-related Behaviour and Attitudes, 2007*. London: Office for National Statistics; 2008. *http://www.statistics.gov.uk/downloads/theme_health/smoking2007.pdf; Accessed 09.01.09.*

26. *World Health Organization*. The World Health Report 2008http://www.who.int/whr/2008/en/index.html; Accessed 08.01.09.

27. Centers for Disease Control and Prevention (CDC). Smoking-attributable mortality, years of potential life lost, and productivity losses—United States, 2000–2004. *MMWR Morb Mortal Wkly Rep*. 2008;57(45):1226–1228.

28. CDC Fact Sheet. Tobacco-Related Mortality (updated September 2006). http://www.cdc.gov/tobacco/data_statistics/fact_sheets/health_effects/tobacco_related_mortality.htm; Accessed 11.01.09.

29. Venn A, Britton J. Exposure to secondhand smoke and biomarkers of cardiovascular disease risk in never-smoking adults. *Circulation*. 2007;115(8):990–995.

30. Kawachi I, Colditz GA, Stampfer MJ, et al. Smoking cessation and time course of decreased risks of coronary heart disease in middle-aged women. *Arch Intern Med*. 1994;154(2):169–175.

31. Kawachi I, Colditz GA, Stampfer MJ, et al. Smoking cessation and decreased risk of stroke in women. *JAMA*. 1993;269 (2):232–236.

32. Shankar PS. Recent advances in the assessment and management of chronic obstructive pulmonary disease. *Indian J Chest Dis Allied Sci.* 2008;50(1):79–88.

33. Izquierdo JL, Barcina C, Jiménez J, Muñoz M, Leal M. Study of the burden on patients with chronic obstructive pulmonary disease. *Int J Clin Pract.* 2009;63(1):87–97.

34. Ozlü T, Bülbül Y. Smoking and lung cancer. *Tuberk Toraks.* 2005;53 (2):200–209.

35. Ames BN, Gold LS. Environmental pollution, pesticides, and the prevention of cancer: misconceptions. *FASEB J.* 1997;11 (13):1041–1052.

36. Mehta H, Nazzal K, Sadikot RT. Cigarette smoking and innate immunity. *Inflamm Res.* 2008;57 (11):497–503.

37. Harris JE, Thun MJ, Mondul AM, Calle EE. Cigarette tar yields in relation to mortality from lung cancer in the cancer prevention study II prospective cohort, 1982-8. *BMJ.* 2004;328(7431):72.

38. Tomatis L. Environmental cancer risk factors. *Acta Oncol.* 1988;27:465–472.

39. Ross RK, Bernstein L, Garabrandt D, Henderson BE. Avoidable nondietary risk factors for cancer. *Am Fam Physician.* 1988;38:153–160.

40. Department of Health. *Statistical Bulletin 2003/21: Statistics on smoking: England, 2003.* Last modified date: 8 February 2007. http://www.dh.gov.uk/en/ Publicationsandstatistics/Statistics/ StatisticalWorkAreas/ Statisticalpublichealth/ DH_4082243; Accessed 09.01.09.

41. Doll R, Peto R, Whetley K, Gray R, Sutherland I. Mortality in relation to smoking: 40 years' observation on male British doctors. *BMJ.* 1994;309:901–911.

42. Peretti-Watel P, Constance J, Guilbert P, Gautier A, Beck F, Moatti JP. Smoking too few cigarettes to be at risk? Smokers' perceptions of risk and risk denial, a French survey. *Tob Control.* 2007;16(5):351–356.

43. Kim JE, Koo KH, Kim YH, Sohn J, Park YG. Identification of potential lung cancer biomarkers using an in vitro carcinogenesis model. *Exp Mol Med.* 2008;40 (6):709–720.

44. Carpagnano GE, Spanevello A, Carpagnano F, et al. Prognostic value of exhaled microsatellite alterations at 3p in NSCLC patients. *Lung Cancer.* 2009;64 (3):334–340.

45. Qiao YL, Tockman MS, Li L, et al. A case-cohort study of an early biomarker of lung cancer in a screening cohort of Yunnan tin miners in China. *Cancer Epidemiol Biomarkers Prev.* 1997;6 (11):893–900.

46. CDC. Fact Sheet—Women and Tobacco (updated November 2006). http://www.cdc.gov/ tobacco/data_statistics/fact_sheets/ health_effects/ tobacco_related_mortality.htm; Accessed 11.01.09.

47. Romero FMS, Santillán AL, Olvera HPC, Morales SMA, Ramírez MVL. [Frequency of risk factors in breast cancer.]. *Ginecol Obstet Mex.* 2008;76(11):667–672.

48. Swift M, Lukin JL. Breast cancer incidence and the effect of cigarette smoking in heterozygous carriers of mutations in the ataxia-telangiectasia gene. *Cancer Epidemiol Biomarkers Prev.* 2008;17 (11):3188–3192.

49. Parente RC, Faerstein E, Celeste RK, Werneck GL. The relationship between smoking and age at the menopause: a systematic review. *Maturitas.* 2008;61 (4):287–298.

50. Papaioannou A, Kennedy CC, Cranney A, et al. Risk factors for low BMD in healthy men age 50 years or older: a systematic review. *Osteoporos Int.* 2009;20 (4):507–518.

51. Jackson RD, Donepudi S, Mysiw WJ. Epidemiology of fracture risk in the Women's Health Initiative. *Curr Osteoporos Rep.* 2008;6(4):155–161.

52. Law MR, Hackshaw AK. A meta-analysis of cigarette smoking, bone mineral density and risk of hip fracture: recognition of a major effect. *BMJ.* 1997;315 (7112):841–846.

53. Forsen L, Bjorndal A, Bjartveit K, et al. Interaction between current smoking, leanness, and physical inactivity in the prediction of hip fracture. *J Bone Miner Res.* 1994;9 (11):1671–1678.

54. Albrecht SA, Maloni JA, Thomas KK, Jones R, Halleran J, Osborne J. Smoking cessation counseling for pregnant women who smoke: scientific basis for practice for AWHONN's SUCCESS project. *J Obstet Gynecol Neonatal Nurs.* 2004;33(3):298–305.

55. Jones G, Riley M, Dwyer T. Maternal smoking during pregnancy, growth, and bone mass in prepubertal children. *J Bone Miner Res.* 1999;14(1):146–151.

56. Ebert L, van der Riet P, Fahy K. What do midwives need to understand/know about smoking in pregnancy? *Women Birth.* 2009;22 (1):35–40.

57. Ernster VL, Grady D, Mizke R, et al. Facial wrinkles in men and women, by smoking status. *Am J Public Health.* 1995;85:78–82.

58. Colrain IM, Trinder J, Swan GE. The impact of smoking cessation on objective and subjective markers of sleep: review, synthesis, and recommendations. *Nicotine Tob Res.* 2004;6(6):913–925.

59. Gaughan SE. Developing corporate smoking policies. *AAOHN J.* 1988;36:354–360.

60. CDC. Fact Sheet—Economic Facts about U.S. Tobacco Use and Tobacco Production (updated July 2007). http://www.cdc.gov/ tobacco/data_statistics/fact_sheets/ economics/economic_facts.htm; Accessed 11.01.09.

61. National Cancer Institute. http:// www.cancer.gov/cancertopics/ factsheet/Tobacco/cancer; Accessed 11.01.09.

62. CDC. *Surgeon General's Report— The Health Consequences of Smoking The Benefits of Quitting.* http:// www.cdc.gov/tobacco/ data_statistics/sgr/sgr_2004/ posters/benefits.htm; Accessed 01.11.09.

63. Sneve M, Jorde R. Cross-sectional study on the relationship between body mass index and smoking, and longitudinal changes in body mass index in relation to change in smoking status: the Tromso Study. *Scand J Public Health.* 2008;36 (4):397–407.

64. Flegal KM, Troiano RP, Pamuk ER, Kuczmarski RJ, Campbell SM. The

influence of smoking cessation on the prevalence of overweight in the United States. *N Engl J Med.* 1995;333(18):1165–1170.

65. McGill Jr HC, McMahan CA, Malcom GT, Oalmann MC, Strong JP. Effects of serum lipoproteins and smoking on atherosclerosis in young men and women. *Arterioscler Thromb Biol.* 1997;17:95–106.

66. Bala M, Strzeszynski L, Cahill K. Mass media interventions for smoking cessation in adults. *Cochrane Database Syst Rev.* 2008;(1):CD004704.

67. Thomas RE, Baker P, Lorenzetti D. Family-based programmes for preventing smoking by children and adolescents. *Cochrane Database Syst Rev.* 2007;(1):CD004493.

68. Okuyemi KS, Nollen NL, Ahluwalia JS. Interventions to facilitate smoking cessation. *Am Fam Physician.* 2006;74 (2):262–271.

69. Naughton F, Prevost AT, Sutton S. Self-help smoking cessation interventions in pregnancy: a systematic review and meta-analysis. *Addiction.* 2008;103 (4):566–579.

70. Norman GJ, Velicer WF, Fava JL, Prochaska JO. Cluster subtypes within stage of change in a representative sample of smokers. *Addict Behav.* 2000;25(2):183–204.

71. Anatchkova MD, Velicer WF, Prochaska JO. Replication of subtypes for smoking cessation within the contemplation stage of change. *Addict Behav.* 2005;30 (5):915–927.

72. Tønnesen P. Which drug to be used in smoking cessation? *Pol Arch Med Wewn.* 2008;118(6):373–376.

73. Stead LF, Perera R, Bullen C, Mant D, Lancaster T. Nicotine replacement therapy for smoking cessation. *Cochrane Database Syst Rev.* 2008;(1):CD000146.

74. Cahill K, Stead LF, Lancaster T. Nicotine receptor partial agonists for smoking cessation. *Cochrane Database Syst Rev.* 2008;(3): CD006103.

75. Cheong Y, Yong HH, Borland R. Does how you quit affect success? A comparison between abrupt and gradual methods using data from the International Tobacco Control Policy Evaluation Study. *Nicotine Tob Res.* 2007;9(8):801–810.

76. Becker LA. Helping patients quit smoking. *J Fam Pract.* 1998;46:195–196.

77. Ockene JK. Physician delivered interventions for smoking cessation: strategies for increasing effectiveness. *Prev Med.* 1987;16:723–737.

78. Stead LF, Bergson G, Lancaster T. Physician advice for smoking cessation. *Cochrane Database Syst Rev.* 2008;(2):CD000165.

79. Bao Y, Duan N, Fox SA. Is some provider advice on smoking cessation better than no advice? An instrumental variable analysis of the 2001 National Health Interview Survey. *Health Serv Res.* 2006;41 (6):2114–2135.

Alcohol

Points to Ponder !

- The blood alcohol level for legal drunkenness varies with geography rather than physiology.
- You may still be over the legal driving limit the morning after a heavy night of drinking – despite numerous cups of coffee.

Alcohol is a good example of a socially acceptable drug which, when abused, has dire personal and community consequences. Alcohol is the intoxicating ingredient in beer, wine and spirits. Grapes are used to produce wine, apples are the raw material for cider, and grains are the source of beer and various distilled liquors. Wines, ciders and beers result from the fermentation of the fruit or grain, hard liquors undergoing a further distillation. Brandy is derived from wine, rum from molasses (sugar cane), vodka from wheat, rye, corn or potato, and whisky from barley. Ethanol is produced by anaerobic metabolism or fermentation of carbohydrate.

Once absorbed, alcohol is broken down by the liver, which can cope with 15 mL (0.5 oz) of ethanol per hour. In other words, a healthy liver takes an hour to remove one standard drink from the bloodstream. Women's blood alcohol concentration will be higher after drinking the same amount of alcohol as men. One reason for this is that women absorb about one-third more alcohol from a similar size drink than do males. The male stomach contains more alcohol dehydrogenase, which breaks down a percentage of the alcohol ingested. Women also have more body fat than men. As alcohol is water-soluble, men, with their higher water content, achieve better dilution.

Carbonated alcohol passes more rapidly through the stomach. More alcohol is absorbed from sparkling wines and champagne than from non-carbonated drinks with equivalent alcohol content. Wine drinkers can drink more than champagne drinkers and remain below a blood alcohol concentration of 0.05.

The health dose–effect relationship of alcohol and beyond

The emphasis on the blood level of alcohol reflects the dose–effect relationship of this drug. At a blood alcohol concentration of 0.05, inhibitions are relaxed, judgement is impaired, and mood is altered. At a blood alcohol level of 0.1, coordination is impaired, reaction time delayed, peripheral vision impaired and emotions exaggerated. Heavier drinking may result in a hangover, the symptoms of which include headache, nausea, shakiness and possibly vomiting.

Overall mortality rates drop 18% in women who have one drink daily and in men who have up to two drinks daily; intakes of more than two drinks daily in women or three drinks daily in men is associated with increased mortality in a dose-dependent fashion.[1] Men who abstain from smoking, maintain their body mass index under 25 kg/m^2, exercise 30 or more minutes daily and eat a healthy diet can further reduce their risk of a heart attack by drinking one or two alcoholic drinks daily.[1] The consumption of one to two standard drinks, i.e. 10–20 g alcohol each day, is regarded as being largely beneficial as alcohol has antithrombotic properties and increases high-density lipoprotein levels. While moderate alcohol consumption is not associated with any significant morbidity; three or more drinks (>30 g) daily is associated with hypertriglyceridaemia, cardiomyopathy, hypertension, and stroke.[2] This dose–response relationship has also been shown with respect to cancer. Consuming at least one glass of red wine per day is associated with a 60% reduced risk of lung cancer, a benefit that extends to smokers.[3] On the other hand, meta-analysis found high consumption of beer and liquors may be associated with increased lung cancer risk.[4] This study identified that both the dose and type of drink are important. Whereas averaging one drink of beer or liquor daily increases the relative risk of lung cancer more than 1.2 fold, a similar level of wine consumption reduces the relative risk to 0.78!

The potential health benefits of wine have been linked to resveratrol, a powerful polyphenol and antifungal chemical that occurs naturally under the skin of red grapes. Nearly all dark red wines – merlot, cabernet, zinfandel, shiraz and pinot noir – contain resveratrol. The amount of resveratrol in a bottle varies between 0.2 and 5.8 mg per litre depending on the type of grape and growing season. Compared with white wine and other alcoholic drinks, red wine has higher levels of bioflavonoids rich in antioxidant, antiplatelet, and antiendothelin-1 effects.[1]

The frequency of alcohol intake is relevant. Daily alcohol intake provides superior health benefits than less frequent consumption.[1] In one large study, those who drank on 5 to 7 days a week had less risk of a heart attack than those who drank less than once a week. On the other hand, binge drinking, defined as three or more drinks within 1 or 2 hours, put persons who had had a previous heart attack at greater risk than those who abstained.[5] In this study, binge drinking doubled the risk regardless of whether the drink chosen was wine, beer or liquor. The dose, the type and the pattern of the alcohol intake all appear critical.[6]

Alcohol abuse: the statistics

Alcohol abuse is the third largest preventable cause of death in the US.[7] In 2005, 51.8% of Americans 12 years and over used alcohol; 22.7% were binge drinkers and 6.6% heavy drinkers.[8] During the 12 months before the 2007 national Youth Risk Behavior Survey, 75% of high school students in the US had drunk alcohol.[9] Alcohol use is similarly high in the UK. In 2005, 22% of pupils in England aged 11–15 reported drinking alcohol in the week prior to interview, while in 2004, 74% of men and 59% of women reported drinking alcohol on at least one day in the week prior to interview.[10] In 2006, 41% of all men and 33% of all women had drunk more than the recommended amounts of no more than four units for men and no more than three units for women on at least 1 day in the past week.[11] In fact, men who drank within the past 7 days consumed an average of 8.1 units on the day they drank most; women consumed an average of 5.5 units. Australians fare no better. In 2004, around 84% of the Australian population aged 14 years and over had consumed at least one full serve of alcohol in the last 12 months.[12] Of more concern is the finding that 35% of Australians aged 14 years and over consumed alcohol in a manner that puts them at increased risk of alcohol-related harm in the short term on at least one occasion in the last 12 months. Ten percent of Australians consume alcohol at levels that are considered risky or high risk for alcohol-related harm in the long term.

Using the terminology of drug abuse,[13] consuming 40–60 g alcohol daily is harmful drinking. 'Harmful use' indicates that there is evidence use of a substance has adverse physical and/or psychological consequences. Alcohol consumption in excess of 60 g per day is considered hazardous. The hazardous use of a substance implies that the quantity and/or pattern of use is placing the user at risk of tissue damage and other disabilities. Tissue damage and related disorders are inevitable in persons drinking in excess of 120 g daily. As previously explained, the dose–effect consequences of alcohol differ between males and females. In males, regular consumption of up to 40 g each day is safe, 40–60 g per day is hazardous and over 60 g per day is regarded as harmful. This translates into hazardous behaviour when the person is drinking four to six standard drinks each day or 28–42 each week. Harmful drinking is defined as six or more standard drinks per day or 42 or more per week. In females, the regular consumption of up to 20 g each day is safe; 20–40 g daily is hazardous and over 40 g a day is harmful. Drinking is considered hazardous when two to four standard drinks are consumed each day or 14–28 each week. Harmful drinking for women is defined as four or more standard drinks daily or 28 or more weekly. This gender discrepancy is further reflected in the liver damage threshold for alcohol being 40 g a day in women and 80 g in men. As a generalization, 40–60 g of alcohol daily appears to increase the risk of liver cirrhosis and oesophageal, oral and pharyngeal cancer and markedly increases the age-adjusted risk of death from cancer and cardiovascular disease.

A standard drink contains 10 g alcohol. For mid-strength beer (3.5% alcohol), a standard drink is equal to one schooner (375 mL); for full-strength beer (4.9% alcohol), it equals one middie (285 mL). A standard drink of wine is found in one small 100-mL glass, and one of fortified wines such as port or sherry in one 60-mL glass. A standard drink of spirits is 30 mL. One bottle of wine contains seven standard drinks; that of port or sherry, 11.

When 'safe' intake levels may be risky

Persons on prescription medicines may be at increased risk due to the propensity for alcohol to interact adversely with various drugs. Persons being treated for angina or high blood pressure may experience an unacceptable drop in blood pressure when they drink. Alcohol increases the likelihood analgesics such as aspirin will cause gastrointestinal bleeding. A delayed reaction time, impaired motor coordination and impaired judgement result when alcohol is combined with antihistamines, sedative-hypnotics (e.g. barbiturates) or benzodiazepines (e.g. Valium and Librium). Cross-tolerance can develop between alcohol and other sedative/hypnotic drugs.

In pregnancy, the consumption of no more than 10 g alcohol each day is regarded as safe. Abstinence is preferrable. Women of childbearing age are more likely to drink alcohol than smoke or use illicit drugs.[14] Alcohol used during pregnancy can harm the unborn baby: it has been linked with a higher risk of miscarriage, stillbirth, premature birth, and birth defects, the most serious outcome being fetal alcohol syndrome. The effects of fetal alcohol syndrome range from mild to severe and commonly include a lower birth weight, a small head and flattened facial features. Central nervous system damage can result in intellectual disability, poor coordination and inadequate movement skills. Birthmarks, heart defects, curvature of the spine and cleft palate are other potential consequences. Following birth, the baby may demonstrate alcohol withdrawal symptoms varying from tremors, irritability, and fits, to a bloated stomach. Women who give birth to fetal alcohol syndrome babies average at least six drinks a day during their pregnancy. The risk to the fetus is greatest during the first 3 months of pregnancy, so total abstinence during this period is preferable. Women who are contemplating pregnancy should consider cutting down or avoiding alcohol altogether.

Alcohol abuse

Alcohol abuse is a major cause of mortality and is associated with psychiatric conditions, neurologic impairment, cardiovascular disease and malignant neoplasms.[15,16] Heavy drinking is a potent cause of gastrointestinal disorders ranging from gastritis and chronic diarrhoea to hepatic and pancreatic disease. Psychiatric consequences of heavy drinking include depression, phobias, generalized anxiety disorder and suicide. In fact, habitual alcohol abuse results in a clearly defined syndrome: Korsakoff's psychosis in malnourished alcoholics presents with a gross disturbance of recent memory and confabulation. Confabulations – false descriptions – are created to conceal the memory gaps. The effects on the central nervous system range from cognitive impairment to peripheral neuropathy, from epilepsy to cerebellar ataxia. Hypertension, cardiomyopathy, proximal muscle wasting and weakness are also encountered. Family difficulties, poor work performance, financial difficulties and legal problems often follow.

People who drink regularly may develop tolerance due to induction of liver enzymes accelerating alcohol catabolism. Regular drinkers can become alcohol dependent, requiring larger amounts of alcohol to achieve the desired effect. If alcohol is unavailable, anxiety or even panic may be experienced. Alcohol withdrawal results in sweating, tremors, vomiting, convulsions and hallucinations.

Alcohol overdose may result in stupor or coma, a cold and clammy skin, low body temperature, depressed breathing and an increased heart rate. Deaths from suicide and accidents most typically result from a combination overdose of alcohol and sedatives.

Safe drinking

Despite the disadvantages of alcohol consumption, prudent drinking does confer a health advantage. The mechanism whereby alcohol achieves a health benefit remains unclear. Nonetheless, a J-shaped association between alcohol intake and uric acid, C-reactive protein, homocysteine, fibrinogen, triglycerides, apolipoproteins A1 and B, HDL and total cholesterols, blood glucose levels, leukocyte count and arterial blood pressure levels has been identified.[17] The cost:benefit dose of alcohol consumption may be, at least in part, related to the antioxidant:pro-oxidant balance of the total beverage. Certainly, moderate wine consumption increases HDL-cholesterol and decreases various inflammatory markers. Red wine has more pronounced anti-inflammatory effects than has white wine, probably because of its higher polyphenol content.[18] Although the major benefit of alcohol may be linked to its polyphenol content, this is not the sole mechanism involved. While polyphenol-rich alcoholic beverages such as red wine have a more pronounced anti-inflammatory effect, polyphenol-free alcoholic beverages, e.g. gin, also have anti-inflammatory properties.[19]

In view of the potential for alcohol to confer a health advantage, awareness of safe drinking behaviour is encouraged. In view of uncertainty as to who is likely to be susceptible to alcohol dependence, non-drinking patients should be advised to adopt health-promoting behaviours other than moderate alcohol consumption. However, individuals who already use alcohol should be advised as follows:

- men should not exceed 4 units or 40 g absolute alcohol per day on a regular basis, or 28 units per week. One unit is taken as half a pint of beer, one measure of spirits or one glass of sherry or wine

- women should not exceed 2 units or 20 g alcohol per day on a regular basis, or 14 units per week. Abstinence during pregnancy is highly desirable

- people who undertake hazardous activities or drive should not drink. In order to stay safely below 0.05, drivers are advised to limit their drinking. Men should drink no more than two standard drinks in the first hour and no more than one standard drink every hour after that. Similarly, women should drink no more than one standard drink in the first hour and no more than one standard drink every hour after that. To stay under 0.02, however, it is best to avoid drinking altogether: just one standard drink can put some people over the limit.

To facilitate limiting alcohol intake to safe levels on social occasions, various strategies can be employed (see **Handout 17.1**).

Clinical recognition and management of alcoholism

It is desirable to recognize an incipient alcohol problem early. Drinkers are encouraged to be aware of their drinking behaviour. A number of approaches are available[20,21] – see **Handout 17.2**. Two questions that are an invaluable guide to alcohol abuse are: 'In the past year, have you ever drunk more than you meant to?' and 'Have you felt that you wanted or needed to cut down on your drinking in the past year?'. A single positive response has around an 81% sensitivity and specificity for current substance use disorders. **Handout 17.3** lists some 'red flags' for alcohol abuse and **Handout 17.4** draws attenton to important facts and mistaken beliefs about the 'benefits' of alcohol. A definitive diagnosis of alcohol abuse can be obtained by measuring actual alcohol intake. A 'red flag' for alcohol consumption in men is more than 14 drinks a week or four drinks on any one occasion. In women, the equivalent intakes are seven drinks a week or three on any one occasion. A diary can be used to document actual alcohol use more accurately. The volume and type of alcohol consumed on each occasion should also be noted – candour can be a problem. It is also helpful to record the occasions on which alcohol is drunk as this can alert the individual to drinking triggers and heighten awareness of when to exercise caution.

All patients who drink alcohol may benefit from being aware of the characteristics of responsible drinking behaviour (see **Handout 17.1**). Awareness of the impact of alcohol abuse is also important. **Handout 17.5** provides an overview of some of the physical, lifestyle and emotional consequences of uncontrolled drinking. Patients who have a drinking problem and have developed dependence will develop withdrawal symptoms on becoming abstinent. **Handout 17.6** describes the clinical manifestations of delirium tremens. In view of the potentially serious physical consequences of alcohol withdrawal, medical supervision is recommended. Attendance at an abstinence-based treatment programme such as Alcoholics Anonymous is also advocated as this can increase, even double, the recovery rate.

Handout 17.7 is a template for safe alcohol use.

In perspective

Alcohol is a popular socially acceptable drug that carries a substantial physical, psychological and socioeconomic cost for those susceptible to its abuse. However, unlike tobacco, which is always detrimental to health, moderate alcohol consumption affords a health benefit. Nonetheless, this benefit can be derived from sources free of the risk of dependence!

References

1. O'Keefe JH, Bybee KA, Lavie CJ. Alcohol and cardiovascular health: the razor-sharp double-edged sword. *J Am Coll Cardiol.* 2007;50 (11):1009–1014.

2. Saremi A, Arora R. The cardiovascular implications of alcohol and red wine. *Am J Ther.* 2008;15(3):265–277.

3. Chao C, Slezak JM, Caan BJ, Quinn VP. Alcoholic beverage intake and risk of lung cancer: the California Men's Health Study. *Cancer Epidemiol Biomarkers Prev.* 2008;17(10):2692–2699.

4. Chao C. Associations between beer, wine, and liquor consumption and lung cancer risk: a meta-analysis. *Cancer Epidemiol Biomarkers Prev.* 2007;16(11):2436–2447.

5. Mukamal KJ, Maclure M, Muller JE, Mittleman MA. Binge drinking and mortality after acute myocardial infarction. *Circulation.* 2005;112 (25):3839–3845.

6. Ellison RC. Importance of pattern of alcohol consumption. *Circulation.* 2005;112:3818–3819.

7. Gunzerath L, Faden V, Zakhari S, Warren K. National Institute on Alcohol Abuse and Alcoholism report on moderate drinking. *Alcohol Clin Exp Res.* 2004;28:829–847.

8. National Centre for Health Statistics. *Health, United States, 2007. With Chartbook on Trends in the Health of Americans.* Hyattsville, MD: US Department of Health and Human Services; 2007.

9. Eaton DK, Kann L, Kinchen S, et al. Centers for Disease Control and Prevention (CDC). Youth risk behavior surveillance—United States, 2007. *MMWR Surveill Summ.* 2008;57(4):1–131.

10. NHS Information Centre. *Statistics on Alcohol: England, 2006.* <http://www.ic.nhs.uk/statistics-and-data-collections/health-and-lifestyles/alcohol/statistics-on-alcohol>; Accessed 02.01.09.

11. NHS Information Centre. Health Survey for England 2006. <http://www.ic.nhs.uk/statistics-and-data-collections/health-and-lifestyles-related-surveys/health-survey-for-england/health-survey-for-england-2006:-cvd-and-risk-factors-adults-obesity-and-risk-factors-children>; Accessed 02.01.09.

12. Australian Institute of Health and Welfare. *Statistics on Drug Use in Australia 2004.* Drug Statistics Series No. 15. AIHW Cat. No. PHE 62. Canberra: AIHW; 2005.

13. Schorling JB, Buchscaum DG. Screening for alcohol and drug abuse. *Med Clin North Am.* 1997;81:845–865.

14. Floyd RL, Jack BW, Cefalo R, et al. The clinical content of preconception care: alcohol, tobacco, and illicit drug exposures. *Am J Obstet Gynecol.* 2008;199 (6 suppl 2):S333–S339.

15. Li TK. Quantifying the risk for alcohol-use and alcohol-attributable health disorders: present findings and future research needs. *J Gastroenterol Hepatol.* 2008;23 (suppl 1):S2–S8.

16. Cargiulo T. Understanding the health impact of alcohol dependence. *Am J Health Syst Pharm.* 2007;64(5 suppl 3):S5–S11.

17. Chrysohoou C, Panagiotakos DB, Pitsavos C, et al. Effects of chronic alcohol consumption on lipid levels, inflammatory and haemostatic factors in the general population: the 'ATTICA' Study. *Eur J Cardiovasc Prev Rehabil.* 2003;10 (5):355–361.

18. Sacanella E, Vázquez-Agell M, Mena MP, et al. Down-regulation of adhesion molecules and other inflammatory biomarkers after moderate wine consumption in healthy women: a randomized trial. *Am J Clin Nutr.* 2007;86 (5):1463–1469.

19. Vázquez-Agell M, Sacanella E, Tobias E, et al. Inflammatory markers of atherosclerosis are decreased after moderate consumption of cava (sparkling wine) in men with low cardiovascular risk. *J Nutr.* 2007;137(10):2279–2284.

20. Russell M, Martier SS, Sokol RJ, et al. Screening for pregnancy risk – drinking. *Clin Exp Res.* 1994;18:1156–1161.

21. Brown RL, Leonard T, Saunders LA, Papasouliotis O. A two-item conjoint screen for alcohol and other drug problems. *J Am Board Fam Pract.* 2001;14(2):95–106.

Stress

- The health impact of stress is determined more by how the individual responds than by the situation itself.
- Stress can be managed.

The construct of homeostasis evolved from the notion of a need to maintain a relatively constant internal cellular environment. Homeostasis is achieved when physiological systems maintain biological variables within a set of acceptable ranges of values. However, it appears there is no single ideal setpoint for steady-state conditions in life. It has therefore become necessary to transform homeostasis to accommodate this novel perception. Allostasis is the process whereby complex physiological systems adapt to physical, psychosocial and environmental challenges. It is a dynamic regulatory process, continuously adjusting physiology in response to stressors.[1,2] Allostasis encompasses those active, adaptive processes that attempt to maintain an apparent steady state. Stress occurs when allostatic processes are strained.

Psychosocial stress

Detection of a discrepancy between information and a homeostatic set point activates a physiological response to reduce the divergence. The response patterns from the sympathetic nervous, adrenomedullary and hypothalamic–pituitary–adrenocortical systems depend on the stressor. Failure to adapt to stressors results in accumulation of an allostatic load. The allostatic load mediates the adverse effects of psychosocial stress on health.

The allostatic load

An allostatic load is the total physiological burden resulting from dysregulation across multiple physiological systems. When the frequency, duration, and/or intensity of adaptation efforts are excessive, the body may gradually lose the ability to maintain its physiological parameters within normal operating ranges. This accumulated dysregulation across physiological systems results in an allostatic load detected as pathophysiological changes. Frequent or chronic arousal has been associated with ultimate dysregulation, amongst others, of the hypothalamic–pituitary–adrenal axis, and the sympathetic nervous and immune systems.

Adverse health may be a consequence of an allostatic load. A composite allostatic load score constructed from cardiovascular markers and neuroendocrine hormones has been shown to predict a variety of health outcomes in high-functioning elderly individuals. The allostatic score used reflected the resting activity of major physiological systems. It was based on 10 biological markers: the waist-to-hip circumference ratio; systolic and diastolic blood pressure; urinary cortisol, noradrenaline and adrenaline; and serum dehydroepiandrosterone sulphate, glycosylated haemoglobin, high-density lipoprotein and total cholesterol. Although none of the 10 markers exhibited substantial individual association with health outcomes, a summary measure of the allostatic load was found to be significantly associated with incident cardiovascular events, decline in both physical and cognitive functioning, and total mortality in high-functioning older adult.[3]

Stimulus or stressor?

Psychosocial stress is an established health risk. It can lead to accumulation of an allostatic load. Psychosocial stress is a physical and psycho-emotional state of excessive or unwanted arousal. The stimulus causing the arousal reaction can be a person, event or object. Stress results when there is an imbalance between the stimulus and the individual's coping strategies. The stress reaction is a physical and psychoemotional expression of this imbalance. Stress is considered to encompass:

- an undesirable stimulating observable event (stressor) that influences an individual in a harmful way
- a condition in which an external or internal demand exceeds a person's coping abilities
- the body's response or adaptation to a stressor.

The magnitude of the stimulus does not itself determine distress. Although stress can result from major events, it is important to appreciate that continual exposure to minor irritations is a potent cause of stress.

Stimuli that can cause stress may be physiological or psychological, arising from one's thoughts or social interaction. Stimuli are stressors when they cause overload. A stimulus becomes a stressor when it overwhelms one's ability to cope. Physical, chemical, social and cultural demands may upset physical, psychological or emotional balance. Examples of physical stressors are environmental pollution, cigarette smoking, and excessive coffee and/or alcohol. Psychological stressors include negative thoughts (self-talk), erroneous beliefs and inaccurate perceptions. Viewing a situation as a problem is conducive to a stressful response; however, welcoming that same situation as a challenge provokes a different reaction. Lifestyle stimuli are stressors when they are *perceived* to be a threat, likely to cause loss or produce unwanted change. In fact, higher levels of perceived stress, but not stressful life events, were shown to be associated with an impaired immune response in women with cervical dysplasia.[4]

The stress response

Stress can be considered from three different perspectives: the stressful event or stressor, the individual's appraisal of the situation, and their pathophysiological response. The stressor may be physical or psychosocial. The former stressor can be objectively measured, the latter is subjectively evaluated. Regardless of the nature of the stressor, pathophysiological responses are similar. Both physical and psychosocial stressors activate a physiological fight–flight response. While this is an appropriate response to a physical threat, it is an inept reaction to a psychosocial stressor. Psychosocial stress appears to adversely affect autonomic and hormonal homeostasis, resulting in metabolic abnormalities, inflammation, insulin resistance, and endothelial dysfunction.[5] Furthermore, while physical stressors have a fairly predictable impact on most individuals, psychological stimuli are processed differently by each individual. This profound difference is due to the unique personal meaning ascribed to an event by the individual.

The psychosocial stress response reflects the individual's reaction to the stimulus rather than the stimulus itself. While temperament and habits may have some impact, individual differences in appraisal and coping effectiveness are the major determinants of individual differences in the magnitude of physiologic responses to stressors.[6] In fact, modifying one's beliefs can reduce psychological stress levels. Furthermore, because stimuli are not appraised in isolation, different stress states result from similar psychological stimuli. Each stimulus is appraised in the light of one's previous experience, thoughts and feelings. Prior positive experience plays a key role in both behavioural and neurophysiological responses.[7] Conditioning, i.e. previous experience, and verbal suggestion, i.e. expectation, influence placebo and nocebo outcomes.

Personal appraisal and efficacy expectations are cognitive mediators of stress reactions. Any stress responses are mediated by the individual's appraisal of the possible impact of an event and how they may cope with any possible changes. Change, especially when associated with a lot of uncertainty, is stressful. When change is anticipated to cause a loss or is perceived as a threat, then change is stressful. Threat is anticipated harm. Harm is psychological damage already done and/or irrevocable loss. On the other hand, when change is anticipated and the individual feels confident they can adapt using effective coping resources, then change is stimulating and welcomed as a challenge.

Stress is not inherently bad – some stress is necessary, even desirable! Stress is damaging when it causes distress by overwhelming the person's ability to cope or adapt to change. However, depending on how an event is perceived, arousal may be pleasurable rather than distressing. Stressors can stimulate growth. Stress is good when it stimulates growth and psychosocial development. See **Handout 18.1**.

Optimal stimulation: superior functioning

The aim of good stress management is not to eliminate all stress, but to change the stress experience into something that is productive rather than destructive. Too much stimulation leads to burn out and impaired function. The consequences of distress are felt at all levels: physical illness, low energy, low self-esteem, dissatisfaction, interpersonal conflict, and poor productivity. Too little stimulation leads to boredom; sensory deprivation leads to serious psychological and physical difficulty. The right amount of stimulation leads to optimal function. The right amount of stimulation is unique to each individual.

Different people function optimally at different levels of stimulation. Depending on their level of arousal, performance may be enhanced or impaired. The Yerkes–Dodson Law identifies an inverted U-shaped relationship between performance and arousal. Performance is impaired if the stress level is too high or too low. If level of arousal is compared to the tension in an elastic bangle, then boredom results when the bangle is too loose and slips off; whereas stimulus overload results in a too tight bangle painfully constricting the wrist. Performance, health and life satisfaction are enhanced at optimum stress or 'eustress' levels. A snugly fitting bangle equates to 'eustress'. Individuals function best when they achieve a 'eustress' level of arousal. To operate in one's zone of positive stress, it is necessary to avoid situations that cause either stimulus overload or underload. This means having a strategy to cope with situations in which one's stimulus level falls outside the eustress range. The level of arousal at which optimal performance is achieved differs between individuals. Some people are thrill seekers, others opt for a quiet life. Some people have a narrow stress range, others can function well at both relatively low and high levels of stimulation. In general, introverts function better at lower levels of arousal than extroverts.

Undesirable stimulation: substandard functioning

Stress causes disease through persistent arousal overload or tonal exhaustion. Disease may result when the body's arousal 'homeostat' gets set at a level at which the capacity of the individual to adapt to change is severely hampered. The reticular activating system receives motor and sensory information from the body. The hypothalamus primes body 'tone' according to the intensity of stimulation from the reticular activating system. This basal tone is modified according to the information supplied from the limbic (emotional) and cortical (thinking) areas. Our thoughts and feelings can alter our body tone! The hypothalamus sets body tone through its control of the autonomic nervous and endocrine systems. See Figure 18.1.

The autonomic nervous system sets tonal homeostasis in any particular individual by enhancing either sympathetic (intensifies) or parasympathetic (reduces) nervous activity. The general response to sympathetic stimulation is to provoke the stress reaction or the fight/flight response. See **Handout 18.2**. The sympathetic nervous system (systemic sympathetic and adrenomedullary systems), along with the hypothalamic–pituitary axis, is the peripheral limb of an arousal system whose main function is to maintain both basal and stress-related homeostasis.[8] Through direct neural stimulation of tissues and release of adrenaline from the adrenal gland, sympathetic stimulation increases respiratory and heart rate, elevates blood pressure, mobilizes fat stores and increases cellular metabolism. The individual is primed to escape physical danger. In stressful psychosocial situations, instead of the individual actively responding, the socially acceptable response is often to contain rather than release pent-up energy. Instead of physically dispelling energy, frustration accumulates. The result is an increase in 'tone' (allostatic load) or level of arousal. Instead of speeding away, the individual is like a racing car revving in the blocks. Prolonged exposure to stimuli perceived as stressful or persistent use of inappropriate responses to life events leads to a chronic

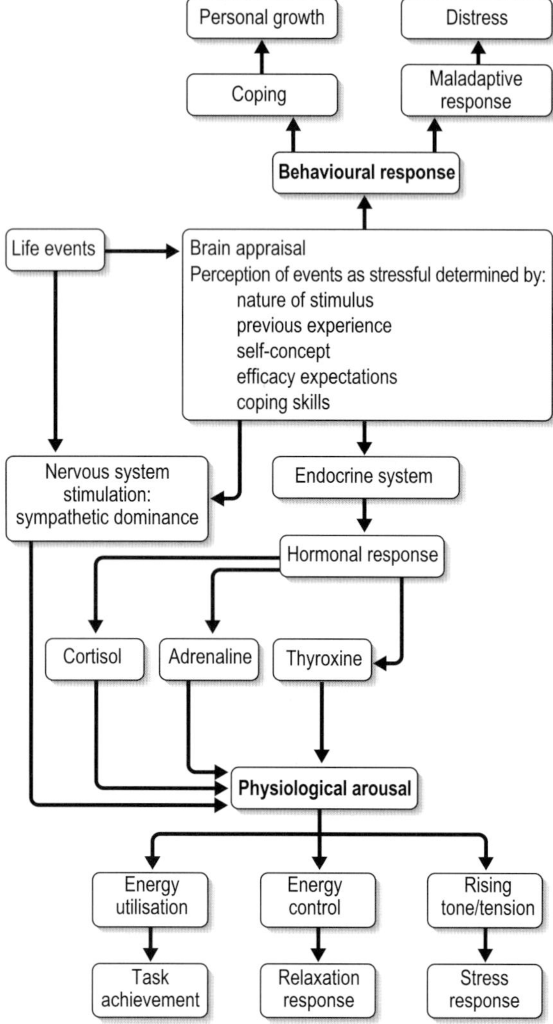

Figure 18.1 • Mind–body interaction.

stress response. Continual stimulation of the sympathetic nervous system and the hypothalamic–pituitary–adrenal axis due to chronic stress can produce a cascade of negative pathophysiological consequences.[9] Enhanced sympathetic nervous system activation evoked under conditions of chronic stress appears to produce an intrinsic increase in 'cardiovascular reactivity' with increased heart rate and blood pressure fluctuations. **Handout 18.3** shows the multidimensional impact of stress.

When homeostasis is disturbed by internal or external challenges, the hypothalamic–pituitary axis become activated, increasing peripheral levels of glucocorticoids. Normally, elevations of cortisol associated with acute stress downregulate

hypothalamic–pituitary–adrenal function through a negative feedback mechanism. However, under chronic stress, cortisol binds to central nervous system receptors, resulting, paradoxically, in a continued secretion of cortisol. This hypercortisolaemia is associated with a loss in the normal physiological plasticity of the hypothalamic–pituitary–adrenal interaction manifest as reduced variability in cortisol secretion. In the short term, increased cortisol secretion enhances the availability of glucose from protein and glycogen; in the long term, it suppresses the immune system and causes muscle wasting.

Physiological responses to acute psychosocial stress may lead to pathological changes upon chronic exposure. A recent meta-analysis confirmed that acute stress responsiveness changes with chronic psychosocial stress exposure.[10] The integrated stress response pattern of hypo- or hyperactivity appears to depend on the specific nature of the psychosocial background in which exposure to an acute stimulus occurs. Chronic psychosocial exposures include job stress; general life stress; depression or hopelessness; anxiety, neuroticism, or negative affect; hostility, aggression, or type-A behaviour; fatigue, burnout, or exhaustion. The heightened output from the sympathetic nervous system and the hypothalamic–pituitary axis associated with chronic stress produces changes conducive to increased inflammation, central obesity, hyperinsulinaemia, diabetes, hypertension, and endothelial dysfunction.

Stress management

When body 'tone' is set too high, i.e. the individual is carrying an allostatic load, the capacity of the body to adapt is impaired and organ reserves are depleted. Stress management aims to minimize allostatic load and enhance resilience. Resilience represents successful allostasis.

It has been postulated that three interrelated factors promoting healthy psychological functioning are vitality, emotional flexibility, and coping flexibility.[9] Vitality is a positive and restorative emotional state associated with a sense of enthusiasm and energy. Chronic stress and negative emotions can individually invoke a 'chronic stress response' and diminish vitality. Vitality is necessary to maintain flexibility. Flexibility is related to the ability both to regulate emotions effectively and to cope effectively with challenging daily experiences. Emotional flexibility *is* the ability to flexibly regulate emotions across a wide range of situations. The regulation of negative emotions involves various skills ranging from the ability to positively reappraise stimuli to being able to efficiently process one's emotional experiences. Failure to express emotions is associated with the buildup of negative thoughts, a tendency to ruminate and decreased ability to achieve emotional closure. Coping flexibility involves the ability to accurately appraise stressors as controllable or not, to flexibly adjust goals to changing life circumstances, and to appropriately select coping strategies. Emotional and coping flexibility are seen as key indicators of one's ability to successfully manage negative emotions and solve problems. Vitality, emotional flexibility, and coping flexibility form a dynamic and complex system of psychological functioning. People who always use the same pattern when responding to stress are rigid responders. People who do not respond in a predictable pattern are random responders. Random responders demonstrate flexibility, rigid responders are more at risk of organ system fatigue and disease. Stress management programmes are best tailored to meet individual needs. See **Handout 18.1**.

As the physicochemical response to mental stimuli does not discriminate between mental imagery and life events, thoughts influence whether a stimulus is perceived as a stressor. Beliefs or enduring thought patterns are a screen through which all social stimuli are filtered. An individual's arousal in response to a stimulus is modified by their beliefs. Stress management programmes should therefore include cognitive measures. However, while emotions are not immediately responsive to intellectual reasoning, they do respond to behaviour. The emotional response can be influenced by behaviour. Breathing and walking slowly contributes to feeling calm in stressful situations! Stress management programmes should therefore take a global approach and target the stressor, the individual's beliefs and thinking processes, as well as the physical response. Psychosocial stress management requires biopsychosocial intervention.

Stressful events

While eliminating stressors is not a major objective of stress management, it does deserve consideration. Before it is possible to reduce exposure to stressful stimuli, it is necessary to identify the stimuli that are inherently stressful or perceived to be stressful by particular individuals. Holmes and Rahe developed a scale to measure stress-provoking events in terms of 'life change units'.[11] Death of a partner was allocated a rating of 100 life change units; death of a close family member or a jail term received 63; marital reconciliation or retirement, 45; a change in responsibility at work or trouble with the in-laws, 29; and a vacation or minor violations of the law, around 12 life change units. The life change units were then totalled and used to ascertain the risk of future illness. A score in excess of 300 life change units is associated with an 80% risk of minor illness in the near future. A score of under 150 carries a 30% risk. Illness is most likely to occur within 3 months of experiencing the life change. The probability and severity of illness correlates with the score. The number of stressful life events is deemed a significant predictor at 12 months of quality of life for cancer patients.[12] It is furthermore noteworthy that persistent minor stresses can have an equal or even greater impact on health than short-term exposure to a major stressor. Although a good stress management strategy may be to avoid stressors once they have been identified, it is not always possible to avoid stressful environments. Other strategies are needed.

Event appraisal and processing

Modern stress management focuses on optimizing the individual's response to a stressor and not the nature of the stimulus itself. The response of an individual to stress seems to be less influenced by the nature or intensity of an event than by their appraisal of the stimulus and their efficacy and outcome expectations. The physical effects of stress are more closely linked to how the individual views the event and the confidence they have in their ability to cope, than to the situation itself. Behaviour and feelings are based upon a subjective interpretation of events. Adaptation is mediated through psychosocial coping measures which include cognitive appraisal of the event, evaluation of coping resources, and physiological responses mediated by the autonomic and neuroendocrine systems. Events perceived as stressful can induce chemical and histological changes that may progress to disease (see Figure 18.1). Developing effective stress management techniques at this level involves restructuring faulty psychological defences and supporting healthy coping mechanisms.

Good stress management can be enhanced by helping the patient to change their perception of:

- self. This involves changing self-concept. Self-confidence and self-esteem can be learned. Persons can improve their self-concept and their resistance to stress by becoming resourceful and taking more control of their health behaviour[13]
- specific stressors. This requires looking at problems from diverse angles. Humour is a useful tool for helping to get things into perspective. Laughter not only reduces stress, it also improves NK cell activity.[14] Low NK cell activity is linked to decreased resistance to disease
- general life situation. This includes reviewing feelings and self-talk. Self-talk is self-fulfilling and can be self-regulated. It is important for individuals to analyse and optimize self-talk.

Discriminating between fact and inference can avoid perceptual errors.

Stress management also requires that cognitive skills are improved. Task-oriented coping is characterized by moving through the stages of defining the problem, working out alternative solutions, implementing the chosen intervention, and evaluating the outcome. Problem solving is aided by creative thinking.[15] Cognitive therapy recognizes that by focusing on patterns of thinking and beliefs, feelings and behaviour can be changed. A stress management cycle can be initiated or a stress-provoking cycle can be intercepted.[16] The guiding principles of such cognitive–behavioural intervention strategies suggest that:[17]

- rather than responding directly to the environment, humans respond primarily to cognitive representations of the environment
- a large part of human behaviour is mentally mediated
- cognitions (thoughts), emotions (feelings) and behaviours (actions) are causally interrelated
- understanding patient's problems and the benefits of clinical communication are enhanced by attention to cognitive activators such as expectations, beliefs, self-statements and attributions.

Particular techniques for creating a thinking environment conducive to stress alleviation include thought blocking, visualization and affirmative self-talk. See **Handout 18.4**. Thought stopping is recommended when negative or unhelpful thoughts are persistently revisited. The aim is to identify the intrusive thought, deliberately put it aside and focus on something positive.

Visualization uses the senses to imagine a relaxing scenario. The rules for effective visualization include being specific in the image pictured and using colour, sound, taste, touch, smell and sight to imagine taking positive action. Effective affirmations use 'I' statements, are positively worded and do not contradict the current experience. Coping self-talk has calming and coaching elements.[18] Calming self-talk is helpful before an anxiety-provoking event. Calming self-talk involves telling oneself to stay calm and affirms that one can cope. Coaching self-talk involves setting clear goals, breaking tasks into manageable components and concentrating on the task at hand. Coaching self-talk is improved by focusing on problem solving and creative thinking skills.

Changing the physiology

Breathing and muscle relaxation techniques are integral components of any stress management programme.[19] See **Handout 18.5**. Breathing helps to focus the mind and relax muscles. Focused breathing involves focusing on breathing slowly and deeply and using the diaphragm. In diaphragmatic breathing, the ribcage is held as still as possible and movement of the abdomen is noted with each breath. As muscle tension is an early indicator of stress and muscle tension itself exacerbates feelings of tension, muscle relaxation is a good strategy to break the stress–tension cycle. Various techniques can be used to reduce muscle tension. They usually involve repeated tensing and relaxing of diverse muscle groups. Particular note is taken of the decrease in tension upon relaxation. In progressive deep muscle relaxation, sequential tightening and relaxation of all muscle groups coupled with deep, usually diaphragmatic, breathing and conscious letting go of mental distractions combine to generate awareness of inner peace. See **Handouts 18.6**.

A number of user-friendly books which may benefit patients are available.[19]

Coping can be directed towards:

- distress prevention. On recognizing that particular events are stressful, one may attempt to eliminate the stressor or change one's perception of the event

- health promotion. This is achieved by improving the baseline health status of the body. The body can be primed so as to function with maximum efficiency by paying attention to diet, to thought and communication patterns, to rest and exercise. Refer to handouts in Part 2; take particular note of those in Chapter 14

- disease prevention. Unacceptably high levels of arousal following exposure to potentially stressful events can be counteracted with mental and physical relaxation strategies to effectively dispel or modify distress. This involves detection and management of acute and persistent stress.

Managing acute stress

When exposed to short-term periods of extreme stress, it is important to keep things in perspective – how important will this problem be in 20 years, 2 years, 2 months or even in 2 days? Stress impedes clear thinking and decreases efficiency. It is a good idea to have a standard plan that can be routinely implemented at times of peak stress. **Handout 18.2** identifies the characteristics of an acute stress reaction and **Handout 18.3** provides additional information on how to identify the dimensions being most affected. **Handout 18.5** provides easy to implement strategies for coping with acute stress reactions.

Minor life adjustments often help adaptation during particularly stressful periods. Figure 18.2 outlines a standard strategy for minimizing the disruptive effects of short-term stress.[16]

In formulating a stress management programme, the most effective protocol is one that suits the individual concerned. No single strategy is most effective. In general, it is a good idea to start by selecting one or more techniques that particularly target the area of greatest vulnerability. Persons whose predominant stress response is physical may benefit most from physically orientated stress relaxation techniques. See **Handouts 18.6** and **18.7**.

▪ Review goals and examine current demands. ▪ List the tasks which need to be completed to fulfill identified goals. Tasks are ranked according to their urgency. ▪ Make lists and reminders. Stress impairs memory and concentration. ▪ Put aside some planning time each day. Stress impairs time management and decision making. ▪ Set aside enough time for sleep. Stress drains energy. ▪ Take time to relax and exercise. Take a break. ▪ Eat properly. Uncontrolled experiments suggest that carbohydrate-rich, protein-poor food in high stress subjects may increase personal control, probably under the influence of higher levels of brain tryptophan and serotonin.[20] ▪ Actively attempt to solve problems. Indecisiveness and procrastination are signs of stress. Unresolved problems become urgent and increase stress. Tackle the small problems first! ▪ Be satisfied with your efforts. You don't have to be perfect. ▪ Ask for help. Let people know you are feeling pressured. ▪ Spend time with someone who cares. ▪ Look for the funny side. Having a laugh can help to keep things in perspective and release tension.

Figure 18.2 • Minimizing the disruptive effects of short-term stress.

Similarly, those who respond with pronounced emotional lability should try to change their perceptions. See **Handout 18.4**. After initially focusing on the area in which the person is experiencing most distress, a more comprehensive approach may be useful. **Handout 18.8** provides an overview of various stress management options. Evidence of long-term distress suggests the desirability of committing to a lifelong stress management programme.

In perspective

Psychosocial stress is an inescapable aspect of modern life. It is increasingly being acknowledged as a recognized health hazard. Good stress management techniques would seem an indispensable asset in any personal wellness programme.

References

1. Goldstein DS. Computer models of stress, allostasis, and acute and chronic diseases. *Ann N Y Acad Sci.* 2008;1148:223–231.

2. Logan JG, Barksdale DJ. Allostasis and allostatic load: expanding the discourse on stress and cardiovascular disease. *J Clin Nurs.* 2008;17(7B):201–208.

3. Karlamangla AS, Singer BH, Seeman TE. Reduction in allostatic load in older adults is associated with lower all-cause mortality risk: MacArthur studies of successful aging. *Psychosom Med.* 2006;68 (3):500–507.

4. Fang CY, Miller SM, Bovbjerg DH, et al. Perceived stress is associated

with impaired T-cell response to HPV16 in women with cervical dysplasia. *Ann Behav Med.* 2008;35 (1):87–96.

5. Das S, O'Keefe JH. Behavioral cardiology: recognizing and addressing the profound impact of psychosocial stress on cardiovascular health. *Curr Hypertens Rep.* 2008;10(5):374–381.

6. Holmes SD, Krantz DS, Rogers H, Gottdiener RJ, Contrada RJ. Mental stress and coronary artery disease: a multidisciplinary guide. *Prog Cardiovasc Dis.* 2006;49 (2):106–122.

7. Colloca L, Tinazzi M, Recchia S, et al. Learning potentiates neurophysiological and behavioral placebo analgesic responses. *Pain.* 2008;139(2):306–314.

8. Elenkov IJ, Wilder RL, Chrousos ES, Vizi ES. The sympathetic nerve – an integrative interface between two supersystems: the brain and the immune system. *Pharmacol Rev.* 2000;52(4):595–638.

9. Rozanski A, Kubzansky LD. Psychologic functioning and physical health: a paradigm of flexibility.

10. Chida Y, Hamer M. Chronic psychosocial factors and acute physiological responses to laboratory-induced stress in healthy populations: a quantitative review of 30 years of investigations. *Psychol Bull.* 2008;134(6):829–885.

11. Holmes TH, Rahe RH. The social adjustment rating scale. *J Psychosom Res.* 1967;11:2133–2138.

12. Golden-Kreutz DM, Thornton LM, Wells-Di Gregorio S, et al. Traumatic stress, perceived global stress, and life events: prospectively predicting quality of life in breast cancer patients. *Health Psychol.* 2005;24(3):288–296.

13. Rosenbaum M. The role of learned resourcefulness in the self-control of health behavior. In: Rosenbaum M, ed. *Learned Resourcefulness: On Coping Skills, Self-Control and Adaptive Behavior.* New York: Springer; 1990:3–30.

14. Bennett MP, Zeller JM, Rosenberg J, McCann J. The effect of mirthful laughter on stress and natural killer cell activity. *Altern Ther Health Med.* 2003;9(2):38–45.

Psychosom Med. 2005;67(suppl 1): S47–S53.

15. De Bono E. *Serious Creativity.* London: Harper Collins; 1995.

16. Butler G, Hope T. *Managing Your Mind: The Mental Fitness Guide.* New York: Oxford University Press; 1995.

17. Kendall PC, Turk DC. Cognitive-behavioral strategies and health enhancement. In: Matarazzo JD, Weiss JA, Herd JA, Miller NE, Weiss SM, eds. *Behavioral Health: A Handbook Of Health Enhancement And Disease Prevention.* New York: John Wiley; 1984:393–394.

18. Nelson-Jones R. *Effective Thinking Skills.* London: Cassell Educational; 1989.

19. Wilson P. *Instant Calm.* Ringwood, Victoria: Penguin Books; 1995.

20. Markus CR, Panhuysen G, Tuiten H, Koppeschaar H, Fekkes ML, Peters ML. Does carbohydrate-rich, protein-poor food prevent a deterioration of mood and cognitive performance of stress-prone subjects when subjected to a stressful task? *Appetite.* 1998;31(1):49–65.

Accidents

In 2003, unintentional injuries or accidents ranked as the fifth most common cause of death in the US.[1] In 2005, 39.7 in every 100,000 Americans died due to accidents. In 2004, 7% of all deaths in the US resulted from injury.[2] Accidents are the leading cause of death for those under 35 years of age. In 2000, the estimated cost of injury-related death and disability totalled more than $400 billion in medical expenses and lost productivity.[2] The five major causes that account for 81% percent of all injury deaths are motor vehicle traffic, firearms, poisoning, falls, and suffocation.[1]

The risk of premature morbidity or mortality due to accidents is increased by poor behavioural choices. Accidents involve a sequence of events that produce unintended injury. Prevention programmes are based upon two principles. One focuses on the environment, the other on the individual. Intervention strategies range from education, through legislation to better product design. Environmental intervention aims to prevent contact between the hazard and the susceptible individual. Examples include the legal proscription that persons under a certain age may not drive a motor vehicle, operate powered equipment such as meat slicers or circular saws, or work on demolition sites. Fifteen-year-olds may not work on a ladder or scaffold. Prevention may also be achieved at the level of the individual, by either enhancing personal resistance or reducing susceptibility. Education can improve knowledge and skills, while protective clothing can decrease vulnerability. High-risk behaviours for unintentional injuries range from failing to use bicycle/motorcycle helmets or seat belts to riding in a car with a driver who has used marijuana or alcohol. The 2007 US Youth Risk Behavior Survey found that, in the 30 days prior to the survey, 11.1% of high school students had never or rarely worn a seat belt when being driven; 29.1% had been a passenger in a vehicle driven by someone who had been drinking alcohol; and 18.0% had carried a weapon.[3] Behaviours increasing the risk of intentional injuries include carrying a weapon, engaging in physical fighting and attempting suicide. In the US, 72% of all deaths among persons aged 10–24 years result from four causes: motor vehicle accidents, other unintentional injuries, homicide, and suicide.[3] While risk reduction may be achieved through behaviour change resulting from changing attitudes and beliefs by improving knowledge and skill, such intervention is often found to be more effective when combined with legislation. Successful combination interventions include those pertaining to the use of bicycle helmets, child restraints, and smoke detectors.[4]

Prevention is better than cure. Prevention of accidents and injury can be targeted at:[5]

- primary intervention. In the pre-event phase the aim is to prevent an incident or accident that could lead to injury. An approach may be to

Prevent creation of the hazard
- Reduce the amount of hazard present
- Prevent the release of a hazard that already exists
- Modify the rate or spatial release of hazard from the source
- Separate, in time and space, the hazard and that which needs to be protected
- Interpose a physical barrier between the hazard and that being protected
- Reduce the noxious potential of the hazard
- Increase the resistance of the potential 'host'
- Counter damage done by the hazard
- Stabilize, repair and rehabilitate the object of damage

Figure 19.1 • Important steps for injury prevention.

separate the hazard from the individual, e.g. use of a swimming pool fence, not drinking alcohol and driving

- secondary prevention. In secondary intervention the event or accident is not prevented but injury is avoided. Interventions include protection given by bicycle helmets or seat belts
- tertiary intervention. This is damage limitation. The post-event phase attempts to minimize the extent of injury, e.g. by first aid training for motorists.

Figure 19.1 lists important steps for injury prevention. Another key to success is sustained use of surveillance systems and implementation of a range of interventions.

Home safety

Nearly 40% of self-reported episodes of non-fatal injuries occur during sports or leisure activities and 44% occur in or around the home.[1]

In England and Wales, home accidents have decreased, with deaths due to falls and poisoning dropping over 10% since 1995.[6] Serious injuries dropped by over one-third and slight injuries by over 12%. Coupling general practitioner advice with access to low-cost equipment for low-income families increases safety in the home.[7] Home safety education has been shown to effectively increase the proportion of families keeping hot water temperature in a safe range, having functional smoke alarms, storing medicines and cleaning products out of reach, having syrup of ipecac and poison control centre numbers accessible, fitting stair gates, covering electrical sockets, and storing sharp objects out of reach.[8] Despite a lack of evidence showing home safety education reduces the rate of thermal

injuries, poisoning or a range of injuries, when care-givers provide a safe environment a reduced level of risk-taking behaviours in children has been observed.[9]

Handout 19.1 provides a checklist of factors that increase and reduce the risk of accidents in the home. **Handout 19.2** provides a list of additional safeguards for households with children under the age of 5 years. Injuries are the leading cause of mortality and morbidity in preschool and school-age children.

Burns and scalds

Scalds occur as a result of burns from hot liquids. In children under 5 years of age, scalds may result from tap water, hot cooking utensils (e.g. kettles), hot beverages or opening a microwave oven.[10] Boys are more commonly affected and up to 67% of scalds occur in children under 2 years of age.[11] Saunas are another potential source of scalds. Saunas should not be used after strenuous exercise. The time in a sauna should be limited and the sauna vacated if lightheadedness is experienced. The whirlpool should be used at a temperature under 105°C.

House fires are an important source of burns and other injuries. Smoking is a risk factor for death from residential fires.[12] An estimated 30% of deaths due to fire in the US and 10% globally are tobacco related. Smoking is believed to cause around one in four home fire deaths in the US,[13] with smoking-related fire costs amounting to $6.95 billion in 1998.[14] Fire risk is greatest late at night and early in the morning. The risk of fatal injury is highest in mobile homes and homes with fewer safety features, such as a smoke detector or a telephone. **Handout 19.3** provides information for reducing the risk of home fires. Safety is enhanced when householders minimize the risk of a fire starting, know what to do once a fire starts, and are able to treat minor burns. First-degree burns result in red, slightly swollen skin. First aid for minor burns is to immediately immerse the area in cold water and keep the area immersed until pain is relieved. Ice cubes may be added to keep the water cold. When treating blisters, first sterilize a needle by holding it for 10 seconds in a flame, then puncture the side of the blister and gently squeeze out the accumulated fluid. The overlying skin is left and the area is covered with antibiotic ointment and sterile gauze. Minor chemical burns should be treated by immediately flushing the burnt area with plenty of cold running water. The area should then be covered with a thick layer of manuka honey and a loose protective bandage.

Another potential household hazard is electricity. **Handout 19.4** provides tips on how electrical hazards can be minimized. In cases of accidents, disconnect the power before attempting to help if the victim is touching live equipment. If necessary, separate the victim from live equipment with a long dry stick. Be sure you are dry!

Household poisons

Unintentional poisoning is responsible for 8 in every 100,000 American deaths.[1] Poisoning is the leading means of injury-related death for Americans 34–53 years of age, and in 2004 was the second leading age-adjusted cause of death.[2] Non-hazardous personal care products include bubble bath, soap, lipstick, hand lotion, suntan lotion, perfume, cosmetics and deodorants. Ink, crayons, chalk, candles and erasers are also non-toxic. Common household items such as chlorine bleach and acidic cleaning products are health hazards unless appropriately used. Caustic substances, bleach, and kerosene were the agents mainly involved in producing the adverse and toxic effects reported by 27% respondents in a recent survey.[15] Most respondents reported mixing and discarding cleaning product leftovers and their containers improperly. They were also found to use suboptimal storage places. Another study confirmed products common in poisoning were often stored at low elevations – as were prescription medications.[16] In this study, 19% indicated they transferred cleaning items, usually bleach, to other containers; even more (29%) transferred prescription medications. A South American study found the main causes of childhood poisoning were products being within the child's reach, storage in soft drink bottles, mixing food with rodenticides, incorrect product use, and using kitchen utensils for measuring cleaning products.[17] **Handout 19.5** provides tips on how to reduce household poisoning.

Poisons may be ingested, inhaled, injected or absorbed through the skin. The most frequent exposure routes are ingestion, followed by inhalation, skin contact and eye contact. Important considerations in ingested poisoning include the patient's age, weight and gender. Identifying the poison and establishing the quantity, time and route of exposure are important management considerations. Physical signs following ingestion of stimulants may include dilated pupils, tremors, tachycardia, irritability and even convulsions. Commonly ingested stimulants include cocaine, amphetamines, caffeine, and antihistamines. Physical findings produced by depressants include lethargy, decreased responsiveness to stimulation, constricted pupils and even coma. Common sedatives include alcohol, benzodiazepines and barbiturates.

In cases of ingested poisoning, dilute the poison by immediately drinking water or milk. Activated charcoal may be used to adsorb certain toxins. Activated charcoal is not used when caustic acids or alkalis, alcohols, lithium or heavy metals have been ingested. The usual dosage is 1 to 2 g/kg and the charcoal is mixed with water in a ratio of 1:4 or 1:8 to form a slurry. Vomiting should not be induced if the ingested poison is unknown or if a corrosive or petroleum product is suspected. Gastric emptying is most effective when used within 1 hour of ingesting the poison. It cannot be justified beyond 4 hours following toxin ingestion except in patients with concretions, massive ingestions, or ingestion of substances that markedly decrease gastric motility. The stomach may be emptied by gastric lavage or by inducing emesis with syrup of ipecac. A potential complication is aspiration. Gastric emptying is beneficial when used early in the treatment of potentially severe poisoning. Whole bowel irrigation using isosmotic cathartic solutions to flush and cleanse the bowel is another option.

Food safety

Food poisoning presents a particular health hazard. In rare cases it is necessary to globally recall products, as was the case with melamine contamination of foods produced in China. Melamine is a useful addition to a variety of building materials, fire retardant materials and commercial cleaning products. It is harmful if ingested, absorbed or inhaled. The addition of melamine to inflate readings for protein levels in the milk used in manufacturing infant formulas resulted in a number of deaths, tens of thousands of illnesses and several thousand hospitalizations in China in 2008.[18]

While chemical additives may cause global problems, natural toxins may result in local outbreaks (see Tables 19.1 and 19.2). In many cases the food is consumed in small quantities, so the natural food toxin does not constitute a health hazard,

Table 19.1 Natural toxicants in plants

Toxicant	Major food source	Clinical manifestations
Caffeine	Coffee, tea, cocoa, cola-type beverages	Diuresis; cardiac, CNS and gastric acid secretion stimulant; smooth muscle relaxant; animal teratogen
Cucurbitacins	Melons, squash, zucchini (bitter varieties)	Cramps, diarrhoea
Cyanogenic glycosides		
Amygdalin	Kernels/seeds of apples, apricots, bitter almonds	
Dhurin	Sorghum (high concentration in leaves)	
Linamarin	Cassava	Cyanide poisoning, tropical ataxic neuropathy (myelopathy, optic atrophy, deafness, polyneuropathy). A deterrent is the bitter taste.
Favism-causing compounds	Broad beans (*Vicia faba*)	Acute haemolytic anaemia (pallor, breathlessness, tachycardia)
Glycoalkaloids	Potatoes	Gastrointestinal upsets, vomiting, diarrhoea, abdominal pain; drowsiness, confusion, coma. An 11 mg% concentration – bitter taste
Glucosinolates	Brussels sprouts, cabbage, cauliflower, mustard, turnip	Goitrogenic activity; enlarged thyroid, risk of hypothyroidism
Hypoglycin	Akee fruit	Acute hypoglycaemia, vomiting
Lathyrogens	*Lathyrus sativus* (lathyrus pea, chickling vetch)	Spastic paralysis, lower limbs. Probably only occurs in vitamin C deficiency
Nitrate/nitrite	Cabbage, celery, lettuce, spinach	Methaemoglobinaemia in infants; ? gastric cancer via N-nitrosamine formation
Oxalic acid	Rhubarb, spinach, tea	Gastroenteritis, renal damage, decreased calcium absorption
Pyrrolizidine alkaloids	Comfrey (a plant source of vitamin B12)	Liver disease, cancer

e.g. lathyrism only occurs when the chickpea makes up one-third of the diet and is consistently eaten over 3–6 months. In other cases, food preparation procedures ensure that only minimal amounts of toxin are ingested, e.g. cassava is soaked and boiled; hydrogen cyanide is leeched out into the water and lost to the atmosphere during boiling. Traditional food selection practices also ensure that toxins are avoided, e.g. the growing leaves of sorghum are rich in cyanogenic glycosides and these are discarded while the relatively safe seeds are widely consumed. Consumer rejection of bitter foods, e.g. apple seeds with amygdalin or potatoes rich in glycoalkaloids, provides another protective food selection mechanism. The fish toxins outlined in Table 19.2 are resistant to cooking, freezing, drying and smoking; ichthyosarcotoxic fish are not distinguishable by appearance or smell. No field test is available for recognition of these fish; neither is there an antidote to neutralize the toxin.

Food poisoning can also result from ingestion of toxins produced by microbial contamination of food. Poor food-handling practices are an important source of microbial food contamination. Food handlers who fails to properly wash hands, inadequate cleaning of processing or preparation equipment or utensils, cross-contamination of ready-to-eat foods by contaminated raw ingredients, and failure to

Table 19.2 Fish poisoning

Toxicant grouping	Ciguatera	Tetrodotoxism	Clupeoid	Scomboid
Suspect fish	Spanish mackerel Spotted mackerel Red Emperor Sweetlip Emperor Red bass Coral trout (NB: Tropical waters, Northern Australia – coral reefs	Puffer fish Toad fish Blow fish (Fish with large teeth, inflatable bodies and 'no' scales)	Sardine Herring Anchovies	Anchovies Mackerels Sardines Tuna Pilchards
Time lapse between ingestion and symptom onset	5–6 hours; occasionally 30	10–15 minutes	Short	Short
Clinical presentation	Abdominal pain Nausea Diarrhoea Reversed temperature sensation Pruritus Paraesthesia Arthralgia	Abdominal pain Nausea and vomiting Tingling of parts of the body in contact with the poisonous fish Generalized paralysis	Metallic taste Dry mouth Gastrointestinal upsets Cardiovascular collapse	Headache Hypotension Bronchoconstriction Nausea Abdominal pain
Postulated pathogenesis	Fish ingestion of dinoflagellate; notable after disturbance of coral reefs	Toxin in gonads, intestine, liver and skin of fish	Unknown Sporadic unpredictable outbreaks	Histamine intoxication – fish spoilage under non-chilled storage

prepare food at the temperature required to destroy pathogens are all recognized risks.[19] The most frequently reported risk scenario, however, is bare hand contact with the food by an asymptomatic disease carrier. The pathogens most likely to be transmitted by food workers are norovirus, hepatitis A virus, *Salmonella* species, *Shigella* species, and *Staphylococcus aureus*.[20] Some pathogens appear to be able to infect at doses as low as 1 to 100 units.

Staphyloccal food poisoning may result when meat, dairy and bakery products are contaminated. *Staphylococcus aureus* is carried in the nose and throat and can be transmitted by droplets or on the hands of food handlers. If the organism contaminates food and is allowed to multiply, it produces a heat-resistant toxin. Conditions that favour multiplication of the organism and toxin production are warmth and moisture. Heating the food to 65°C for 30 minutes kills the organisms but the toxin remains stable, even at 100°C for 3 minutes. Vomiting, and sometimes diarrhoea, occur some 2–8 hours after eating the food. Another organism causing vomiting is *Bacillus cereus*. This bacterium, found in rice and cereals, produces vomiting within 1 to 3 hours after eating.

Botulism is a form of food poisoning that results from ingestion of toxin produced by *Clostridium botulinum*. Spores are found in soil and may contaminate fruit, vegetables and other food products. Adequate cooking of contaminated food kills all vegetative forms of the organism but will not destroy the spores. Bottling food creates the anaerobic environment under which spores germinate and produce toxin. Persons eating the food present with paralysis, double vision and difficulty with swallowing. The food looks, tastes and smells good. Swollen cans are a red flag for toxin production and should be discarded. In general, the danger lies in home bottling. The canning industry overcomes the problem by preparing food at temperatures of 120°C.

Bacteria are responsible for a number of other foodborne infections. Cholera is spread in water and food and causes profound diarrhoea. Dehydration, especially if patients are unable to drink due to vomiting, may cause death. The incubation period is 24 to 72 hours. Salmonella is spread in dairy products, custards and eggs. Egg nogs are a particular risk. The organism, present in the hen's faeces, is deposited on the shell of the newly laid egg. As the egg cools, the organism is drawn through the porous shell. Once cool, the shell is impermeable and the organism is trapped in a moist nutritious environment. Eating raw contaminated eggs causes diarrhoea, sometimes with vomiting, within 8 to 48 hours. Shigella is spread by food and direct contact. Infection may result from transferring organisms from contaminated toilet doors to the mouth. Within 24 to 48 hours following exposure, malaise, fever, abdominal cramps and diarrhoea or dysentery (bloodstained diarrhoea) develop. Abdominal pain, diarrhoea and fever may also result from food, especially milk, contaminated by *Yersinia enterocolitica*. Symptoms occur within 3 to 8 hours after consuming the suspect food and may persist for months. Campylobacter causes abdominal pain, malaise, diarrhoea and vomiting. but only lasts for 24 to 72 hours. Seafood contaminated by *Vibrio parahaemolyticus* causes diarrhoea and vomiting 6 to 96 hours after eating contaminated fish. Diarrhoea starts abruptly and may last for 3 days. Although food heated to above 64°C is usually safe, exceptions to this rule occur when food such as the centre of a roast has not reached this temperature, or when heat-resistant spores are involved. **Handout 19.6** provides guidelines for avoiding food poisoning.

Travellers are at particular risk of *E. coli* infection. Communities adapt to the local strain of the organism, but visitors to the region present with diarrhoea 24 to 72 hours after exposure to local water and food. Microbial standards require that no more than 100 colonies of bacteria be present in 1 mL of water; that no more than 10 coliforms be present in 100 mL of water; and that no *E. coli* be present in any 100 mL of water tested. Bacterial counts are used as a means of determining faecal pollution of water. Safe water is an important prerequisite to avoiding diarrhoea when travelling and adequate hydration is an important rule in treatment. Up to 50% of travellers to developing countries experience one or more episode of diarrhoea. Water and food are the major sources of infection. **Handout 19.7** provides prevention guidelines and **Handout 19.8** provides therapeutic guidelines for travellers.

Another food-related health risk is choking. If the person can continue to speak, then air is still reaching the lungs and the situation is not critical. Persons who cannot talk should immediately have the obstruction removed. **Handout 19.9** provides first aid advice for restoring the airway.

Drowning and water accidents

Obstruction to airflow occurs in both choking and drowning. When food or other foreign objects lodge in the upper airway, choking results; when water is inhaled, laryngospasm occurs. In both cases, air cannot reach the lungs and suffocation results. During 2003 there were 381 drownings in the UK, with 38% occurring in rivers or streams, 24% in the sea and 14% in lakes or reservoirs.[6]

Drowning may occur in boating accidents. Cold water temperature is a significant factor in North American drowning, yet a survey found the majority of respondents underestimated the time available for survival during ice water immersion.[21] It takes more than 30 minutes to become hypothermic, and for cooling to become life threatening takes over an hour. With 2007 persons dying of cold-water immersion in Canada between 1991 and 2000, it is also important that the public be made aware that swimming is a viable option for self-rescue during accidental cold-water immersion.[22] Swimming failure develops earlier than systemic hypothermia. Swimming failure results not from general hypothermia as previously believed, but rather from muscle fatigue of the arms as a consequence of arm cooling.[22] Studies conducted in water between 10°C and 14°C indicate that people can swim in cold water for between 800 and 1500 m before being incapacitated by the cold. Furthermore, although subjects are usually successful at deciding their swimming strategy early in the immersion, after about 30 minutes, decision-making ability becomes impaired. It therefore seems wise to formulate a survival plan early during immersion, directly after the cold shock responses ceases. Anoxic encephalopathy is the most dreaded consequence of submersion accidents; respiratory involvement is very common in these patients.

Improvement of lung injury following near-drowning in seawater is rapid in most cases, with hypoxaemia resolving in three-quarters and radiographic findings in two-thirds of cases by day 4.[23] The duration of hospitalization varies from 2 to 14 days.

In 2005, apart from boating incidents, there were 10 deaths daily from drowning in the US.[24] Despite a decline, fatal drowning remains the second-leading cause of unintentional injury-related death for children aged 1 to 14 years. More than one in four fatal-drowning victims are children 14 and younger, and for every child who dies from drowning, another four receive emergency department care for non-fatal submersion injuries. Children may drown by falling into water while playing, swimming or even bathing.

In 2005 in the US, of all children 1 to 4 years old who died, almost 30% died from drowning. It is necessary for children to be watched at all times when around water. Children under 1 year most often drown in bathtubs, buckets, or toilets. Among children aged 1 to 4 years, most drowning occurs in residential swimming pools.[24] In general, three groups of causative factors – environmental, parent-related and victim-related – have been identified. Environmental causes can often be addressed by legislation. Installation of a 4-foot or higher fence with self-closing and self-latching gates that completely isolates the pool is legally required in certain countries. **Handout 19.10** provides a checklist of swimming pool requirements and child safety recommendations.[25] Parent-related causes are non-supervision of a child and lack of first aid training. Victim-related factors include a child reaching for interesting objects in or on the water and the inability to swim. Removing balls and toys from the area and teaching children to swim is a good start to prevention. Approved personal flotation devices can be lifesaving. Air-filled or foam toys, such as 'water wings', 'noodles', or inner-tubes do not suffice.

Most drownings in those over 15 years of age occur in natural water settings.[23] Alcohol use is involved in up to half of adolescent and adult deaths associated with water recreation and about one in five reported boating fatalities. Risk can be reduced by checking local weather conditions, using approved life jackets when boating, and watching for dangerous waves and signs of rip currents when swimming. Persons caught in a rip current should swim parallel to shore and once free of the current, swim toward shore.

Being able to perform cardiopulmonary resuscitation may be lifesaving.

Handout 19.10 provides a checklist for remaining safe near water.

Motor vehicle accidents

Except for children under 2 years of age, motor vehicle accidents are the leading cause of injury-related death in the US.[2] In 2005, 153 in every million Americans died in motor vehicle accidents.[1] Major factors in motor vehicle accidents are alcohol, speed, the condition of the vehicle and the road. Despite a decrease in motor vehicle accidents overall and a decrease in the number of legally intoxicated drivers, alcohol accounted for one-third of fatally injured drivers in 2004.[2] There is a significant relationship between driver age and injury severity, manner of collision, speed and alcohol involvement.[26]

Motor vehicle traffic death rates were highest for young people 18–21 years of age, with a lower secondary peak for older adults.[2] Medical conditions are an important risk factor in the elderly; driver fatigue is a major risk in younger people. Fifty-five percent of accidents due to sleeping at the wheel occur in persons 25 years of age or younger, with a peak age occurrence at 20 years.[27] Fatigue is thought to play a role in one in five accidents. Crashes due to drivers falling asleep usually take place at higher speeds, i.e. over 50 mph (80 kph), and involve the vehicle being driven off the road.

Sleep deprivation is an important risk factor. Extended wakefulness significantly decreases psychomotor vigilance tasks and driving performance.[28] The duration of driving is another significant cause of fatigue-related accidents. The fatigue caused by driving for extended periods acutely impairs driver alertness and performance and can compromise safety. A study which quantitatively measured the progression of driver fatigue found sleepiness ratings, poor reaction time and unstable driving performance significantly increased over time.[29] It appears that 80 minutes is the safe limit for monotonous highway driving. Crashes occur primarily during two danger periods.[27] Accident risk due to sleepiness peaks between midnight to 7.00 a.m. and during the mid-afternoon 'siesta' time around 3.00 p.m. Both disturbance of the sleep–wake cycle and the duration of the drive are important determinants of sleepiness at the wheel. The only safe counter measure to driver sleepiness is to stop driving. Taking a 15- to 30-minute nap plus a strong cup of coffee somewhat reduces driver risk. Compared with alcohol-related motor vehicle accidents, which carry a fatality rate of 2.1%, the fatality rate associated with the driver falling asleep is 1.4%.[27]

In addition to the state of the driver influencing fatal crashes, seating in the vehicle impacts on passenger risk. The rear middle seat is safer than any other position in a fatal crash.[30] However, restrained occupants over the age of 50 in frontal crashes have a higher risk of injury in the rear seat than in the front. This problem may be overcome with seat belt modification. Modifications introducing a retractor pretensioner and a progressive force-limiter on rear seat belts may provide injury-reducing benefit to rear seat occupants in moderate to high severity frontal crashes.[31] Seat belts are the single most effective means of reducing deaths in motor vehicle crashes. Primary enforcement seat belt laws which allow police to stop a motorist solely for being unbelted are most effective.[32] Among children under age 5, in 2006, an estimated 425 lives were saved by car and booster seat use.[33]

Child safety seats, used correctly, reduce the risk of death in passenger cars by 71% for infants, and by 54% for toddlers up to 4 years of age. However, child restraint systems are often used incorrectly and misused booster seats can increase a child's risk of injury during a crash. In the US during 2005, an average of four children 14 years old and younger died and 504 were injured in motor vehicle accidents each day.[33] The National Highway Traffic Safety Administration estimates annual savings of $50 billion with safety belt use, $1.94 billion from airbags, and $670 million with motorcycle helmet use.[34] A further potential saving is estimated at $13 billion annually if speed limits were to be restricted to 65 mph.[34]

The risk of motorcycle accidents and fatalities are increased by excessive speed, less crash protection, inclement weather and being poorly visible to other motorists. When motorcycle accidents involve other motorists, left turns into the path of oncoming vehicles and failure to yield have been identified as the most risky procedures. Injuries can be minimized by wearing a helmet and protective bright clothing with long sleeves. Knowledge of road rules and proper use of protective clothing also applies to bicycle riders.

In addition to environmental measures such as improved roads and the manufacture of safer vehicles, measures to reduce motor vehicle accidents and fatalities rely on legislation and education. Legislation enforces speed, seat belt and helmet use, and drunk driving laws. Education enhances awareness of safe driver, passenger and pedestrian behaviour, including the use of protective measures such as seat belts, airbags and helmets. **Handout 19.11** provides a road safety checklist.

Falls

Falls are the leading cause of non-fatal injury.[35] While overall the leading cause of fatal injury is motor-vehicle-occupant injuries,[35] falls are the leading cause of injury death for elderly people over 72 years of age[2] and the leading cause of non-fatal unintentional injuries for infants.[36] In 2005, falls were responsible for the death of 6.6 out of every 100,000 Americans.[1]

Falls are a particular problem in the elderly. Every 18 seconds, an older American is treated in an emergency department for a fall, and every 35 minutes someone in this population dies as a result of their injuries.[37]

In 2000, the total direct cost of all fall injuries for people 65 and older exceeded $19 billion; a figure expected to increase to $54.9 billion by 2020 as the population ages.[37] One in three adults 65 and older falls each year and fractures are the most common and most costly type of non-fatal injuries. Owing to their reduced bone mass and bone fragility, falls in the elderly create a serious health hazard.

Handout 19.12 lists risk factors related to falls in the elderly. Environmental factors may be responsible for up to half of the falls in the elderly. An Australian study found that 80% of homes in which persons over 70 years of age resided had at least one hazard and 39% had more than five hazards.[38] The bathroom was identified as the most hazardous room; particularly with respect to floor surfaces and the absence of appropriate grab- or handrails. In contrast to home safety intervention in the elderly, environmental factors, other than stair-gate use, have little impact on successfully reducing childhood falls.[39] While reduced baby-walker use may be helpful, there is little evidence that increased possession of window locks, screens, or windows with limited opening or of non-slip bath mats reduces the risk of children falling.[39]

Older persons are at increased risk due to physiological changes of ages. A recent study of risk factors for falling which examined medication, balance and mobility, fear of falling, orthostatic hypotension, mood, high risk of osteoporosis, impaired vision, and urinary incontinence, found medication and failing vision had greatest clinical validity.[40] The risk of falling was increased both by the type of drug, chiefly sedative, psychoactive, antihypertensive and/or antidiuretic medication, as well as by the number (four or more) of medications. Vision impairment, with respect to either substantially reduced eyesight over the last 6 months or the inability to read the newspaper without glasses, also significantly increased risk. To cope with deteriorating vision and information-processing ability, elderly individuals seemed to have developed a strategy of stiffening and freezing their lower legs during upright standing.[41] Clinically detected abnormalities of gait or balance are the most consistent predictors of future falls.[42] Another risk factor is alcohol. A New Zealand study reported that approximately 20% of falls at home in adults of any age were associated with consumption of two or more alcoholic drinks in the preceding 6 hours.[43]

Effective multifactorial interventions may reduce the frequent falling rate of older patients by over 30%. The risk of injury can furthermore be reduced by falling 'carefully'. Tips for falling 'safely' are to:

- fold your arms around your head
- try to roll forward
- relax your body
- attempt to land on a well-padded area, e.g. buttocks, thigh, shoulder.

The relative risk of a fracture is increased 17.3-fold if five or more of the risk factors listed in **Handout 19.13** are present or 11.8-fold if more than one vertebral fracture has been sustained.[44] Other factors that suggest the presence of osteoporosis and indicate an increased relative risk of fractures in excess of fivefold are tobacco use, a body mass index of less than 23 and one previous vertebral facture.[44]

Suicide – intentional self-injury

In 2003, suicide was the 11th and homicide the 15th most common cause of death in the US.[1] Suicides outnumbered homicides by 2 to 1. Every 16 minutes an American takes his or her own life.

In 2008, suicide was the cause of 1.3% of deaths in the US; in 2006 it was responsible for almost 1% of all deaths in the UK; and in 2005 it accounted for 1.6% of deaths in Australia.[45–47] Overall, suicide rates are highest among young Americans and those over 65 years of age. In 2007, 6.9% of high school students reported making at least one suicide attempt in the previous 12 months. Amongst adults, the suicide rate peaks in males 75 years and older and in women around 50 years of age.[45] Men are four times more likely than women to die from suicide but women are three times more likely to attempt suicide.[45] There is one suicide for every 25 attempted suicides. Attempted suicide employs self-injury as a cry for help. American males most commonly commit suicide with firearms, women prefer poisoning.[45] In Australia, the most frequent methods of suicide in 2005 were by hanging (including strangulation and suffocation; 51%), drug overdose (12%), other poisons (16%) and firearms (7%).[47] Other causes were drowning and jumping from a high place.

Several risk factors for attempting or committing suicide have been identified. Red flags include: previous suicide attempt(s), a history of depression or other mental illness, alcohol or drug abuse, a family history of suicide or violence, physical illness and social isolation. Some 95% of suicides are committed by people with one or more psychological disorders; mood disorders are important predictors.[48] Depression is characterized by a pervasive depressed mood and loss of interest or pleasure for a period of 14 days or more (see Figure 19.2). A sleep disturbance, changes in appetite and weight, psychomotor retardation or agitation, feelings of worthlessness/guilt, impaired thinking, and autonomic nervous system problems are all encountered.[49] Social anxiety, post-traumatic stress and generalized anxiety disorders are each predictive of suicide attempts.[48] Smoking, alcohol and drug use are associated with an increased risk for suicidal ideation, attempted suicide, and completed suicide;[50] however, whether this is a causative association or merely reflects self-destructive behaviour is unknown.

Handout 19.14 considers the risk of suicide from various angles. It lists several factors predisposing to suicide[51] and identifies risk factors for completed suicide. The best predictor of completed suicide is a history of attempted suicide. The relationship between suicide and suicidal ideation is less clear.

DIAGNOSE DEPRESSION IF TWO OF THE FOLLOWING ARE POSITIVE:
- Do you feel depressed?
- Has there been a change in your self-esteem?
- Are you more self-critical than usual?

Additional findings may include:
- feeling helpless/hopeless
- a sense of giving up
- feeling guilty
- being pessimistic about the future

DIAGNOSE PHYSIOLOGICAL DEPRESSION IF:
- The depression is of less than 14 days duration
- There is no significant mood disturbance or social impairment

DIAGNOSE CLINICAL DEPRESSION IF:
- The depression has lasted longer than 14 days
- There is significant mood disturbance or social impairment

Non-melancholic depression is diagnosed:
- in the absence of observable psychomotor disturbance
- the mood is reactive, often improving during the consultation

Psychotic melancholia (endogenous depression) is diagnosed in cases of:
- severe psychomotor disturbance (poverty of movement and ideas, agitation may occur)
- psychotic features (delusions, hallucinations)
- no diurnal mood variation
- constipation

Non-psychotic melancholia is considered in cases with:
- moderate psychomotor disturbance
- diurnal variation in mood
- diurnal variation in energy
- no psychotic features

Figure 19.2 • The clinical recognition of depression.

In perspective

Household and recreational safety can reduce the risk of accidents and injury. **Handout 19.15** provides some tips and access to useful accident prevention websites. Prevention is better than cure.

References

1. CDC. *FastStats – Accidents or Unintentional Injuries.* http://www.cdc.gov/nchs/FASTATS/acc-inj.htm; Accessed 16.01.09.

2. CDC. *Injury in the United States. Chartbook.* http://www.cdc.gov/nchs/data/misc/injury2007.pdf; Accessed 16.01.09.

3. Eaton DK, Kann L, Kinchen S, et al. Centers for Disease Control and Prevention (CDC). Youth risk behavior surveillance—United States, 2007. *MMWR Surveill Summ.* 2008;57(4):1–131.

4. Dowswell T, Towner EM, Simpson SN, Jarvis SN. Preventing childhood unintentional injuries— what works? A literature review. *Inj Prev.* 1996;2(2):140–149.

5. Ozanne-Smith J, Vulcan P. Injury control. In: McNeil JJ, King RWF, Jennings JW, Powles JW, eds. *A Textbook of Preventive Medicine.* Melbourne: Edward Arnold; 1990:213–229.

6. *RoSPA. General Accident Statistics.* www.rospa.com/factsheets/general_accident.pdf; Accessed 16.01.09.

7. Clamp M, Kendrick D. A randomised controlled trial of general practitioner safety advice for families with children under 5 years. *BMJ.* 1998;316(7144):1576–1579.

8. Kendrick D, Coupland C, Mulvaney C, et al. Home safety education and provision of safety equipment for injury prevention. Cochrane Database Syst Rev. 2007;(1):CD005014.

9. Hong J, Min J, Kong KA, et al. Comparison of the risk-taking behaviours of children and the practices adopted by their caregivers for improving home safety. *Public Health.* 2008;122(10):1079–1088.

10. Lowell G, Quinlan K, Gottlieb LJ. Preventing unintentional scald burns: moving beyond tap water. *Pediatrics.* 2008;122(4):799–804.

11. Warda L, Tenenbein M, Moffatt ME. House fire injury prevention update. Part I. A review of risk factors for fatal and non-fatal house fire injury. *Inj Prev.* 1999;5 (2):145–150.

12. Diekman ST, Ballesteros MF, Berger RS, Caraballo RS, Kegler SR. Ecological level analysis of the relationship between smoking and residential-fire mortality. *Inj Prev.* 2008;14(4):228–231.

13. Ahrens M. Smoking and fire. *Am J Public Health.* 2004;94 (7):1076–1077.

14. Leistikow BN, Martin DC, Milano CE. Fire injuries, disasters, and costs from cigarettes and cigarette lights: a global overview. *Prev Med.* 2000;31(2 Pt 1):91–99.

15. Sawalha AF. Storage and utilization patterns of cleaning products in the home: toxicity implications. *Accid Anal Prev.* 2007;39(6):1186–1191.

16. Smolinske SC, Kaufman MM. Consumer perception of household hazardous materials. *Clin Toxicol (Phila).* 2007;45(5):522–525.

17. Presgrave Rde F, Camacho LA, Villas Boas MH. A profile of unintentional poisoning caused by household cleaning products, disinfectants and pesticides. *Cad Saude Publica.* 2008;24 (12):2901–2908.

18. Yang VL, Batlle D. Acute renal failure from adulteration of milk with melamine. *ScientificWorldJournal.* 2008;8:974–975.

19. Todd EC, Greig JD, Bartleson CA, Michaels BS. Outbreaks where food workers have been implicated in the spread of foodborne disease. Part 3. Factors contributing to outbreaks and description of outbreak categories. *J Food Prot.* 2007;70 (9):2199–2217.

20. Todd EC, Greig JD, Bartleson CA, Michaels BS. Outbreaks where food workers have been implicated in the spread of foodborne disease. Part 4. Infective doses and pathogen carriage. *J Food Prot.* 2008;71 (11):2339–2373.

21. Giesbrecht GG, Pretorius T. Survey of public knowledge and responses to educational slogans regarding cold-water immersion. *Wilderness Environ Med.* 2008;19(4):261–266.

22. Ducharme MB, Lounsbury DS. Self-rescue swimming in cold water: the latest advice. *Appl Physiol Nutr Metab.* 2007;32(4):799–807.

23. Gregorakos L, Markou N, Psalida V, et al. Near-drowning: clinical course of lung injury in adults. *Lung.* 2009;187(2):93–97.

24. CDC. *Water-Related Injuries. Fact Sheet.* http://www.cdc.gov/ncipc/factsheets/drown.htm; Accessed 19.01.09.

25. Hwang MY, Glass RM, Molter J. Practicing water safety. *JAMA.* 1999;281:2260.

26. Abdel-Aty MA, Chen CL, Schott JR. An assessment of the effect of driver age on traffic accident involvement using log-linear models. *Accid Anal Prev.* 1998;30(6):851–861.

27. Pack AI, Pack AM, Rodgman E, Cucchiara DF, Dinges DF, Schwab CW. Characteristics of crashes attributed to the driver having fallen asleep. *Accid Anal Prev.* 1995;27(6):769–775.

28. Baulk SD, Biggs SN, Reid KJ, van den Heuvel CJ, Dawson D. Chasing the silver bullet: measuring driver fatigue using simple and complex tasks. *Accid Anal Prev.* 2008;40 (1):396–402.

29. Ting PH, Hwang JR, Doong JL, Jeng MC. Driver fatigue and highway driving: a simulator study. *Physiol Behav.* 2008;94(3):448–453.

30. Mayrose J, Priya A. The safest seat: effect of seating position on occupant mortality. *J Safety Res.* 2008;39(4):433–436.

31. Forman J, Michaelson J, Kent R, Kuppa O, Bostrom O. Occupant restraint in the rear seat: ATD responses to standard and pre-tensioning, force-limiting belt restraints. *Annu Proc Assoc Adv Automot Med.* 2008;52:141–154.

32. Shults RA, Elder RW, Sleet DA, Thompson JL, Nichols JL. Primary enforcement seat belt laws are effective even in the face of rising belt use rates. *Accid Anal Prev.* 2004;36(3):491–493.

33. CDC. *Child passenger safety.* http://www.cdc.gov/ncipc/factsheets/childpas.htm; Accessed 20.01.09.

34. Shafi S, Parks J, Gentilello L. Cost benefits of reduction in motor vehicle injuries with a nationwide speed limit of 65 miles per hour (mph). *J Trauma.* 2008;65 (5):1122–1125.

35. Vyrostek SB, Annest JL, Ryan GW. Surveillance for fatal and nonfatal injuries—United States, 2001. *MMWR Surveill Summ.* 2004;53 (7):1–57.

36. Mack KA, Gilchrist J, Ballesteros MF. Injuries among infants treated in emergency departments in the United States, 2001–2004. *Pediatrics.* 2008;121 (5):930–937.

37. CDC. *Preventing falls among older adults.* http://www.cdc.gov/ncipc/duip/preventadultfalls.htm; Accessed 20.01.09.

38. Carter SE, Campbell EM, Sanson-Fisher S, Redman S, Gillespie WJ. Environmental hazards in the homes of older people. *Age Ageing.* 1997;26(3):195–202.

39. Kendrick D, Watson MC, Mulvaney CA, et al. Preventing childhood falls at home: meta-analysis and meta-regression. *Am J Prev Med.* 2008;35 (4):370–379.

40. Boele van Hensbroek P, van Dijk N, van Breda GF, et al. Combined Amsterdam and Rotterdam Evaluation of FALLs (CAREFALL) study group. The CAREFALL Triage instrument identifying risk factors for recurrent falls in elderly patients. *Am J Emerg Med.* 2009;27 (1):23–36.

41. Benjuya N, Melzer I, Kaplanski J. Aging-induced shifts from a reliance on sensory input to muscle cocontraction during balanced standing. *J Gerontol A Biol Sci Med Sci.* 2004;59(2):166–171.

42. Ganz DA, Bao Y, Shekelle PG, Rubenstein LZ. Will my patient fall? *JAMA.* 2007;297(1):77–86.

43. Kool B, Ameratunga S, Robinson E, Crengle R, Jackson R. The contribution of alcohol to falls at home among working-aged adults. *Alcohol.* 2008;42(5):383–388.

44. Ullom-Minnich P. Prevention of osteoporosis and fractures. *Am Fam Physician.* 1999;60:194–202.

45. CDC. *Suicide.* http://www.cdc.gov/ncipc/dvp/Suicide/default.htm; Accessed 20.01.09.

46. *Office for National Statistics. Suicides in the UK – National Statistics Online.* http://www.statistics.gov.uk/cci/nugget.asp?id=1092; Accessed 20.01.09.

47. *Australian Bureau of Statistics. Suicides, Australia.* http://www.abs.gov.au/AUSSTATS/abs@.nsf/mf/3309.0/; Accessed 20.01.09.

48. Cougle JR, Keough ME, Riccardi N, Sachs-Ericsson N. Anxiety disorders and suicidality in the National Comorbidity Survey-Replication. *J Psychiatr Res.* 2009;43(9):825–829.

49. Ballenger JC, Davidson JR, Lecrubier DJ, Nutt DJ. A proposed algorithm for improved recognition and treatment of the depression/anxiety spectrum in primary care. *Prim Care Companion J Clin Psychiatry.* 2001;3(2):44–52.

50. Wilcox HC. Epidemiological evidence on the link between drug use and suicidal behaviors among adolescents. *Can Child Adolesc Psychiatr Rev.* 2004;13(2):27–30.

51. Hall RC, Platt DE, Hall RC. Suicide risk assessment: a review of risk factors for suicide in 100 patients who made severe suicide attempts. Evaluation of suicide risk in a time of managed care. *Psychosomatics.* 1999;40(1):18–27.

Environmental risk exposure

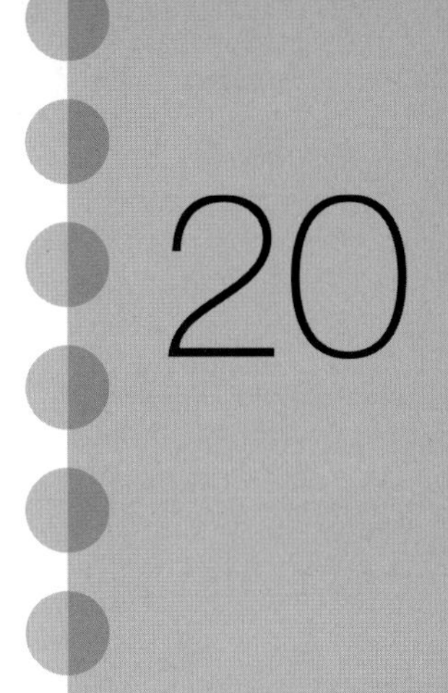

20

Governments attempt to reduce their citizens' exposure to environmental hazards through both legislation and education. This chapter examines some of the environmental hazards that governments try to minimize. While legislation can provide a safety net, it only provides a minimum standard of protection. Individual choices determine whether minimum or maximum health benefits are enjoyed. This chapter considers some government initiatives and demonstrates how the efficacy of these measures is influenced by individual choices.

Reducing the risk of environmental hearing loss

Although most hearing loss is attributable to ageing, noise-related hearing loss is preventable. Noise is unwanted sound. Sound level is expressed in decibels (dBA). Noise may be continuous, intermittent, or impact as in a gun shot. The more intense the noise, the shorter the safe exposure period; it is permissible to be exposed to 90 dBA for 8 hours, to 95 dBA for 4 hours, to 100 dBA for 2 hours and to 110 dBA for 30 minutes.[1] Permissible exposure time to impact noise at 140 dBA is less than 0.1 second. The decibel scale is a logarithmic one and most noise standards recognize a three-decibel 'exchange rate'. The exchange rate is the decibel level that equals a doubling of energy, i.e. a 3-dBA increase doubles the sound pressure while a 3-dBA decrease halves it. The National Institute for Occupational Health and Safety has selected a 3-dBA exchange rate for continuous time exposure, assuming no more than an 8-hour work shift.[2] In contrast, the Occupational Safety and Health Administration rule of a 5-dBA exchange rate is less protective and assumes interruptions in work exposure.[1] Occupational monitoring is required where noise levels may exceed 85 dBA.[1]

Any individual who is exposed to noise which averages 85 dBA or greater over an 8-hour period is at risk of hearing impairment. This level of noise is similar to being in heavy traffic and needing to raise one's voice to be heard by somebody 1 metre away. In environments with noise in excess of 85 dBA, there is a gradual loss of hearing starting at about 21,111 Hertz (Hz). Major noise-induced hearing loss occurs in the 3111–6111 Hz range. Loss in this high-frequency range is similar to turning down the treble on a sound system. Hearing loss attributable to noise exposure usually shows greater loss in the 4111 Hz than in the 8111 Hz frequency. Once hearing loss enters the speech range (3111 Hz), communication becomes difficult with words sounding similar. Speaking louder does not help. Most difficulty is experienced talking on the telephone and in social settings.

Occupational noise exposure, which probably accounts for less than 10% of the burden of adult hearing loss in the US, is largely attributable to unprotected exposures above 95 dBA.[3] Impairment becomes clinically significant in middle age, when occupational noise exposure has ceased but age-related threshold shifts are imposed upon prior noise-induced shifts. Occupational noise may be reduced through the use of engineering controls, work practices, and personal protective equipment. Noise can be decreased at the source by enclosing noisy machinery, installing mufflers on mechanical tools, fitting sound-absorbing materials, and increasing the distance between the work area and the noise source. Workers can be rotated, limiting periods in noisy work areas. Use of personal protective equipment such as earmuffs or earplugs can be required. A study of occupational noise exposure expressed concern about the adequacy of prevention, regulation, and enforcement strategies in the US insofar as most companies studied gave limited or no attention to noise controls, relying on hearing protection – which 38% of employees failed to use.[4]

It is not only persons exposed to occupational noise that fail to appreciate the potential for noise exposure to cause irreversible hearing loss, those who listen to loud music are also at risk. A survey of persons using portable music players, including MP3 players, found they mistakenly felt that noise-induced hearing loss is a medically reversible condition.[5]

Handout 20.1 provides information on how behaviours, based upon informed decisions, can reduce the risk of environmental hearing loss. Legislative safeguards need to be complemented by informed consumers making sensible choices.

Safe air

Governments are concerned about the quality of both indoor and outdoor air.[6,7] The prevalence of community air pollution changes with the season and prevailing wind conditions. The major impact of air pollution is on the respiratory system, where symptoms include a cough, mild dyspnoea, and nasal and throat irritation. Natural pollution occurs as a result of dust, erupting volcanoes, bush fires and lightning discharges. Manmade pollution occurs daily from the burning of fossil fuels. The major types of community pollution are:

- the combustion of fossil fuel. Burning of sulphur-containing fossil fuels results in emission of sulphur dioxide, particulate matter and other chemical reducing agents. Sources include household heating units, coal and oil-fired power plants

- photochemical air pollution. Motor vehicle emissions are rich in nitrogen oxides and hydrocarbons. These chemicals can be activated by sunlight to product ozone, nitrogen compounds and aldehydes. Photochemical smog is rich in highly reactive oxidizing agents

- point source emission. Communities in the vicinity of certain industrial areas may be subject to abnormally high levels of particular pollutants, e.g. hydrogen sulphide from oil refineries.

Primary air pollutants are largely the product of incomplete combustion. Secondary air pollutants, including photochemical smog, SO_2, NO_2, particles and ozone, have been associated with increases in mortality and hospital admissions due to respiratory and cardiovascular disease.[8,9] Environmental Protection Agencies monitor air pollution. Measurable air pollutants include: ozone, hydrocarbons, CO, SO_2, hydrogen sulphides, NO_2, NO and the airborne particle index. Each of these items has a potentially adverse effect on human health. The air pollution index is calculated by measuring each of these pollutants and incorporating the concentration present into a formula. Based upon the result, air is classified as clean or as light, significant, heavy or severe pollution. Important constituents of air pollution include:

- Particles. Particles are visible as dust, smoke or haze. The potential toxicity of airborne particles appears related to the size and composition of the particle as well any gaseous or liquid-phase pollutants that coexist with the particles. Particles with a diameter of 1–11 μm in diameter penetrate and remain in the lower respiratory tract. These particles may exert a direct toxic effect or may passively carry biologically active hydrocarbons or inorganic metals in a thin film of absorbed material. Persons who are particularly susceptible can wear masks in high-risk areas.

- Ozone. Total oxidants are often determined by measuring nitrogen oxides and ozone. Ozone is produced as a result of sunlight acting upon oxides, nitrogen and hydrocarbons. Solar radiation interacting with discharges from motor vehicles and high-voltage electrical equipment are an important source. Ozone, like nitrogen oxides, cause irritation of mucous membranes and aggravate respiratory conditions. Although it is unclear whether a threshold concentration exists for ozone below which no effects on health are likely, effects have been seen at very low levels of exposure.[8] Depending on individual sensitivity and activity level, exposure to ozone in concentrations of 120 parts per million (ppm) over a 7-hour period may impair respiratory function, decrease athletic performance and increase respiratory symptoms.

- Sulphur oxides. Sulphur dioxide and other sulphur oxides irritate bronchial mucosa and damage cilia. Sulphur dioxide provokes bronchoconstriction in asthmatics and may cause coughing in non-asthmatics. Control of oxides of sulphur can, to a certain extent, be achieved by permitting only combustion of coal with a low sulphur content. Acid rain results when sulphur oxides interact with atmospheric moisture. Acid rain erodes statues and historic buildings, and adversely affects fish and plant life. Plants exposed to sulphur dioxide pollution or acid rain take up less selenium. Up to half the selenium content of food is determined by the selenium content of the soil and consequently the selenium content of fodder. Animals and shellfish are major sources of dietary selenium. Metal toxicity may also be linked with acid rain.

- Nitrogen oxides. The principal constituents of photochemical smog are nitrogen oxides, especially nitrogen dioxide. Nitrogen oxides are formed primarily from oxidation of atmospheric nitrogen at high temperatures. The concentration of oxides of nitrogen cannot be controlled by careful selection of the fuel source. As a group, nitrogen oxides have been shown to cause bronchial irritation, ciliary stasis and impairment of the alveolar reticuloendothelial/immune defences. It has been postulated that nitrogen oxides may directly initiate fibrosis and cause alveolar destruction.

- Hydrocarbons. Hydrocarbons are derived from incomplete combustion of fossil fuel and from evaporation of liquids, e.g. household solvents. Certain ring and straight-chain hydrocarbons can be photochemically oxidized to form aldehydes. These, like other oxidants, cause irritation of mucous membranes and the conjunctiva. In addition to accelerating the production of ozone, certain hydrocarbons, e.g. benzene and other polycyclic ring structures, are known to be carcinogenic. Adsorption of polycyclic aromatic hydrocarbons onto the surface of particulate matter may result in the transfer of carcinogenic substances into the lower respiratory tract.

- Carbon monoxide. Carbon monoxide is a product of incomplete hydrocarbon combustion. Carbon monoxide competes successfully with oxygen for combination with haemoglobin. When carboxyhaemoglobin levels increase three- to six-fold, irritability, restlessness, and delayed reaction time result. These blood levels of carboxyhaemoglobin may be reached at busy intersections during peak hours!

While government legislation can control industrial emissions, it cannot prevent air pollution. Monitoring provides an advanced warning system alerting those with respiratory conditions to consider remaining indoors on days of extreme pollution. Indoor pollution, however, can also prove a hazard.

Smoking tobacco or marijuana is an important source of indoor pollution. Secondhand smoke contains more than 50 carcinogens and causes cardio-respiratory disease in non-smoking adults. Eliminating smoking in indoor spaces is the only way to fully protect non-smokers. Substantial progress has been made in the number and restrictiveness of state laws regulating smoking in private-sector worksites, restaurants, and bars.[10] Meeting the nationwide Healthy People 2010 objectives for making these venues smoke-free looks promising! Steps can be taken to reduce one's personal risk. See **Handout 20.2**.

Legislation can seek to provide safe air for the community, however it cannot control for the idiosyncratic genetic predisposition of certain individuals to allergy. Control of airborne allergens requires individual action. Homes cannot be made allergen-free, but exposure to the major indoor allergens can be reduced.[11] Dust mites, pollen, moulds and animal dander are all potential allergens. Risk reduction is based on the principle of reducing or isolating the source. Dust mite allergen largely settles with house dust but can be environmentally controlled. A concentration of 2 µg of dust mite allergen per gram of house dust creates a risk of sensitization and development of bronchial hyperresponsiveness. At concentrations of 11 µg of dust mite allergen per gram of house dust, there is a risk of an asthma attack in susceptible persons. Mites feed on human skin and animal dander. They breed best in damp sealed environments. House dust mite avoidance measures include fitting allergen-proof mattress and pillow encasings, washing bedding regularly, and reducing humidity.[11] Wet and steam cleaning removes soluble mite allergens from carpets more efficiently than dry vacuuming. The benefit of wet/steam cleaning lasts less than a month and only 66% of allergens are removed. Animal allergens float on the air and permeate the whole house. Once the animal has been banished, it takes about 4 months of thorough and repeated cleaning before animal allergen decreases significantly. Washing pets frequently and isolating the pet from a bedroom are usually ineffective alternatives. Cockroach allergen avoidance begins with effective pest control, followed by thorough and repeated cleaning; 1 to 2 months are required to eliminate roaches, and an additional 4 to 6 months are required to remove residual allergen. Once allergen levels have been reduced, continued efforts are necessary to maintain the home free of allergen sources.

As airborne allergens are not the sole source of bronchospasm, a health diary may be helpful in identifying sources of personal risk. A diary will help to identify if an ingested rather than inhaled allergen is involved. Foods – including cow's milk, eggs, nuts, wheat, corn, soy, tomatoes, berries and seafood – drugs, e.g. aspirin, and food additives may all cause asthma.

General measures to control airborne allergens can be helpful. See **Handout 20.3**.

Reducing the risk of food-mediated disease

Despite governments legislating to regulate the sale, labelling and safety of food, foodborne illness remains a problem, even in developed countries. In the USA in 1995, it was estimated that annual outbreaks of between 3.3 million and 12 million cases of foodborne illness caused by seven pathogens cost US $6.5–35 billion.[12] The medical costs and the value of the lives lost during just five foodborne outbreaks in England and Wales in 1996 were estimated at £300–700 million and the cost of the estimated 11,500 daily cases of food poisoning in Australia was calculated at A$2.6 billion annually.[12] Microorganisms and chemicals pose the major risk of foodborne illness. Individuals can take measures to reduce their personal risk (see **Handouts 19.6** and **19.7**). Chemical contaminants in food include natural toxicants such as mycotoxins and marine toxins, environmental contaminants such as mercury, lead, radionuclides and dioxins, and naturally occurring chemicals in plants, such as glycoalkaloids in potatoes. See Tables 19.1 and 19.2.

Problems can also arise from deliberate or inadvertent contamination of food during production, processing, packaging, transportation, and preparation. Food additives, micronutrients, pesticides and veterinary drugs can be used at various stages in the food production chain. Certain additives and contaminants are permitted in food; the permitted concentration of such substances is, however, clearly specified. Food additives are non-nutritive substances intentionally added, usually in small quantities, to foods with the intention of improving appearance, taste and/or texture, prolonging shelf life or facilitating processing. Contaminants are substances that are unintentionally or accidentally included in foods. The maximum amount of a contaminant permitted in food is equal to the minimum amount unavoidably incorporated in food with good agricultural or manufacturing practice, provided this level is considered safe. Governments legislate to minimize the risk of foodborne disease at all levels. In the US, the Center for Food Safety and Applied Nutrition is the branch of the Food and Drug Administration responsible for the safety and accurate labelling of nearly all food products in the US.[13] It also provides the public with ready access to information on how to minimize the risk of foodborne illness.[14] It is illegal to sell adulterated food. Food is considered adulterated if it is offensive, dangerous or injurious to health or if it contains more than the permitted amount of particular substances or any prohibited substance. Variables that determine whether an additive, contaminant or toxin present in food will be hazardous to health include:

* the concentration of the substance in the food
* the amount of the food consumed
* individual susceptibility/sensitivity
* interaction of the substance with other components of the food.

Labelling serves to protect and inform the consumers. Labelling aims to prevent deception of the consumer and provide dietary information. See **Handout 9.2**. The 'safety' aspect of food labelling includes legislative specification regarding the purity and identity of food constituents, the technological need for and safety of food additives, consideration of food contaminants and the use of colourings in oral pharmaceuticals and foods.

Factors that determine whether food is microbiologically suitable for human consumption include the nature of any organisms present, the concentration of the organism in the food substance and the growth environment offered to the organism by the food and mode of storage. Prevalent foodborne disease may result from contamination of:

- salads, raw vegetables with *Entamoeba coli*
- shellfish, raw fruit and vegetables with hepatitis A
- cooked rice, meat, vegetables and starchy puddings with *Bacillus cereus*
- cold meats, rice, dairy and bakery products with *Staphylococcus aureus*.

Variables that determine the growth of organisms include nutrient and water availability, temperature, pH, the atmosphere and presence of preservatives. Foods rich in nutrients provide a good growth medium. The water content of food has a profound effect on microbial growth. The water content of food varies from a high in excess of 71% in fruit and vegetables, through 10–20% in cereals, to 5% or less in processed foods such as cornflakes, dried milk powder, whole egg powder, biscuits and rusks. Foods with a low water content provide a poor environment for bacteria, yeasts and moulds. A means of improving food storage and reducing the risk of microbial growth is reducing the water content of foods.

The water content may be absolutely reduced as in drying or the addition of solutes. Reduction of the water available for microbial growth by drying may be achieved by sun drying, e.g. of fruits such as apricots or raisins, by spray drying of milk, eggs or coffee, or by freeze drying with sublimation of ice in high-pressure vacuums. A number of organisms can survive drying, e.g. *Salmonella* species survive in spray-dried milk powders. Adding salt, a saturated sucrose solution or glycerol reduces water available for microbial growth. Curing of a product in a brine mixture of over 13% usually produces a safe product; when a brine mixture of 10% is used, heating is recommended. Though *Staphylococcus aureus* can grow in a 13% brine mixture, the production of enterotoxin is inhibited and food poisoning prevented. The sugar content of jellies, jams and sweetened condensed milk makes them resistant to growing human pathogens.

Although organisms can survive in a temperature range from -15°C to $+90^{\circ}$C; growth of organisms which spoil or make food unsafe usually occurs within a temperature range of 15°C to 40°C. Food spoilage organisms have an optimal temperature range between 18°C and 30°C; pathogens prefer a temperature of between 35°C and 45°C. *Clostridium botulinum* is an exception and can grow at <5°C. Food spoilage organisms such as *Pseudomonas*

species can also multiply in refrigerated meat, eggs and milk. Cooling and freezing are effective at retarding the multiplication of organisms. Cellar storage achieves temperatures of about 15°C; vegetable compartments in domestic refrigerators are between 5°C and 10°C, with temperatures dropping to 0–5°C near the freezer compartment. Commercial freezers chill to -18°C to -23°C. In practice, -12°C is considered the lower limit for microbial growth. It is important to rapidly chill foods, minimizing the time spent in the 5–60°C danger zone. Food should spend no more than 90 minutes in the 5–65°C temperature range.

Heat can be used to kill organisms; however, it may result in an organoleptically unacceptable alteration to foods. Heat may be moist or dry; it may be used as in cooking, scalding, blanching, pasteurization, drying, evaporating, canning or concentrating. It has been suggested that when cooking results in a temperature of over 64°C, pathogens have been destroyed. There are exceptions to this general rule. The first occurs when not all the cooked food has reached this temperature; the internal temperature of a rare roast may reach only 60°C. Spores survive a cooking temperature of 60°C. The heat resistance of *Clostridium perfringens* spores varies from 1 to 60 minutes at 100°C. Toxins previously produced may also survive heating to this temperature. The enterotoxin of *Staphylococcus aureus* is stable to boiling for 30 minutes. Microwaving requires the presence of water to achieve frictional heat. Spices, i.e. dehydrated substances, cannot be sterilized in a microwave.

Sterilization refers to the removal of all organisms. A more realistic term in food processing is pasteurization. This refers to a thermal process in which most organisms are removed as a result of heat treatment up to 100°C. Pasteurization is used in the preparation of beer, vinegar, cured meats, bakery items, eggs and dairy products. Pasteurization of milk at 61.7°C for 30 minutes prevents foodborne spread of mycobacteria. To prevent milk-borne spread of *Coxiella burnetii* (agent for Q fever), milk is now pasteurized at 62.9°C for 30 minutes. Today, milk may also be pasteurized by heating to 71.5°C for 15 seconds. As certain spoilage organisms survive this process, it is important that pasteurized milk be rapidly cooled and stored below 4°C.

Canning involves heating foods to above 100°C. This achieves destruction of all pathogens, including spores. 'Commercial sterilization' or appertization does increase shelf life but does not remove all organisms – thermophils may survive. Canned foods may demonstrate flat sour spoilage due to certain species of the genus *Bacillus*; gas production, including hydrogen sulphide stinkers, is attributable to certain species of the genus *Clostridium*. The time and temperature required to achieve appertization is influenced by the pH of the food. Organisms are more susceptible to heat in highly acidic foods. Nisin, an antibiotic produced by strains of *Streptococcus lactis*, may also be added to canned foods as this increases the organisms' susceptibility to heat.

Most bacteria grow best at a pH of around 7. Yeast grows well at pH 4.5 and moulds have an optimal pH around 3.0. The metabolism of organisms can further alter the pH of food, thereby inhibiting further multiplication while changing the nature of the food, e.g. fermented dairy products. Propionibacteria in Swiss cheese inhibit mould growth by production of propionic acid, thereby altering the pH and flavour of the cheese. Pathogenic and spoilage organisms may be aerobic, micro-aerophilic, anaerobic or facultative. Moulds are only aerobic, while yeasts are aerobic or facultative anaerobes. Storing food in controlled atmospheres may modify microbe growth. Carbon dioxide has proved particularly useful in this regard. The shelf life of meat stored in an atmosphere of 20% carbon dioxide at $0°C$ is prolonged, as is the shelf life of apples stored in an atmosphere of 8% CO_2 and 3% O_2. Ozone treatment has also been effective in inhibiting mould growth on meat, fruits and cheese.

Natural inhibitors and/or preservatives may be added to food to increase microbial resistance. Natural inhibitors in food include lysozyme in egg white and fresh raw milk; phenolic compounds such as allicin in garlic and onions; eugenol in cinnamon and cloves; and oleuropein in olives. Preservatives added to foods include benzoic acid used in carbonated beverages and juices, sorbic acid used in fresh fruit salad and some cheeses, and propionic acid used in bread and pastry. In general, these acids are more potent inhibitors of yeasts and moulds than bacteria. Sulphur dioxide is used as a preservative; the bisulphite ion form is effective against enzymatic browning. The use of preservatives may affect nutrients in food. The addition of sulphur dioxide with subsequent generation of the bisulphite ion results in loss of thiamine. The use of preservative may also constitute a health hazard for particular individuals. Preservatives such as sodium benzoate, sulphur dioxide and tartrazine, and food additives such as monosodium glutamate and sulphites (SO_2) in white wine, dried fruit or cordials may cause asthma. To minimize such risks, legislation in the US and European Union mandates use of labelling of ingredients derived from commonly allergenic sources, even when present in small amounts.[15]

The aim of labelling is not limited to alerting consumers to potential adverse reactions to additives; it also aims to provide consumers with information about the nutrient content of foods. See **Handout 9.2**. Ingredient labelling requires a listing of constituents in order of concentration, except for water, which may be listed last. Any nutritional claims are rigorously controlled. As scientific evidence accumulates, governments review and modify current food labelling legislation. With the scientific evidence associating *trans* fatty acids with an increased risk of heart disease, the US Food and Drug Administration ruled that the amount of *trans* fatty acid present in foods, including dietary supplements, be included on the nutrition label by January 1, 2006.[16] It was estimated that the addition of *trans* fatty acid to the nutrition label could annually prevent 600–1200 cases of coronary heart disease, 240–480 deaths and save $900 million to $1.8 billion annually in medical costs, lost productivity, and pain and suffering.[16]

Legislation to provide populations with a safe food is a health priority. Education can enable consumers to make safe food choices. See **Handout 20.4**. Unfortunately, legislation cannot protect consumers against the major health hazard posed by food. The greatest health risk associated with food is attributed to unhealthy dietary habits. Education can make individuals aware of healthy food alternatives, but ultimately choice remains an individual prerogative.

Safe water

In 2005, 89.5 million Americans got their tap water from a community or municipal water system that used ground water, while some 45 million regularly depended on private ground water wells.[17] The Environmental Protection Agency was given the authority to set safe water standards by the Safe Drinking Water Act.[18] The primary standard is legally enforceable and applies to public water systems. Primary standards protect drinking water quality by limiting the levels of specific contaminants that can adversely affect public health which are known, or anticipated, to occur in water. They specify Maximum Contaminant Levels for both microbes and chemicals, e.g. arsenic, radon and radionuclides. Laws that regulate the levels of contaminants allowed in drinking water supplied by public water systems do not apply to privately owned wells. Private well owners are responsible for ensuring their well water is safe from contaminants causing health concerns. Wells should be checked and tested annually for mechanical problems, cleanliness, and the presence of contaminants, including coliform bacteria, nitrates/nitrites, and any impurities of local concern.[17] In addition to primary standards, the Environmental Protection Agency has a list of secondary standards, which are non-enforceable guidelines regarding contaminants that may cause cosmetic effects (such as skin or tooth discoloration) or aesthetic effects (such as taste, odour or colour) in drinking water.[18]

Reclaimed water is increasingly being recognized as a sustainable water resource. It is derived from treated municipal wastewater. The treatment processes used for production of reclaimed water involve multiple barriers (biological treatment, physical removal, and chemical disinfection) to control pathogens. Reclaimed water, currently used for non-potable applications such as irrigation, cooling water, industrial process water, and environmental enhancement, is increasingly being considered as a drinking water source in drought-affected areas. A major goal of both wastewater reclamation facilities and ground water suppliers is to reduce pathogen loads in order to decrease public health risks. The presence of certain microbes in water is deemed unacceptable. During treatment, water may be passed through the stages of straining, sedimentation and filtration. Depending on the aperture, straining may remove particles as small as algae. Sedimentation may be assisted mechanically by vertical flow hopper tanks, chemically by coagulation with lime or by altering the pH using an electrical charge or chemicals such as alum, iron salts, or silica. Rapid or slow filtration through sand or through diatomaceous earth may further remove fine suspended matter and improve water quality by oxidizing organic matter. Filtration can remove 95–99.9% of bacteria. Microbial safety of water may be achieved by disinfection.

Chlorine is the most common disinfectant used. Chlorine added to water combines with organic material. It combines with ammonia released from the breakdown of nitrogenous organic matter in polluted water to form chloramines. Chloramines are far weaker bactericidal agents than free chlorine.

Once chloramines have formed, addition of further chlorine destroys the chloramines and at breakpoint chlorination, no bactericidal chlorine (free or combined) is detectable in the water. Any additional chlorine beyond breakpoint is free residual chlorine with full bactericidal potency. Modern chlorination either adds a little chlorine beyond breakpoint or employs superchlorination after which residual chloride is removed. Dechlorination following superchlorination removes the chlorine taste. A more expensive alternative to chloride is ozone. Ozone is a powerful bactericide, leaves no residue and gives water a sparkling 'medicated' appearance.

Water treatment may extend to softening and fluoridation. Addition of fluoride to drinking water is somewhat controversial; however, a recent review of the scientific literature concluded fluoridation of drinking water remains the most effective and socially equitable means of achieving community-wide exposure to the caries prevention effects of fluoride. It was recommended that water be fluoridated in the target range of 0.6–1.1 mg/L, depending on the climate, to balance reduction of dental caries and occurrence of dental fluorosis.[19] At 1 ppm, fluoride hardens bone and tooth enamel, increasing resistance to caries; at 3 ppm, early mottling and orange discoloration of enamel occurs; at 10 ppm, severe tooth mottling, chalky soft patches in enamel and bone mottling are noted.

In instances when individuals find themselves in situations when water is not safe to drink, certain steps can be taken to reduce one's personal risk of waterborne disease. See **Handout 20.5**.

Safe sun exposure

Education, rather than law making, is the major tool for solar risk reduction. Solar ultraviolet radiation (UVR) is a human carcinogen. In the US, approximately 60,000 diagnoses of invasive melanoma and 8000 deaths from melanoma were expected in 2007.[20] Melanoma is now the second most common cancer in 15–34 year-olds in the UK, increasing by 49% in 1991–2000.[21] In Australia, it is estimated that up to 95% of cutaneous melanomas, and 99% of squamous and basal cell carcinomas, are caused by sun exposure.[22]

The degree of sun exposure in a particular area of the earth's surface is determined by various factors.[22] Radiation increases in summer due to the shorter zenith angle, and at higher altitudes. There is a 15% increase in radiation for every 1000 m above sea level. Radiation is reduced by clouds, smoke, dust, haze and ozone. The amount of stratospheric ozone varies with latitude, season and time of day. Ozone tends to absorb radiation. Ozone completely absorbs short wave radiation with wavelengths of less than 290 nm, it only partially absorbs UVA long wave radiation of 320–340 nm. The dose of radiation is inversely proportional to the latitude and is influenced by the time of day. About 60% of the total radiation dose is received between 10:00 to 14:00 hours. Surface reflectivity is also important. Snow has a reflectance of 85% while water's reflectance is 5%. White sand, concrete and shiny materials are surfaces with increased reflectance.

Exposure of skin to both UVA (320–400 nm) and UVB (290–320 nm) stimulates melanin production with increased pigment being produced within 24–48 hours and being dispersed over 5 to 10 days. The epidermis thickens with an increased cell turnover over a similar period. Excess short-term exposure may lead to sunburn. In the event of sunburn, soaking in a bath of cool water, a cool shower or cool compresses over the burnt area may relieve discomfort. Blisters should not be broken. Sunburn increases the risk of melanoma.

Long-term exposure to sunlight hastens skin ageing and increases the risk of squamous and basal cell carcinomas. Exposure of the eye to UVB (290–320 nm) produces ocular disorders such as cataract, acute solar retinopathy, age-related macular degeneration, choroidal melanoma, pterygium, pinguecula, acute photokeratitis, and corneal and/or conjunctival dysplasia. Reduced sun exposure reduces or even prevents these conditions.

Measures to reduce sun exposure and prevent skin changes include:[22]

- avoiding sunlight between 10:00 and 14:30 hours
- wearing clothing sufficiently dense to block out UVR. The density of the weave, not the fabric, determines how effectively clothing will prevent sun exposure of clad skin. Fabrics which are good sunscreens cast a shadow when held up to visible light. Dark clothes absorb more radiation than light clothes
- sporting a legionnaire-style cap or wide-brimmed (10 cm) hat
- staying in shade created by umbrellas, awnings or tree canopies. This may not be helpful if sitting near water, sand, snow or concrete, which reflect more than half the UVR onto the skin

- using sunscreen. Sunscreens that protect maximally against UVB and the more energetic lower wavelengths of UVA should be selected. Broader spectrums give better protection. Para-aminobenzoic acid (PABA) esters and cinnamates absorption range is UVB; benzophenones and salicylates are effective in the UVA absorption range. Persons at risk of skin cancer should select a sunscreen with a solar protection factor (SPF) of at least 15. Although it is generally unnecessary for those with skin type 5 (never-burn olive skin) or type 6 (black skin) to wear sunscreen, those with skins types 3 and 4 should wear SPF 8 to 15 in summer while those with skin type 1 require SPF of 25 to 30. Sunscreens should be applied at least 30 minutes before expected exposure and reapplied every 2–3 hours thereafter. Sunscreen needs to be applied more frequently on hot days when sweating or swimming, i.e. in instances of water exposure. Sunscreen should also be applied on overcast days as 70–80% of UVR penetrates the cloud layer. The amount of sunscreen applied also influences the protection afforded. However, thickly applying sunscreen SPF 8+ every few hours and/or avoiding sun exposure prevents dermal production of vitamin D3. Oral contraceptives, tetracyclines and certain cosmetics enhance ultraviolet exposure.

Sunglasses should be worn to protect the eyes against UVR. Select close-fitting and wrap-around UV-absorbing sunglasses with plastic (CR39) lenses, or glass lenses with a UV-blocking coating. Check that sunglasses are properly labelled by health authorities as meeting the local standard. Preferably use sunglasses labelled 'blocks 100% of UV below 400 nm.'

While avoiding sun exposure reduces the risk of skin cancer, it also increases the likelihood of vitamin D deficiency. Vitamin D deficiency is now recognized as a pandemic. Cholecalciferol is produced in the skin on exposure to UVB radiation (290 to 320 nm). Skin pigment, sunscreen use, ageing, time of day, season and latitude dramatically affect previtamin D3 synthesis.[23] The duration and time of sun exposure can limit damage. In January, across Australia, 2–14 minutes of sun three to four times per week at 12:00 is sufficient to ensure recommended vitamin D production in fair-skinned people with 15% of the body exposed.[22] However, erythema can occur in as little as 8 minutes. By contrast, at 10:00 or 15:00, there is a greater difference between exposure time to produce erythema and that to produce recommended vitamin D levels, thereby reducing the risk of sunburn from overexposure. From October to March, around 10–15 minutes of sun exposure at around 10:00 or 15:00 three to four times per week should be enough for fair-skinned people across Australia to synthesize recommended vitamin D levels. Longer exposure times are needed from April to September, particularly in southern regions of Australia. A circulating level of 25-hydroxyvitamin D of >75 nmol/L, or 30 ng/mL, is required to maximize vitamin D's beneficial effects for health. In the absence of adequate sun exposure, at least 800–1000 IU vitamin D3 daily may be needed to achieve this in children and adults.[24] Food fortification is another source of vitamin D.

Handout 20.6 provides advice on sun exposure.

Immunization status – exposure to infections

Organisms may be transmitted in air, food, water or by sexual contact. To live in an environment persistently exposed to microorganisms without becoming ill requires a competent immune system. Immunization seeks to stimulate an individual's immunity to particular organisms without risking the disease caused by that pathogen. Successful immunization implies that the individual or host acquires active immunity so that future exposure to a realistic biological challenge infection does not result in the clinical manifestations of disease. The use of immunization is restricted to increasing the individual's immunity to those diseases with significant mortality, morbidity, or economic consequences.

Active stimulation of the host's immune system without the risk of disease may be achieved by exposing the person to:

- an extract of the organism responsible for the disease
- the killed organism
- a live, attenuated strain of the organism.

Virulence is a measure of the propensity of an organism to cause disease. The virulence of an attenuated organism is markedly reduced. Contraindications to the use of live vaccines include acute fevers, acute systemic viral infections, immune deficiency, corticosteroid or other immunosuppressant therapy, malignant disease, pregnancy, hypersensitivity to constituents of the vaccine, and passive immunity. If the person receiving the live vaccine has had a transfusion of antibodies, these will inactivate the organism in the vaccine and the individual's own immune system will not be stimulated. Unless the host's immune system is stimulated, no active immunity can be achieved to protect the host on subsequent exposure.

Immunization using live, attenuated organisms provides lifelong immunity. The potential problem inherent in this type of immunization is the risk of clinical infection by the attenuated organism should the host's immune system be depressed by, for example, HIV/AIDS or corticosteroid therapy. Whereas extracts and killed organisms do not carry the risk of vaccine-related infection, immunization with these antigens requires booster doses to ensure lifelong immunity.

The World Health Organization monitors outbreaks of infectious diseases and publishes an immunization schedule for persons of all ages and for travellers.[25] In addition, individual countries publish their own immunization schedule, and Americans, UK residents and Australians are well advised to refer to these as they are continually updated.[26–28] In general, immunization starts at birth with boosters of individual vaccines given at 4 months, 6 months, 12 months, 18 months, 4 years and 15–17 years of age. Immunizations recommended most often include hepatitis B, measles, mumps, rubella, diphtheria, tetanus and acellular pertussis, *Haemophilus influenzae* type b, inactivated poliomyelitis, pneumococcal conjugate, rotavirus, meningococcal C and varicella. Immunization against human papillomavirus is recommended for 12–13-year-olds. Hepatitis A, influenza, pneumococcal polysaccharide and BCG (against tuberculosis) are recommended for high-risk groups. There are as yet no effective immunizations against malaria, tuberculosis or HIV/AIDS.

While the advantages of immunization outweigh the risks in the vast majority of instances, certain vaccines remain problematic. The likelihood of side effects and complications, furthermore, vary with the vaccine used. Concern persists about possible side effects of whooping cough immunization despite refinements in vaccine production.[29]

Contraindications to immunization include:

- significant acute illnesses – immunization of sick children should be delayed
- triple antigen, monovalent pertussis vaccine or any vaccine containing pertussis is contraindicated in children who have had a major reaction following DTP (diphtheria, tetanus, pertussis) or who are known to have active progressive neurological disease
- measles/mumps/rubella and/or oral polio vaccine are contraindicated during pregnancy and in cases with high fever, a malignancy especially of the reticuloendothelial system, or an impaired immune system including that due to corticosteroid or immunosuppressive therapy
- allergy to yeast in the case of hepatitis B vaccine.

While no vaccine is completely safe or effective, the appropriate use of immunization offers a useful and natural means of providing an individual with protection against certain virulent wild organisms. Along with better nutrition, sanitation, and housing, immunization is attributed with the successful reduction of age-specific mortality statistics characteristic of this century. Successful immunization programmes are so highly regarded that certain vaccinations have been made compulsory in much of the US and Australia.[30] Most states in the US and Australia have legislation requiring a child be immunized against measles, mumps, rubella, diphtheria, tetanus, whooping cough and polio before starting school. Conscientious objectors, who sign a form stating that they object to immunization on personal, philosophical, or religious beliefs, may enrol in school but their children are not allowed to attend during an outbreak of a relevant disease. Medical exemptions are also permitted for vaccine contraindications. Immunization is not compulsory in the UK and much of the European Union. **Handout 20.7** identifies some issues that need to be taken into consideration when making personal decisions about immunization.

In perspective

Governments can enact laws to protect individuals but ultimately individual choice determines the effectiveness of any government initiative. Governments attempt to provide clean air, and a safe water and food supply. People choose the food they eat and may decide to add pollutants to the air they inhale. Governments require that cigarette packets carry health warning signs, are substantially taxed and restrict smoking opportunities. Personal choice determines whether the warnings are heeded and smoking zones are avoided. Making healthy choices and avoiding risky ones not only benefits individuals, it also has profound economic repercussions for society.

References

1. AFSCM. Noise. http://www. afscme.org/issues/1324.cfm Accessed 21.01.09.
2. NIOSH. Occupational noise exposure. http://www.cdc.gov/ niosh/docs/9-126/chap3.html#33 Accessed 21.01.09.
3. Dobie RA. The burdens of age-related and occupational noise-induced hearing loss in the United States. *Ear Hear.* 2008;29(4):565–577.
4. Daniell WE, Swan SS, McDaniel MM, Camp JE, Cohen MA, Stebbins JG. Noise exposure and hearing loss prevention programmes after 20 years of regulations in the United States. *Occup Environ Med.* 2006;63(5):343–351.
5. Shah S, Gopal B, Reis J, Novak M. Hear today, gone tomorrow: an assessment of portable entertainment player use and hearing acuity in a community sample. *J Am Board Fam Med.* 2009;22(1):17–23.
6. CDC. Air pollution and respiratory health. http://www.cdc.gov/nceh/ airpollution/; Accessed 21.01.09.
7. UK/EU Legislation air quality control. http://www.ace.mmu.ac. uk/eae/air_quality/Older/ Legislation.html; Accessed 21.01.09.
8. Brunekreef B, Holgate ST. Air pollution and health. *Lancet.* 2002;360(9341):1233–1242.
9. Saez M, Ballester F, Barceló MA, et al. A combined analysis of the short-term effects of photochemical air pollutants on mortality within the EMECAM project. *Environ Health Perspect.* 2002;110 (3):221–228.
10. Centers for Disease Control and Prevention (CDC). State smoking restrictions for private-sector worksites, restaurants, and bars— United States, 2004 and 2007. *MMWR Morb Mortal Wkly Rep.* 2008;57(20):549–552.
11. Eggleston PA. Improving indoor environments: reducing allergen exposures. *J Allergy Clin Immunol.* 2005;116(1):122–126.
12. WHO. Food safety. http://www. who.int/foodsafety/publications/ general/global_strategy/en/ Accessed 21.01.09.
13. Centre For Food Safety And Applied Nutrition. http://www. cfsan.fda.gov/~lrd/cfsan4.html Accessed 21.01.09.
14. FDA. Consumer advice and publications on food safety, nutrition and cosmetics. http:// www.cfsan.fda.gov/~lrd/advice. html#prepare; Accessed 21.01.09.

15. Taylor SL, Hefle SL. Food allergen labeling in the USA and Europe. *Curr Opin Allergy Clin Immunol.* 2006;6(3):186–190.

16. Moss J. Labeling of trans fatty acid content in food, regulations and limits—the FDA view. *Atheroscler Suppl.* 2006;7(2):57–59.

17. CDC. Drinking water. http://www.cdc.gov/Features/GroundWater/; Accessed 21.01.09.

18. U.S. Environmental protection Agency. Safe drinking water. http://www.epa.gov/safewater/; Accessed 21.01.09.

19. Yeung CA. A systematic review of the efficacy and safety of fluoridation. *Evid Based Dent.* 2008;9(2):39–43.

20. Wartman D, Weinstock M. Are we overemphasizing sun avoidance in protection from melanoma? *Cancer Epidemiol Biomarkers Prev.* 2008;17(3):469–470.

21. Hedges T, Scriven A. Sun safety: what are the health messages? *J R Soc Health.* 2008;128(4):164–169.

22. Samanek AJ, Croager EJ, Gies P, et al. Estimates of beneficial and harmful sun exposure times during the year for major Australian population centres. *Med J Aust.* 2006;184(7):338–341.

23. Holick MF. Sunlight, UV-radiation, vitamin D and skin cancer: how much sunlight do we need? *Adv Exp Med Biol.* 2008;624:1–15.

24. Holick MF, Chen TC. Vitamin D deficiency: a worldwide problem with health consequences. *Am J Clin Nutr.* 2008;87(4):1080S–1086S.

25. WHO. WHO recommendations for routine immunization – summary tables. http://www.who.int/immunization/policy/immunization_tables/en/index.html; Accessed 22.01.09.

26. Centers for Disease Control and Prevention (CDC). Recommendations and Guidelines: 2009 Child & Adolescent Immunization Schedules. http://www.cdc.gov/vaccines/recs/schedules/child-schedule.htm#printable; Accessed 22.01.09.

27. NHS. Immunisation Information. http://www.immunisation.nhs.uk/Immunisation_Schedule Accessed 22.01.09.

28. Australian Government, Department of Health and Ageing. Immunise: Australia program. http://www.immunise.health.gov.au/internet/immunise/publishing.nsf/Content/nips; Accessed 22.01.09.

29. Zieliński A, Rosińska M. Comparison of adverse effects following immunization with vaccine containing whole-cell vs. acellular pertussis components. *Przegl Epidemiol.* 2008;62(3):589–596.

30. Salmon DA, Teret SP, MacIntyre CR, Salisbury D, Burgess MA, Halsey NA. Compulsory vaccination and conscientious or philosophical exemptions: past, present, and future. *Lancet.* 2006;367(9508):436–442.

PART 4

Red flags: signalling health hazards ahead

Points to Ponder !

- Wellness is most successfully achieved when particular attention is paid to an individual's vulnerabilities or specific predisposition to disease.
- Red flags are danger signs indicating an urgent need for intervention.

The road to optimal health and longevity is marked by green flags. The road towards disease is signposted by orange and an ever-growing number of red flags. The body puts out distress signals as individuals accumulate orange flags. When an organism is physiologically stressed, it attempts to restore homeostasis. When red flags appear, the organism's equilibrium has moved out of the physiological range of function into the pathological sphere. Active screening for red flags or disease markers offers a penultimate opportunity to intercept the progression of pathology. Biomarkers which act as warning flags of impending disease vary depending on the pathophysiological process involved and nature, intensity and duration of exposure to the stressor(s). See Figure P4.1.

In an effort to re-establish homeostasis, an organism under chronic stress modifies their neuroendocrine, immune/inflammatory and cardiovascular system function. Chronic stress causes biomarkers to fall outside their optimal range of function. Aberrant levels of cortisol, adrenaline, noradrenaline, serum dehydroepiandrosterone sulphate, insulin-like growth factor 1, interleukin-6, C-reactive protein, albumin, systolic blood pressure, diastolic blood pressure, waist–hip ratio, total cholesterol–HDL ratio, HDL cholesterol, and/or glycosylated haemoglobin are all red flags for impending health problems. Raised inflammatory cytokines are present early in postmenopausal osteoporosis; they are also raised in atherosclerosis and arthritis. Non-specific biomarkers, detected early in the pathogenesis of a variety of disorders, are very early warning signs or orange flags. Orange/red flags indicating inflammation are elevated well in advance of overt disease.

High-sensitivity C-reactive protein (hsCRP) is elevated years in advance of first-ever myocardial infarction (MI) or thrombotic stroke and is highly predictive of recurrent MI, recurrent stroke, diabetes, and cardiovascular death.[1] When interpreted within the context of usual risk factors, levels of hsCRP <1, 1–3, and >3 mg/L denote lower, average, and higher relative risk for future vascular events.[1] Knowledge of hsCRP has led to correctly reclassifying a substantial proportion of 'intermediate-risk' individuals into clinically relevant higher- or lower-risk categories.[2] However, while hsCRP may

	HEALTH ———————————————————————————————► DISEASE				
FUNCTIONAL SPECTRUM	Optimal function	Reversible dysfunction		Irreversible dysfunction	
PATHO-PHYSIOLOGICAL CHANGES	Optimal energy/ Function	Chemical changes	Histological changes		Structural modification
ASSESSMENT	Wellness triggers	Health hazard appraisal	Case finding/screen	Disease diagnosis	Screen for complications
CLINICAL CLUES	Healthy lifestyle choices	Lifestyle risks exposures	Subclinical disease markers	Symptoms	Signs
SCREENING TO DETECT	Green flags	Orange flags	Covert red flags http://www.mayoclinic.com/health/health-screening/WO00112	Overt red flags http://www.healthcentral.com/symptom-checker/?ic=506039	

Figure P4.1 • Stages to disease.

participate in atherogenesis and is well recognized as a robust independent risk marker for predicting primary and secondary adverse cardiovascular events,[3] questions remain as to whether reducing inflammatory biomarkers will alter the clinical outcome. Vitamin D deficiency is another orange/red flag of interest. More than one in three healthy adults in the US is vitamin D deficient.[4] Evidence is accumulating to suggest vitamin D deficiency may precipitate or exacerbate osteopenia, osteoporosis, muscle weakness, fractures, common cancers, autoimmune diseases, infectious diseases and cardiovascular diseases. As data are derived from cross-sectional studies, cause–effect links have yet to be adequately established.

Due to prognostic uncertainty, interventions other than lifestyle modification based on the detection of orange flags are somewhat problematic. While high levels of C-reactive protein and interleukin-6, correlate significantly with poor physical performance and muscle strength in older persons,[5] it is unclear whether their detection should initiate active intervention. In contrast, recognition that the capacity of ageing skin to produce vitamin D on sun exposure is impaired, and as adequate vitamin D levels depend on fortified food and sun exposure, health authorities have increased the recommended daily intake of vitamin D to 600 IU for those over 70 years of age.[6] As a general principle, intervention should seek to return risk markers to within a 'normal' range. Ideally, this is achieved initially through healthy lifestyle choices and only where this is not feasible is medication, e.g. vitamin D supplementation, contemplated. As bright red flags emerge later in the progression of the disease, cause–effect links are more clearly established and more radical intervention measures are justified.

Red flags are useful for predicting the probability of developing a particular disease. They may denote functional or structural change. High levels of cross-linked N-telopeptides in the urine is a red flag providing functional evidence of excess bone resorption, while reduced bone mass detected using dual-photon absorptiometry provides structural evidence of osteopenia and a future risk of osteoporosis. Red flags may signify a risk of developing a disease or herald complications. Fasting hyperglycaemia is an early indication of aberrant metabolism and diabetes mellitus; glycosylated haemoglobin is a later sign predicting an increased risk of complications. Hypercholesterolaemia and hypertension are red flags for cardiovascular disease. On a population basis, a reduction of 3 mmHg systolic would reduce stroke mortality by 8%, cardiovascular death by 5% and all-cause mortality by 4%.[7] Identification of bright red flags with a clear cause–effect association with disease requires energetic intervention.

Active screening for and early detection of disease markers alerts carers to the probability that individuals will suffer from a particular condition in future.

The earlier intervention is initiated, the better the prognosis. Although research is needed to evaluate whether reducing hsCRP levels translates into a decreased risk for cardiovascular morbidity, lifestyle interventions have been shown to decrease hsCRP levels in obese individuals with impaired glucose tolerance for up to 1 year.[8] Furthermore, although it remains controversial whether this inflammatory marker is integral to the pathogenesis of cardiovascular disease,[2] it is recognized that half of all heart attacks and strokes in the US occur among those without hyperlipidaemia, and between 15% and 20% occur among individuals who additionally do not smoke or suffer from hypertension or diabetes.[9] As research clarifies cause–effect relationships, orange/red flags may be transformed into bright red flags and more extreme intervention justified. While hsCRP currently enjoys the status of an orange/red flag, it may be upgraded to a bright red flag should future research demonstrate clinical benefit from reducing its levels.

This chapter considers how early detection and modification of six red flags could impact on wellness. Figure P4.2 provides a six-step approach to tackling potential problems. While detection and modification of red flags is health enhancing, wellness is most effectively and safely achieved by making prudent lifestyle choices. A population making healthy dietary and exercise choices minimizes risks associated with engineered wellness interventions. Contrived interventions may have untoward repercussions. Folic acid fortification programmes successfully reduce the risk of neural tube

Step 1: Identify orange flags:
- personal genetic predisposition to the condition
- risky lifestyle choices.

Identify red flags

Step 2: List strategies targeting risk factors amenable to change.

Step 3: Rank possible interventions according to patient acceptability.

Step 4: Implement selected health promotion, disease prevention and therapeutic strategies.

Step 5: Monitor adherence to the selected program and indices of the condition.

Step 6: Modify the program as necessary.

Figure P4.2 • Promoting health in the presence of disease.

defects but may marginally increase the risk of colon cancer. While an adequate intake of folate appears to offer cancer protection, giving individuals who harbour a pre-cancerous or cancerous tumour additional folate may instead facilitate the promotion of cancer.[9] Obtaining additional folic acid, the natural form of the vitamin, from the diet does not appear to carry this risk. High oral doses of folic acid may overwhelm intestinal wall conversion of folic acid to 5-methyltetrahydrofolate, the naturally circulating form of folate. Unlike naturally occurring co-enzymatic folate, circulation of the oxidized, non-substituted folic acid form of this vitamin might be detrimental.[10] Wellness, and consequently disease prevention, is best achieved through initiating a healthy lifestyle in childhood well before orange and red flag risk markers emerge!

References

1. Ridker PM, Silvertown JD. Inflammation, C-reactive protein, and atherothrombosis. *J Periodontol.* 2008;79(8 Suppl):1544–1551.

2. Ridker PM. C-reactive protein and the prediction of cardiovascular events among those at intermediate risk: moving an inflammatory hypothesis toward consensus. *J Am Coll Cardiol.* 2007;49 (21):2129–2138.

3. Devaraj S, Singh U, Jialal I. The evolving role of C-reactive protein in atherothrombosis. *Clin Chem.* 2009;55(2):229–238.

4. Holick MF. High prevalence of vitamin D inadequacy and implications for health. *Mayo Clin Proc.* 2006;81(3):353–373.

5. Cesari M, Penninx BW, Pahor M, et al. Inflammatory markers and physical performance in older persons: the InCHIANTI study. *J Gerontol A Biol Sci Med Sci.* 2004;59(3):242–248.

6. Office of Dietary Supplements, National Institutes of Health. Dietary Supplement Fact Sheet. Vitamin D. http://ods.od.nih.gov/factsheets/vitamind.asp#h2 Accessed 25.01.09.

7. Taubert D, Roesen R, Lehmann C, Jung N, Schömig E. Effects of low habitual cocoa intake on blood pressure and bioactive nitric oxide: a randomized controlled trial. *JAMA.* 2007;298(1):49–60.

8. Andersson J, Boman K, Jansson JH, Nilsson TK, Lindahl B. Effect of intensive lifestyle intervention on C-reactive protein in subjects with impaired glucose tolerance and obesity. Results from a randomized controlled trial with 5-year follow-up. *Biomarkers.* 2008;13(7):671–679.

9. Hirsch S, Sanchez H, Albala C, et al. Colon cancer in Chile before and after the start of the flour fortification program with folic acid. *Eur J Gastroenterol Hepatol.* 2009;21(4):436–439.

10. Mason JB. Folate, cancer risk, and the Greek god, Proteus: a tale of two chameleons. *Nutr Rev.* 2009;67:206–212.

Hypertension: a red flag for strokes

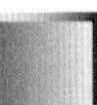

Points to Ponder !

- High blood pressure can cause irreversible damage in people unaware they have the condition.
- Raised blood pressure is an important red flag heralding an increased stroke risk.
- Lifestyle choices can lower raised blood pressure.

- numbness or weakness of the face or limbs, especially when restricted to one side of the body
- confusion, difficulty understanding or speaking
- visual impairment
- trouble walking, dizziness, loss of balance or coordination
- severe headache with no known cause.

Stroke: a disease endpoint for hypertension

Stroke is the third leading cause of death and the leading cause of serious long-term disability in the US and UK.[1,2] In 2005, the direct and indirect cost of stroke in the US was around $57 billion, in the UK the NHS spent an estimated £2.8 billion, and in Australia the cost was A$2.14 billion.[1–3] Every 10 minutes an Australian has a stroke. The risk of having a stroke doubles every decade after the age of 55. Three in four strokes occur in persons 65 years of age and older. A stroke is a focal neurological deficit lasting longer than 24 hours and is caused by a vascular event. Strokes may result from thrombosis in cerebral vessels, emboli to or haemorrhage into the brain. Transient ischaemic attacks (TIA) last less than 24 hours and are often described as mini-strokes. A stroke in evolution is an enlarging neurological deficit, presumably due to infarction, that increases over 24–48 hours. The clinical presentation is influenced by the cause of the stroke. Nonetheless, the five major signs of a stroke are the sudden onset of:

Hypertension: a modifiable red flag/risk marker

Although smoking, asymptomatic carotid stenosis, atrial fibrillation, coronary artery disease, hyperlipidaemia and diabetes all indicate increased risk, the strongest predictor of a stroke is hypertension. High blood pressure ranked third, after obesity and tobacco, as a major health risk faced by Australians in 2006.[4] About 60 million people in the US have hypertension, and in 2006 a survey in England and Wales reported that 31% of men and 28% of women had raised blood pressure.[1,5] On a population basis, a reduction of 3 mmHg systolic would reduce stroke mortality by around 8% and all-cause mortality by 4%. As changes in blood pressure have a substantial impact on the risk for strokes, it is important that individuals appreciate the potential of lifestyle choices to modulate raised blood pressure. See **Handout 21.1**.

The higher the blood pressure, the greater the health risk (see Table 21.1). A healthy blood pressure is today considered to be less than 120/80 mmHg; a high-normal level is 120–139 mmHg

Table 21.1 The risk of stroke relative to blood pressure level

Category	Systolic (mmHg)	Diastolic (mmHg)	Relative risk		
			Stroke	CHD	Renal failure
Optimal	<120	<80	<1	<1	<1
Normal	120–129	80–84	1	1	1
High normal	130–139	85–89			
Hypertension Stage 1	140–159	90–99	3.6	2.3	2.8
Hypertension Stage 2	160–179	100–109	6.9	3.2	5
Hypertension Stage 3	180–209	110–119	9.7	4.6	8.4
Hypertension Stage 4	>209	>119	19.2	6.9	12.4

CHD, coronary heart disease

Table 21.2 Diagnosing hypertension

Outdated system for diagnosing hypertension in adults

Interpretation	Systolic pressure (mmHg)	Diastolic pressure (mmHg)
Borderline hypertension	140–159	90–94
Definite hypertension	>159	>94
Mild hypertension	160–179	95–104
Significant hypertension	Varies with age	Varies with age
Malignant hypertension	Target organ damage	120 or higher

Current diagnostic levels for hypertension

Interpretation	Systolic pressure (mmHg)	Diastolic pressure (mmHg)	Screening frequency
Normotensive	<120	<80	24 months
Prehypertension	120–139	80–89	12 months
Stage 1 hypertension	140–159	90–99	2 months
Stage 2 hypertension	160–179	100–109	<1 month
Stage 3 hypertension	180–209	110–119	1–7 days
Isolated systolic hypertension	140 or higher	<90	1–7 days

systolic and 80–89 mmHg diastolic.[5] The frequency of blood pressure checks varies with the base reading (see Table 21.2). The level at which hypertension is diagnosed and therapy initiated has been lowered because:[6]

- the risk of cardiovascular disease begins at 115/75 mmHg and doubles with each increment of 20/10 mmHg
- mild hypertension is responsible for over 50% of the excess mortality attributable to hypertension

- individuals who are normotensive at age 55 have a 90% lifetime risk for developing hypertension
- individuals with prehypertension benefit from health-promoting lifestyle modifications to prevent cardiovascular disease.

Healthy choices for optimizing blood pressure

Everybody, and particularly those in the high-normal or prehypertension range, should reduce their risk of developing hypertension by:[6]

- Physical activity. Doing 30 minutes of moderate-intensity physical activity on most, if not all, days of the week reduces both systolic and diastolic blood pressure. Systolic pressure may drop by up to 9 mmHg. Sporadic exercise, especially if extremely vigorous in an otherwise sedentary individual, should be avoided in favour of moderate-level activities performed consistently.
- Quitting. One study found that daily cigarette smoking increased the risk of a fatal stroke 3.5-fold.[7] The risk of a stroke is influenced by the number of cigarettes smoked, increasing among heavy smokers. Both active and passive smoking are independent risk factors. In Germany, passive smoking may account for 774 stroke-related deaths and 1837 incident first-ever strokes annually.[8] Women and those over 65 years of age are at greatest risk.
- Maintaining a healthy body weight. A BMI of less than 25, or preferably 22, is desirable. BMI is the anthropological measure that shows the highest correlation with systolic blood pressure. Weight loss of 10 kg can achieve a 5–20 mmHg decrease in systolic blood pressure. Weight gain over a 1–2-month period is associated with a predictable rise in arterial pressure, and weight loss of as little as 4 or 5 kg may normalize blood pressure. During periods of weight loss, reductions of blood pressure are evident within 2–3 weeks. The greatest reduction in blood pressure occurs early in a weight loss programme. Overweight increases the risk of stroke; however, clinical trials to assess the effect of weight reduction on stroke risk are still lacking.
- Avoiding a 'beer' belly. Males should aim for a waist measurement of no more than 94 cm and females should target a waist circumference of less than 80 cm.

- Limiting sodium. Restrict salt to 4 g/day or less. By reducing dietary sodium intake to no more than 100 mmol per day (2.4 g sodium or 6 g sodium chloride) systolic blood pressure can drop by 2–8 mmHg. This in household measures is a little over 1 teaspoon of salt. Taste adapts to sodium restriction within about 2 months. A diet of less than 0.3 g/day of salt is unpalatable. **Handout 21.2** provides tips on how to eat a low-sodium diet. A high-sodium diet increases and a low-sodium diet decreases both systolic and diastolic blood pressure. The results of a dietary feeding study suggested that women, the elderly and persons with hypertension are most sodium sensitive.[9]
- Limiting alcohol. Systolic blood pressure decreases 2–4 mmHg in men who restrict their alcohol intake to two or fewer standard drinks daily or women who limit their intake to one standard drink or less. Drinking with meals appears to provide further protection. Alcohol's pressor effect becomes apparent when 30 g of alcohol or more are regularly consumed. The hypertensive effect of alcohol is probably reversed in 7–28 days. Blood pressure medication is more effective in light than heavy drinkers, and 'binge' drinkers are at increased risk of having a stroke.

Handout 21.1 provides access to lifestyle tips for lowering raised blood pressure.

Predicting a stroke: assessing risk factors

The risk of a stroke multiplies as blood pressure increases. If the risk is taken as 1 in persons with prehypertension, it increases 3.6-fold in those with stage 1 hypertension, 6.9-fold in those with stage 2 hypertension, and 9.7-fold in those with stage 3 hypertension (see Table 21.1). One in five persons with a systolic pressure in excess of 209 mmHg is likely to have a haemorrhagic stroke. While diastolic pressure tends to remain stable or decline after the age of 40, systolic pressure tends to rise until the age of 70 or 80 years! The level of systolic blood pressure bears a direct relationship to the risk of a cerebrovascular event.[10] The frequency of screening for raised blood pressure increases both with increasing blood pressure levels and with age. Screening is recommended at 4-yearly intervals for normotensive persons between 20 and 40 years, every 2 years between 40 and 60 years, and annually thereafter. Age is an important non-modifiable risk that impacts on the predictive value of hypertension. Persons 75 years and older have a 15% risk of a cardiovascular event within 5 years; in the presence of existing cardiovascular disease this escalates to over 20%.[5]

The presence of additional stroke risk factors – an indication for more frequent screening – increases the probability of a cerebrovascular accident. More accurate prediction of outcome is achieved when a number of risk markers are used as indicators. See **Handout 21.3**. Single risk factors are poor predictors of stroke. In men aged 40 to 59, a simple cumulative risk scoring system was able to predict more than 80% of all strokes occurring within 5 years in the top fifth of the score distribution.[11] The risk of stroke escalates as the number of risk factors present increases. The relative risk of a stroke escalates from 1.4-fold to 4.3-fold as a smoker becomes overweight and develops hypertension, hypercholesterolaemia and diabetes.[12] A stroke risk formula was derived using age, systolic blood pressure, current cigarette consumption, and evidence of angina. The formula devised to calculate the risk of stroke is:

$$\text{Stroke risk score} = \text{age} + \text{systolic blood pressure} + \text{angina} + \text{smoking habit}$$

These variables are loaded by multiplying individual risk factors as follows:

$$\text{Stroke risk score} = 9(\text{age in years}) + 2.85(\text{systolic pressure}) + 1(70 \text{ if angina is present}) + 1(90 \text{ if } 1\text{–}20 \text{ cigarettes are smoked each day}) \text{ or } 1(130 \text{ if over } 20 \text{ cigarettes are smoked each day})$$

Persons who score over 1000 need intervention.

Predicting the type of stroke: refining risk assessment

Strokes can also be more accurately predicted when the pathology of strokes is considered. Different types of strokes are the result of diverse risk factors.[12,13]

An increased risk of a haemorrhagic stroke is associated with:

- raised blood pressure. Persons with borderline hypertension are at a 1.5-fold greater risk than normotensive individuals. Blood pressure

reduction reduces this risk. The risk of a stroke is estimated to be almost halved by a 7.5 mmHg reduction in diastolic pressure, and to be reduced by one-third on successful treatment of isolated systolic hypertension. The treatment target for persons with a history of stroke or TIAs is lower than 130/80
- hypocholesterolaemia. In haemorrhagic strokes, serum cholesterol levels of at least 5.5 mmol/L are protective
- anticoagulant therapy. The risk with respect to anticoagulant therapy is dose dependent
- high alcohol intake in the preceding week. Only heavy alcohol consumption is linked to an increased risk of stroke. The risk may be mediated through raised blood pressure levels.

Risk factors for a haemorrhagic stroke correlate better with intracerebral than subarachnoid haemorrhage.

Atheroma, emboli and thrombosis may cause an ischaemic stroke. An increased risk of ischaemic stroke is associated with:

- diabetes mellitus
- transient ischaemic attacks. A TIA increases the 5-year risk of stroke by 33%. At least half occur within the first year after the initial atttack
- hypercholesterolaemia. Cholesterol has diverse effects on different types of stroke. In contrast to ischaemic stroke, the risk of haemorrhagic stroke is increased by hypocholesterolaemia.[14]

In addition to identifying the risk of an initial stroke, the presence of certain risk markers and risky behaviours predict an increased risk of a second or subsequent stroke. Within 48 hours of an index stroke, the risk of stroke recurrence is:[13]

- 2.5 times higher in alcohol abusers
- 1.6 times higher in patients requiring drug therapy for hypertension
- 1.2 times higher in patients with elevated blood glucose.

Stroke prevention

Primary prevention of stroke through controlling risk factors is very effective.[15]

It is widely accepted that strokes can be substantially reduced by an active lifestyle, cessation of smoking and a healthy diet.[16] See **Handout 21.4**. A prospective cohort study over 10 years of apparently healthy women of 45 years of age and older found a healthy lifestyle was associated with a significantly reduced risk of total and ischaemic stroke, but not of haemorrhagic stroke.[17] Healthy behavior was defined as: never smoking; alcohol consumption between 4 and 10.5 drinks per week; exercising four or more times per week; body mass index less than 22; a diet high in cereal fibre, folate, and omega-3 fatty acids, a high polyunsaturated:saturated fat ratio, low in *trans* fat and a low glycaemic load. A second prospective cohort study confirmed a low-risk lifestyle was beneficial in the prevention of stroke, especially ischaemic stroke, in both men and women.[18] While healthy lifestyle choices are recommended regardless of blood pressure readings, more rigorous attention to lifestyle measures is required for those with diagnosed hypertension.

The Dietary Approaches to Stop Hypertension (DASH) eating plan, which is low in sodium and rich in potassium, calcium and vitamin D, lowers systolic pressure by 8–14 mmHg. The DASH diet emphasizes fruits and vegetables (9.6 servings per day at 2100 kcal) and low-fat dairy foods (2.7 servings per day at 2100 kcal). Americans eating this diet increase their intake of whole grains (4.1 servings per day), fish (0.5 servings per day), and nuts and seeds (0.6 servings per day), and decrease their consumption of fats (2.5 servings per day), red meat (0.5 servings per day), and sweets (0.5 servings per day).[19] A high intake of fruit and vegetables has repeatedly been shown to be beneficial.[20] Eating more than five servings of fruit and vegetables each day is considered likely to cause a major reduction in strokes.[21] A plant-rich diet increases the intake of potassium, magnesium and fibre, each of which independently decreases blood pressure. Dietary fibre supplementation of 14 g per day achieves an overall mean reduction of systolic pressure of 1.2 mmHg and diastolic 1.8 mmHg in hypertensive persons.[22] In addition to the benefits offered by following the DASH diet, persons with hypertension may also need to consider dietary supplementation.

Fish oil supplementation may reduce systolic and diastolic blood pressure by 1.5 mmHg and 1.0 mmHg, respectively.[23] It appears that docosahexaenoic acid may more effectively lower blood pressure and heart rate and improve vascular function than eicosapentaenoic acid.[24] Omega-3 fatty acids appear particularly protective against ischaemic strokes. Isoflavones, present in soy products, enhance synthesis of nitric oxide, leading to muscle relaxation, reduced blood pressure and a lower risk of strokes.[25] Calcium intake is also believed to

be inversely associated with risk of stroke. A prospective study suggested that those consuming most calcium have a reduced risk of both total and ischaemic stroke.[26] The source of calcium was dairy products. Milk peptides have been shown to lower blood pressure through inhibition of angiotensin-converting enzyme and may also have opioid-like activities, and mineral-binding and antithrombotic properties.[27] Fortified dairy products are another source of vitamin D. Low vitamin D status has been found to be prevalent in women with hypertension,[28] and low levels of this vitamin are independently predictive for fatal strokes.[29] Given the prevalence of low vitamin D status, particularly among the elderly, vitamin D supplementation deserves consideration to promote health and prevent strokes. Vitamin D is not the only vitamin that may be protective. A review of eight randomized trials with stroke as one of the endpoints concluded that folic acid supplementation could effectively reduce the risk of stroke in primary prevention.[30]

Exercise prescription for hypertensive patients can be refined. Eight weeks of aerobic exercise has been shown to benefit those with stage 1 and stage 2 hypertension.[31] Exercising for 61–90 minutes each week was shown to most effectively reduce systolic blood pressure, while exercising anywhere between 1 and 2 hours weekly had a similar impact on diastolic blood pressure.

While lifestyle measures may suffice for those with prehypertension, once hypertension is diagnosed, lifestyle changes need to be combined with drug intervention. For those with uncomplicated stage 1 hypertension, diuretics are recommended; for those with stage 2 hypertension, a two-drug combination is required.[32] For those with isolated systolic hypertension, the onset of grade 3 hypertension or associated target organ damage, more vigorous intervention is required.

In addition to the brain, target organs at particular risk of raised blood pressure are the heart and kidney. Compared with normotensive individuals, the relative risk of coronary heart disease increases 2.3-fold in stage 1 hypertension, 3.2-fold in stage 2 hypertension, and 4.6-fold in stage 3 hypertension. Compared with normotensive individuals, the relative risk of renal failure increases 2.8-fold in stage 1 hypertension, 5-fold in stage 2 hypertension, and 8.4-fold in stage 3 hypertension (see Table 21.1). Both the level of blood pressure and the presence of microalbuminuria are useful prognostic indicators in patients with hypertension. Microalbuminuria is directly related to the level of systolic blood pressure. It provides evidence that hypertension has caused vascular damage. Vascular damage in hypertensive patients indicates an increased risk of a major new vascular event such as a stroke.

When primary prevention fails, early diagnosis can be lifesaving. Recognizing that an individual who suddenly has difficulty smiling, lifting their arms or talking may be having a stroke, may be lifesaving.

In perspective

Hypertension is a significant modifiable risk factor for stroke. Blood pressure screening should start at an early age – in 2003/04, one in three Americans over the age of 20 years had hypertension.[33] Lifelong monitoring of blood pressure is recommended. Risk increases proportionally with increasing blood pressure and even persons with prehypertension are at increased risk. A systolic blood pressure of 135 mmHg is equivalent in risk to a diastolic pressure of 90 mmHg; after middle age, a systolic of 160 mmHg is more risky than a diastolic of 95 mmHg. Lifestyle intervention suffices for persons with prehypertension, while those with diagnosed hypertension require more vigorous lifestyle changes and drug therapy. The Heart Foundation's *Guide to management of hypertension 2008* provides a good overview.[34] With cerebrovascular disease taking the lives of 46.6 in every 100,000 Americans in 2005,[33] intervention is a priority. Individuals would be well advised to actively pursue a personal stroke prevention and risk assessment programme. See **Handout 21.5**.

Hypertension is not only a major risk marker for strokes; it is also a red flag for coronary artery disease.

References

1. *CDC. Stroke.* http://www.cdc.gov/Stroke/stroke_facts.htm; Accessed 24.01.09.

2. *The Stroke Association.* http://www.stroke.org.uk/media_centre/facts_and_figures/index.html; Accessed 24.01.09.

3. *Stroke Foundation.* http://www.strokefoundation.com.au/facts-figures-and-stats; Accessed 24.01.09.

4. *AIHW. Australia's health 2006.* http://www.AIHW.gov.au/publications/index.CFM/title/10321; Accessed 12.11.07.

5. *Heart Foundation. Guide to Management of Hypertension 2008.* http://www.heartfoundation.org.au/Professional_Information/Clinical_Practice/Hypertension/Pages/default.aspx; Accessed 24.01.09.

6. *National High Blood Pressure Education Program.* Seventh Report of the Joint National Committee on Prevention, Detection, Evaluation, and Treatment of High Blood Pressure JNC 7 Express. US Department Of Health And Human Services; 2003. http://www.nhlbi.nih.gov/guidelines/hypertension/jncintro.htm; Accessed 24.01.09.

7. Haheim LL, Holme I, Hjermann I, Leren P. Smoking habits and risk of fatal stroke: 18 years follow up of the Oslo Study. *J Epidemiol Community Health*. 1996;50 (6):621–624.

8. Heuschmann PU, Heidrich J, Wellmann J, Kraywinkel K, Keil U. Stroke mortality and morbidity attributable to passive smoking in Germany. *Eur J Cardiovasc Prev Rehabil*. 2007;14(6):793–795.

9. He J, Gu D, Chen J, et al. GenSalt Collaborative Research Group. Gender difference in blood pressure responses to dietary sodium intervention in the GenSalt study. *J Hypertens*. 2009;27(1):48–54.

10. Neaton JD, Wentworth D. Serum cholesterol, blood pressure, cigarette smoking, and death from coronary heart disease. Overall findings and differences by age for 316,099 white men. Multiple Risk Factor Intervention Trial Research Group. *Arch Intern Med*. 1992;152:56–64.

11. Coppola WG, Whincup PH, Papacosta O, Walker M, Ebrahim S. Scoring system to identify men at high risk of stroke: a strategy for general practice. *Br J Gen Pract*. 1995;45(393):185–189.

12. Yusuf HR, Giles WH, Croft JB, Anda RF, Casper ML. Impact of multiple risk factor profiles on determining cardiovascular disease risk. *Prev Med*. 1998;27(1):1–9.

13. Sacco RL, Shi T, Zamanillo M, Kargman DE. Predictors of mortality and recurrence after hospitalized cerebral infarction in an urban community: the North Manhattan Stroke Study. *Neurology*. 1994;44:626–634.

14. Palmer A, Bulpitt C, Beevers G, et al. Risk factors for ischaemic heart disease and stroke mortality in young and old hypertensive patients. *J Hum Hypertens*. 1995;9:695–697.

15. Rubenstein LZ. Update on preventive medicine for older people. *Generations*. 1996;20 (4):47–53.

16. Galimanis A, Mono ML, Arnold M, Nedeltchev K, Mattle HP. Lifestyle and stroke risk: a review. *Curr Opin Neurol*. 2009;22(1):60–68.

17. Kurth T, Moore SC, Gaziano JM, et al. Healthy lifestyle and the risk of stroke in women. *Arch Intern Med*. 2006;166(13):1403–1409.

18. Chiuve SE, Rexrode KM, Spiegelman D, Logroscino G, Manson JE, Rimm EB. Primary prevention of stroke by healthy lifestyle. *Circulation*. 2008;118 (9):947–954.

19. Karanja N, Lancaster KJ, Vollmer WM, et al. Acceptability of

sodium-reduced research diets, including the Dietary Approaches to Stop Hypertension diet, among adults with prehypertension and stage 1 hypertension. *J Am Diet Assoc.* 2007;107:1530–1538.

20. Utsugi MT, Ohkubo T, Kikuya M, et al. Fruit and vegetable consumption and the risk of hypertension determined by self measurement of blood pressure at home: the Ohasama study. *Hypertens Res.* 2008;31 (7):1435–1443.

21. He FJ, Nowson CA, MacGregor GA. Fruit and vegetable consumption and stroke: meta-analysis of cohort studies. *Lancet.* 2006;367(9507):320–326.

22. He J, Whelton PK, Klag MJ. Dietary fibre supplementation and blood pressure reduction: a meta-analysis of controlled clinical trials. *Am J Hypertens.* 1996;9:74A (abstract).

23. Appel LJ, Miller ER, Seidler AJ, et al. Does supplementation of diet with 'fish oil' reduce blood pressure? A meta-analysis of controlled clinical trials. *Arch Intern Med.* 1993;153:1429–1438.

24. Mori TA. Omega-3 fatty acids and hypertension in humans. *Clin Exp Pharmacol Physiol.* 2006;33 (9):842–846.

25. Si H, Liu D. Genistein, a soy phytoestrogen, upregulates the expression of human endothelial nitric oxide synthase and lowers blood pressure in spontaneously hypertensive rats. *J Nutr.* 2008;138 (2):297–304.

26. Umesawa M, Iso H, Ishihara J, et al. Dietary calcium intake and risks of stroke, its subtypes, and coronary heart disease in Japanese: the JPHC Study Cohort I. *Stroke.* 2008;39 (9):2449–2456.

27. Jauhiainen T, Korpela R. Milk peptides and blood pressure. *J Nutr.* 2007;137(3 suppl 2):825S–829S.

28. Hintzpeter B, Mensink GB, Thierfelder W, et al. Vitamin D status and health correlates among German adults. *Eur J Clin Nutr.* 2008;62(9):1079–1089.

29. Pilz S, Dobnig H, Fischer JE, et al. Low vitamin D levels predict stroke in patients referred to coronary angiography. *Stroke.* 2008;39 (9):2611–2613.

30. Wang X, Qin X, Demirtas H, et al. Efficacy of folic acid supplementation in stroke prevention: a meta-analysis. *Lancet.* 2007;369(9576):1876–1882.

31. Ishikawa-Takata K, Ohta T, Tanaka H. How much exercise is required to reduce blood pressure in essential hypertensives: a dose-response study. *Am J Hypertens.* 2003;16(8):629–633.

32. Goldstein LB, Adams R, Alberts MJ, et al. Primary prevention of ischemic stroke: a guideline from the American Heart Association/American Stroke Association Stroke Council. *Stroke.* 2006;37(6):1583–1633.

33. *National Centre for Health Statistics. Health, United States, 2007 With Chartbook on Trends in the Health of Americans.* Hyattsville, MD; 2007. *http://www. cdc.gov/nchs/data/hus/hus07.pdf; Accessed 26.01.09.*

34. *Heart Foundation. Guide to management of hypertension 2008.* http://www.heartfoundation.org. au/Professional_Information/ Clinical_Practice/Hypertension; Accessed 02.02.09.

Hyperlipidaemia: a red flag for heart attacks

22

The World Health Organization (WHO) estimates that 8% of the total disease burden in the developed world is due to raised blood cholesterol levels.[1] High cholesterol is estimated to be responsible for 56% of ischaemic heart disease globally.[1] Although persons with a normal cholesterol level can have coronary heart disease, hypercholesterolaemia is an important red flag signalling an increased risk for a heart attack. Familial hypercholesterolaemia is an inherited condition in which cholesterol levels are high at birth. About 85% of men with familial hypercholesterolaemia have a heart attack by age 60.[2] Persons with normal cholesterol levels at birth, through risky lifestyle choices, can raise their blood cholesterol levels and risk a heart attack. Compared to those with normal lipid levels, the risk of a heart attack increases threefold in persons with hyperlipidaemia.

Overall, 10% of Americans between the ages of 20 and 64 years had undiagnosed high cholesterol levels in 1999–2004. In 2002/04, 17% of Americans had hypercholesterolaemia and 26% of women in the 65–74 age group had levels in excess of 6.15 mmol/L. In 2006, 57% of men and 61% of women in Britain had cholesterol levels of 5.0 mmol/L or more.[3] The mean total cholesterol level was 5.3 mmol/L for British men and 5.4 mmol/L for women.[3] In 1999–2000, around half of all Australians 25 years of age and over had blood cholesterol levels exceeding 5.5 mmol/L.[4] Over 60% of heart attacks and possibly 40% of ischaemic strokes in developed countries are attributable to total cholesterol levels in excess of 3.8 mmol/L.[1]

Although the proportion of Americans with high cholesterol levels is dropping, primarily due to drug therapy, 144.4 in every 100,000 Americans died from a heart attack in 2005.[5] Coronary heart disease (CHD) is the most common cause of death in the UK: despite declining death rates, the 2008 statistics report that one in five men and one in seven women in the UK die from CHD.[3] Furthermore, 19% of premature deaths in men and 10% in women are due to heart attacks.[3] Similarly, in Australia, despite CHD death rates falling by 45% in males and 44% in females between 1996 and 2006, in 2006, heart attacks – at 17% – were the most common cause of death.[6] Older people are more susceptible to CHD: 7.5% of Australians aged 55–64 years have CHD, increasing to 20.3% for those aged 75 years or older.[6] Men are more commonly affected than women; the male to female ratio in the US is 1.68:1.[5] Given the prevalence of heart attacks, periodic screening for the major risk factors listed in **Handout 22.1** is advisable.

Determining risk

The three major lifestyle modifiable risk factors routinely assessed are smoking, hypertension and blood cholesterol levels. **Handout 22.2** lists some

Table 22.1 Cholesterol levels: determining risk

Level of risk	Total cholesterol		LDL cholesterol	
	mmol/L	mg/dL	mmol/L	mg/dL
Optimal	<5.13	<200	<2.56	<100
Near-above optimal			2.56–3.3	100–129
Borderline high	5.13–6.13	200–239	3.3–4.0	130–159
High	>6.13	>239	4.0–4.8	160–189
Very high			>4.8	>189

of the many other risk factors shown to influence the risk of a heart attack. Although total blood cholesterol level is routinely measured (see Table 22.1), it is an inferior risk indicator as it reflects the sum of low-density lipoprotein (LDL) and high-density lipoprotein (HDL) cholesterol. High levels of LDL cholesterol and/or low levels of HDL cholesterol increase the risk of coronary heart disease; conversely, low LDL and high HDL levels are protective. The NIH's Adult Treatment Panel recommendation is thus that in all adults aged 20 years or older, a fasting lipoprotein profile, including total, LDL and HDL cholesterol and triglyceride, should be obtained every 5 years.[7] If a non-fasting test is performed and total cholesterol is over 5.13 mmol/L (200 mg/dL) or HDL cholesterol is under 1 mmol/L (40 mg/dL), a follow-up lipoprotein profile to assess appropriate management based on the LDL cholesterol level is needed. A fasting blood sample is required for accurate triglyceride assessment. Triglycerides, at levels in excess of 200 mg/dL (2.3 mmol/L), become a risk factor in patients with a reduced HDL cholesterol. Hypertriglyceridaemia impairs flow-induced arterial vasodilation and increases blood viscosity. Triglycerides are an independent risk factor for coronary artery disease.

The relationship between LDL cholesterol levels and cardiac risk is continuous over a broad range of LDL levels from low to high. This association, although continuous, is not linear but J-shaped, with risk rising more steeply as LDL concentration increases. This curvilinear, or log-linear, relationship means that at any level of LDL, for a given millimole per litre change in the LDL level, the change in relative risk is the same as at any other LDL level. In practice, regardless of the initial LDL level, persons with an equivalent risk of a heart attack (due to the presence of other risk factors) benefit equally from each mmol/L cholesterol is lowered. On the other hand, comparing persons with equal absolute risk, those with higher LDL levels benefit more than those with low levels when LDL is reduced. While the LDL level below which further reduction fails to provide benefit has yet to be clarified, various serum cholesterol levels have been deemed desirable and excessive. See Table 22.1. In addition to total and LDL cholesterol, HDL levels are important. Epidemiological studies have shown levels of HDL under 1.0 mmol/L (40 mg/dL) to be an independent determinant of increased cardiovascular risk.[7,8] High levels of HDL are considered to be 1.54 mmol/L (60 mg/dL) and over.[7] Studies suggest that for every 0.03 mmol/L (1.0 mg/dL) increase in HDL, cardiovascular risk is reduced by 2–3%.[8]

Setting therapeutic targets for LDL

Improving an unfavourable cholesterol profile is a central strategy in the prevention of coronary heart disease. Lifestyle choices can alter cholesterol levels as well as the ratio of HDL to LDL. Although low HDL levels are identified as a cardiovascular risk factor, it is LDL that has been designated a therapeutic target.[7] Lowering LDL reduces total mortality, coronary mortality, major coronary events, coronary artery procedures, and stroke in persons with established ischaemic heart disease. The therapeutic targets established for LDL levels vary depending on the presence of associated coronary heart disease risks. Table 22.2 identifies targets applicable to those at greatest risk and Table 22.3

Table 22.2 The radical perspective

Lipid moiety	Desirable mg/dL (mmol/L)	Dietary therapy mg/dL (mmol/L)	Consider drug therapy mg/dL (mmol/L)
Total cholesterol	<170 (<4.40)	170–199 (4.4–5.15)	≥200 (≥5.15)
LDL cholesterol	<110 (<2.85)	110–29 (2.85–3.35)	≥130 (≥3.35)
HDL cholesterol	>62 (>1.6)	<39 (<1.0)	<35 (<0.9)
Triglycerides*	160 (1.8)	200 (2.3)	400 (4.6)

*Acceptable level of triglyceride is influenced by HDL cholesterol level

Table 22.3 Controlling blood cholesterol: the Step I and II diet

The Step I diet is the initial dietary target to achieve desired LDL and total cholesterol goals

The Step II diet is introduced if the Step I diet fails to achieve the desired goals

	Step I diet	Step II diet
Dietary cholesterol	<300 mg/day	<200 mg/day
Total calories	As required to achieve and maintain normal body weight	As required to achieve and maintain normal body weight
Total fat	<30%	<30%
Saturated fatty acids	<10%	<7%
Polyunsaturated fatty acids	Up to 10%	Up to 10%
Monounsaturated fatty acids	10–15%	10–15%
Carbohydrates	50–60%	50–60%
Protein	10–20%	10–20%

demonstrates how lipid dietary intake targets may be modified to meet various blood cholesterol goals.

Both modifiable and non-modifiable risk factors affect the clinical impact of lowering LDL. Two important non-modifiable risk factors that impinge on LDL treatment targets are inheritance and age. A genetic predisposition should be considered in persons with high levels of lipoprotein(a) [Lp(a)] or a family history of premature coronary heart disease, viz. a heart attack in either a male first-degree relative under 55 or a female first-degree relative under 65 years. From the age of 45 and 55 years, respectively, men and women are at increased risk. The beneficial effects of reducing serum cholesterol are age related. A reduction of 0.06 mmol/L of serum cholesterol achieves:[9]

- a 54% decrease of ischaemic heart disease at 40 years of age
- a 39% decrease at 50 years of age
- a 27% decrease at 60 years of age.

Modifiable red flags are cigarette smoking, blood pressure of 140/90 mmHg or greater, taking anti-hypertensive medication, and an HDL cholesterol level under 1 mmol/L (40 mg/dL). An HDL level of 1.54 mmol/L (60 mg/dL) is protective and is considered to 'neutralize' one risk factor from the overall total risk count. Other life 'choice' orange flags include obesity, physical inactivity and an atherogenic diet. Emerging risk factors include lipoprotein(a), homocysteine, prothrombotic and pro-inflammatory factors, impaired fasting glucose, and evidence of subclinical atherosclerotic disease.[7] An individual's risk of a heart attack is a function both of the LDL cholesterol level and the presence of associated risk factors. The more associated risks, the lower the acceptable LDL level.

An individual with no more than one risk factor for heart disease and a LDL of 4.0 mmol/L (160 mg/dL) or less is judged to have no more than a 1 in 10 chance of a coronary event within the next 10 years. Such persons require no further risk analysis. Persons with more than one risk factor require a 10-year risk assessment. Framingham scoring is used. This divides persons with multiple risk factors, such as age, total cholesterol, HDL cholesterol, blood pressure, and cigarette smoking, into those with a 10-year risk for heart disease of over 20%, 10–20%, and less than 10%. An acceptable LDL level in persons with two or more risk factors is 3.3 mmol/L (130 mg/dL). In those with coronary heart disease risk equivalents such as diabetes, other clinical forms of atherosclerotic disease or multiple risk factors that increase the 10-year risk to over 20%, the acceptable LDL level falls to 2.56 mmol/L (100 mg/dL). Other clinical forms of atherosclerotic disease include peripheral arterial disease, abdominal aortic aneurysm and symptomatic carotid artery disease. Lifestyle changes are indicated when these LDL cholesterol levels are breached. Therapeutic lifestyle changes require increased physical activity, weight control and a reduced intake of saturated fat and cholesterol. **Handout 22.3** provides general dietary guidelines for limiting unhealthy fat choices and **Handout 22.4** provides lifestyle information on how to target particular risk factors. Lipid-lowering drugs are highly effective. Drug therapy needs to be considered if LDL cholesterol reaches 4.8 mmol/L (190 mg/dL) in those with no more than one risk factor or 3.3 mmol/L (130 mg/dL) in those with heart disease risk equivalents.[7] See also Table 22.2.

Cholesterol reviewed: is LDL the best choice?

While risk factors predictive of hazardous LDL have been identified (see **Handout 22.5**), before considering how cholesterol levels can be modified it is necessary to take a closer look at serum cholesterol. Serum cholesterol is composed of several different moieties. LDL cholesterol levels reflect both the less harmful, large buoyant LDL and the more atherogenic small-density LDL (sdLDL) particles.[10] Not only does the total LDL cholesterol value fail to distinguish between its more and less atherogenic components, it also fails to consider other atherogenic cholesterol elements such as very-low-density lipoprotein (VLDL) and intermediate-density lipoprotein (IDL). Apolipoprotein B (apoB), on the other hand, provides an indication of the cholesterol content in LDL, VLDL and IDL. ApoB is the major apolipoprotein in all potentially atherogenic lipoprotein particles. The most abundant apoB particle is the sdLDL, which constitutes about 90% of the whole apoB population. Non-HDL cholesterol, i.e. the total of LDL, IDL and VLDL, correlates with apoB with r-values about 0.8–0.9.[10] ApoB provides a sound measure of atherogenic potential.

Although unproven, it is widely accepted that increased HDL is protective, with epidemiologic associations repeatedly suggesting that raising HDL prevents coronary artery disease. Serum HDL transports phospholipids, triacylglycerol and cholesterol scavenged from peripheral tissues back to liver.[11] The liver converts this cholesterol into bile acids, bile salts, and esterifies the rest, secreting them into bile. High-density lipoproteins are complex macromolecules consisting of a core of hydrophobic lipids (cholesteryl esters and triglycerides), an envelope of phospholipids and some unesterified (free) cholesterol, and apolipoproteins. The apolipoproteins ensure structural integrity, serve as ligands for protein (and possibly lipid) receptors, act as coactivators of enzymatic reactions, and are involved in the cellular secretion of the lipoprotein. Serum apolipoprotein A-I (apoA-I), the major protein moiety of HDL particles, reflects diverse circulating HDL particles. ApoA-I is the major apolipoprotein in HDL particles. ApoA-I manifests several anti-atherogenic effects.[10] ApoA-I is a major initiator and driver of reverse cholesterol transport, it displays antioxidant and anti-inflammatory effects, stimulates endothelial production of nitric oxide and release of prostacyclin from the endothelium.

Atherosclerosis is triggered when foam cells are formed by oxidized LDL being taken up by scavenger receptors on activated macrophages. Various cytokines are produced by macrophages within the developing atheromatous plaque in response to modified LDL. Production and activation of vascular cell adhesion molecules and intercellular adhesion molecules bind increasing numbers of mononuclear cells to the surface of endothelial cells. Together, modified LDL and these activated molecules form a potentially escalating inflammatory cascade.

In patients with atherosclerosis and/or inflammatory conditions, HDL can paradoxically increase recruitment and activation of macrophages, upregulate the expression of endothelial cell adhesion molecules, and participate in the oxidation of low-density lipoproteins.[12,13] Contrary to conventional thinking, it is now recognized that very high plasma levels of HDL and very large HDL particles are associated with an increased risk of heart disease![12] Instead of limiting phospholipid oxidation in LDL, paradoxically, modified HDL can promote oxidation of LDL, enhancing production of monocyte chemoattractant protein, and increasing expression of cellular adhesion molecules and recruitment of mononuclear cells. Not only may modified HDL become pro-inflammatory, its ability to promote reverse cholesterol transport can become impaired. Under normal circumstances, HDL inhibits the oxidation of LDL through a combination of antioxidant enzymes and apoA-I. The apoA-I component of HDL remains protective even at higher HDL levels. ApoA-I more accurately reflects the atheroprotective capacity of this lipoprotein fraction.[12]

As each one of LDL, IDL and VLDL particles carries only one apolipoprotein B-100 molecule, the total apoB value represents the total number of potentially atherogenic lipoproteins.[14] ApoA-I, even when corrected for HDL cholesterol and apoB, remains cardioprotective.[15] Current opinion favours the use of apoA-I and apoB values as estimates of cardiovascular risk and as treatment goals in patients undergoing treatment for hyperlipidaemia.[14]

Intervention strategies

Therapeutic lifestyle changes and drug therapy can effectively reduce blood cholesterol levels. Trials have found that statin therapy can reduce total cholesterol by 32%, LDL cholesterol by 45% and increase HDL cholesterol by almost 10%.[16] By inhibiting 3-hydroxy-3-methylglutaryl coenzyme A reductase, statins can successfully lower LDL. Statins can achieve a reduction in the risk of major cardiovascular events of 21% for every 1 mmol/L (39 mg/dL) decrease in LDL.[8] A randomized study reported that the reduction in LDL levels in patients with hypercholesterolaemia given a diet based upon red yeast, rice and fish oil was comparable to that achieved with standard drug therapy.[16] Another study found that persons on a diet very low in saturated fat, based on milled whole-wheat cereals and low-fat dairy foods and a statin achieved a 30.9% reduction in LDL cholesterol, while those on a diet high in plant sterols (1.0 g/1000 kcal), soy protein (21.4 g/1000 kcal), viscous fibres (9.8 g/1000 kcal), and almonds (14 g/1000 kcal) achieved a 28.6% reduction.[17] Not only are therapeutic lifestyle changes effective, they are a more cost-effective means of controlling heart disease.

The diet recommended to lower LDL is one that permits 25–35% of its total calorie content to be derived from fat, 50–60% from carbohydrate and around 15% from protein. Less than 7% of the total calorie intake should be contributed by saturated fat, up to 10% of energy may be contributed by polyunsaturated fat and up to 20% may be derived from monounsaturated fat. *Trans* fatty acids raise LDL levels and should be avoided. Intake should be limited to less than 1% of total energy. Less than 200 mg/day of dietary cholesterol is permitted. By favouring foods rich in complex carbohydrates such as whole grains, fruits, and vegetables, a desirable daily level of 20–30 g of fibre may be achieved. In all instances, energy intake and expenditure should ensure achieving and maintaining a desirable body weight.

While HDL levels are not used as a therapeutic marker, it is well recognized that HDL levels can be increased through lifestyle changes such as regular aerobic exercise, smoking cessation, lowered alcohol consumption, weight loss and dietary manipulation; and/or drug intervention with niacin, fibrates, thiazolidinediones or bile acid sequestrants.[8] What is less clear is the character of the particles contributing to the increased HDL levels. In view of mounting evidence of the adverse impact of high levels of large HDL particles, clarification as to which interventions increase small rather than large, cholesterol-rich HDL particles is needed.[15]

A regimen of high-fibre grains, increased vegetables and fruits, decreased saturated fat, increased plant/fish protein sources, and exercise reduces LDL and HDL levels. Although HDL levels decline, the characteristics of the HDL particles improve substantially.[16] Compared with a diet rich in saturated fat, one primarily including polyunsaturated fat reduces production of adhesion cell molecules, provoking a beneficial change in the nature of the resultant HDL particles. Altering dietary fat composition improves HDL's anti-inflammatory function,[17] as does drug therapy. Niacin and simvastatin lower LDL by around 42%, and raise HDL2 by 65% and apoA-I by 76%. HDL2 is one of the two major subclasses of HDL. Its major role appears to be as a final receptor in the reverse cholesterol transport, a process involving HDL moving cholesterol from peripheral tissues back to the liver where it is broken down and excreted as bile.

When LDL lowering is used as the therapeutic yardstick, statin therapy, with or without long-acting formulations of nicotinic acid to elevate HDL and reduce Lp(a) levels, provides the most effective and best tolerated pharmacological strategy.[8] Intensive high-dose statin therapy, with or without therapeutic lifestyle changes, can lower LDL levels to below 2.6 mmol/L (100 mg/dL). Nonetheless, the risk of a major cardiovascular event in patients with established coronary artery disease remains close to 9% annually.[8] It is possible cardiovascular risk management may be more effective if risk assessment relied on more precise measurements of the total atherogenic potential. Comparing apoB levels with the actual protective potential of HDL by measuring apoA-I levels achieves this. Cardiovascular risk may be more precisely determined in the future using the more accurate indices of apoB and apoA-I. In the interim, recommendations must rely on studies using changes in LDL and HDL levels as their intervention endpoint.

Therapeutic lifestyle changes

The two major approaches to neutralizing the risk of a heart attack posed by dyslipidaemia are either to improve the lipid profile, i.e. lower LDL and increase HDL cholesterol levels, or to prevent oxidation of cholesterol.

Adjusting lipid levels

The major lifestyle strategies for improving blood cholesterol levels are diet and exercise. Dietary changes focus largely, but not exclusively, on dietary fats.

Dietary cholesterol is not the major determinant for blood cholesterol levels. In fact, if dietary cholesterol falls too low, hepatic synthesis of cholesterol is stimulated to ensure sufficient levels of cholesterol are available for synthesis of steroid hormones and vitamin D. A daily cholesterol intake not exceeding 300 mg is generally recommended. This is reduced to 200 mg for persons with a risky cholesterol profile. Animals and animal products, particularly shellfish, eggs and dairy products, are rich dietary sources of cholesterol. As a single egg contains about 210 mg of cholesterol, eating fewer than four egg yolks per week is generally recommended. However, a study in healthy adults found that adding an egg each day to their basic diet for a period of 12 weeks significantly increased HDL without a meaningful decrease in the total cholesterol:HDL ratio.[18] Furthermore, in addition to dietary cholesterol appearing to only increase plasma cholesterol in around 3 in 10 people, egg intake has been shown to promote a less atherogenic LDL profile.[19] Animal studies have confirmed that egg markedly lowers the lymphatic absorption of cholesterol under in vivo conditions.[20] The inhibitory effect may be attributable to phosphatidylcholine in egg yolk. Furthermore, as dietary cholesterol may downregulate the activity of HMG CoA reductase, the enzyme involved in the synthesis of endogenous cholesterol, egg consumption may modulate rather than raise blood cholesterol. A double-blind, crossover study found that eating one extra egg daily did not have a negative impact on blood lipids or inflammation markers.[21] Furthermore, consumption of omega-3-enriched eggs results in higher levels of apoA-I, a lower apoB/apoA-I ratio and lower plasma glucose.[21] Based on these findings, it is possible omega-3-enriched eggs may reduce the risk for cardiovascular mortality! Despite concerns, epidemiological data suggest that cholesterol intake is associated with only, at worst, a modest increase in the risk of coronary events.[22] In fact, 70% of the population experiences a mild increase or no alteration in plasma cholesterol concentrations when challenged with high amounts of dietary cholesterol; the remainder increase both their HDL and LDL levels.[23]

Rather than cholesterol, the major dietary stimulus to raised blood cholesterol levels are saturated fatty acids. Increasing energy consumed as saturated fats by 1% elevates serum cholesterol levels by around 2.7 mg/dL.

In order, the most atherogenic fats are butter, lard (beef fat), cocoa butter and olive oil. Metabolic studies have shown that different classes of saturated fatty acids have different effects on plasma lipid and lipoprotein levels.[24] Saturated fatty acids with 12–16 carbon atoms tend to increase total and LDL cholesterol levels. Myristic acid (C14) is a potent elevator of blood cholesterol. Dairy products, and coconut and palm kernel oils are a source of myristic acid. Palmitic acid (C16), the most common saturated fat in plants and animals, elevates cholesterol only in people whose blood cholesterol is already elevated. Stearic acid is plentiful in fats, oils and cocoa butter. Stearic acid (C18), rather than raising total cholesterol, tends to lower HDL while increasing apoA concentration. One-third of the lipid in cocoa butter is stearic acid. While the effect of stearic acid is neutral, the high concentration of flavonoids in dark chocolate implies cardioprotection – when eaten in small quantities![25] With few exceptions, avoiding animal in favour of plant sources of fats decreases the intake of saturated and increases the intake of polyunsaturated and monounsaturated fatty acids.

Replacing saturated fat with omega-6 polyunsaturated fat reduces plasma total cholesterol by 19%, LDL by 22%, and HDL by 14%. Replacing saturated with monounsaturated fat decreases total cholesterol by 12%, LDL by 15%, and HDL by 4%.[26] Olive oil, a good source of monounsaturated fatty acid, is one reason why the Mediterranean diet is cardioprotective.[27] The health benefits of the Mediterranean diet can be further enhanced by adding nuts.[28] Nuts are rich sources of monounsaturated fats. Macadamia nuts, a rich source of monounsaturated fats (oleic and palmitoleic acids) and polyphenol compounds, were found to reduce plasma biomarkers of oxidative stress, coagulation and inflammation in hypercholesterolaemic males.[29]

The North American diet is typically high in linoleic acid (n-6), which, despite having a cholesterol-lowering effect, favours oxidative modification of LDL.[23] Nonetheless, replacing saturated fat with linoleic acid decreases the risk for coronary events.[30] However, while the proportion of serum linoleic acid is inversely related, an increase in dihomo-gamma-linolenic acid, a metabolite of linoleic acid, is directly related to cardiovascular mortality.[31] In contrast, alpha linolenic acid (n-3) has been found in several studies to reduce the risk of dying from a heart attack. The ratio of omega-6 to omega-3 fatty acids in Western diets promotes the pathogenesis of many chronic diseases, including cardiovascular disease.[32] Increased dietary intake of linoleic acid (n-6), in addition to increasing oxidized LDL, enhances platelet aggregation and interferes with the incorporation of essential fatty acids into cell membrane phospholipids. In Western diets, the ratio of n-6 to n-3 is 15:1–16.7:1.[33] In the secondary prevention of cardiovascular disease, a ratio of 4:1 was associated with a 70% decrease in total mortality; a ratio of 2.5:1 reduced rectal cell proliferation in patients with colorectal cancer; a ratio of 2–3:1 suppressed inflammation in patients with rheumatoid arthritis; and a ratio of 5:1 benefited patients with asthma. A high intake of ocean fish, particularly coldwater fish, increases dietary omega-3 fatty acids.[34]

One study found that, compared with placebo, omega-3 fatty acids had a statistically significant effect, reducing levels of triacylglycerol, VLDL-cholesterol and VLDL-triacylglycerol, although increasing LDL by 5.7%.[35] Another found that, compared with placebo, omega-3 fatty acid supplementation decreased triglycerides by 7%, increased LDL by 3%, but did not benefit HDL or LDL particle size.[36] Long-chain omega-3 fatty acids, especially DHA, are consistently and significantly reduced in patients experiencing ischaemic heart disease events.[37] A daily intake of omega-3 fatty acids between 250 and 500 mg is believed to reduce the risk of heart disease.

In contrast to a healthy heart diet emphasizing nutrient-rich plant foods and fatty fish, a diet rich in *trans* fatty acids is associated with an increased risk of heart attacks due to impaired cholesterol metabolism.[38] *Trans* fatty acids increase LDL and lower HDL cholesterol levels. They appear to carry an even greater risk than saturated fatty acids. The effect of *trans* fatty acids on total cholesterols is double that of saturated fatty acids![38] *Trans* fats may adversely effect thrombogenesis and Lp(a) levels, high blood levels of which have been independently linked with an increased risk of coronary heart disease.[39] There is definitive evidence that *trans* fatty acids have adverse effects on blood lipids, near definitive evidence that *trans* fatty acids increase inflammatory markers in blood, and strong evidence from prospective epidemiologic studies that high *trans* fatty acid intake is associated with elevated risks of coronary heart disease.[40] A high intake of *trans* fats can increase the risk of heart disease by over 1.3-fold.[39] A diet in which 2% of calories is provided by *trans* fats increases the risk of ischaemic heart disease by 23%.

Since 1 January 2006, the FDA has required that food labels indicate levels of *trans* fatty acids. Adding information on *trans* fatty acid content to nutrition labels is predicted to prevent 600–1200 cases of coronary heart disease and 240–480 deaths each year, saving between $900 million and $1.8 billion annually in medical costs, lost productivity, and pain and suffering.[41] For the purpose of nutrition labelling, *trans* fatty acids are defined as the sum of all unsaturated fatty acids that contain one or more isolated (i.e. non-conjugated) double bonds in a *trans* configuration. Prior to regulation, McDonald's French fries in the US had 21% *trans* and 21% saturates.[42] In the Netherlands, where a major reduction in the *trans* fatty acid content of retail foods was achieved in the 1990s, McDonald's French fries have 4% *trans* and 24% saturates.[42] Some 40% of the *trans* fatty acids in the US diet are derived from baked goods such as cakes, pastries, crackers and bread; 21% from animal products, and 17% from margarine.[43] *Trans* fats are formed when vegetable oils are hydrogenated to form spreads.[44]

Both saturated and *trans* fatty acids raise cholesterol levels; *cis*-polyunsaturated fatty acids decrease total cholesterol by decreasing LDL and HDL cholesterol levels. Monounsaturated fatty acids do not achieve an equivalent lowering of total cholesterol but are more cardioprotective than polyunsaturated fats as they lower LDL and raise HDL.[10] Long-chain omega-3 fatty acids are cardioprotective. Selective use of functional foods and dietary supplementation can offer further protection. Placing mildly hypercholesterolaemic patients on a low-fat diet reduces total cholesterol, HDL, LDL, apoA-I and apoB; when this diet was supplemented daily with 3.3 g of plant sterols, reductions in total cholesterol, LDL and apoB were noted without affecting HDL or apoA-I.[45] Plant sterols further reduce the atherogenicity of the cholesterol profile in hypercholesterolaemic patients on a low-fat diet. An average intake of 2.15 g of phytosterols per day was linked to a reduction in LDL levels of 0.34 mmol/L; a decline which extrapolates to an 8.8% drop in heart disease.[46] Although no significant differences in outcome were detected between sterols or stanols, fat-based or non-fat-based, dairy or non-dairy food formats, solid foods in doses over 2 g per day did appear to offer an advantage over liquid foods.[46] Multiple rather than single daily intakes also seemed more effective. Benecol and Unilever, under the Flora Pro.activ brand, have a range of cholesterol-lowering products.

Beta-glucan, a soluble fibre, also decreases LDL levels. A daily dose of 6 g of concentrated oat beta-glucan has been shown to significantly reduce total and LDL cholesterol in hypercholesterolaemic patients.[47] Fruit is rich in pectin and pectin enhances faecal excretion of bile acids and cholesterol. Apples 400 g/day lower blood cholesterol up to 11%; 200 g of fresh carrots daily achieves an 11% drop, guava 0.5–1 kg/day an 8% drop, and prunes 100 g/day a 5% decline.[48] Whole fruits rather than juices are recommended. Indeed, care must be exercised choosing a diet rich in refined carbohydrate. For every 15-unit increase in the glycaemic index, the HDL concentration drops by 0.06 mmol/L.[49] Dietary choices rich in simple sugars, e.g. bread, pasta, cornflakes, potato, bananas, honey and fruit juice, create a high glycaemic load and should be limited. Dietary choices with a low glycaemic index, e.g. apples, peaches, legumes, barley, oat bran cereals, milk and yoghurt, are preferable options. Using plant stanols/sterols and soluble fibre as therapeutic dietary options is routinely encouraged to enhance lowering of LDL cholesterol. A less generally supported option is supplementation with ginger. Ginger capsules, 3 g daily, have been shown to significantly reduce triglycerides and LDL cholesterol while increasing HDL.[50]

Although 'dietary interventions have much better luck in lowering blood cholesterol levels' than physical activity,[51] exercise does reduce the risk of coronary heart disease. Adoption of a physically active lifestyle reduces coronary heart disease risk through diverse mechanisms including decreased blood pressure, dampened inflammation and a modified lipid profile.[51–53] Compared with sedentary women, those engaging in vigorous, leisure-time physical activity have a less atherogenic risk factor profile and potentially reduce their coronary heart disease risk by up to 30%.[54] The intensity, duration and frequency of exercise required to achieve a meaningful change in blood lipids is unclear.

One study found that significant changes in total and LDL cholesterol were only observed with high-intensity exercise.[55] High-intensity training was shown to be more effective in improving the lipid profile than moderate-intensity training of equal energy cost. Another prospective randomized study found that higher amounts of exercise resulted in greater improvements in lipoprotein variables but that these improvements were related to the amount of activity, and not the intensity of exercise or improvement in fitness.[56] A third study reported a dose–response relationship between exercise duration and HDL levels in postmenopausal women.[57] It appears that the minimal weekly exercise for increasing HDL may be 900 kcal of energy expenditure or 120 minutes of exercise each week.[58] Every additional 10 minutes of exercise per session appears to be associated with an approximately

1.4-mg/dL (0.036-mmol/L) increase in the HDL level. This study reported no significant association between exercise frequency or intensity.[58] Exercise was more effective in subjects with initially high total cholesterol levels or low body mass index.

Increased exercise frequency has been associated with higher HDL and apoA-I and lower total and LDL cholesterol, triglycerides and blood pressure.[54] A later study confirmed that almost all blood lipids were inversely associated with physical activity status; however, after adjustments for age, smoking habits, body mass index and dietary intake were made, only HDL and apoA-I concentrations were significantly affected by exercise in women.[59] While it has been suggested that substantial independent increases in HDL and apoA-I concentrations may be limited to women,[51] a recent meta-analysis intimates that aerobic exercise reduces total cholesterol and triglycerides and increases HDL in adult men.[60] A second meta-analysis reported aerobic exercise increased HDL2 in adults.[61] Small HDL (nascent HDL) is rich in apoA-I, phospholipids and free cholesterol. Esterification of small HDL by lecithin: cholesterol acyltransferase generates small HDL3 particles and, in turn, large HDL2 particles; the latter of which can be reconverted to HDL3 through a number of steps.[62] Of the two major HDL subfractions, HDL2, a final receptor in the reverse cholesterol transport, appears to provide greater protection against heart disease than HDL3. A low level of HDL is strongly and inversely related to coronary heart disease. Low circulating levels of HDL cholesterol might be associated with the functionally defective small HDL particles of abnormal structure and composition.[63] Small, dense HDL possesses potent antioxidative activity but this is compromised under conditions of atherogenic dyslipidaemia.

Antioxidant therapy

Natural LDL is recognized by LDL receptors in the liver, which expedite its removal from the blood by LDL-cholesterol catabolic pathways. LDL receptors fail to recognize oxidized cholesterol. In addition to the amount of dietary cholesterol consumed, consideration therefore needs to be given to the nature of circulating cholesterol. As oxidized cholesterol is atherogenic and the antioxidant capacity of apoA-I can be compromised in those at risk, sound biological reasoning would suggest that antioxidant therapy offers some protection against coronary heart disease.

Nutritional oxidative stress denotes a disturbance of the redox state resulting from an excessive oxidative load or from a diet favouring pro-oxidant reactions.[64] Low intake or impaired availability of dietary antioxidants, including vitamins E and C, carotenoids, polyphenols, and micronutrients such as selenium, weakens the antioxidant network. Postprandial oxidative stress, a subcategory of nutritional oxidative stress, arises from sustained postprandial hyperlipidaemia and is associated with a higher risk for atherosclerosis. Dietary unsaturated fatty acids and lipid hydroperoxides that escape from the gastrointestinal barrier can be incorporated into plasma lipoproteins, leading to a modified form of LDL.[65] In hyperlipidaemic subjects, endothelium-dependent vasodilation is impaired in the postprandial state, making postprandial oxidative stress an important factor modulating cardiovascular risk. However, postprandial oxidative stress is attenuated when dietary antioxidants are supplied together with a meal rich in oxidized or oxidizable lipids. Ingestion of dietary polyphenols, e.g. from wine, cocoa or tea, reduces endothelial dysfunction and lowers susceptibility of LDL lipids to oxidation.[64] Red wine polyphenols have been shown to effectively inhibit absorption of cytotoxic lipid peroxidation products.[66] Mandarin juice (500 mL/day) has been shown to improve the antioxidant status of hypercholesterolaemic children,[67] while 400 mL tomato juice and 30 mg tomato ketchup daily increased LDL resistance to oxidation in healthy normocholesterolaemic adults.[68] Cranberry juice has a similarly beneficial effect.[69] Selenium supplementation has been shown to prevent meal-induced increases in both modified LDL and LDL susceptibility to oxidation.[65]

Although dietary intervention favourably alters the redox state, it has not been proven to reduce the risk of coronary heart disease by decreasing oxidation of cholesterol. Although oxidative stress is significantly increased in the majority of ischaemic heart disease patients, one study failed to find any association between total antioxidant activity and the lipid profile.[70] Furthermore, recent studies have shown that commonly used antioxidant vitamin regimens do not prevent cardiovascular events.[71] In fact, it now appears that the addition of antioxidant vitamins to simvastatin–niacin therapy substantially blunts the expected rise in the protective HDL2 and apoA-I subfractions of HDL.[71] Supplementing statin therapy with antioxidant vitamins may enhance rather than intercept the progression of coronary artery disease. As antioxidants beta-carotene and vitamins E and C, alone or in combination, do not protect against cardiovascular disease and may blunt the protective HDL2 response to HDL cholesterol-targeted therapy, they are potentially harmful in this setting! While a diet rich in antioxidants is recommended for general wellness, antioxidant vitamin supplementation appears contraindicated for persons on drug therapy to lower their cholesterol levels. Antioxidants are best obtained from a diet rich in fruits, vegetables and whole grains.

Looking ahead

Currently, management targets are set using LDL levels; advances in laboratory diagnosis may change this in the future. More accurate assessment of coronary heart disease risk is already possible using the apoB:apoA-I ratio. Other emerging diagnostic markers are high-sensitivity C-reactive protein (hs-CRP) and lipoprotein-associated phospholipase A_2 (Lp-PLA$_2$), both of which are useful in reclassifying intermediate-risk patients. Compared with CRP, which reflects systemic inflammation, Lp-PLA$_2$ has high specificity for vascular inflammation and a directly causal role in plaque inflammation. Lp-PLA$_2$ resides mainly on and travels with LDL particles in plasma, although it is also associated with HDL particles, lipoprotein(a), and remnant lipoproteins.[72] Lp-PLA$_2$ is highly upregulated in atherosclerotic plaques. Through hydrolysis of oxidized LDL particles, Lp-PLA$_2$ generates two pro-inflammatory mediators: lysophosphatidylcholine and oxidized fatty acid.[72] Unlike hs-CRP, with which the cardiac risk is markedly attenuated as more traditional risk factors are taken into consideration, trials demonstrate generally consistent correlations between elevated Lp-PLA$_2$ levels and an increased risk for cardiovascular events.[72,73] Furthermore, lipid-modifying therapies combining a statin with niacin or a statin with omega-3 fatty acids significantly lower Lp-PLA$_2$, even when the statin has already lowered LDL cholesterol to optimal levels.[73] Increasingly sophisticated laboratory investigations are likely to further clarify the association between exercise, diet, drugs, blood cholesterol levels and coronary heart disease.

In perspective

Hypercholesterolaemia is a traditional major modifiable risk marker for ischaemic heart disease. Other factors being equal, individuals on a diet rich in animal products with its high content of saturated fatty acids and cholesterol have higher blood cholesterol levels and are at greater risk of atherosclerosis than those on a diet rich in plant foods and vegetable oils. Persons on a diet rich in polyunsaturated fats have lower total blood cholesterol levels but are more at risk of heart attacks than those on a high monounsaturated fatty acid diet. Polyunsaturated fatty acids lower both LDL and HDL levels. Monounsaturated fatty acids are more protective of HDL levels. **Handout 22.3** provides dietary advice consistent with these guidelines.

Hypercholesterolaemia, however, is but one modifiable risk factor of coronary heart disease. **Handout 22.2** lists some other recognized risk factors. Risk factor analysis using age, sex, obesity, smoking, alcohol intake, hypertension, diabetes mellitus, serum uric acid; total, LDL and HDL cholesterol; triglyceride, and atherogenic indices was found to predict coronary artery disease with a sensitivity of 75.8%, a specificity of 68.5%, and a predictive accuracy of 71.5% in the test group.[74] Quitting tobacco use, lowering raised blood pressure and maintaining an ideal body weight also reduce the risk of atheroma formation. Furthermore, atheromatous plaque formation is but one part of the heart attack equation – the critical event may be precipitated by coronary vasospasm or thrombus formation. Low vitamin E, high fibrinogen, plasma S-adenosylhomocysteine and psychosocial stress are all recognized risk factors. Rather than limiting prevention to controlling the lipid profile, good clinical care embraces a more holistic approach. **Handout 22.6** suggests behaviours conducive to a healthy heart. One study found that improvements in dietary fat intake, exercise, and stress management were individually, additively and interactively related to reducing coronary risk.[75] Reductions in dietary fat intake predicted reductions in weight and total and LDL cholesterol; and interacted with increased exercise to predict reductions in perceived stress. Increased exercise predicted improvements in total cholesterol and exercise capacity in women. Stress management reduced hostility, weight, triglycerides and total:HDL cholesterol in men. Adherence to a Mediterranean-style diet is also effective. It reduces the risk of death from cardiovascular disease by 22% in men and 12% in women.[76] The Mediterranean diet improves lipid and glucose metabolism, reduces blood pressure, and positively modulates the antithrombotic profile, endothelial function and inflammation/oxidative stress. Conformity with the Mediterranean dietary pattern is associated with high antioxidant capacity and low concentrations of oxidized LDL cholesterol.[75] **Handout 22.7** outlines a self-care protocol to reduce the risk of coronary heart disease.

The last word

A plant-based diet, a low intake of saturated and *trans* fatty acids, exercise and drug intervention to lower raised cholesterol, as required, remain the mainstay of therapy. Primary prevention offers the greatest opportunity for reducing the burden of coronary heart disease in developed countries. Blood cholesterol in its various forms remains an important red flag signalling an increased risk in apparently healthy individuals.

References

1. World Health Organization. WHO Report 2002. http://www.who.int/whr/2002/en/; Accessed 26.01.09.
2. CDC. Prevention Research Centres. http://www.cdc.gov/prc/research-projects/special-interest-projects/diagnosis-treatment-familial-hypercholesterolemia.htm; Accessed 27.01.09.
3. British Heart Foundation. Coronary Heart Disease Statistics 2008. http://www.heartstats.org/datapage.asp?id=7998; Accessed 27.01.09.
4. Australian Institute of Health and Welfare. http://www.aihw.gov.au/riskfactors/cholesterol.cfm Accessed 27.01.09.
5. National Centre for Health Statistics. Health, United States, 2007 With Chartbook on Trends in the Health of Americans. Hyattsville, MD; 2007. http://www.cdc.gov/nchs/data/hus/hus07.pdf; Accessed 26.01.09.
6. Australian Institute of Health and Welfare. http://www.aihw.gov.au/cvd/coronary_disease.cfm Accessed 27.01.09.
7. NIH. Third Adult Treatment Panel (ATP) Report High Blood Cholesterol. http://www.nhlbi.nih.gov/guidelines/cholesterol/index.htm Accessed 26.01.09.
8. Hausenloy DJ, Yellon DM. Targeting residual cardiovascular risk: raising high-density lipoprotein cholesterol levels. *Heart*. 2008;94 (6):706–714.
9. Law MR, Wald NJ, Thompson SG. By how much and how quickly does a reduction in serum cholesterol concentration lower risk of ischaemic heart disease. *BMJ*. 1994;308:67–373.
10. Walldius G, Jungner I. Is there a better marker of cardiovascular risk than LDL cholesterol? Apolipoproteins B and A-I—new risk factors and targets for therapy. *Nutr Metab Cardiovasc Dis*. 2007;17(8):565–571.
11. Gupta S, Rajagopal G. The significance of plasma high density lipoprotein cholesterol (hdlc). *Nepal Med Coll J*. 2007;9 (3):212–214.
12. van der Steeg WA, Holme IH, Boekholdt SM, et al. High-density lipoprotein cholesterol, high-density lipoprotein particle size, and apolipoprotein A-I: significance for cardiovascular risk: the IDEAL and EPIC-Norfolk studies. *J Am Coll Cardiol*. 2008;51:634–642.
13. Ansell BJ. Targeting the anti-inflammatory effects of high-density lipoprotein. *J Am Coll Cardiol*. 2007;100:S3–S9.
14. Andrikoula M, McDowell IF. The contribution of ApoB and ApoA1 measurements to cardiovascular risk assessment. Diabetes. *Obes Metab*. 2008;10(4):271–278.
15. Genest J. The Yin and Yang of high-density lipoprotein cholesterol. *J Am Coll Cardiol*. 2008;51:643–644.
16. Becker DJ, Gordon RY, Morris PB, et al. Simvastatin vs therapeutic lifestyle changes and supplements: randomized primary prevention trial. *Mayo Clin Proc*. 2008;83 (7):758–764.
17. Nicholls SJ, Lundman P, Harmer JA, et al. Consumption of saturated fat impairs the anti-inflammatory properties of high-density lipoproteins and endothelial function. *J Am Coll Cardiol*. 2006;48:715–720.
18. Mayurasakorn K, Srisura W, Sitphahul P, Hongto PO. High-density lipoprotein cholesterol changes after continuous egg consumption in healthy adults. *J Med Assoc Thai*. 2008;91 (3):400–407.
19. Fernandez ML. Dietary cholesterol provided by eggs and plasma lipoproteins in healthy populations. *Curr Opin Clin Nutr Metab Care*. 2006;9(1):8–12.
20. Jiang Y, Noh SK, Koo SI. Egg phosphatidylcholine decreases the lymphatic absorption of cholesterol in rats. *J Nutr*. 2001;131 (9):2358–2363.
21. Ohman M, Akerfeldt T, Nilsson I, et al. Biochemical effects of consumption of eggs containing omega-3 polyunsaturated fatty acids. *Ups J Med Sci*. 2008;113 (3):315–323.
22. Kritchevsky SB, Kritchevsky D. Egg consumption and coronary heart disease: an epidemiologic overview. *J Am Coll Nutr*. 2000;19 (5 suppl):549S–555S.
23. Fernandez ML. Dietary cholesterol provided by eggs and plasma lipoproteins in healthy populations. *Curr Opin Clin Nutr Metab Care*. 2006;9(1):8–12.
24. Khor GL. Dietary fat quality: a nutritional epidemiologist's view.

Asia Pac J Clin Nutr. 2004;13 (suppl):S22.

25. Ding EL, Hutfless SM, Ding X, Girotra S. Chocolate and prevention of cardiovascular disease: a systematic review. *Nutr Metab (Lond)*. 2006;3(1):2.

26. Hodson L, Skeaff CM, Chisholm WA. The effect of replacing dietary saturated fat with polyunsaturated or monounsaturated fat on plasma lipids in free-living young adults. *Eur J Clin Nutr*. 2001;55 (10):908–915.

27. de Lorgeril M, Salen P. The Mediterranean diet: rationale and evidence for its benefit. *Curr Atheroscler Rep*. 2008;10 (6):518–522.

28. Salas-Salvadó J, Fernández-Ballart J, Ros E, et al. PREDIMED Study Investigators. Effect of a Mediterranean diet supplemented with nuts on metabolic syndrome status: one-year results of the PREDIMED randomized trial. *Arch Intern Med*. 2008;168 (22):2449–2458.

29. Garg ML, Blake RJ, Wills RB, Clayton EH. Macadamia nut consumption modulates favourably risk factors for coronary artery disease in hypercholesterolemic subjects. *Lipids*. 2007;42 (6):583–587.

30. Harris WS. Linoleic acid and coronary heart disease. *Prostaglandins Leukot Essent Fatty Acids*. 2008;79(3–5):169–171.

31. Warensjö E, Sundström J, Vessby B, Cederholm T, Risérus U. Markers of dietary fat quality and fatty acid desaturation as predictors of total and cardiovascular mortality: a population-based prospective study. *Am J Clin Nutr*. 2008;88 (1):203–209.

32. Simopoulos AP. The omega-6/ omega-3 fatty acid ratio, genetic variation, and cardiovascular disease. *Asia Pac J Clin Nutr*. 2008;17 (suppl 1):131–134.

33. Simopoulos AP. The importance of the omega-6/omega-3 fatty acid ratio in cardiovascular disease and other chronic diseases. *Exp Biol Med (Maywood)*. 2008;233 (6):674–688.

34. Lockheart MS, Steffen LM, Rebnord HM, et al. Dietary patterns, food groups and myocardial infarction: a case-control study. *Br J Nutr*. 2007;98 (2):380–387.

35. Hartweg J, Farmer AJ, Perera R, Holman RR, Neil HA. Meta-analysis of the effects of n-3 polyunsaturated fatty acids on lipoproteins and other emerging lipid cardiovascular risk markers in patients with type 2 diabetes. *Diabetologia*. 2007;50 (8):1593–1602.

36. Hartweg J, Farmer AJ, Holman RR, Neil A. Potential impact of omega-3 treatment on cardiovascular disease in type 2 diabetes. *Curr Opin Lipidol*. 2009;20(1):30–38.

37. Harris WS, Poston WC, Haddock CK. Tissue n-3 and n-6 fatty acids and risk for coronary heart disease events. *Atherosclerosis*. 2007;193(1):1–10.

38. Mensink RPM, Katan MB. Effect of dietary trans fatty acids on high-density and low-density lipoprotein cholesterol levels in healthy subjects. *N Engl J Med*. 1990;323:439–445.

39. Murray S, Flegel K. Chewing the fat on trans fats. *CMAJ*. 2005;173 (10):1158–1159.

40. Willett WC. The scientific basis for TFA regulations—is it sufficient? Comments from the USA. *Atheroscler Suppl*. 2006;7(2):69–71.

41. Moss J. Labeling of trans fatty acid content in food, regulations and limits—the FDA view. *Atheroscler Suppl*. 2006;7(2):57–59.

42. Katan MB. Regulation of trans fats: the gap, the Polder, and McDonald's French fries. *Atheroscler Suppl*. 2006;7(2):63–66.

43. *FDA*. http://www.fda.gov/FDAC/ features/2003/503_fats.html; Accessed 30.01.09.

44. Bu SY, Mashek DG. Trans fats: foods, facts, and biology. *Minn Med*. 2008;91(10):41–44.

45. Chen SC, Judd JT, Kramer M, Meijer GW, Clevidence BA, Baer DJ. Phytosterol intake and dietary fat reduction are independent and additive in their ability to reduce plasma LDL cholesterol. *Lipids*. 2009;44 (3):273–281.

46. Demonty I, Ras RT, van der Knaap HC, et al. Continuous dose-response relationship of the LDL-cholesterol-lowering effect of phytosterol intake. *J Nutr*. 2009;139(2):271–284.

47. Queenan KM, Stewart ML, Smith KN, Thomas W, Fulcher RG, Slavin JL. Concentrated oat beta-glucan, a fermentable fiber, lowers serum cholesterol in hypercholesterolemic adults in a randomized controlled trial. *Nutr J*. 2007;6:6.

48. Robertson J, Brydon WG, Tadesse K, Wenham P, Walls A, Eastwood MA. The effect of raw carrot on serum lipids and colon function. *Am J Clin Nutr*. 1979;32 (9):1889–1892.

49. Adler AJ, Holub BJ. Effect of garlic and fish-oil supplementation on serum lipid and lipoprotein concentrations in hypercholesterolemic men. *Am J Clin Nutr*. 1997;65(2):445–450.

50. Alizadeh-Navaei R, Roozbeh F, Saravi M, et al. Investigation of the effect of ginger on the lipid levels. A double blind controlled clinical trial. *Saudi Med J*. 2008;29 (9):1280–1284.

51. Skoumas J, Pitsavos C, Panagiotakos DB, et al. Physical activity, high density lipoprotein cholesterol and other lipids levels, in men and women from the ATTICA study. *Lipids Health Dis*. 2003;2:3.

52. Panagiotakos DB, Pitsavos C, Chrysohoou C, Kavouras S, Stefanadis C. ATTICA Study. The associations between leisure-time physical activity and inflammatory and coagulation markers related to cardiovascular disease: the ATTICA Study. *Prev Med*. 2005;40 (4):432–437.

53. Kokkinos P, Manolis A, Pittaras A, et al. Exercise capacity and mortality in hypertensive men with and without additional risk factors. *Hypertension*. 2009;53(3):494–499.

54. Ashton WD, Nanchahal K, Wood DA. Leisure-time physical activity and coronary risk factors in women. *J Cardiovasc Risk*. 2000;7 (4):259–266.

55. O'Donovan G, Owen A, Bird SR, et al. Changes in cardiorespiratory fitness and coronary heart disease risk factors following 24 wk of moderate- or high-intensity exercise of equal energy cost. *J Appl Physiol*. 2005;98(5):1619–1625.

56. Kraus WE, Houmard JA, Duscha BD, et al. Effects of the amount and intensity of exercise on plasma lipoproteins. *N Engl J Med.* 2002;347(19):1483–1492.

57. Dalleck LC, Allen BA, Hanson BA, Borresen EC, Erickson ME, De Lap SL. Dose-response relationship between moderate-intensity exercise duration and coronary heart disease risk factors in postmenopausal women. *J Womens Health (Larchmt)*. 2009;18 (1):105–113.

58. Kodama S, Tanaka S, Saito K, et al. Effect of aerobic exercise training on serum levels of high-density lipoprotein cholesterol: a meta-analysis. *Arch Intern Med.* 2007;167(10):999–1008.

59. Panagiotakos DB, Pitsavos C, Chrysohoou C, et al. Effect of leisure time physical activity on blood lipid levels: the ATTICA study. *Coron Artery Dis.* 2003;14 (8):533–539.

60. Kelley GA, Kelley KS. Aerobic exercise and lipids and lipoproteins in men: a meta-analysis of randomized controlled trials. *J Mens Health Gend.* 2006;3(1):61–70.

61. Kelley GA, Kelley KS. Aerobic exercise and HDL2-C: a meta-analysis of randomized controlled trials. *Atherosclerosis.* 2006;184(1):207–215.

62. Kontush A, Chapman MJ. *Antiatherogenic effects of small HDL and therapeutic roles: normal, functional HDL.* http://www. medscape.com/viewarticle/ 525041_2; Accessed 30.01.09.

63. Kontush A, Chapman MJ. Antiatherogenic small, dense HDL–guardian angel of the arterial wall? *Nat Clin Pract Cardiovasc Med.* 2006;3(3):144–153.

64. Sies H, Stahl W, Sevanian A. Nutritional, dietary and postprandial oxidative stress. *J Nutr.* 2005;135(5):969–972.

65. Natella F, Fidale M, Tubaro F, Ursini F, Scaccini C. Selenium supplementation prevents the increase in atherogenic electronegative LDL (LDL minus) in the postprandial phase. *Nutr Metab Cardiovasc Dis.* 2007;17 (9):649–656.

66. Gorelik S, Ligumsky M, Kohen R, Kanner J. A novel function of red wine polyphenols in humans: prevention of absorption of cytotoxic lipid peroxidation products. *FASEB J.* 2008;22 (1):41–46.

67. Codoñer-Franch P, López-Jaén AB, Muñiz P, et al. Mandarin juice improves the antioxidant status of hypercholesterolemic children. *J Pediatr Gastroenterol Nutr.* 2008;47(3):349–355.

68. Silaste ML, Alfthan G, Aro A, Antero Kesäniemi Y, Hörkkö S. Tomato juice decreases LDL cholesterol levels and increases LDL resistance to oxidation. *Br J Nutr.* 2007;98(6):1251–1258.

69. Ruel G, Pomerleau S, Couture P, Lemieux S, Lamarche B, Couillard C. Low-calorie cranberry juice supplementation reduces plasma oxidized LDL and cell adhesion molecule concentrations in men. *Br J Nutr.* 2007;99:352–359.

70. Maharjan BR, Jha JC, Adhikari D, et al. Oxidative stress, antioxidant status and lipid profile in ischemic heart disease patients from western region of Nepal. *Nepal Med Coll J.* 2008;10(1):20–24.

71. Brown BG, Cheung MC, Lee AC, Zhao XQ, Chait A. Antioxidant vitamins and lipid therapy: end of a long romance? *Arterioscler Thromb Vasc Biol.* 2002;22 (10):1535–1546.

72. Anderson JL. Lipoprotein-associated phospholipase A2: an independent predictor of coronary artery disease events in primary and secondary prevention. *Am J Cardiol.* 2008;101 (12A):23F–33F.

73. Lerman A, McConnell JP. Lipoprotein-associated phospholipase A2: a risk marker or a risk factor? *Am J Cardiol.* 2008;101 (12A):11F–22F.

74. Kambara H, Imoto A, Owada C, Tamaki S, Fudo T, Maetani S. Coronary risk factors used to predict coronary artery disease by logistic regression analysis. *Jpn Circ J.* 1992;56:1199–1205.

75. Daubenmier JJ, Weidner G, Sumner MD, et al. The contribution of changes in diet, exercise, and stress management to changes in coronary risk in women and men in the multisite cardiac lifestyle intervention program. *Ann Behav Med.* 2007;33(1):57–68.

76. Mitrou PN, Kipnis V, Thiebaut ACM, et al. Mediterranean dietary pattern and prediction of all-cause mortality in a US population – eesults from the NIH-AARP Diet and Health Study. *Arch Intern Med.* 2007;167:2461–2468.

Abdominal obesity: a red flag for type 2 diabetes

Globally, more than one billion adults are overweight and at least 300 million are clinically obese. The mean body mass index (BMI) of adults in North America and Europe is now in the overweight range of 25–27 kg/m^2.[1] **Handout 23.1** lists orange flags for obesity, provides information on how increasing adiposity is a health hazard and gives tips on weight control. As shown in Tables 23.1 and 23.2, the risk of disease increases progressively once BMI levels exceed 20 to 22. In a study of women aged 30 years and over who had never smoked and whose weight had recently been stable, it was found that the relative risk of death from all causes was 1.0 in those with a BMI under 19, 1.2 for a BMI of 19–24.9, 1.3 for a BMI of 25–26.9, 1.6 for a BMI of 27–28.9, 2.1 for a BMI of 29–31.9, and 2.2 for a BMI in excess of 32.[2] Due to the adverse metabolic effect of overweight and obesity on insulin resistance, blood lipids and blood pressure, increased BMI progressively increases the risk for type 2 diabetes mellitus (formerly called NIDDM, type II or adult-onset), coronary heart disease and ischaemic stroke. Raised BMI also increases the risk

for cancer of the breast, colon, prostate, endometrium, kidney and gallbladder. Chronic overweight and obesity contribute significantly to osteoarthritis, a major cause of disability in adults. **Handout 23.2** provides information on how to assess overweight and obesity.

Obesity rates have risen threefold or more since 1980 in North America, Europe and Australia.[1] With 67% of men and 57% of women overweight or obese, the number of people with diabetes in the UK is predicted to reach 4 million by 2025.[3] In 2003, 67% of Americans over 20 years of age had a BMI of 25 or over, with 34% in the obese range; in 2005, 19% of those 20 years or younger were overweight.[4] Diabetes, prediabetes, or the metabolic syndrome is present in approximately one in every three American adults and two of three patients who present with symptomatic ischaemic heart disease.[5] In 2006, diabetes ranked as the seventh leading cause of death in the US. In 2004, heart disease was reported in 68% and stroke in 16% of diabetes-related death certificates among people aged 65 years or older.[6] In 2007, the estimated prevalence of diabetes was 2.6% in 20–39-year-olds, 10.8% in 40–59-year-olds and reached 23.8% in those over 60 years of age.[6] The lifetime risk for Americans to develop diabetes is in excess of 30%.[6] In the 2000 AusDiab study, 39.1% of adult Australians were overweight and a further 20.5% were obese.[7] The prevalence of diabetes in this population aged 25 years and older was 7.5%, rising from 2.5% in those 35 to 44 years of age to 23.6% in those 75 years and over. For every known case of diabetes, there was one undiagnosed case.

Table 23.1 Disease risk relative to normal weight and waist circumference

*BMI = Wt(kg)/ Ht²(m)	Classification	Disease risk	Waist circumference Male = <102 cm (<40 in) Female = <88 cm (<35 in)	Waist circumference Male = >102 cm (>40 in) Female = >88 cm (>35 in)
<18.5	Underweight	Low		
18.5–24.9	Normal	Average		
25.0–29.9	Overweight	Increased	Increased	High
30.0–34.9	Level 1 obesity	Moderate	High	Very high
35.0–39.9	Level 2 obesity	Severe	Very high	Very high
≥40	Level 3 obesity	Very severe	Extremely high	Extremely high

*Refine 'normal' body mass index (BMI) by body frame using wrist size.
Assess wrist size by clasping your wrist in your hand:

- small body frame, i.e. the middle finger and thumb overlap, BMI around 20
- medium frame, middle finger and thumb meet, BMI 22.5
- large frame, middle finger and thumb fail to meet, BMI 25.

Almost one in four Australians 25 years and over has either diabetes or a condition of impaired glucose metabolism.[7] Diabetes shortens life expectancy by up to 15 years and its annual cost to Australia exceeds $1.2 billion.[7] Its annual cost to the US in 2007 was $174 billion: $116 billion for direct medical costs and $58 billion for indirect costs attributable to disability, work loss, premature mortality etc.[6] After adjusting for population age and sex differences, the average medical expenditure on diagnosed diabetics is 2.3 times higher than on non-diabetics.[6]

Understanding obesity

Obesity has long been thought to be a behavioural disorder resulting from eating too much and/or exercising too little.[8] Studies now suggest that body weight is under substantial genetic control, accounting for around 33% of the variation in body mass.[9] Genes appear to influence body fat distribution,[10] weight gain in response to overeating,[11] and individual differences in basal metabolic rate.[12] An *ob* gene in mice produces leptin, a protein secreted by adipose tissue, which acts on central neural networks regulating eating behaviour and energy balance.[13] Leptin increases energy expenditure and body temperature and decreases body weight and appetite. It circulates at levels proportional to body fat, increasing when adipose mass increases and decreasing on a low-energy diet. Leptin stimulates oxidation of fatty acids in skeletal muscle and liver, but not adipose tissue. High leptin levels are associated with increased energy expenditure.[14] Mitochondrial uncoupling enhances heat rather than energy production.[15] As most obese people have high leptin levels,[16] it has been suggested that obese individuals may be insensitive to leptin, in the same manner that persons with type 2 diabetes mellitus are insensitive to insulin.[17]

In man, autonomic nervous system regulation of body weight appears to be controlled by feedback mechanisms influencing energy intake, energy expenditure and appetite. Weight loss both alters substrate oxidation in a manner that favours lipid storage and improves the co-morbidities of obesity such as hypertension, dyslipidaemia, insulin resistance and type 2 diabetes. An increase in 24-hour dietary fat oxidation was detected following weight loss, despite a slight reduction in total fat oxidation for the 5 hours after the experimental meal.[18] This suggests that the increase in dietary fat being used for immediate energy resulting from a successful diet and exercise weight loss programme is more than offset by a reduction in the oxidation of endogenous fatty acids. The difference between fat oxidation at 5 and 24 hours could be due to enhanced insulin-mediated suppression of free fatty acid

Table 23.2 Obesity-related health risks*

Health condition	Odds ratio of BMI (kg/m^2) categories with health conditions			
	<25	25–29	30–33	35+
History of serious diseases				
Coronary artery disease	1.0	1.4	2.1	2.7
Congestive heart failure	1.0	1.5	2.5	5.6
Stroke	1.0	1.3	1.4	1.8
Cardiovascular disease risk factors				
Hypercholesterolaemia	1.0	1.9	2.6	2.5
Hypertension	1.0	1.9	3.3	5.4
Physician-diagnosed medical conditions				
Diabetes	1.0	2.3	5.2	12.5
Depression	1.0	1.4	1.7	2.3
Gastro-oesophageal reflux disease	1.0	1.7	2.4	2.6
Diabetes	1.0	2.3	5.2	12.5
Gallbladder removal	1.0	1.8	3.1	4.9
Osteoarthritis	1.0	1.3	1.7	2.4
Knee replacement	1.0	2.3	5.4	11.7
Health complaints				
Hip replacement	1.0	1.2	1.4	1.7
Fatigue/lack of energy	1.0	1.5	2.3	3.7
Chronic insomnia	1.0	1.5	2.2	3.5
Indigestion or heartburn	1.0	1.7	2.3	2.4

*Modified from Patterson RE, Frank LL, Kristal AR, White E. A comprehensive examination of health conditions associated with obesity in older adults. *Am J Prev Med.* 2004;27(5):385-390.

availability, which in turn may contribute to the improved tissue sensitivity to insulin following weight loss. Total energy expenditure declines 15% more than the percentage drop in body weight, i.e. a 20% decrease in energy expenditure occurs after a 5% fall in body weight.[19] In overweight individuals, the response to a dietary intervention was not as strong as in lean persons and, moreover, the response among overweight subjects was variable.[20] Weight loss pushes against a feedback mechanism and is not merely a question of willpower. Adipose tissue is a fat storage organ with important metabolic and endocrine functions.

Fatty acid storage in adipose tissue during dietary modification and exercise-induced weight loss favours maintenance of regional body fat distribution.[18] Women with lower body obesity (pears) are more efficient at storing dietary fatty acids around their buttocks than men with upper body obesity (apples). Men store a higher proportion of dietary fat in abdominal subcutaneous regions. As shown in Table 23.3, an android or upper body fat

Table 23.3 Anthropometric indices of metabolic risk

	BMI	Waist circumference	Risk of an obesity-related metabolic complication
Men	25	>90	Increased risk lipid
	25	>94 cm	Increased
	27.9	>99 cm	? Crucial threshold diabetes
	30	>102 cm	Substantial increase
Women	25	>80 cm	Increased
	26	>85 cm	Increased risk lipid
	30	>88 cm	Substantial increase
	29.2	>96 cm	? Crucial threshold diabetes

distribution is an important variable predicting the increased health risks of obesity. Adipose tissue has depot-specific differences. Adipose tissue and dietary saturated fatty acids correlate with an increase in fat cell size and number, but there is no significant association between omega-9 acids content and adipocyte size.[21] Furthermore, omega-9 adipose tissue fatty acid content is inversely associated with fat cell number, suggesting that this type of fatty acid could limit hyperplasia in obese populations. Long-chain fatty acids cross the plasma membrane via a protein-mediated mechanism involving one or more binding proteins. One key long-chain fatty acid transporter in muscle is regulated by insulin. The expression and/or subcellular distribution of this insulin-regulated long-chain fatty acids transporter is altered in obesity and type 2 diabetes. In subcutaneous adipose tissue, its expression is upregulated in obesity and type 2 diabetes.[22] As this transporter's expression is not different in lean, overweight and obese subjects, and was only increased in type 2 diabetics, it is possible that visceral adipose tissue may respond in a less dynamic manner to metabolic disturbances than subcutaneous adipose tissue.

The gene expression profiles of subcutaneous adipose tissue in lean and overweight subjects are distinctly different.[20] Increasing consumption of short-chain omega-3 polyunsaturated fatty acids (C18:2 and C18:3), conjugated linoleic acid and medium-chain triglycerides (C12:0) lowered expression of genes related to energy metabolism in lean subjects. In contrast, in the majority of overweight subjects, expression of lipid metabolism genes was upregulated while expression of inflammatory genes was downregulated.[20] Genes involved in energy metabolism and/or in encoding mitochondrial proteins are expressed at a higher level in adipose tissue from lean compared to overweight subjects. On the other hand, genes involved in defence response, intracellular signalling and cell adhesion are expressed at higher levels in adipose tissue from overweight compared to lean subjects.[20] Expression of inflammation-related genes and leptin are higher and expression of adiponectin is lower in adipose tissue from overweight than from lean subjects. Adiponectin and leptin perform complementary actions and can have additive effects. Adiponectin, a hormone produced and secreted exclusively by adipocytes, influences lipid and glucose metabolism, the body's response to insulin and has an anti-inflammatory effect.

It has been suggested that obesity corresponds to a subclinical inflammatory condition that promotes production of pro-inflammatory factors involved in the pathogenesis of insulin resistance.[23] In most obese patients, obesity is associated with low-grade inflammation of white adipose tissue resulting from chronic activation of the innate immune system. Several factors, including leptin, tumour necrosis factor-alpha (TNF-alpha) and interleukin-6, derived from adipocytes and macrophages infiltrating adipose tissue, are overproduced during obesity and probably contribute to the pathogenesis of insulin resistance. Conversely, expression and plasma levels of adiponectin are downregulated during obesity. Adiponectin inhibits liver neoglucogenesis, promotes fatty acid oxidation in skeletal muscle and counteracts the pro-inflammatory effects of TNF-alpha on the arterial wall. Weight loss is associated with a reduction in macrophage infiltration of adipose tissue and an improvement in the genetically determined inflammatory profile.[23] Chronic low-grade inflammation in adipose tissue could lead to insulin resistance, impaired glucose tolerance and diabetes.

Individual responses to dietary lipids in overweight subjects are variable and correlate more closely to obesity phenotype markers such as waist–hip ratio and fat percentage than to BMI.[20] Dietary intervention in two overweight subjects with a similar BMI upregulated expression of mitochondrial genes in the one with the lowest waist–hip ratio, and downregulated expression in the one with the highest waist–hip ratio. Individuals, classified as overweight on the basis of their BMI, are heterogeneous in their response to dietary intervention. Waist–hip ratio and waist circumference are more specific markers for body fat distribution and presence of central or upper body obesity. These phenotype markers appear to offer a more precise link between body fat distribution and response to nutritional intervention than BMI.

The metabolic syndrome is a common and complex disorder combining abdominal obesity, insulin resistance, dyslipidaemia and hypertension. More than one in five adult Americans have the metabolic syndrome,[24] and in those over 50 years of age the prevalence approaches 50%.[25] Over 50% of Australian adults have at least one component of this dangerous quartet.[7] The metabolic syndrome with its constellation of interrelated metabolic risk factors appears to directly promote the development of diabetes and cardiovascular disease.

Abdominal obesity

It has been postulated that the metabolic syndrome may be an adipose tissue disease different from obesity and characterized by inflammation. Clinically detectable systemic inflammatory markers such as high-sensitivity C-reactive protein and insulin resistance are postulated to reflect histological changes in adipose tissue.[26] Abdominal obesity, a characteristic of the metabolic syndrome, has subcutaneous and visceral components. Loss of visceral fat improves metabolic control in type 2 diabetes and reduces the risk of cardiovascular complications, while abdominal subcutaneous fat, although less lipolytically active than visceral fat, may be an important contributor to insulin resistance. In addition to abdominal obesity, the metabolic syndrome features atherogenic dyslipidaemia, hypertension, insulin resistance, with or without glucose intolerance, and a prothrombotic and pro-inflammatory state. Hyperinsulinaemia coupled with an atherogenic dyslipidaemia is characterized by low levels of HDL and increased in-vivo LDL oxidation, higher levels of circulating oxidized LDL and small LDL particles plus elevated triglyceride.[27] The metabolic syndrome is a primary risk factor for diabetes and cardiovascular disease.

Severe obesity is associated with suppressed expression of both adiponectin and its receptors in subcutaneous and visceral adipose tissue.[28] In visceral adipose tissue, the expression of adiponectin and its receptors are specifically linked with hyperinsulinaemia and dyslipidaemia.[28] Abdominal obesity identifies a subgroup of overweight and obese persons at particular risk. Waist circumference provides an indication of abdominal obesity; it predicts cardiovascular and coronary artery disease better than BMI.[29]

Abdominal obesity is present when waist circumference, measured round the umbilicus, exceeds the maximum measurement around the hips. A larger waist circumference identifies people at increased cardiovascular risk independent of body weight. Both BMI and waist circumference are positively associated with diastolic blood pressure and total and LDL cholesterol levels, and negatively associated with HDL cholesterol.[30] In fact, BMI, waist to hip circumference ratio, and waist circumference are all powerful independent predictors of type 2 diabetes (see Table 23.4). The risk of chronic disease increases as BMI and abdominal obesity increase. In addition to BMI and waist circumference, other anthropometric measures may also be used.[30] An increased waist to hip ratio and waist to height ratio, like a high BMI and/or enlarged waist circumference, correlate with increased glycaemia, especially after an oral glucose load. Waist circumference shows the strongest correlation with fasting glycaemia in woman; BMI the strongest relationship in men. Glycaemia, 2 hours after a glucose load, correlates best with BMI and weight–height ratio. Weight–height ratio is the most useful diagnostic tool in the risk assessment of impaired glucose tolerance, but waist circumference offers the better diagnostic choice for risk assessment of diabetes type 2. On the other hand, waist–hip ratio

Table 23.4 Anthropometric indices for type 2 diabetes
Guesstimates of the best cut-off points suggesting higher diabetes type 2 risk:

	Men	Women
BMI	27.9	29.2
Waist to hip ratio	0.97	0.91
Waist to height ratio	0.57	0.62
Waist circumference	99 cm	96 cm

See also Waist:hip ratio http://www.healthcalculators.org/calculators/waist_hip.asp

has the highest sensitivity, specificity and accuracy to predict cardiovascular risk factors. The usefulness of various indices varies in different population groups. Waist–height is the more valuable obesity index for predicting diabetes, hypertension and lipidaemia in Bangladesh.[31]

The optimal cut-offs to predict diabetes, hypertension or dyslipidaemia are at variance in different population groups. In Mexicans these are:[32]

- BMI 25.2 to 26.6 kg/m^2 in both men and women
- waist circumference 90 cm in men; 85 cm in women
- waist–hip ratio about 0.90 in men; 0.85 in women
- waist–height ratio 52.5 in men; 53–53.5 in women.

In Taiwan, optimal cut-off points of anthropometric indices in men and women respectively are:[33]

- BMI of 23.6 and 22.1
- waist circumference 80.5 and 71.5 cm
- waist–hip ratio 0.85 and 0.76
- waist–height ratio 0.48 and 0.45.

Tables 23.3 and 23.4 suggest cut-off points that may be helpful for Western society. It should be noted that some increase in adiposity is considered acceptable with increasing age. However, in European populations, men with a waist circumference of 94 cm and women with a waist circumference of 80 cm should gain no further weight, and men with a waist circumference of 102 cm and women with a waist circumference of 88 cm or more should actively reduce their weight. Overall, reasonable target anthropometric parameters may be BMI 22.6 kg/m^2 in men and 21.1 kg/m^2 in women; waist circumference 95 cm or less in men and 80 cm or less in women; and a waist–hip ratio under 0.9 for men and under 0.85 for women. Definitive risk assessment requires a blood glucose assessment. Anthropometric measures are red flags for diabetes; the disease is present when blood glucose levels exceed specified limits. Diabetes is diagnosed when a blood sugar level of over 126 mg/dL (7 mmol/L) is found on at least two occasions after an overnight fast. Fasting sugar levels run between 70 and 110 mg/dL in normoglycaemic people. In addition to random and fasting blood sugar assessments, an oral glucose tolerance test can be performed to confirm the diagnosis. See Table 23.5. In a diabetic, glucose levels rise and fall more rapidly than normal.

The prevalence of cardiovascular risk factors increases with increasing blood glucose levels. In normoglycaemic Australians, the prevalence of:[34]

Table 23.5 Interpreting blood glucose levels

Interpretation	Blood glucose	
	mg/dL	mmol/L
Normal	110 or less	6.1 or less
Impaired fasting glucose (IFG)	>110 but <126	>6.1 but <7
Impaired glucose tolerance 2 hours postprandial 75 g glucose	140 or more but <200*	≥7.8–<11*
Diabetes	200 or more* 126 or more†	11.0 or more* 7.0 or more†
Gestational diabetes‡	> 165	>9.2

*On two occasions of casual readings; consideration is being given to lowering the upper level to 180 mg/dL
†Fasting reading on two occasions
‡Fasting blood glucose >105 mg/dL (5.8 mmol/L), 1 hour >190 mg/dL (10.5 mmol/L) and 3 hour >145 mg/dL (8.0 mmol/L)
Escalating risk for:
- retinopathy – fasting plasma glucose level >116 mg/dL (6.45 mmol/L)
- other complications – fasting plasma glucose level >126 mg/dL (7.0 mmol/L)
Blood glucose treatment targets:
- FBG test: < 5.6 mmol/L (100 mg/dL)
- OGTT test: <7.8 mmol/L. (140 mg/dL)

- obesity is 16.2%, increasing to 46.2% in diabetics
- hypertension is 21.1%, increasing to 68.6% in diabetics
- an LDL cholesterol of 3.5 mmol/L or greater is 47.3%, increasing to 63.8% in diabetics
- HDL cholesterol levels under 1.0 mmol/L is 4.9%, increasing to 39.1% in diabetics
- triglycerides equal to or greater than 2.0 mmol/L is 19.6%, increasing to 56.7% in diabetics.

Intervention

Individuals who are obese in middle age have a higher risk of hospitalization and mortality from diabetes and ischaemic heart disease as they age than do those who are normal weight.[35] As shown in Table 23.2, health risk escalates as weight increases. Health benefits accrue as weight is lost. Weight loss is a primary intervention target offering health benefits beyond metabolic improvements.[36] Persons with a BMI of over 25 kg/m^2, by losing 5 kg (2 BMI units), reduced their later onset of knee osteoarthritis by 50% if female, or 25% if male.[37] Weight reductions of as little as 4 or 5 kg may normalize blood pressure;[38] on the other hand, weight gain over a 1- to 2-month period is associated with a predictable rise in arterial pressure. Over 80% of type 2 diabetes and ischaemic heart disease cases could potentially be prevented by changes in lifestyle factors such as maintaining an ideal body weight, diet and physical activity.[39] Unfortunately, American physicians rate treatment of obesity as significantly less effective than therapies for 90% of chronic conditions.[40] The success of weight loss programmes can nonetheless be increased by formulating a personalized weight management programme that enhances self-efficacy for specific behaviour changes and encourages self-monitoring.[41,42] **Handout 23.2** outlines various methods for determining current body weight and **Handout 23.3** provides information on the health implications of being overweight or obese and outlines intervention options. **Handout 23.4** provides the information needed to determine the energy required to achieve weight loss. As shown in Table 23.6, the basal energy requirement is

Table 23.6 Adjusted energy requirements

Basal energy requirement (kilojoules) (BER) = 100 × ideal body weight for females

Basal energy requirement (kilojoules) (BER) = 110 × ideal body weight for males

Age-adjusted energy requirements

Younger persons are judged to require more energy than older persons

Age (years)	Basal kJ adjustment	
	Males	Females
25	×1.1	×1.1
45	×1.0	×1.0
65	×0.8	×0.85

Activity-adjusted energy requirements

Energy requirements differ depending on the individual's lifestyle

Activity level	Adjustment to basal kJ requirement
Sedentary	+30%
Moderately active	+50%
Strenuous	+100%

Energy requirements adjusted for body frame

Persons with a large body frame have a greater energy requirement than those with small frames. Energy intake therefore needs to be adjusted according to one's stature

Wrist measurement*	Body frame	Adjustment to basal kJ
Middle finger and thumb overlap	Small	−10%
Middle finger and thumb meet	Medium	−
Middle finger and thumb fail to meet	Large	+10%

*Assess wrist size by clasping your wrist in your hand.

modified by body frame, age and activity levels. Weight loss is essentially achieved through dietary and exercise lifestyle changes. **Handout 23.5** provides general guidelines on prudent eating choices, while **Handouts 23.6** and **23.7** outline a comprehensive weight loss regimen. **Handout 23.6** has been developed for those who wish to achieve weight loss by focusing predominantly on reducing their energy intake. **Handout 23.7** has been developed for those who wish to achieve weight loss by focusing predominantly on increasing their energy expenditure. Both handouts provide guidance on how to determine weight loss goals, set safe weekly weight loss targets, and use diet and exercise to achieve weight loss goals. **Handout 23.6** includes a diary for monitoring food intake and output; **Handout 23.7** includes a diary for monitoring energy expenditure. In either case, a combination of dietary vigilance and increased exercise should be observed. Regardless of the preferred dominant weight loss strategy, awareness of food nutrient and energy density in food selection (Table 23.7) should be combined with an appreciation of the relationship between various activities and energy expenditure (Table 23.8). Starting off using a self-awareness diary to determine baseline behaviours provides a good baseline for programme development. The self-monitoring diaries provide a record of progress.

Dietary strategies

An independent relationship between risk factors of the metabolic syndrome and habitual dietary patterns has been identified.[43] The habitual dietary patterns of women were designated Heart Healthier, Lighter Eating, Wine and Moderate Eating, Higher Fat, and Empty Calories. The diet with the strongest association with the metabolic syndrome was the Empty Calories diet with its high levels of refined grains, desserts, high-fat animal proteins (including meats and mixed-protein dishes), whole milk, eggs, animal fats, sweets, and salty snacks and the minimal levels of low- and non-fat dairy products. The Empty Calories diet is rich in energy-dense, and deficient in nutrient-dense, foods (see Table 23.7).

Dietary patterns

While it is clear that a high-fat, refined carbohydrate, empty-calorie diet is not conducive to weight loss or health promotion, it is less clear which diet

Table 23.7 Nutrient-dense and energy-dense foods

Nutrient-dense foods

Nutrient density	Food sources
Very high	Eggs, green leafy and yellow vegetables, liver, milk, oysters
High	Beans, cheese, oranges, pork
Medium	Bread, chicken, fish, steak
Low	Apples, beer, margarine
Very low	Butter, polished rice, soft drinks, spirits, sugar, wine

Energy-dense foods

Energy density	Food sources
Very high (>2000 kJ/100 g or 100 mL)	Cream-filled biscuits, butter, cooking oil, margarine, nuts
High (1000–1999 kJ/100 g or 100 mL)	Plain biscuits and cakes, cheese, grilled sausages, fatty lamb or steak, honey, sugar, spirits, confections
Medium (400–999 kJ/100 g or 100 mL)	Boiled egg, bread, fried fish, grilled lean lamb or steak, canned salmon, spaghetti, boiled rice
Low (200–399 kJ/100 g or 100 mL)	Apple, fruit salad, avocado, creamed soup, milk, jelly, potato, steamed fish
Very low (<200 kJ/100 g or 100 mL)	French beans, broccoli, carrot, marrow, pumpkin, skimmed milk, clear soup, beer

4.2 kJ =1.0 calorie (kcal)

most effectively achieves these ends. Comparison of the Atkins diet (high in protein plus restricted carbohydrate) with the Zone macronutrient balanced diet (energy ratio of carbohydrate:fat:protein of 40:30:30), the calorie-restricted diet of Weight Watchers, and the fat-restricted Ornish diet, found that all the diets modestly reduced body weight and several cardiac risk factors without significant changes in blood glucose or blood pressure at 1 year.[44] Furthermore, adherence to all four diets was low. As weight control is a lifelong endeavour,

Table 23.8 Energy and exercise

Activity	Energy utilization per minute	
	Kilojoules	Calories (kcal)
Sleeping	4	0.9
Sitting	6	1.4
Standing	10	2.4
Light gardening	10–20	2.4–2.8
Household work with modern appliances	10–20	2.4–2.8
Gymnastics	10–20	2.4–2.8
Slow walking	10–20	2.4–2.8
Golf/bowling	10–20	2.4–2.8
Heavy gardening	20–30	4.8–7.2
Ballroom dancing	20–30	4.8–7.2
Fast walking	20–30	4.8–7.2
Tennis/cycling/swimming	20–30	4.8–7.2
Jogging	30–40	7.2–9.6
Climbing stairs	30–40	7.2–9.6
Country dancing	30–40	7.2–9.6
Fast swimming	40	9.6
Hill climbing	40	9.6
Cross-country running	40	9.6

good dietary adherence is essential. One diet that repeatedly demonstrates good adherence is the Mediterranean diet.

The typical Mediterranean-type diet includes daily consumption of non-refined cereals and grains, vegetables (2–3 serves), fruits (6), olive oil and dairy products (1–2); a weekly intake of fish (4–5), poultry (3–4), olives, pulses, and nuts (3), potatoes, eggs and sweets (3–4); and each month 4 or 5 serves of red meat/meat products. There is increasing evidence of health benefits from diets rich in fruits, vegetables, legumes, and whole grains which include fish, nuts, and low-fat dairy products. The Mediterranean diet is associated with reduced odds of having hyper-cholesterolaemia, hypertension, diabetes and obesity

among elderly people.[45] Compared with a non-Mediterranean diet, firm adherence to the Mediterranean diet is associated with a 51% lower risk of obesity and a 59% lower risk of central obesity.[46] Insulin sensitivity, total cholesterol and systolic blood pressure are independently, albeit modestly, correlated with Mediterranean diet in people with excess body weight.[47] The Mediterranean diet is a good choice for diabetics and prediabetics. Although the inverse association between a Mediterranean diet and indices of glucose homeostasis are only observed in normoglycaemic people,[48] adding extra nuts or olive oil to the standard diet can further reduce the prevalence of the metabolic syndrome.[49] After 1 year, the prevalence of the metabolic syndrome was reduced by 2% in those on the Mediterranean diet, 13.7% in those who added 30 g of mixed nuts daily, and 6.7% in those who supplemented the Mediterranean diet with 1 litre of olive oil weekly. It has been suggested that Mediterranean-type diets could serve as an anti-inflammatory dietary pattern helping counteract diseases related to chronic inflammation, including visceral obesity, type 2 diabetes and the metabolic syndrome.[50]

Energy considerations

Whatever diet is followed, the basic requirement for successful weight loss is that energy output exceeds energy intake. A moderate decrease in energy intake (−2.5 MJ/day) could result in slow sustained weight loss of around 2.5 kg a month. Small changes in energy intake and output seem to have a major impact on obesity risk. Increasing daily energy intake by a single can of a sweetened carbonated drink (0.50 MJ) over a 10-year period in a constant environment could theoretically add 50 kg of weight.[51] Conversely, reducing daily intake by a nominal amount of energy may help to prevent weight gain. It has been suggested that reducing energy intake by eliminating the equivalent of one can of sugar-sweetened carbonated drink daily would prevent excessive weight gain in most adult Americans.[52] The impact on weight gain is reduced when diet sodas are chosen, as they incorporate artificial sweeteners (see Table 9.1). It is worth being aware that 1 g of fat, regardless of whether it is of animal or vegetable origin, provides 39 kJ (9 kcal). The energy density of alcohol is 29 kJ/g (7 kcal/g); of carbohydrates, 16 kJ/g (4 kcal/g); and of protein, 17 kJ/g (4 kcal/g). It has been suggested that hypocaloric weight-loss diets should be moderate in carbohydrate (35% to 55% of total energy), rich in fibre (25 g/day), and moderate in fat (25% to 35% of energy) and protein (25% to 30% of energy).[53]

Protein appears to promote short-term weight loss, possibly due to increased satiety. A systematic review of randomized investigations on the effects of high-protein diets on dietary thermogenesis, satiety, body weight and fat loss concluded that there is convincing evidence that a higher protein intake increases thermogenesis and satiety compared with diets of lower protein content.[54] The weight of evidence also suggests that high-protein meals lead to reduced subsequent energy intake. Although the effect of chronic high protein intake on glucose metabolism is inconclusive, randomized, controlled trials continue to show comparable, if not superior, effects of high-protein diets compared with lower-protein diets on weight loss, preservation of lean body mass and improvement in several cardiovascular risk factors for up to 12 months.[55] High-protein diets produce more favourable cholesterol ratios. Excessively high-protein diets are not without risk. Kidney damage due to excretion of high levels of sulphur-containing amino acids may occur. Particularly at-risk individuals may be those with obesity, metabolic syndrome and type 2 diabetes mellitus.[56] Compliance is also an issue.

Specific food choices

While no dietary supplements have convincingly been proven to achieve and maintain weight loss over the long term, certain foods deserve consideration in a weight-loss regimen. Isocaloric substitution of yoghurt (calcium content 1100 mg/day) for other foods may augment fat loss and reduce central adiposity during energy restriction.[57] Meta-analysis confirms higher calcium intake consistently results in lower body fat and/or body weight, and reduced weight gain at midlife.[58] A fairly consistently dose–response effect was reported, with each 300-mg increment in regular calcium intake resulting in a 2.5–3.0 kg lower body weight in adults and approximately 1 kg less body fat in children. Increasing calcium intake by the equivalent of two dairy servings per day may reduce the risk of overweight substantially. Dairy products are frequently fortified with vitamin D, and plasma 25(OH)D concentrations are inversely associated with fasting plasma glucose and insulin concentrations.[59] Vitamin-D-fortified products may therefore be particularly beneficial choices for reducing the risk of type 2 diabetes. Grapefruit is another good dietary choice. A 12-week study found that half a fresh grapefruit eaten before meals was associated with significant weight loss (1.6 kg compared to 0.3 kg with placebo) and insulin resistance was improved.[60] Another 12-week study of overweight and obese adults found that those receiving supplements of oligofructose lost an average of 1 kg, compared with an average gain of almost 0.5 kg in the placebo group.[61] Although levels of ghrelin were suppressed and peptide YY levels increased, no effects were observed on the satiety hormone glucagon-like peptide 1. Prebiotic fibres have been associated with lower levels of the hunger hormone ghrelin, and higher levels of a hormone in the gut, peptide YY (PYY), linked to increased feelings of fullness (satiety). Certainly, the oligofructose group reported a reduction in caloric intake, in addition to decreased levels of glucose and a mirroring effect on insulin concentrations.

Due to the complexity of chronic conditions like the metabolic syndrome, tailored dietary approaches beyond macronutrient ratio modification may be necessary – the success of the Mediterranean diet may be attributable not only to its macronutrient content but also to its rich content of phytochemicals.[62] Prudent eating choices that tend to decrease the intake of high-energy foods and increase the intake of nutrient-rich foods are listed in **Handout 23.5**. Hot lifestyle tips are to eat breakfast, take smaller serves, don't snack between meals, chew food well and avoid grocery shopping when hungry. **Handout 23.8** suggests wise choices when eating at home and **Handout 23.9** makes suggestions for dining out.

Overall, studies have shown:[63]

- A diet that is individually planned to help create a deficit of 500 to 1000 kcal/day should be part of any programme to achieve a weekly weight loss of 0.5–1 kg (1–2 lb). An average weight-loss goal of 10% is recommended for obese patients.

- Low-energy diets are effective, reducing waist circumference and total body weight by an average of 8% over a period of 6 months.

- Reducing both dietary fat and carbohydrate facilitates calorie reduction.

- Herbal products and dietary supplements promoted for weight loss currently lack sufficient supporting efficacy and safety data for any to be recommended.

- Physical activity is useful, indeed essential, in weight control.

Physical activity

To maintain weight, energy input must balance energy output; to lose weight, energy output must exceed energy intake. Energy intake is modified by dietary consumption and energy output by physical activity. There are basically two approaches: those of programmed and lifestyle exercise.[63]

Programmed exercise

In programmed exercise, patients implement a regular exercise regimen of walking, swimming, or cycling.[63] In general, 30 to 45 minutes of exercise 3 to 5 days each week is recommended, although more exercise at greater intensity affords additional benefits. To expend 420 kJ/day (100 kcal/day), it is necessary to walk slowly for an hour or briskly for 30 minutes. Thirty minutes of moderate-intensity activity on most days of the week, or the equivalent of expending approximately 1000 kcal in activity weekly, does not appear sufficient for weight loss and maintenance. Data from epidemiologic studies and randomized trials suggest the daily activity requirement to maintain reduced body weight is 60 to 90 minutes of moderate-intensity, totalling a weekly activity energy expenditure of 2500 to 2800 kcal.[64] Furthermore, the duration of exercise (at least 150 minutes/week of walking) may be more important than exercise intensity for achieving/maintaining weight loss.[65] In sedentary women, the threshold of energy expenditure required for weight maintenance appears to be 80 minutes/day of moderate activity or 35 minutes/day of vigorous activity.[66]

A compendium has been developed that provides a system linking energy expenditure with activity.[67] Energy expenditure can be expressed in metabolic equivalent tasks (MET). Energy expenditure per kilogram body weight can be estimated for specific activities by type or MET intensity. Physical activities and their intensity are defined as the ratio of work metabolic rate to a standard resting or basal metabolic rate (BMR). One (1) MET represents the energy used when sitting quietly and is roughly equivalent to the BMR. The duration of activity required to use 150 kcal (630 kJ) is 150 METs. Moderate-intensity physical activity refers to any activity that burns 3.5 to 7 kcal per minute. These levels are equal to the energy a healthy individual might expend while walking briskly, mowing the lawn, dancing, swimming for recreation, or bicycling. Vigorous-intensity physical activity refers to any activity that burns more than 7 kcal/minute. These levels are equal to the energy a healthy individual might burn while jogging, engaging in heavy yard work, participating in high-impact aerobic dancing, swimming continuous laps, or bicycling uphill.[68] See Table 23.8. The MET system, although a useful guide, is imperfect. A study on 12-year-old girls found body weight was a statistically significant predictor of the MET for walking but not the MET of sitting or standing.[69] The use of average MET values to estimate the energy cost of walking could result in an underestimation of their energy cost in heavier girls and an overestimation in lighter girls.

Lifestyle exercise

In addition to programmed exercise, lifestyle exercise or physical activity levels need to be considered.[62] Given the increasing pace of technological change, modern man is becoming increasingly inactive. This causes concern as studies suggest inactivity initiates unique cellular processes that are qualitatively different from the exercise responses. It seem likely that there are unique molecular, physiologic, and clinical effects of too much sitting (inactivity physiology) that are disparate from the responses caused by structured exercise (exercise physiology).[70] There is a dose–response relationship between the sedentary time and health risk; interrupting sedentary time reduces metabolic risk.[71,72] Regardless of their physical activity level, the risk of the metabolic syndrome is positively associated with the time women 45 years of age and older spend watching television or doing computer activities.[73] Maintaining a high daily level of low-intensity activity is emerging as important. Independently of undertaking moderate–vigorous physical activity, sedentary behaviour increases the risk for type 2 diabetes, triglyceridaemia and low HDL levels.[70]

Skeletal muscle lipoprotein lipase is an important protein for controlling plasma triglyceride catabolism, HDL cholesterol, and other metabolic risk factors. Low lipoprotein lipase has been associated with blunted plasma triglyceride uptake and reduced plasma HDL levels and may affect the metabolic syndrome, diabetes-induced dyslipidaemia, hypertension and coronary artery disease. Lipoprotein lipase helps to prevent diet-induced adiposity and insulin resistance in transgenic rabbits. Skeletal muscle lipoprotein lipase increases following short-term exercise training in humans and animals. Furthermore, experimentally reducing normal spontaneous standing and ambulatory time has a much greater effect on lipo-protein lipase regulation than adding vigorous exercise training on top of the normal level of non-exercise activity. The sum of daily muscular contractions during non-exercise activity requires a greater energy demand than a bolus of continuous exercise. There is a wide range in the energy demand of non-exercise activity thermogenesis. Even brisk walking 5 days a week or running 35 miles a week produces less energy expenditure (and fewer muscle contractions) than intermediate amounts of non-exercise activity thermogenesis. The energy expenditure of 'standing workers' is at least double that of seated workers. Estimations from prolonged TV and computer time led to the conclusion that too much sitting can more than double the risk for metabolic syndrome. Each extra hour of TV viewing each day correlates with a 26% increase in the prevalence of metabolic syndrome in women. The negative effect of an extra hour of sedentary TV viewing roughly neutralizes the positive effect of 30 minutes of extra physical activity.[74] Whereas total physical activity of at least 2.5 hours weekly is associated with a reduced prevalence of both insulin resistance and dyslipidaemia, TV viewing in excess of 14 hours a week is associated with an increased risk of insulin resistance, obesity and dyslipidaemia in both men and women.[74] Weight gain following a successful weight loss programme is positively associated with time spent watching television.[65] Furthermore, while the association between TV viewing and waist circumference in preschoolers and young adults may be partially explained by food and beverage consumption during TV viewing,[75] it cannot be explained by a reduction in overall leisure-time physical activity.[76] Substituting even light-intensity activity for television viewing or other sedentary time may be a practical and achievable preventive strategy to reduce the risk of type 2 diabetes and cardiovascular disease.[77] Metabolic syndrome, excessive adiposity, weight gain and poor glucose management in diabetes are all directly related to sitting time and inversely related to a lack of non-exercise activity.[73] Independent of moderate–vigorous physical activity, maintaining a high daily level of low-intensity activity is emerging as important for a number of metabolic risk factors, including type 2 diabetes, triglycerides and HDL.[73]

An integrated approach is needed. Regardless of sedentary time, moderate to vigorous leisure-time physical activity remains inversely associated with the risk of the metabolic syndrome.[71] Since both behavioural changes might provide additional effects, efforts should be made to reduce sedentary behaviour while promoting moderate to vigorous physical activity.[78] Overall physical activity can be increased by lifestyle measures such as using the stairs rather than an elevator and avoiding the use of a car for short distances. Three 10-minute periods of activity have about the same benefit as two 15-minute periods or one 30-minute period.[73] Furthermore, a combined diet-plus-exercise programme provides greater long-term weight loss than a diet-only programme.[79] Regrettably, both diet-only and diet-plus-exercise programmes are associated with partial weight regain.

Benefit: risk ratio of weight loss

Weight loss carries a substantial risk of regaining weight. Weight cycling or yo-yo dieting is associated with greater weight gain, less physical activity, and a higher prevalence of binge eating.[80] In some people, subsequent weight loss is more difficult and weight more readily regained.[81] Weight cycling is strongly and consistently linked with negative health outcomes, particularly all-cause mortality and mortality from coronary heart disease.[81,82] Whereas weight stability is associated with higher natural killer (NK) cell cytotoxicity, weight cycling alters the number and proportion of NK cells.[83] Loss of 10 lb or more on more than one occasion predictably results in decreased NK cytotoxicity. Skeletal damage is a major concern. Weight fluctuations of 5 or 6 kg alter bone mass and produce permanent micro-architectural damage.[84] Weight loss, even without recycling, of 10% or more from maximum weight among both middle-aged and older women is recognized as an important risk factor for hip fractures.[85] Weight cycling may have negative psychological and behavioural consequences ranging from psychological maladjustment to disordered eating behaviour.[81]

In long-term follow-up, weight fluctuations are a major risk factor for all-cause mortality in middle-aged men; however, stable obesity does not appear to further increase mortality in men aged 55–74 years.[86] Risks associated with weight cycling can be minimized by controlling weight through a lifestyle change rather than a temporary weight loss diet. Furthermore, modification of lifestyle that controls weight improves health.[87] Concerns about weight fluctuation and excess mortality do not override the potential benefits of weight loss in obese patients.[88] The benefits of prudent weight loss outweigh the risks. A major benefit of weight loss is modulation of the metabolic syndrome with a reduced risk of diabetes type 2, ischemic heart disease and hypertension.

Diabetes

Type 2 diabetes mellitus is characterized by varying degrees of insulin resistance in peripheral tissue and an insulin secretory defect of the beta cell. In the US, complications of diabetes include:[6]

- Death. Diabetes was the seventh leading cause of death listed on US death certificates in 2006. Overall, the risk for death among people with diabetes is about twice that of people without diabetes of similar age.
- High blood pressure. In 2003–2004, 75% of adults with self-reported diabetes were on antihypertensive medication or had blood pressure greater than or equal to 130/80 mmHg.
- Blindness. Diabetes is the leading cause of new cases of blindness among adults aged 20–74 years.
- Kidney disease. Diabetes is the leading cause of kidney failure, accounting for 44% of new cases in 2005.
- Nervous system damage is present in 60% to 70% of people with diabetes. Almost 30% of people with diabetes aged 40 years or older have impaired sensation in their feet.
- Amputations. More than 60% of nontraumatic lower-limb amputations occur in people with diabetes.

Diabetes screening

Tailored lifestyle intervention can prevent progression of diabetes in at least 60% of cases; however, as type 2 can go undetected for 12 years, 50% of diabetics present with complications of the disease.[3] Although overweight children have a higher prevalence of risk factors for adverse health such as insulin resistance, elevated blood lipid levels, increased blood pressure, and impaired glucose tolerance, the U.S. Preventive Services Task Force (USPSTF) felt there was insufficient evidence to recommend routine screening of children and adolescents for overweight.[89] The USPSTF, however, does recommend that asymptomatic adults with sustained blood pressure (treated or untreated) of over 135/80 should be screened for type 2 diabetes by their clinicians. Furthermore, a plasma glucose test for everybody at age 45, repeated every 3 years thereafter, is suggested.[89] More frequent testing is recommended if one or more of the following risk factors is present:[89]

- obesity: $\geq$120% of desirable body weight or BMI $\geq$27 kg/m^2. Waist measurements of over 100 cm for men and over 90 cm for women are also of concern[66]
- having a first-degree relative with diabetes mellitus
- membership of high-risk ethnic group (black, Hispanic, Native American, Asian)
- a personal history of gestational diabetes mellitus or delivering a baby weighing more than 4032 g (9 lb)
- raised blood pressure ($\geq$140/90 mmHg)
- low HDL cholesterol level ($\leq$35 mg/dL [0.90 mmol/L]) and/or raised triglyceride level ($\geq$250 mg/dL [2.83 mmol/L])
- a history of impaired glucose tolerance (IGT) or impaired fasting glucose (IFG) on prior testing.

People with prediabetes have impaired fasting glucose and/or impaired glucose tolerance. They are at increased risk of developing type 2 diabetes, heart disease and stroke.[6]

Any patient with two fasting plasma glucose levels of 126 mg/dL (7.0 mmol/L) or greater is considered to have diabetes mellitus.[90] Complications rise rapidly above these cut-off points. The risk of retinopathy increases once fasting plasma glucose rises above 109 to 116 mg/dL (6.05 to 6.45 mmol/L) or when the result of a 2-hour postprandial glucose test is higher than 150 to 180 mg/dL (8.3 to 10.0 mmol/L). A random or fasting blood glucose under 100 mg/dL (5.5 mmol/L) probably excludes diabetes.

Therapy is indicated for all persons diagnosed with diabetes on venipuncture. The targets for blood sugar control are:

- a fasting blood sugar of 4.4–6.1 mmol/L
- a postprandial blood sugar level of 4.4–8.0 mol/L
- a glycosylated haemoglobin (HbA$_{1c}$) of less than 6.5%. Glycosylated haemoglobin is used as a guide to the nature of intervention required. In diabetics, an HbA$_{1c}$ level below 7.0% would generally be treated with diet and exercise, regardless of the diagnosis of blood glucose levels. An HbA$_{1c}$ level of 7.0% or higher usually requires pharmacological intervention. The presence of ketones in the urine suggests the need for insulin therapy.

Improved glycaemic control in type 2 diabetes reduces complications. In general, every percentage point drop in HbA_{1c} blood test results (e.g. from 8.0% to 7.0%) reduces the risk of microvascular complications by 40%.

Risk reduction

Age, followed by weight, is the major predictor of type 2 diabetes. Age aggravates the complications of diabetes (see Table 23.9). Unlike age, weight is a modifiable risk factor! The prevalence of type 2 diabetes in obese adults is three to seven times that in normal-weight adults, and those with a BMI of 35 are 20 times as likely to develop diabetes as are those with a BMI between 18.5 and 24.9.[91] Furthermore, weight gain during adulthood is directly correlated with an increased risk of type 2 diabetes. Weight gain of 5.0 to 7.9 kg over an 18-year period increases the risk of diabetes 1.9-fold in women; a weight increase of 8.0 to 10.9 kg increases the risk of diabetes 2.7-fold.[92] On the other hand, weight loss over 5.0 kg halves the risk of this disease. These findings were independent of a family history of diabetes.

Early detection of, and lifestyle modification to rectify, abdominal obesity can reduce the prevalence of type 2 diabetes. **Handout 23.10** lists orange and red flags for diabetes type 2.

Diabetes prevention

About 80% of type 2 diabetics are or have been obese. One of the major benefits of weight loss is modulation of the metabolic syndrome, with a reduced risk of diabetes, ischaemic heart disease and hypertension. Despite a lack of knowledge regarding effective and safe interventions to promote weight management for those who have already developed type 2 diabetes, lifestyle modification remains the foremost strategy for preventing and controlling this disorder.[93] Overall, weight loss strategies using dietary, physical activity, or behavioural interventions produce significant improvements in weight among persons with prediabetes and a significant decrease in diabetes incidence.[94] Multicomponent interventions are particularly promising.[95] Behavioural modification of lifestyle, especially self-control over daily energy balance, plays a crucial role in long-term success of weight management.[96] Self-monitoring of weight, dietary intake, and daily physical activity on a regular basis are important determinants of weight loss maintenance. A consistent eating pattern, including regularly eating breakfast, influences the outcome of weight management. Compared to standard dietary and exercise advice, intensive lifestyle intervention to reduce body weight, dietary energy and saturated fat and to increase physical activity and dietary fibre achieved a 43% reduction in relative risk of developing diabetes or its complications.[97] In general, the cost of preventing type 2 diabetes using low-fat diets plus exercise programmes, with or without behaviour therapy, is comparable to that of drug treatments for individuals at risk of obesity-related illness.[98] For maximum benefit, standard weight loss programmes need to be modified for prediabetic and type 2 diabetes management.

Exercise

Physical activity of moderate intensity, 30 minutes or more in duration, performed 5 days a week contributes 0.5 kg of weight loss each month.[96] Daily exercise without caloric restriction achieves substantial reduction in insulin resistance and total, abdominal and visceral fat in women.[99] Physical fitness, even without weight loss, is associated with a substantial reduction in total and abdominal obesity.

Table 23.9 The impact of age on diabetes complications							
Age (years)	Macro vasc dis	Micro vasc dis	IHD	PVD	Retinopathy	Neuropathy	Albuminuria
40–60	1:3	1:2	1:5	1:4	1:3	1:7	1:3
>60	2:3	2:3	1:2	1:3	1:2	1:4	1:3

IHD, ischaemic heart disease; PVD, peripheral vascular disease.

A highly sedentary lifestyle is an independent risk for at least a number of metabolic risks. Physical activity efforts to decrease health risks contingent on the metabolic syndrome should include an increase in both moderate to vigorous exercise and non-exercise physical activity.[100] Regular exercise decreases the risk of developing diabetes by 40% in men of normal weight and 60% in overweight men.[101]

Dietary pattern

The American Diabetes Association recommends limiting saturated fats to less than 7% of total calories and to minimize the intake of *trans* fat. Although a diet rich in omega-3 fatty acids reduces cardiometabolic health risks, a high intake of fish oil moderately increases blood glucose level and decreases insulin sensitivity in type 2 diabetics.[96] Diabetics are well advised to follow coronary heart disease prevention guidelines with respect to fat intake (see Chapter 22). This also applies to *trans* fatty acids. Animal studies suggest a diet rich in *trans* fatty acids enhances intra-abdominal deposition of fat, even in the absence of caloric excess, and increases insulin resistance, possibly by impairing post-insulin receptor binding signal transduction.[102] Whereas the intake of saturated fats is limited to less than 10% of energy intake, mono-unsaturated fatty acids and carbohydrates combined should provide 60–70% of daily energy intake, with individual flexibility in the respective proportions.[103] This is not dissimilar to a Palaeolithic-type diet, based on lean meat, fish, fruits, vegetables, root vegetables, eggs and nuts, which appears to improve glucose tolerance independently of decreased waist circumference.[104] The type of carbohydrate in the diet of diabetics is important. Overweight or obese people on ad libitum low glycaemic index (GI) diets have been shown to reduce body mass, total fat mass, BMI, total cholesterol and LDL cholesterol more successfully than those on conventional restricted-energy low-fat diets.[105] The glycaemic index measures how quickly foods release polysaccharide, raising blood glucose levels. It compares the increase in blood glucose following ingestion of a food with the amount blood glucose would rise following eating an equivalent amount of glucose. Whole foods, particularly those rich in soluble fibre, are absorbed more slowly and produce lower blood glucose levels.

Food: the GI perspective

More refined, high GI foods cause blood sugar levels to rise more rapidly. Improved glycaemic control through diet could minimize medications, lessen the risk of diabetic complications, improve quality of life, and increase life expectancy and glycaemic control in diabetes without compromising hypoglycaemic events.[106] The aim is to keep the fasting blood sugar between 4.4 and 6.1 mmol/L and prevent postprandial blood sugar exceeding 8.0 mmol/L. Good blood glucose control prevents complications. Dietary intervention aims to prevent excessive blood glucose fluctuation and peaks. Compared with high GI diets, low GI diets are associated with lower fasting plasma glucose values and lower glycated protein values. GI has been shown to be independently related to glycosylated haemoglobin (HbA_{1c}) and a lower dietary GI is related to lower HbA_{1c} concentrations.[107] In diabetics, an HbA_{1c} level below 7.0% can be treated by diet and exercise, regardless of the blood glucose levels.

Foods with a GI of less than 55 are desirable. Good choices are apples, grapefruit, beans, lentils, dense grainy bread and bran cereals. Energy-rich low-GI food such as chocolate (GI = 49), ice cream (GI = 61) and potato crisps (GI = 54) are not recommended.[66] Dietary fibre influences the GI level and the diabetic diet should provide 25–50 g/day of dietary fiber (15–25 g/1000 kcal).[108] The efficacy of dietary fibre differs with respect to dietary sources (fruits, legumes or cereals) and specific chemical structure. The chemical composition of fibre is responsible for the physical properties of fibre, e.g. its gel-forming capacity and its fermentation capacity in the lower part of the gut.[109]

Soluble fibre forms a gel in the intestine, slowing absorption, effectively lowering the GI and, with prolonged use, decreasing serum cholesterol levels. Per 100 g of edible portion, foods rich in soluble fibre are peanuts (6.4 g), wholewheat bread (6 g), kidney and white beans (5.7 g), fresh pears (5 g), peas (4.5 g), cooked corn (4.3 g), potatoes with skin (2.5 g), carrots (2.2 g), green beans (1.9 g), peaches (1.5 g) and banana (1.1 g). Oats and barley are good sources of beta-glucan, a non-starch polysaccharide and soluble fibre that reduces the glycaemic response.[110] The reduction in glycaemic response is enhanced by combining resistant starch and soluble fiber.[111] Soluble fibre appears to have a greater effect on postprandial insulin response, while glucose reduction is greater after eating resistant starch from high-amylose cornstarch.[111] Starches can be divided into three groups: rapidly digestible starch (digested within 20 minutes), slowly digestible starch (digested in 20 to 120 minutes), and resistant starch. Maize starch consists of 53% slowly digestible starches, 22.4% rapidly digested starch and 22.6% resistant starch.[112] Potato starch contains less slowly digested starch (15%) and is considered a high GI food. The GI also varies depending on the species of potato and preparation method.[113]

Whereas consumption of foods rich in resistant starch and soluble fibre improve glucose metabolism in normal and overweight women,[111] the combination of a high glycaemic load and a low intake of cereal fibre further increases the risk of diabetes.[66] Diabetics should favour whole grains in their diet. Compared with women who eat fewer than one serve weekly, those who have one or more daily serves of whole grains lower their risk of diabetes by 31%.[112] As magnesium acts as a co-factor for enzymes involved in the metabolism of glucose, or possibly on insulin secretion, the magnesium content of whole grains may be beneficial. Whole grain cereals are good sources of plant lignans, an indigestible fibre which is metabolized in the colon by microflora into enterodiol and enterolactone. A recent study found that women with the highest enterolactone concentrations have a better metabolic profile, higher insulin sensitivity and lower adiposity measures. Lignin gives strength to the cell wall of plants.[114] Foods with a low GI value keep the body's blood sugar levels relatively steady throughout the day, regulating appetite and reducing the tendency to snack. Short-term studies (1 day) suggest the low GI foods or meals have higher satietogenic effect than high GI foods or meals.[115] Low GI meals suppress appetite and enhance feelings of fullness both by raising blood sugar more slowly due to protracted digestion and by increasing the release of the gut hormone glucagon-like peptide 1 (GLP-1) in the bloodstream. Low GI foods tend to be more fibre-rich and levels of GLP-1 were found to be significantly higher following 40 compared to 25 chews.[116]

In diabetic subjects, moderate-carbohydrate high-fibre diets, as compared with moderate-carbohydrate low-fibre diets, are associated with significantly lower values for postprandial plasma glucose; total, LDL and HDL cholesterol; and triglycerides.[108] These measures are also lower in persons on high-carbohydrate high-fibre diets compared to moderate-carbohydrate low-fibre diets. Adherence to low GI and/or low glycemic load (GL) diets is independently associated with a reduced risk of certain chronic diseases.[117] In subjects consuming diets with the lowest GI and/or GL, the rate ratios for various chronic diseases were as follows: type 2 diabetes (GI rate ratio: 1.40; GL rate ratio: 1.27); coronary heart disease (GI rate ratio: 1.25); gallbladder disease (GI rate ratio: 1.26; GL rate ratio: 1.41); breast cancer (GI rate ratio: 1.08); all diseases combined (GI rate ratio: 1.14; GL rate ratio: 1.09).[117]

The dairy option

While diabetics should limit fat, particularly saturated fats, dairy products may be beneficial. A prospective study over 10 years found that each serving-per-day increase in dairy intake was associated with a 4% lower risk of type 2 diabetes in middle-aged or older women.[118] Altered vitamin D and calcium homeostasis may play a role in the development of type 2 diabetes. Observational studies show a relatively consistent association between low vitamin D status, calcium or dairy intake, and prevalence of type 2 diabetes and the metabolic syndrome.[119] There is also an inverse association with incident type 2 diabetes and the metabolic syndrome when comparing highest versus lowest intakes of vitamin D plus calcium.

Evidence-based guidelines for the treatment of type 2 diabetes mellitus focus on three areas:[120]

- intensive lifestyle intervention that includes at least 150 minutes per week of physical activity, an initial weight loss goal of 7%, and a low-fat, reduced-calorie diet
- aggressive management of cardiovascular risk factors with drugs such as aspirin, statins, and angiotensin-converting enzyme inhibitors
- normalization of blood glucose levels and HbA_{1c} levels less than 7%.

In perspective

Diabetes is increasing at an alarming rate in developed societies. Obesity, particularly abdominal obesity, is a red flag for diabetes type 2 – a condition which can often be successfully prevented and controlled by lifestyle choices.

References

1. World Health Organization. WHO Report 2002. http://www.who.int/whr/2002/en/; Accessed 27.01.09.

2. Mason JE, Willett WC, Stampfer MJ, et al. 1995 Body weight and mortality among women. *N Engl J Med.* 1995;333:677–685.

3. Diabetes UK. http://www.diabetes.org.uk/About_us/Our_Views/Position_statements/; Accessed 01.02.09.

4. National Centre for Health Statistics. *Health, United States, 2007 With Chartbook on Trends in the Health of Americans.* Hyattsville, MD; 2007. http://www.cdc.gov/nchs/hus.htm; Accessed 26.01.09.

5. Conaway DG, O'Keefe JH, Reid KJ, Spertus J. Frequency of undiagnosed diabetes mellitus in patients with acute coronary syndrome. *Am J Cardiol.* 2005;96:363–365.

6. CDC. *Diabetes.* http://www.cdc.gov/Diabetes/pubs/general07.htm#gen_a; Accessed 01.02.09.

7. Diabesity and associated disorders in Australia – 2000 AusDiab study. http://www.aph.gov.au/LIBRARY/INTGUIDE/SP/obesity.htm; Accessed 02.01.09.

8. Flegal KM, Carroll MD, Kuczmarski RJ, Johnson CL. Overweight and obesity in the United States: prevalence and trends, 1960–1994. *Int J Obes.* 1988;22:39–47.

9. Bouchard C. Human variation in body mass: evidence for a role of the genes. *Nutr Rev.* 1997;55(pt 2):S21–S30.

10. Bouchard C, Pérusse L, Rice T, Rao DC. The genetics of human obesity. In: Bray GA, Bouchard C, James WPT, eds. *Handbook of Obesity.* New York: Marcel Dekker; 1998:157–190.

11. Bouchard C, Tremblay A, Després JP, et al. The response to long-term overfeeding in identical twins. *N Engl J Med.* 1990;322:1477–1482.

12. Rice T, Tremblay A, Dériaz O, Pérusse L, Rao DC, Bouchard C. A major gene for resting metabolic rate unassociated with body composition: results from the Québec Family Study. *Obes Res.* 1996;4:441–449.

13. Campfield LA, Smith FJ, Burn P. The OB protein (leptin) pathway: a link between adipose tissue mass and central neural networks. *Horm Metab Res.* 1996;28:619–632.

14. Ezzell C. Fat times for obesity research: tons of new information, but how does it all fit together? *J NIH Res.* 1995;7:39–43.

15. Fleury C, Neverova M, Collins S, et al. Uncoupling protein-2: a novel gene linked to obesity and hyperinsulinemia. *Nat Genet.* 1997;15:223–224.

16. Wadden TA, Considine R, Foster GD, Anderson DA, Sarwer DB, Caro J. Short- and long-term changes in serum leptin in dieting obese women: effects of caloric restriction and weight loss. *J Clin Endocrinol Metab.* 1998;83:214–218.

17. Caro JF, Sinha MK, Kolaczynski JW, Zhang PL, Considine RV. Leptin: the tale of an obesity gene. *Diabetes.* 1996;45:1455–1462.

18. Santosa S, Hensrud DD, Votruba SB, Jensen MD. The influence of sex and obesity phenotype on meal fatty acid metabolism before and after weight loss. *Am J Clin Nutr.* 2008;88(4):1134–1141.

19. Aronne LJ. Obesity. *Med Clin North Am.* 1998;82:161–181.

20. van Erk MJ, Pasman WJ, Wortelboer HM, van Ommen B, Hendriks HF. Short-term fatty acid intervention elicits differential gene expression responses in adipose tissue from lean and overweight men. *Genes Nutr.* 2008;3(3–4):127–137.

21. Garaulet M, Hernandez-Morante JJ, Lujan J, Tebar FJ, Zamora S. Relationship between fat cell size and number and fatty acid composition in adipose tissue from different fat depots in overweight/obese humans. *Int J Obes (Lond).* 2006;30(6):899–905.

22. Bonen A, Tandon NN, Glatz JF, Luiken JJ, Heigenhauser GJ. The fatty acid transporter FAT/CD36 is upregulated in subcutaneous and visceral adipose tissues in human obesity and type 2 diabetes. *Int J Obes (Lond).* 2006;30(6):877–883.

23. Bastard JP, Maachi M, Lagathu C, et al. Recent advances in the relationship between obesity, inflammation, and insulin resistance. *Eur Cytokine Netw.* 2006;17(1):4–12.

24. Keller KB, Lemberg L. Obesity and the metabolic syndrome. *Am J Crit Care.* 2003;12(2):167–170.

25. Anderson JL. Lipoprotein-associated phospholipase A2: an independent predictor of coronary artery disease events in primary and secondary prevention. *Am J Cardiol.* 2008;101(12A):23F–33F.

26. Oda E. The metabolic syndrome as a concept of adipose tissue disease. *Hypertens Res.* 2008;31(7):1283–1291.

27. Holvoet P. Relations between metabolic syndrome, oxidative stress and inflammation and cardiovascular disease. *Verh K Acad Geneeskd Belg.* 2008;70(3):193–219.

28. Nannipieri M, Bonotti A, Anselmino M, et al. Pattern of expression of adiponectin receptors in human adipose tissue depots and its relation to the metabolic state. *Int J Obes (Lond).* 2007;31(12):1843–1848.

29. Welborn TA, Dhaliwal SS, Bennett SA. Waist-hip ratio is the dominant risk factor predicting cardiovascular death in Australia. *Med J Aust.* 2003;179(11–12):580–585.

30. Lopatynski J, Mardarowicz G, Szczesniak G. A comparative evaluation of waist circumference, waist-to-hip ratio, waist-to-height ratio and body mass index as indicators of impaired glucose tolerance and as risk factors for type-2 diabetes mellitus. *Ann Univ Mariae Curie Sklodowska [Med].* 2003;58(1):413–419.

31. Sayeed MA, Mahtab H, Latif ZA, et al. Waist-to-height ratio is a better obesity index than body mass index and waist-to-hip ratio for predicting diabetes, hypertension and lipidemia. *Bangladesh Med Res Counc Bull.* 2003;29(1):1–10.

32. Berber A, Gomez-Santos R, Fanghanel G, Sanchez-Reyes L. Anthropometric indexes in the prediction of type 2 diabetes mellitus, hypertension and dyslipidaemia in a Mexican population. *Int J Obes Relat Metab Disord*. 2001;25(12):1794–1799.

33. Lin WY, Lee LT, Chen CY, et al. Optimal cut-off values for obesity: using simple anthropometric indices to predict cardiovascular risk factors in Taiwan. *Int J Obes Relat Metab Disord*. 2002;26(9):1232–1238.

34. Shaw JE, Chisholm DJ. Epidemiology and prevention of type 2 diabetes and the metabolic syndrome. *Med J Aust*. 2003;179 (7):379–383.

35. Yan LL, Daviglus ML, Liu K, et al. Midlife body mass index and hospitalization and mortality in older age. *JAMA*. 2006;295 (2):190–198.

36. Patterson RE, Frank LL, Kristal AR, White E. A comprehensive examination of health conditions associated with obesity in older adults. *Am J Prev Med*. 2004;27 (5):385–390.

37. Meisler JG, St Jeor S. Foreword. *Am J Clin Nutr*. 1996;63 (suppl):409S–411S.

38. McCarron DA, Reusser ME. Body weight and blood pressure regulation. *Am J Clin Nutr*. 1996;63:423S–425S.

39. Puska P. Nutrition and global prevention on non-communicable diseases. *Asia Pac J Clin Nutr*. 2002;11(suppl 9):S755–S758.

40. Foster GD, Wadden TA, Makris AP, et al. Primary care physicians' attitudes about obesity and its treatment. *Obes Res*. 2003;11(10):1168–1177.

41. Byrne NM, Meerkin JD, Laukkanen R, Ross R, Fogelholm M, Hills AP. Weight loss strategies for obese adults: personalized weight management program vs. standard care. *Obesity (Silver Spring)*. 2006;14(10):1777–1788.

42. Krummel DA, Semmens E, Boury J, Gordon PM, Larkin KT. Stages of change for weight management in postpartum women. *J Am Diet Assoc*. 2004;104(7):1102–1108.

43. Sonnenberg L, Pencina M, Kimokoti R, et al. Dietary patterns and the metabolic syndrome in obese and non-obese Framingham women. *Obes Res*. 2005;13 (1):153–162.

44. Dansinger ML, Gleason JA, Griffith JL, Selker HP, Schaefer EJ. Comparison of the Atkins, Ornish, Weight Watchers, and Zone diets for weight loss and heart disease risk reduction: a randomized trial. *JAMA*. 2005;293(1):43–53.

45. Panagiotakos DB, Polystipioti A, Papairakleous N, Polychronopoulos E. Long-term adoption of a Mediterranean diet is associated with a better health status in elderly people; a cross-sectional survey in Cyprus. *Asia Pac J Clin Nutr*. 2007;16(2):331–337.

46. Panagiotakos DB, Chrysohoou C, Pitsavos C, Stefanadis C. Association between the prevalence of obesity and adherence to the Mediterranean diet: the ATTICA study. *Nutrition*. 2006;22 (5):449–456.

47. Tzima N, Pitsavos C, Panagiotakos DB, et al. Mediterranean diet and insulin sensitivity, lipid profile and blood pressure levels, in overweight and obese people; the Attica study. *Lipids Health Dis*. 2007;6:22.

48. Panagiotakos DB, Tzima N, Pitsavos C, et al. The association between adherence to the Mediterranean diet and fasting indices of glucose homoeostasis: the ATTICA Study. *J Am Coll Nutr*. 2007;26(1):32–38.

49. Salas-Salvado J, Fernandez-Ballart J, Ros E, et al. Effect of a Mediterranean diet supplemented with nuts on metabolic syndrome status: one-year results of the PREDIMED randomized trial. *Arch Intern Med*. 2008;168 (22):2449–2458.

50. Giugliano D, Esposito K. Mediterranean diet and metabolic diseases. *Curr Opin Lipidol*. 2008;19(1):63–68.

51. Ebbeling CB, Pawlak DB, Ludwig DS. Childhood obesity: public-health crisis, common sense cure. *Lancet*. 2002;360:473–482.

52. Hill JO, Wyatt HR, Reed GW, Peters JC. Obesity and the environment: where do we go from here? *Science*. 2003;299:853–857.

53. Schoeller DA, Buchholz AC. Energetics of obesity and weight control: does diet composition matter? *J Am Diet Assoc*. 2005;105 (5 suppl 1):S24–S28.

54. Halton TL, Hu FB. The effects of high protein diets on thermogenesis, satiety and weight loss: a critical review. *J Am Coll Nutr*. 2004;23 (5):373–385.

55. Brehm BJ, D'Alessio DA. Benefits of high-protein weight loss diets: enough evidence for practice? *Curr Opin Endocrinol Diabetes Obes*. 2008;15(5):416–421.

56. Soenen S, Westerterp-Plantenga MS. Proteins and satiety: implications for weight management. *Curr Opin Clin Nutr Metab Care*. 2008;11(6):747–751.

57. Zemel MB, Richards J, Mathis S, Milstead A, Gebhardt L, Silva E. Dairy augmentation of total and central fat loss in obese subjects. *Int J Obes (Lond)*. 2005;29(4):391–397.

58. Heaney RP, Davies KM, Barger-Lux MJ. Calcium and weight: clinical studies. *J Am Coll Nutr*. 2002;21(2):152S–155S.

59. Liu E, Meigs JB, Pittas AG, et al. Plasma 25-hydroxyvitamin d is associated with markers of the insulin resistant phenotype in nondiabetic adults. *J Nutr*. 2009;139(2):329–334.

60. Fujioka K, Greenway F, Sheard J, Ying Y. The effects of grapefruit on weight and insulin resistance: relationship to the metabolic syndrome. *J Med Food*. 2006;9 (1):49–54.

61. Parnell JA, Reimer RA. Weight loss during oligofructose supplementation is associated with decreased ghrelin and increased peptide YY in overweight and obese 62 adults. *Am J Clin Nutr*. 2009;89:1751–1759.

62. Minich DM, Bland JS. Dietary management of the metabolic syndrome beyond macronutrients. *Nutr Rev*. 2008;66(8):429–444.

63. Lang A, Froelicher ES. Management of overweight and obesity in adults: behavioral intervention for long-term weight loss and maintenance. *Eur J Cardiovasc Nurs*. 2006;5 (2):102–114.

64. Johannsen DL, Redman LM, Ravussin E. The role of physical activity in maintaining a reduced weight. *Curr Atheroscler Rep*. 2007;9(6):463–471.

65. Chambliss HO. Exercise duration and intensity in a weight-loss program. *Clin J Sport Med*. 2005;15 (2):113–115.

66. *National Guide*. <http://www. diabetesaustralia.com.au/For-Health-Professionals/Diabetes-National-Guidelines/>; Accessed 01.02.09.

67. Ainsworth BE, Haskell WL, Whitt MC, et al. Compendium of physical activities: an update of activity codes and MET intensities. *Med Sci Sports Exerc*. 2000;32(9 suppl):S498–S504.

68. CDC. *General physical activities defined by level of intensity*. http:// www.cdc.gov/nccdphp/dnpa/ physical/recommendations/adults. htm; Accessed 22.11.06.

69. Spadano JL, Must A, Bandini LG, Dallal GE, Dietz WH. Energy cost of physical activities in 12-y-old girls: MET values and the influence of body weight. *Int J Obes Relat Metab Disord*. 2003;27 (12):1528–1533.

70. Hamilton MT, Hamilton DG, Zderic TW. Role of low energy expenditure and sitting in obesity, metabolic syndrome, type 2 diabetes, and cardiovascular disease. *Diabetes*. 2007;56 (11):2655–2667.

71. Healy GN, Dunstan DW, Salmon J, et al. Breaks in sedentary time: beneficial associations with metabolic risk. *Diabetes Care*. 2008;31(4):661–666.

72. Lakka TA, Laaksonen DE. Physical activity in prevention and treatment of the metabolic syndrome. *Appl Physiol Nutr Metab*. 2007;32 (1):76–88.

73. Wijndaele K, Duvigneaud N, Matton L, et al. Sedentary behaviour, physical activity and a continuous metabolic syndrome risk score in adults. *Eur J Clin Nutr*. 2009;63(3):421–429.

74. Dunstan DW, Salmon J, Owen N, et al. Associations of TV viewing and physical activity with the metabolic syndrome in Australian adults. *Diabetologia*. 2005;48 (11):2254–2261.

75. Manios Y, Kourlaba G, Kondaki K, Grammatikaki E, Anastasiadou A, Roma-Giannikou E. Obesity and television watching in preschoolers in Greece: the GENESIS Study. *Obesity (Silver Spring)*. 2009;17 (11):2047–2053.

76. Cleland VJ, Schmidt MD, Dwyer T, Venn AJ. Television viewing and abdominal obesity in young adults: is the association mediated by food and beverage consumption during viewing time or reduced leisure-time physical activity? *Am J Clin Nutr*. 2008;87(5):1148–1155.

77. Healy GN, Dunstan DW, Salmon J, et al. Objectively measured light-intensity physical activity is independently associated with 2-h plasma glucose. *Diabetes Care*. 2007;30(6):1384–1389.

78. Schmidt WD, Biwer CJ, Kalscheuer LK. Effects of long versus short bout exercise on fitness and weight loss in overweight females. *J Am Coll Nutr*. 2001;20 (5):494–501.

79. Wu T, Gao X, Chen M, van Dam RM. Long-term effectiveness of diet-plus-exercise interventions vs. diet-only interventions for weight loss: a meta-analysis. *Obes Rev*. 2009;10(3):313–323.

80. Field AE, Manson JE, Taylor CB, Willett WC, Colditz GA. Association of weight change, weight control practices, and weight cycling among women in the Nurses' Health Study II. *Int J Obes Relat Metab Disord*. 2004;28 (9):1134–1142.

81. Brownell KD, Rodin J. Medical, metabolic, and psychological effects of weight cycling. *Arch Intern Med*. 1994;154(12):1325–1330.

82. Diaz VA, Mainous 3rd AG, Everett CJ. The association between weight fluctuation and mortality: results from a population-based cohort study. *J Community Health*. 2005;30(3):153–165.

83. Shade ED, Ulrich CM, Wener MH, et al. Frequent intentional weight loss is associated with lower natural killer cell cytotoxicity in postmenopausal women: possible long-term immune effects. *J Am Diet Assoc*. 2004;104(6):903–912.

84. Meyer HE, Tverdal A, Falch JA. Changes in body weight and incidence of hip fracture among middle aged Norwegians. *BMJ*. 1995;311(6997):91–92.

85. Langlois JA, Mussolino ME, Visser M, Looker AC, Harris T, Madans J. Weight loss from maximum body weight among middle-aged and older white women and the risk of hip fracture: the NHANES I epidemiologic follow-up study. *Osteoporos Int*. 2001;12(9):763–768.

86. Rzehak P, Meisinger C, Woelke G, Brasche S, Strube G, Heinrich J. Weight change, weight cycling and mortality in the ERFORT Male Cohort Study. *Eur J Epidemiol*. 2007;22(10):665–673.

87. Amigo I, Fernández C. Effects of diets and their role in weight control. *Psychol Health Med*. 2007;12(3):321–327.

88. Muls E, Kempen K, Vansant G, Saris W. Is weight cycling detrimental to health? A review of the literature in humans. *Int J Obes Relat Metab Disord*. 1995;19(suppl 3):S46–S50.

89. *U.S. Preventive Services Task Force*. http://www.ahrq.gov/clinic/uspstf/ uspsobes.htm Accessed 06.02.09.

90. Mayfield J. Diagnosis and classification of diabetes mellitus: new criteria. *Am Fam Physician*. 1998;58(6):1355–1362, 1369–1370.

91. Klein S, Sheard NF, Pi-Sunyer X, et al. Weight management through lifestyle modification for the prevention and management of type 2 diabetes: rationale and strategies. A statement of the American Diabetes Association, the North American Association for the Study of Obesity, and the American Society for Clinical Nutrition. *Am J Clin Nutr*. 2004;80(2):257–263.

92. Sowers JR. Modest weight gain and the development of diabetes: another perspective. *Ann Intern Med*. 1995;122(7):548–549.

93. Wu L, While A. Weight management in people with type 2 diabetes. *Br J Community Nurs*. 2007;12(9):390–397.

94. Norris SL, Zhang X, Avenell A, Gregg E, Schmid CH, Lau J. Long-term non-pharmacological weight loss interventions for adults with prediabetes. *Cochrane Database Syst Rev*. 2005;(2) CD005270.

95. Norris SL, Zhang X, Avenell A, et al. Long-term non-pharmacologic weight loss interventions for adults with type 2 diabetes. *Cochrane Database Syst Rev*. 2005;(2) CD004095.

96. Hainer V, Toplak H, Mitrakou A. Treatment modalities of obesity: what fits whom? *Diabetes Care*. 2008;31(suppl 2):S269–S277.

97. Lindström J, Ilanne-Parikka P, Peltonen M, et al. Finnish Diabetes Prevention Study Group. Sustained reduction in the incidence of type 2 diabetes by lifestyle. Intervention: follow-up of the Finnish Diabetes Prevention Study. *Lancet*. 2006;368 (9548):1673–1679.

98. Avenell A, Broom J, Brown TJ, et al. Systematic review of the long-term effects and economic consequences of treatments for obesity and implications for health improvement. *Health Technol Assess*. 2004;8(21):iii–iv 1–182.

99. Ross R, Janssen I, Dawson J, et al. Exercise-induced reduction in obesity and insulin resistance in women: a randomized controlled trial. *Obes Res*. 2004;12 (5):789–798.

100. Wijndaele K, Duvigneaud N, Matton L, Duquet W, Delecluse C, et al. Sedentary behaviour, physical activity and a continuous metabolic syndrome risk score in adults. *Eur J Clin Nutr*. 2009;63(3):421–429.

101. Keller KB, Lemberg L. Retirement is no excuse for physical inactivity or isolation. *Am J Crit Care*. 2002;11(3):270–272.

102. Kavanagh K, Jones KL, Sawyer J, et al. Trans fat diet induces abdominal obesity and changes in insulin sensitivity in monkeys. *Obesity (Silver Spring)*. 2007;15 (7):1675–1684.

103. Kelley DE. Sugars and starch in the nutritional management of diabetes mellitus. *Am J Clin Nutr*. 2003;78(4):858S–864S.

104. Lindeberg S, Jönsson T, Granfeldt Y, et al. Palaeolithic diet improves glucose tolerance more than a Mediterranean-like diet in individuals with ischaemic heart disease. *Diabetologia*. 2007;50 (9):1795–1807.

105. Thomas DE, Elliott EJ, Baur L. Low glycaemic index or low glycaemic load diets for overweight and obesity. *Cochrane Database Syst Rev*. 2007;(3) CD005105.

106. Thomas D, Elliott EJ. Low glycaemic index, or low glycaemic load, diets for diabetes mellitus. *Cochrane Database Syst Rev*. 2009;(1) CD006296.

107. Buyken AE, Toeller M, Heitkamp G, et al. Glycemic index in the diet of European outpatients with type 1 diabetes: relations to glycated hemoglobin and serum lipids. *Am J Clin Nutr*. 2001;73(3):574–581.

108. Anderson JW, Randles KM, Kendall CW, Jenkins DJ. Carbohydrate and fiber recommendations for individuals with diabetes: a quantitative assessment and meta-analysis of the evidence. *J Am Coll Nutr*. 2004;23(1):5–17.

109. Delzenne NM, Cani PD. A place for dietary fibre in the management of the metabolic syndrome. *Curr Opin Clin Nutr Metab Care*. 2005;8(6):636–640.

110. Behall KM, Scholfield DJ, Hallfrisch J. Comparison of hormone and glucose responses of overweight women to barley and oats. *J Am Coll Nutr*. 2005;24 (3):182–188.

111. Behall KM, Scholfield DJ, Hallfrisch JG, Liljeberg-Elmståhl HG. Consumption of both resistant starch and beta-glucan improves postprandial plasma glucose and insulin in women. *Diabetes Care*. 2006;29 (5):976–981.

112. van Dam RM, Hu FB, Rosenberg L, Krishnan S, Palmer JR. Dietary calcium and magnesium, major food sources, and risk of type 2 diabetes in U.S. Black women. *Diabetes Care*. 2006;29(10):2238–2243.

113. *Diet And Fitness Today: GI potatoes* http://www.dietandfitnesstoday.com/glycemicIndexDetails.php?id=1180; Accessed 06.02.09.

114. Morisset AS, Lemieux S, Veilleux A, Bergeron J, Weisnagel SJ, Tchernof A. Impact of a lignan-rich diet on adiposity and insulin sensitivity in post-menopausal women. *Br J Nutr*. 2009;102(2):195–200.

115. Bornet FR, Jardy-Gennetier AE, Jacquet N, Stowell J. Glycaemic response to foods: impact on satiety and long-term weight regulation. *Appetite*. 2007;49 (3):535–553.

116. Cassady BA, Hollis JH, Fulford AD, Considine RV, Mattes RD. Mastication of almonds: effects of lipid bioaccessibility, appetite, and hormone response. *Am J Clin Nutr*. 2009;89:794–800.

117. Barclay AW, Petocz P, McMillan-Price J, et al. Glycemic index, glycemic load, and chronic disease risk: a meta-analysis of observational studies. *Am J Clin Nutr*. 2008;87(3):627–637.

118. Liu S, Choi HK, Ford E, et al. A prospective study of dairy intake and the risk of type 2 diabetes in women. *Diabetes Care*. 2006;29 (7):1579–1584.

119. Pittas AG, Lau J, Hu FB, Dawson-Hughes B. The role of vitamin d and calcium in type 2 diabetes. A systematic review and meta-analysis. *J Clin Endocrinol Metab*. 2007;92(6):2017–2029.

120. Ripsin CM, Kang H, Urban RJ. Management of blood glucose in type 2 diabetes mellitus. *Am Fam Physician*. 2009;79(1):29–36.

Osteopenia: a red flag for fractures

24

Osteoporosis, described as a systemic skeletal disease characterized by low bone mass and microarchitectural deterioration of bone tissue, increases the risk of fractures. In 2000 there were an estimated 9 million new osteoporotic fractures globally.[1] By 2004 there were an estimated 10 million cases and 34 million persons at risk in the US alone.[2] The National Osteoporosis Foundation anticipates 14 million cases of osteoporosis and over 47 million cases of low bone mass in the US by 2020.[1] The UK estimate for osteoporosis is around the 6.2 million mark, while some 2.2 million Australians are affected.[1,2] The lifetime risk of an osteoporotic fracture for Australians over the age of 50 years is 42% in women and 27% in men;[1] every second woman and every fourth man in America over 50 is predicted to run the risk of having a fracture during their lifetime.[3] In 2005 in the US an estimated $17 billion was spent on treatment of osteoporotic fractures; by 2025, annual fractures and costs are projected to increase by 50% and $25 billion, respectively.[1] In the UK the cost of treating all osteoporotic fractures in postmenopausal women has been predicted to increase to more than £2 billion by 2020, while in Australia the total cost of osteoporosis is AU$7.4 billion per year of which AU$1.9 billion are direct costs.[1] In New Zealand the total cost of care is currently estimated to be over NZ$1.1 billion per year and anticipated to increase by over 30% between 2007 and 2020.[1]

Osteoporosis-related fractures most commonly affect the hip, vertebra and forearm. Globally, by 2050, the worldwide incidence of hip fracture is projected to be between 4.5 million and 6.3 million, with a 310% increase in men and a 240% increase in women.[1] Current trends in the UK suggest hip fracture rates may increase from 46,000 in 1985 to 117,000 in 2016, with every second woman and every fifth man suffering a fracture after the age of 50.[1] At age 50, a white woman has a 17% chance and a white male a 6% chance of sustaining a hip fracture. In the US, the number of hip fractures is anticipated to double or triple by 2040. In Australia, there are 20,000 hip fractures per year, with an annual increase around 4%. The mortality rate for hip fractures can reach 24% in the 12 months following a hip fracture, with the increased risk of dying persisting for 5 years or more. The risk of death due to a hip-related fracture in a 50-year-old woman is 2.8%, equivalent to her risk of death from breast cancer and four times higher than her lifetime risk of endometrial cancer. Hip fractures cause loss of function, with 40% of casualties unable to walk independently; 60% require assistance a year later and 5–10% experience a recurrent hip fracture within 3 to 4 years. Some 90% of hip fractures result from falls and one in three people over age 65 fall annually – 60% of those who fell the previous year will fall again. Approximately 10–15% of falls in the elderly result in a fracture.[1] A 10% loss in hip bone mass increases the risk of a hip fracture 2.5-fold.[3]

In 2005, vertebral fractures represented 27% of total fractures and accounted for 6% of total costs in the US.[1] The lifetime risk of a fractured vertebra for a 50-year-old white woman is 16%; for a man it is 5%. A woman 65 years of age with one vertebral fracture has a one in four chance of another fracture within 5 years.[1] Vertebral fractures can lead to back pain, loss of height, deformity, immobility, an increased number of bed days and reduced pulmonary function. A 10% loss of vertebral bone mass doubles the risk of a vertebral fracture.[3]

Treatment reduces the risk of vertebral fracture by 30–65% and of non-vertebral fracture by 16–70%.[1] Reducing the risk of a first fracture from 8% to 2% can reduce the 5-year fracture incidence from approximately 34% to 10%. Approximately 70% of fractures and 87% of costs are incurred by those over 65 years of age.[1] Diagnosis of osteopenia and treatment before fractures occur will substantially reduce the long-term burden of osteoporosis. In Australia, about 42% of men and 51% of women 60 years of age and older are osteopenic, 11% of men and 27% of women are osteoporotic. Of the estimated 44 million Americans at risk of osteoporosis, 10 million have osteoporosis, 34 million have osteopenia.[3] An estimated 54% of postmenopausal white American women are osteopenic and 30% are osteoporotic.[1] By the age of 80, this ratio is reversed, with 27% of women being osteopenic and 70% osteoporotic. Osteopenia progresses to osteoporosis as age increases – active intervention is required to slow this relentless progression.

Osteopenia: red flag for osteoporosis

Osteoporosis, like type 2 diabetes and hypertension, has a long latent period during which irreversible damage may occur. Over 90% of bone mass is accrued by the age of 20 years. Once peak bone mass has been reached by the age of 30, total skeletal mass and density remain relatively constant until around 50 years of age. Although a number of orange flags for osteopenia have been identified (see **Handout 24.1**), bone fragility is well established before objective clinical evidence verifies an increased fracture risk. Up to 50% of trabecular bone is lost before changes are visible on radiographs. Tests that are more discerning are needed to detect bone mineral density (BMD) at a stage before bone develops the propensity to fracture on exposure to minor trauma. The most widely used techniques used to measure BMD are based on X-ray absorptiometry. Absorption of X-rays is very sensitive to the calcium content of tissue in bone. Dual-energy X-ray absorptiometry (DXA) is the preferred option as it can be used to assess bone mineral content of the whole skeleton as well as specific sites. Techniques include, amongst others: quantitative ultrasound; quantitative computed tomography applied to the spine, hip and appendicular skeleton; peripheral DXA, digital X-ray radiogrammetry and radiographic absorptiometry.[4] Bone density in young healthy adults is approximately normally distributed, irrespective of the measurement technique used.

BMD thresholds for men aged 50 years or more and postmenopausal women using measurements of DXA at the femoral neck are set as follows:[4]

- A BMD value higher than 1 standard deviation (SD) below the young adult female reference mean is considered normal. When SDs are calculated in relation to the mean of a young healthy population, this is referred to as the T-score. A T-score greater than or equal to -1 SD is considered normal.

- A BMD more than 1 SD below the young female adult mean but less than 2.5 SD below this value (T-score <-1 and >-2.5 SD) is classified as low bone mass or osteopenia. By the age of 50 years, the prevalence of osteopenia is 35.5% in women and 21.8% in men. Absolute risk rises markedly with age and the gradient of risk is steeper at 50 than at 80 years.

- A BMD value of 2.5 SD or more below the young female adult mean (T-score ≤-2.5 SD) is diagnostic for osteoporosis.

- A BMD value 2.5 SD or more below the young female adult mean in the presence of one or more fragility fractures is diagnosed as severe or established osteoporosis.

The T-score cannot be used interchangeably with different techniques and at different skeletal sites; furthermore, combining the lowest value for BMD from the femoral neck and lumbar spine, while increasing sensitivity at the expense of specificity, does not increase the predictive ability of BMD tests.[5] The use of the T-score undervalues the contribution of gender and age to risk. The Z-score, which represents the number of SDs that a given value for BMD deviates from the average value for age and gender, provides an unsatisfactory alternative. Subjects diagnosed with osteoporosis by T-score were reclassified as either normal or osteopenic when the Z-score was used.[6] Thresholds recommended for male reference ranges of BMD for osteopenia are:[7] 20–29 years, 0.792 g/cm^2; 30–39 years, 0.770 g/cm^2; 50 years, 0.702 g/cm^2; for osteoporosis they are 0.585, 0.564 and 0.510 g/cm^2, respectively.[7] The female reference threshold ranges for osteopenia are:[6] 20–29 years, 0.740 g/cm^2; 30–39 years, 0.729 g/cm^2; 40–49 years, 0.710 g/cm^2; 50 years, 0.649 g/cm^2; for osteoporosis they are 0.577, 0.556, 0.533 and 0.407 g/cm^2, respectively. Smoking, low weight or weight loss along with advancing age are consistent orange flags for low BMD or bone loss in healthy men aged 50 years or older.[8] Smokers may have lower-calcium diets, less efficient calcium absorption and lower osteocalcin levels, resulting in decreased bone formation and accelerated bone loss. Current smoking is associated with a significantly increased risk of fractures compared to non-smokers; however, low BMD accounts for only 23% of the smoking-related risk of hip fracture.[9] Both age and weight modify the risk of hip fractures. Risk increases to 41% at 70 years and escalates to 71% by the age of 80. The risk of hip fracture is doubled in those who smoke 25 cigarettes daily, as it is in those with a BMI of 20, compared to those with a BMI of 25. The significance of BMI as a risk factor varies according to the level of BMI. BMI assumes greater importance as a risk factor in those with a low body weight.[10] Skeletal loading stimulates bone growth in the young and protects against bone loss in adults. Skeletal loading comes largely from muscles, not body weight.

At any point in life, bone mass represents a balance between the amount of bone laid down during growth and development and the amount of bone lost with ageing. At a cellular level, these changes in bone mass occur as the result of bone remodelling; a process whereby bone-resorbing cells (osteoclasts) and bone-forming cells (osteoblasts) remove and replace packets of bone at discrete points throughout the skeleton. This process is regulated by interaction between genetic factors and environmental influences such as nutrition and exercise. Bone modelling is complete by early adulthood. Instead of the generalized continuous growth in which osteoblasts and osteoclasts adaptively reshape 100% of the bone surface, remodelling attempts to maintain adult skeletal mass and morphology. Each year, 3% of cortical bone, 25% of trabecular bone and 20% of the bone surface is remodelled through the local coupled processes of osteoclastic bone resorption and osteoblastic bone formation. Osteoblasts produce osteoid, i.e. bone matrix, type 1 collagen, and noncollagenous proteins such as osteocalcin, osteonectin and osteopontin. Osteoblasts aid osteoid mineralization and produce local regulatory factors such as cytokines and growth factors. They also regulate the differentiation and activity of osteoclasts. Osteoclasts dissolve osteoid and remove mineral by producing, amongst others, lysosomal enzymes, hydrogen protons and free radicals. Osteoclasts function in skeletal maintenance and electrolyte homeostasis. As the concentration of growth factors precipitated in osteoid declines with advancing age, coupling between bone formation and resorption is impaired. Resorption becomes a prime cause of age-related bone loss. Fractures occur when high bone turnover is combined with frequent impact. Osteopenia is a valuable red flag for osteoporosis as its detection will capture the majority of individuals who will develop osteoporosis in the next 10 years.[4] The risk of osteoporosis and/or fracture within next 10 years is 10% in persons with a BMD T-value under −1.4; this soars to 56% as the BMD drops further into the osteopenic range. By the age of 65 years, the risk ratio increases by 2.94 in men and by 2.88 in women for each SD decrease in BMD.[11]

Figure 24.1 lists risk factors for fractures of the vertebrae and hips.

Red flags for osteoporotic fractures

While the level of bone mass can be estimated by measuring BMD, this measurement alone fails to reflect the overall fracture risk. Variations in BMD between populations appear to be substantially less than differences in fracture risk. While differences in BMD from diverse regions of the world vary by approximately 1 SD, age- and sex-specific risks of hip fracture differ more than 10-fold.[4] Clinically, it is the predictability of a fracture rather than an accurate measure of BMD that is relevant.

Chemical markers of bone metabolism have been shown to be predictive of fracture risk independently of BMD.[12] In healthy adults, rapid bone loss is followed by slow bone loss in bone remodelling cycles that last 4 months. In osteoporosis, the local coupled

Clues to an increased risk of an osteoporotic spinal fracture:
- backache lessened or intensified when not lying down
- restricted spinal movement with flexion reduced more than extension
- a pronounced kyphosis
- loss of height
- a protruding abdomen
- feeling bloated after small meals
- skinfolds overlying the margin of the ribs/pelvis
- decreased exercise tolerance due to postural changes
- an arm span-height difference of over 3 cm (especially if over 70 years of age and less than 160 cm tall)

Clues to an increased risk of an osteoporotic hip fracture:
- low bone mineral density
- history of hip, radius or vertebral fracture in a first-degree relative
- personal history of a fracture after the age of 40
- current cigarette smoking
- low body weight
- certain medications/diseases, e.g. steroids
- hip pain
- the inability of the hip to bear weight
- a shortened externally rotated leg

Figure 24.1 • Osteoporotic fracture: clinical alerts.

process of bone resorption and formation in remodelling is defective. The remodelling cycle is extended to 2 years and the equilibrium between resorption and formation is disrupted, resulting in a net loss of 0.3–0.5% bone annually. Markers of bone turnover can be used to predict the rate of bone loss in post-menopausal women and can also be used to assess the risk of fractures.[13] The most sensitive and specific markers of bone formation include serum bone alkaline phosphatase, total osteocalcin and the procollagen type I N-terminal propeptide assay; those for bone resorption are urinary N- and C-terminal cross-linked telopeptides and serum C-terminal cross-linked telopeptides (CTX). In postmenopausal osteoporosis, levels of bone resorption markers above the upper limit of the premenopausal range are associated with an increased risk of hip, vertebral, and non-vertebral fracture, independent of BMD.[12] The urinary ratio of native (alpha) to isomerized (beta) CTX provides an index of bone matrix maturation which is predictive of fracture risk independently not only of BMD but also of bone turnover.[12] Biochemical markers of bone turnover have the potential to reliably assess

skeletal activity and fracture risk, drug effects and response to therapies, and predict various skeletal parameters including bone loss, BMD and bone mass. Biochemical markers of bone turnover provide a non-invasive method for red flag detection.

Changes in the material property of bone are an important determinant of bone strength. Low BMD, loss of BMD and age are independent risk factors for hip fractures.[14] The incidence of hip fracture increases about 40-fold between the ages of 50 and 80 years in many countries; however, based on BMD changes, hip fractures would be expected to increase only about 4-fold.[4] BMD captures neither micro-architectural organization of bone nor the propensity for falls. Furthermore, bone loss at the femoral neck predicts fracture risk in elderly women, independent of baseline BMD and age.[14] Although the sensitivity of BMD for fracture prediction is low, its specificity is high. Thus, although many fractures will occur in individuals with BMD values in the normal range, the fracture risk is very high in individuals with osteoporosis. An increase of 8% in BMD halves the risk of a fracture,[15] yet despite maintaining a consistent BMD, the risk of a fracture increases 8- or 10-fold between the ages of 45 and 80 years. BMD alone is a poor predictor. Other risk factors needs to be considered. BMD is but one factor contributing to the risk of fractures.

Osteoporosis: genetic condition or lifestyle risk?

The risk of osteoporosis is determined by genetic expression modulated by environmental exposures. The influence of genetic factors differs – genes appear to have a substantial impact on peak bone mass, a modest effect on fracture risk, and make little, if any, impression on bone loss.[16] Evidence from twin and family studies suggests that between 50% and 85% of the variance in peak bone mass is genetically determined.[16] A longitudinal twin study documented that genetic factors explain 44–56% of the between-individual variance in bone loss at the femoral neck, lumbar spine, and forearm in postmenopausal Caucasian women.[17] Age modifies the importance of genetic influence on bone mass and liability to fracture. Less than 20% of the overall age-adjusted fracture variance is explained by genetic variation.[18] Nonetheless, genes have been shown to significantly affect key determinants of osteoporotic fracture risk, including quantitative ultrasound properties of bone, femoral neck geometry, muscle strength, bone turnover markers, and BMI.[16] Furthermore, the influence of genetic expression has been shown to be considerably greater for first hip fractures before 69 years of age than after 79 years of age.[18] Environment assumes increased importance as age increases.

Advancing age both depletes bone mass and increases the risk of falls. Age affects bone architecture by reducing the rate of bone turnover, progressively depleting, predominantly trabecular, bone. During growth, the increasing load placed on bones from body weight and muscle forces augments bone mass and strength. Bone mass and strength adapt to the load demand on bones. After about 30 years of age, muscle strength decreases. In ageing adults, bones that have adapted to stronger young-adult muscles enter a phase of partial disuse and remodelling begins to reduce bone mass and strength.[19] Bone strain can increase bone mass during modelling and conserve bone mass or reduce bone loss during remodelling. Bone strain, increased by weight-bearing exercise, conserves BMD. While bone density may alone be a poor predictor of fractures, its predisposing factors, along with falling, constitute a major risk factor for osteoporotic fractures.

Fractures occur when a weak bone is exposed to an activity that generates a large force. The factor of risk is the ratio of the load on the spine to the failure load of the bone.[20] A high factor of risk results if the bone is weak, i.e. has a low failure load, or from a risk activity that generates a large force. The failure load of the vertebrae depend on the density and architecture of the trabecular bone and the size, shape and organization of the vertebral body. DXA correlates strongly with the compressive failure load. The magnitude of the load applied to the spine depends on the activity. Ranked in order from lowest to highest, activities that place greater loads on the spine are:[21] opening a window with 75 N of force, tying shoes while seated, getting up from the seated position, lifting 15 kg weight with bent knees, lifting 15 kg weight with straight knees, lifting 30 kg weight with bent knees, lifting 30 kg weight with straight knees. Bending and lifting can generate loads that exceed the failure load of vertebrae with very low bone mineral density. Fall mechanics also play an important role in the aetiology of hip fractures.[22] Falls to the side, particularly those with impact on the hip or side of the leg, more often result in hip fractures than do other falls. Weight-bearing exercise protects muscle mass and improves co-ordination. Lifestyle choices become increasingly important determinants of fracture risk with increasing age.[18] While lifestyle choices may have their greatest impact with increasing age, they interact with genes determining skeletal health throughout life. Genetic determinants influence various osteoporosis-related phenotypes including BMD, fragility fractures, postmenopausal bone loss, bone geometry, bone quality, and bone mineralization. Genetic predisposition to osteoporosis is polygenic in nature, being mediated by several genetic variants, each of modest effect size, interacting with environmental factors.[16] Genetic inheritance influences receptors for calcitonin, oestrogen, parathyroid hormone, interleukins 1 and 6, and vitamin D. However, lifestyle choices and drug intervention can modulate the expression of these genes. While genetic polymorphism makes unilinear cause–effect intervention unrealistic, it does provide multiple opportunities for making marginal gains. The relative risk of a fracture is increased:[23] 11.8 times in persons with two or more previous fractures; 5.5 times in persons who use tobacco or have a BMI of less than 23; over 3 times in persons with impaired eyesight; about 2.5 times in persons who have decreased BMD, are postmenopausal or have been on anticonvulsant therapy; and is more than doubled in persons with postural instability or who cannot stand from a sitting position without using their arms. Identification of numerous contributing risks provides a plethora of intervention opportunities. Skeletal health can be enhanced by adequate nutrition, particularly with respect to calcium, an active lifestyle, not smoking and good balance/gait. Lifestyle measures can be complemented by drug therapy, depending on age and the presence of other risk factors.[24]

Reducing risk

The objective and nature of interventions to reduce the risk of osteoporosis and fractures are largely influenced by age. In the young, the aim is to achieve a peak bone mass; in adulthood the objective is to retain bone mass, while in later life the intention is to reduce bone loss. Figure 24.2 provides a questionnaire for evaluating patients' knowledge about this condition. Once awareness has been raised, **Handout 24.2** provides guidelines for promoting skeletal health.

Please answer each of the following questions with True, False, or Don't Know.

1. Osteoporosis leads to an increased risk of bone fractures. ☐ True ☐ False ☐ Don't know
2. Osteoporosis usually causes symptoms (e.g. pain) before fractures occur. ☐ True ☐ False ☐ Don't know
3. Having a higher peak bone mass at the end of childhood gives no protection against the development of osteoporosis in later life. ☐ True ☐ False ☐ Don't know
4. Osteoporosis is more common in men. ☐ True ☐ False ☐ Don't know
5. Cigarette smoking can contribute to osteoporosis. ☐ True ☐ False ☐ Don't know
6. White women are at highest risk of fracture as compared to other races. ☐ True ☐ False ☐ Don't know
7. A fall is just as important as low bone strength in causing fractures. ☐ True ☐ False ☐ Don't know
8. By age 80, the majority of women have osteoporosis. ☐ True ☐ False ☐ Don't know
9. From age 50, most women can expect at least one fracture before they die. ☐ True ☐ False ☐ Don't know
10. Any type of physical activity is beneficial for osteoporosis. ☐ True ☐ False ☐ Don't know
11. It is easy to tell whether I am at risk of osteoporosis by my clinical risk factors. ☐ True ☐ False ☐ Don't know
12. Family history of osteoporosis strongly predisposes a person to osteoporosis. ☐ True ☐ False ☐ Don't know
13. An adequate calcium intake can be achieved from two glasses of milk a day. ☐ True ☐ False ☐ Don't know
14. Sardines and broccoli are good sources of calcium for people who cannot take dairy products. ☐ True ☐ False ☐ Don't know
15. Calcium supplements alone can prevent bone loss. ☐ True ☐ False ☐ Don't know
16. Alcohol in moderation has little effect on osteoporosis. ☐ True ☐ False ☐ Don't know
17. A high salt intake is a risk factor for osteoporosis. ☐ True ☐ False ☐ Don't know
18. There is a small amount of bone loss in the 10 years following the onset of menopause. ☐ True ☐ False ☐ Don't know
19. Hormone therapy prevents further bone loss at any age after menopause. ☐ True ☐ False ☐ Don't know
20. There are no effective treatments for osteoporosis available in Australia. ☐ True ☐ False ☐ Don't know

*Winzenberg TM, Oldenburg B, Frendin S, Jones G. The design of a valid and reliable questionnaire to measure osteoporosis knowledge in women: the Osteoporosis Knowledge Assessment Tool (OKAT). *BMC Musculoskelet Disord*. 2003;4(1):17.

© 2003 Winzenberg et al; licensee BioMed Central Ltd.

http://www.pubmedcentral.nih.gov/articlerender.fcgi?tool=pubmed&pubmedid=12877751 This is an Open Access article: verbatim copying and redistribution of this article are permitted in all media for any purpose, provided this notice is preserved along with the article's original URL.

Figure 24.2 • The Osteoporosis Knowledge Assessment Tool (OKAT).*

Maximizing peak bone mass

Peak bone mass can be achieved by lifestyle choices that ensure an adequate calcium intake, sufficient vitamin D production and weight-bearing exercise (see Figure 24.3). Physical activity and calcium intake are important to the development of BMD, and establishing good bone mineral content, while particularly important during puberty, is also important prepuberty.[25]

Calcium deficiency is thought to explain 15% of the population variance in bone mass.[26] An inadequate calcium intake, particularly during early life when peak bone mass is developing, is a substantial risk marker for future osteoporosis. Daily calcium requirements increase with age. At 0 to 6 months the minimum recommended intake of calcium is 210 mg; at 6 to 12 months, 270 mg; at 1 to 3 years, 500 mg; at 4 to 8 years, 800 mg; at 9 to 18 years it increases to 1300 mg and at 18 to 50 years it is 1000 mg.[27] Table 24.1 suggests even higher intakes deserve consideration.

Adolescents and children who consume two or more servings of dairy on a daily basis achieve higher bone mineral content and density levels.[28] Compared to children with lower intakes, the average bone mineral content of children consuming two servings of dairy a day is 175 g higher. When 4 oz of meat or other non-dairy protein is added to the two daily servings of dairy, bone mineral content is 300 g higher. Another study confirmed that an increased intake of dietary calcium or dairy products significantly increased total body and lumbar spine bone mineral content in children with low baseline intakes, but increasing intake in subjects with normal or near-normal baseline intake had little impact.[29]

As a general rule of thumb, at least 60% of daily calcium intake should come from dairy products. One cup of reconstituted non-fat dry milk contains 375 mg of calcium; a cup of low-fat, skim or whole milk, 290 to 300 mg; one cup of yoghurt, 275 to 400 mg; one cup of low-fat cottage cheese, 154 mg, and one cup of part-skim ricotta cheese, 680 mg. One ounce of Swiss cheese contains 272 mg of

AIM: Maximize peak bone mass

- EXERCISE – High-impact strength-building exercise increases strength, lean body mass and bone mineral density
- SUNLIGHT*
  - outdoor activity >10 min × 5/7days
  - avoid sunburn

Balance cancer risk versus requirement for vitamin D

- DIET
  - Adequate calcium (1.2 g/day): dairy, fish bones
  - Avoid highly salted foods
  - Limit carbonated drinks (girls)

*Thickly applied sunscreen SPF 8+ blocks vitamin D synthesis

Adolescent risky lifestyle choices

- Sedentary lifestyle
- Smoking
- Dietary risks:
  - alcohol
  - low calcium intake
  - high animal protein diet
  - high sodium
  - high caffeine
- Weight recycling

Figure 24.3 • Skeletal care for adolescents.

Table 24.1 Calcium intake

Age group	Recommended calcium intake (mg/day)
Birth to 6 months	400
1–5 years	800
6–10 years	800–1200
11–24 years	1500
Women 25–50 years	1000
Pregnancy, lactation	1200–1500
Postmenopausal women on oestrogen	1000
Postmenopausal women not on oestrogen	1500
Men 25–65 years	1000
Over 65 years	1500

calcium and 1 oz of Cheddar contains 204 mg. Of non-dairy sources, 3 oz of sardines with bones contain 370 mg of calcium, while an equivalent amount of canned salmon with bones contains 285 mg. The best vegetable source is tofu: 4 oz contains 154 mg. In the US, foods that supply 200 mg or more of calcium per serve are labelled 'High in Calcium', 'Rich in Calcium', or 'Excellent Source of Calcium'; those that contain more than 100 mg but less than 200 mg are labelled 'Contains Calcium', 'Provides Calcium', or 'Good Source of Calcium'. There is some overlap with products that contain at least 100 mg per serve and are labelled 'Calcium-Enriched', 'Calcium-Fortified', or 'More Calcium'. Calcium absorption, along with the calcium content of the diet, determines the adequacy of calcium intake. Absorption of calcium from a mixed Western diet is thought to be about 20% on low-calcium diets; the maximum absorption possible is 30%. Lactose in dairy products enhances calcium absorption; however, fibre in plant sources may form complexes with calcium, increasing faecal excretion. Cellulose, phytates and oxalates all impair calcium absorption. Calcium is plentiful in sesame seeds, but better absorbed from canned fish, provided that the bones are eaten. Although data on the effect of dietary fibre on calcium balance are limited and somewhat contradictory,[30] it has been suggested that each 18 g of fibre ingested raises the calcium requirement by 100 mg. Calcium supplementation is also available (see Table 24.2). Calcium absorption can be enhanced by dietary choices. The colon can absorb nutritionally significant amounts of calcium when fermentable substrates, especially inulin-type fructans, are

Table 24.2 Percentage elemental calcium

Calcium compound	% calcium
Calcium carbonate	40
Tribasic calcium phosphate	35
Calcium phosphate	30
Dolomite	24
Calcium amino chelate	20
Calcium lactate	13
Calcium orotate	9
Calcium gluconate	9

plentiful in the diet.[31] Inulin-type fructans are fermented in the large intestine to produce short-chain fatty acids, which lower pH and enhance calcium solubility. While inulin may enhance absorption, vitamin D is a prerequisite for adequate calcium absorption and bone growth.[32]

Vitamin D maintains calcium and phosphorus homeostasis. It binds to DNA promoting transcription of specific mRNA which codes for osteocalcin. Osteocalcin, secreted by osteoblasts, binds calcium to bone. It is involved in the differentiation of stem cells into osteoclasts that facilitate bone resorption. Vitamin D also regulates secretion of parathyroid hormone (PTH) which in turn controls levels of vitamin D. Compared to those with low vitamin D status, 12- to 15-year-old girls with high vitamin D status have significantly greater forearm BMD and lower serum PTH concentrations and bone turnover markers.[33] To maximize peak bone mass it was suggested that adolescent girls maintain serum 25-hydroxyvitamin D [25(OH)D] concentrations above approximately 50 nmol/L (20 ng/mL) throughout the year. For adolescent girls to maintain their serum 25(OH)D concentration over 50 nmol/L (20 ng/mL) requires around 1000 IU vitamin D. A study conducted on apparently healthy 10–17-year-old schoolchildren found vitamin D at doses equivalent to 2000 IU/day for 1 year to be safe and result in desirable vitamin D levels.[34] It may be difficult to meet the recommended intake of vitamin D from dietary sources (see Table 24.3). Food fortification with vitamin D is one option for enhancing serum levels. A randomized, placebo-controlled study has shown that cheese fortified with vitamin D is as bioavailable and effective as liquid vitamin D

supplementation for increasing 25(OH)D levels.[35] Another option is sun exposure. About 12 minutes in the sun at noon on a clear day with 50% of the skin exposed produces around an oral equivalent of 3000 IU vitamin D.[36] The benefits of sun exposure are neutralized by sunscreen. Applying sunscreen SPF 8+ thickly every few hours prevents dermal production of vitamin D3.

In addition to enhancing calcium absorption, serum vitamin D concentration appears positively associated with jump velocity, jump power, jump height, fitness and force.[37] It appears that vitamin D may augment the benefits associated with exercise, at least in adolescent girls. A satisfactory peak bone mass requires bone be physically strained. Exercise provides this stimulatory strain. A systematic review of the effects of exercise on bone mineral accrual in children and adolescents concluded that weight-bearing exercise enhanced bone mineral accrual in children, particularly during early puberty.[38] In fact, exercise emerged as the predominant lifestyle determinant of bone strength for females aged 12 to 22 years.[39] Exercise was a more important determinant of increased BMD and bone bending strength than was increased calcium intake and/or oral contraception. Although it remains unclear as to what constitutes the optimal exercise programme,[38] school-based exercise programmes do increase bone size and enhance the accrual of BMD and content in both prepubertal boys and girls.[40,41] The weight-bearing exercise undertaken during childhood provides bone mineral content, geometric and structural advantages that may be preserved for 40 years![42]

Maintaining bone mass

A high peak bone mass provides a buffer allowing for considerable bone loss prior to reaching the fracture threshold. During early and mid adulthood it is nonetheless important to minimize bone loss. Women at particular risk include those with a family history of osteoporosis, those with a BMI of 23 or under, and/or those who have had a late menarche and early menopause. In addition to having an adequate calcium and vitamin D intake, other dietary considerations include limiting alcohol, animal protein, salt and caffeine.

Alcohol may have a direct inhibitory effect on bone remodelling. It reduces bone resorption, decreasing type I collagen N-telopeptides in urine, and diminishes bone formation, lowering mean

Table 24.3 Sources of vitamin D

Source	Measure	Vitamin D
Cod liver oil	1 teaspoon	1360 IU
Salmon – canned with bones	55 g	343 IU
Sardines – canned with bones	55 g	150 IU
Milk	240 mL	98 IU
Fortified ready-to-eat cereals	30 g	40 IU
Noonday sun 50% exposure	12 minutes	3000 IU*

*Varies with latitude.

serum osteocalcin levels. Men who drink more than 28 standard drinks per week are at increased risk of a hip fracture, especially if their preferred beverage is beer.[43] The alcohol fracture risk threshold is 2 units or less daily. When 2 units a day are exceeded, the risk ratio increases to 1.23 for any fracture, 1.38 for osteoporotic fractures, and 1.68 for hip fractures.[44] Alcohol confers risk beyond that explained by BMD.

Caffeine is believed to compromise calcium balance. Both the amount of caffeine consumed and the associated level of calcium intake seem relevant. One cup of coffee a day (77–103 mg caffeine/day) does not appear to compromise bone development and mineralization in adolescents and young adult women;[45,46] however, two to three servings of brewed coffee may accelerate bone loss from the spine and total body in women with calcium intakes below the recommended dietary allowance of 800 mg.[47] Lifetime caffeinated coffee intake equivalent to two cups per day has been associated with decreased bone density in older women who do not drink milk on a daily basis.[48] Although caffeine has been shown to affect calcium retention, it is probably not a major concern at the level of two cups per day, provided that at least one glass of milk is consumed each day of adult life.[49] Oral doses of caffeine increase the urinary excretion of calcium, magnesium, sodium and chloride for at least 3 hours after consumption.[50] Under optimal conditions, an adequate calcium intake may compensate for increased urinary and intestinal losses.

The mechanism underlying sodium-induced calciuria is postulated to be mediated via PTH activation of vitamin D. Attempts to preserve calcium balance may be facilitated by reducing calcium excretion. The equilibration of calcium absorption and urinary excretion is only normally achieved when the net absorbed calcium equals or exceeds 150 mg; absorption of less than 150 mg of calcium per day results in a negative calcium balance due to obligatory excretion of sodium. One additional teaspoon of salt causes an approximate increase of 100 mmol/day of urinary sodium, which is associated with an obligatory rise of about 1.3 mmol/day of urinary calcium. Although a prospective study failed to find that dietary sodium, in the range measured, reduced bone mineral density,[51] total hip BMD appears to be inversely associated with age, being female, and urinary Na/Cr, and positively associated with BMI, urinary K/Cr and dietary calcium intake.[52] Similarly, links between dietary protein intake, calciuria and

clinical manifestations of osteoporosis remain unclear. High-protein diets increase obligatory calcium excretion. Every gram of protein in the diet is associated with excretion of 1 mg of calcium in the urine. Calciuria induced by high dietary protein may be minimized by consumption of protein-rich foods rich in phosphorus. This is supported by recent clinical evidence which found that the intake of dietary protein, especially from animal sources, is associated with a reduced incidence of hip fractures in postmenopausal women.[53] Dietary phosphorus in a range of 160–2270 mg/day or a calcium:phosphorus ratio of between 1:3 and 3:1 probably has no effect on calcium balance.[54]

Aside from calcium and vitamin D, it is probably energy intake that has the most important impact on skeletal health. Weight cycling damages bone. Weight fluctuations of 5–6 kg alter bone mass and produce permanent micro-architectural damage.[55] A weight reduction of 10% or more below maximum weight among middle-aged women is an important indicator for hip fracture risk.[56]

Weight-bearing exercise is obligatory for maintaining bone mass. Prolonged immobilization depletes bone mineral content; physical activity increases bone mass, strength and density. Women who exercise three times a week have higher bone density than their sedentary counterparts.[57] A randomized controlled study in premenopausal women found that high-impact exercises that load bones with movements involving rapidly rising forces improve skeletal integrity, muscular performance, and dynamic balance.[58] Weight-bearing exercise such as weight lifting, running and jumping appear well suited to protecting bone mass. Case–control and prospective studies have consistently shown that past and current exercise does protect against hip fracture.

Limiting bone loss

Bone mass peaks around the age of 30 years. Thereafter bone mass declines, the rate of which differs depending on the anatomical region.[59] In general, bone loss is around 0.3% to 0.4% annually. This rate accelerates in perimenopausal women, reaching 2–4% of BMD annually for the first 5–10 years after menopause. While biochemical tests are useful for detecting functional changes suggesting an increased future risk of osteoporosis, with advancing age structural changes become detectable. DXA is recommended for high-risk menopausal women.

Hormonal factors

Menopause is a state of sex hormone, particularly oestrogen, deprivation. Oestrogen replacement has a protective effect, probably by reducing bone resorption through inhibiting release of cytokines and removing the cytokine stimulus to osteoclast formation and bone loss. However, osteoblasts have progesterone not oestrogen receptors and progesterone is the significant hormone at the level of bone synthesis. At best, hormone replacement therapy (HRT) slows bone loss. Furthermore, although HRT is a recognized prevention and treatment method for osteoporosis, it is not licensed as a first-line therapy for this condition.[60] Concerns have been raised regarding the side effects of HRT.[61,62] See **Handout 13.11**. Risk intensifies as the dose and duration of use increase. Nonetheless, the effectiveness of low and ultra-low estrogen doses has been demonstrated for the prevention of bone loss.[60] When used, HRT should be taken for the shortest time possible, certainly less than 5 years.

Drugs that inhibit bone resorption constitute the mainstay for the treatment of postmenopausal osteoporosis.[63] Bisphosphonates, such as alendronate, risedronate or ibandronate, are the most commonly used compounds for treating postmenopausal osteoporosis. Raloxifene, a selective oestrogen-receptor modulator, reduces the rate of vertebral fractures but fails to protect against hip fractures. An amino acid fragment of parathyroid hormone (PTH) reduces both spine and non-spinal fractures. PTH peptides exert anabolic effects on the skeleton. Regardless of the drug therapy chosen, this should be combined with prudent lifestyle choices.

Calcium intake

While detection of a red flag may indicate the need for drug therapy, the presence of either an orange or red flag is an indication for lifestyle intervention. Adequate calcium is essential. Calcium supplementation in the early postmenopausal period dampens remodelling as evidenced by reduced markers for both bone resorption, urinary type I collagen cross-linked N-telopeptides, and formation, serum osteocalcin. Postmenopausal women who obtained calcium primarily from the diet had significantly lower ratios of non-oestrogenic to oestrogenic metabolites than did those who obtained calcium primarily from supplements. In fact, BMD was significantly greater in those who obtained calcium primarily from the diet. Calcium, especially that from dietary sources, is associated with a shift in oestrogen metabolism toward the active 16 alpha-hydroxyl metabolic pathway and greater BMD in postmenopausal women.[64] Absorption of calcium in supplements is increased when taken in divided doses. Calcium supplements are best taken 60–90 minutes after meals, unless the patient has achlorhydria, in which case it is best taken with meals. Calcium intake from supplements varies depending on the concentration of elemental calcium and its bioavailability. See Table 24.1. Calcium is better absorbed from lactate, citrate or gluconate than carbonate – this is a particularly important consideration in elderly people and those with hypochlorhydria. A placebo-controlled trial over 4 years on a healthy population with an average age of 61 years found that supplementation with 1200 mg of calcium daily reduced the risk of a fracture by 72%.[65] The 10-year follow-up showed benefit was lost in those who stopped taking the supplement. Twelve months of supplementation with calcium citrate in a dose of 800 mg daily when combined with aerobic, weight-bearing and weight-lifting exercise three times per week increased trochanteric bone mineral density.[66] Meta-analysis indicates that calcium supplements in combination with vitamin D reduce the risk of hip fractures.[63] A decade ago it was estimated that 134,764 hip fractures and $2.6 billion in direct medical costs could have been avoided if individuals aged 50 years of age and older consumed approximately 1200 mg of supplemental calcium daily.[67]

Vitamin D

Pooled data from double-blind randomized trials suggest a daily dose of 400 IU vitamin D may reduce hip fractures by 18%, and non-vertebral fractures by 20%.[68] Dose is important. Treatment was most beneficial when doses of vitamin D equalled or exceeded 400 IU. The benefit of a combined daily intake of vitamin D, 1000 IU, and calcium, 1200 mg, on the skeletal density of elderly women living in a sunny climate is probably mediated by a reduction in bone turnover rate.[69] Given that lower blood concentrations of vitamin D increase the likelihood of hip fractures among menopausal women by up to 70%, it has been suggested that the vitamin D concentration may be more strongly linked to frailty-related fractures.[70]

It should however also be noted that vitamin D deficiency causes muscle weakness, increasing the risk of falls and fractures.[71] Available evidence suggests that the elderly need a mean serum concentration of at least 65 nmol/L (26 ng/mL) of vitamin D to improve muscle performance and reduce the risk of falling and at least 75 nmol/L (30 ng/mL) to reduce the risk of fracture.[72] Vitamin D3, cholecalciferol, is produced in the skin on exposure to UVB radiation (290 to 320 nm); vitamin D2, ergocalciferol, is derived from plants and only enters the body via the diet. Both D3 and D2 precursors are hydroxylated in the liver and kidneys to form 25-hydroxyvitamin D [25(OH)D], the non-active 'storage' form, and 1,25-dihydroxyvitamin D [1,25(OH)$_2$D], the biologically active form that is tightly controlled by the body. Although equally well absorbed, vitamin D2 has been reported to have markedly reduced potency and shorter duration of action than vitamin D3.[73] While sun exposure may produce the most potent and long-acting form of vitamin D, the ability of the skin to synthesize vitamin D3 (cholecalciferol) decreases with age. Even though, a more recent, randomized, placebo-controlled, double-blind study found 1000 IU of either vitamin D2 or D3 daily equally effective in maintaining serum 25 (OH)D and 1,25(OH)$_2$D levels and improving bone health.[74] Diet is unreliable as the sole or primary source of vitamin D for the elderly. Even if 1000 IU of either vitamin D2 or D3 sustain blood levels of 25(OH)D above a mean of 50 nmol/L (20 ng/ mL), 1000 IU is insufficient to raise blood levels above a mean of 70 nmol/L (30 ng/mL) – a level required to reduce the risk of falls.

The benefit of vitamin D can be augmented by vitamin K. Vitamin D3 (0.75 μg/day) plus vitamin K2 (45 mg/day) protects osteoporotic postmenopausal women against lumbar bone loss better than does calcium or either vitamin alone.[75] Vitamin K is essential for the activation of osteocalcin production. It improves bone compression, bending and impact strength, femoral neck width and hip axis length in postmenopausal women. Vitamin K2 increases bone mineral content but not bone mineral density.[76]

While the elderly are well advised to complement their diet and sun exposure with a supplement rich in, at least, calcium and vitamin D, they can also improve their calcium balance by dietary means. A fibre-rich meal impairs calcium absorption. Taking calcium supplements prior to going to bed rather than after eating reduces faecal calcium excretion. Caffeine intake in excess of 300 mg daily (approximately 514 g [18 oz] of brewed coffee) accelerates bone loss in postmenopausal women, a risk attenuated by increasing the calcium intake.[77,78]

Calcium excretion

The ability to limit bone loss is impaired not only by dietary choices that influence calcium absorption but also by dietary factors that enhance calcium excretion. Sodium and protein can induce calciuria. Calcium excretion is compensated for by increased bone resorption, a response probably influenced by the vitamin D receptor genotype.[79]

Animal protein is rich in sulphur-containing amino acids which increase calciuria. Nonetheless, a cross-sectional study found that a higher intake of protein (72 g daily) was associated with a higher BMD in elderly women provided that calcium intake exceeded 408 mg daily.[80] As animal protein tends to be more acidic and vegetable protein more alkali, it is postulated that vegetable protein causes less calciuria and hence less bone loss. In practice, a recent study has reported that 25 g of soy (i.e. vegetable) protein had no added benefit in preventing bone loss or improving physical performance compared to 25 g of milk protein.[81] Dairy products, sources of calcium and vitamin D, are rich in phosphate, which is protective. Soy, on the other hand, is a source of isoflavones. While some reports suggest that isoflavone intervention significantly inhibits bone resorption and stimulates bone formation,[82] others feel that soy isoflavone supplementation is unlikely to have significant favourable effects on BMD.[83]

Sodium enhances calciuria, with every gram of sodium ingested resulting in a compensatory loss of 15 mg of calcium in the urine. Even a moderately high salt intake of 11.2 g daily elicits a marked increase in urinary calcium excretion and significantly affects bone calcium balance in persons on a high calcium diet (1284 mg).[84] On a low calcium intake, the bone calcium balance is negative even on a low salt diet of 3.9 g. Salt has no effect on the efficacy of calcium absorption. It is important that the elderly meet the recommended daily intake of calcium of at least 1200 mg.[27]

BMD and bone fragility are but two factors that predispose the elderly to fractures. Instability or falling is a major health risk.

Physical activity

Physical activity decreases the risk of falling and increases bone mass, strength and density.[85] Exercise improves gait, coordination, balance, proprioception, reaction time and muscle strength. Exercise should be dynamic, not static; exceed a threshold intensity as well as a threshold strain frequency; be relatively brief but intermittent; impose an unusual loading pattern on the bones and be supported by unlimited nutrient energy, adequate calcium and cholecalciferol (vitamin D3).[86] Exercise devoid of loading fails to exceed intensity and strain thresholds and is considerably less effective. Although still beneficial, exercise limited to brisk walking alone only marginally slows rather than prevents bone loss.[87] In addition to regulating bone maintenance and stimulating bone formation, exercise strengthens muscles and improves balance and coordination. Physical activity increases bone diameter, diminishing the risk of fractures by mechanically counteracting the bone thinning and increased bone porosity associated with ageing. Exercise improves balance, reducing postural sway.

Risk factors predisposing to falls in osteoporotic persons include poor general health, impaired integration of sensory inputs, increased response time to unexpected perturbation, visual impairment, reduced tactile sensitivity and decreased lower limb proprioception.[88] Three primary predictors of falls are body balance deficit, insufficient quadriceps muscle strength and a history of falls. Imbalance and increased postural sway are important predictors of falls and fractures in osteoporotic persons. There is an inverse relationship between the level of physical activity and postural sway both with respect to mediolateral deviation and range of sway.[88] Postural stiffness, a fundamental variable controlling balance, generates corrective signals through monitoring and rapidly acquiring and integrating sensory data to refine posture.[88] A sedentary lifestyle and ageing lead to a decrease of postural stiffness, particularly affecting mediolateral sway. When the frequency of corrective signals is reduced, information may be insufficient to detect and react to unexpected challenges, resulting in imbalance and falls. As little as a 10% increase in mean response times can produce a fivefold increase in falls.[88]

A negative correlation has also been reported between bone density and postural sway. Supplementation with calcium plus vitamin D results in a significant decrease in the number of first falls, a significant improvement in quadriceps strength of 8% and a decrease in body sway of 28%.[89] An exercise station training programme for osteopenic women improved balance, decreasing sway and increasing the strength of the hip muscles, quadriceps and trunk extensors.[90] Persons with osteoporosis tend to change their posture from the normal ankle strategy in quiet standing to rely on a hip strategy. A programme that strengthens hip muscles may be protective.

Visual impairment is another sensory deficit that challenges standing posture. On a compliant surface, sway is affected with all of the visual measures, quadriceps strength and reaction time.[91] Contrast sensitivity, depth perception and quadriceps strength are significant independent predictors of total sway when standing on a compliant surface. In contrast, on a firm surface sway only varies significantly with proprioception in the lower limbs.

The risk of osteoporotic fractures not only relates to the quality and quantity of bone, it is also affected by the propensity for falling. This in turn is influenced by intrinsic and extrinsic factors. See **Handouts 19.12** and **19.13**.

Handout 24.3 can be used to alert individuals to the factors associated with an increased risk for an osteoporotic fracture; **Handout 24.4** to increase awareness of the red flags for a current fracture. **Handout 24.5** provides a self-care programme for skeletal protection.

In perspective

Given the demographics of an ageing population, osteoporosis will predictably take an increasing toll. Lifestyle choices that establish a high peak bone mass are most effective when implemented in childhood and maintained throughout life. Osteopenia, suspected by the presence of orange and red flags, can be confirmed using markers of bone turnover. Anti-resorptive and anabolic therapy, when triggered by early warning of bone depletion, may reduce bone resorption markers by up to 70% and increase bone formation markers by up to 50%.[92]

Lifestyle choices increase or reduce personal risk. Healthy lifestyle choices, early detection of orange and red flags, and active intervention are the key to controlling this epidemic.

References

1. International Osteoporosis Foundation. http://www.iofbonehealth.org/facts-and-statistics.html; Accessed 08.02.09.

2. *Statistics by Country.* http://www.wrongdiagnosis.com/o/osteoporosis/stats-country.htm; Accessed 09.02.09.

3. NIAMS. Osteoporosis. http://www.niams.nih.gov/Health_Info/Bone/Osteoporosis/default.asp; Accessed 02.08.09.

4. Kanis JA, McCloskey EV, Johansson H, Oden A, Melton 3rd LJ, Khaltaev N. A reference standard for the description of osteoporosis. *Bone.* 2008;42(3):467–475.

5. Kanis JA, Johnell O, Oden A, et al. The use of multiple sites for the diagnosis of osteoporosis. *Osteoporos Int.* 2006;17:527–534.

6. Carey JJ, Delaney MF, Love TE, et al. Dual-energy X-ray absorptiometry diagnostic discordance between Z-scores and T-scores in young adults. *J Clin Densitom.* 2009;12(1):11–16.

7. Kanis JA, Johnell O, Oden A, Jonsson B, De Laet C, Dawson A. Risk of hip fracture according to the World Health Organisation criteria for osteopenia and osteoporosis. *Bone.* 2000;27:585–590.

8. Papaioannou A, Kennedy CC, Cranney A, et al. Risk factors for low BMD in healthy men age 50 years or older: a systematic review. *Osteoporos Int.* 2009;20(4):507–518.

9. Kanis JA, Johnell O, Oden A, et al. Smoking and fracture risk: a meta-analysis. *Osteoporos Int.* 2005;16(2):155–162.

10. De Laet C, Kanis JA, Oden A, et al. Body mass index as a predictor of fracture risk: a meta-analysis. *Osteoporos Int.* 2005;16(11):1330–1338.

11. Johnell O, Kanis JA, Oden A, et al. Predictive value of BMD for hip and other fractures. *J Bone Miner Res.* 2005;20(7):1185–1194.

12. Garnero P. Biomarkers for osteoporosis management: utility in diagnosis, fracture risk prediction and therapy monitoring. *Mol Diagn Ther.* 2008;12(3):157–170.

13. Eastell R, Hannon RA. Biomarkers of bone health and osteoporosis risk. *Proc Nutr Soc.* 2008;67(2):157–162.

14. Nguyen TV, Center JR, Eisman JA. Femoral neck bone loss predicts fracture risk independent of baseline BMD. *J Bone Miner Res.* 2005;20(7):1195–1201.

15. Eastell R. Commentary: Bone density can be used to assess fracture risk. *BMJ.* 1999;318:864–865.

16. Ralston SH, de Crombrugghe B. Genetic regulation of bone mass and susceptibility to osteoporosis. *Genes Dev.* 2006;20(18):2492–2506.

17. Zhai G, Andrew T, Kato BS, Blake GM, Spector TD. Genetic and environmental determinants on bone loss in postmenopausal Caucasian women: a 14-year longitudinal twin study. *Osteoporos Int.* 2009;20(6):949–953.

18. Michaëlsson K, Melhus H, Ferm H, Ahlbom A, Pedersen NL. Genetic liability to fractures in the elderly. *Arch Intern Med.* 2005;165(16):1825–1830.

19. Frost HM. On our age-related bone loss: insights from a new paradigm. *J Bone Miner Res.* 1997;12(10):1539–1546.

20. Myers EF, Wilson SE. Biomechanics of osteoporosis and vertebral fracture. *Spine.* 1997;22:25S–31S.

21. Larcos G. Predicting clinical discordance of bone mineral density. *Mayo Clin Proc.* 1998;73(9):824–828.

22. Slemenda C. Prevention of hip fractures: risk factor modification. *Am J Med.* 1997;103(2A):65S–71S.

23. Ullom-Minnich P. Prevention of osteoporosis and fractures. *Am Fam Physician.* 1999;60(1):194–202.

24. Gass M, Dawson-Hughes B. Preventing osteoporosis-related fractures: an overview. *Am J Med.* 2006;119(4 suppl 1):S3–S11.

25. Ondrak KS, Morgan DW. Physical activity, calcium intake and bone health in children and adolescents. *Sports Med.* 2007;37(7):587–600.

26. Heaney RP. Calcium intake in the osteoporotic fracture context: introduction. *Am J Clin Nutr.* 1991;54:242S–244S.

27. 2004 Surgeon General's Report on Osteoporosis. http://www.nlm.nih.gov/medlineplus/osteoporosis.html#cat1; Accessed 08.02.09.

28. Moore LL, Bradlee ML, Gao D, Singer MR. Effects of average childhood dairy intake on adolescent bone health. *J Pediatr.* 2008;153(5):667–673.

29. Huncharek M, Muscat J, Kupelnick B. Impact of dairy products and dietary calcium on bone-mineral content in children: results of a meta-analysis. *Bone.* 2008;43(2):312–321.

30. Wardlaw G. The effects of diet and lifestyle on bone mass in women. *J Am Diet Assoc.* 1988;88:17–25.

31. Coxam V. Current data with inulin-type fructans and calcium, targeting bone health in adults. *J Nutr.* 2007;137(11 suppl):2527S–2533S.

32. Lamberg-Allardt CJ, Viljakainen HT. 25-Hydroxyvitamin D and functional outcomes in adolescents. *Am J Clin Nutr.* 2008;88(2):534S–536S.

33. Cashman KD, Hill TR, Cotter AA, et al. Low vitamin D status adversely affects bone health parameters in adolescents. *Am J Clin Nutr.* 2008;87(4):1039–1044.

34. Maalouf J, Nabulsi M, Vieth R, et al. Short- and long-term safety of weekly high-dose vitamin D3 supplementation in school children. *J Clin Endocrinol Metab.* 2008;93(7):2693–2701.

35. Wagner D, Sidhom G, Whiting SJ, Rousseau D, Vieth R. The bioavailability of vitamin D from fortified cheeses and supplements is equivalent in adults. *J Nutr.* 2008;138(7):1365–1371.

36. Mohr SB, Garland CF, Gorham ED, Grant WB, Garland FC. Relationship between low ultraviolet B irradiance and higher breast cancer risk in 107 countries. *Breast J.* 2008;14:255–260.

37. Ward KA, Das G, Berry JL, et al. Vitamin D status and muscle function in post-menarchal

adolescent girls. *J Clin Endocrinol Metab*. 2009;94(2):559–563.

38. Hind K, Burrows M. Weight-bearing exercise and bone mineral accrual in children and adolescents: a review of controlled trials. *Bone*. 2007;40 (1):14–27.

39. Lloyd T, Petit MA, Lin HM, Beck TJ. Lifestyle factors and the development of bone mass and bone strength in young women. *J Pediatr*. 2004;144(6):776–782.

40. Linden C, Ahlborg HG, Besjakov J, Gardsell P, Karlsson MK. A school curriculum-based exercise program increases bone mineral accrual and bone size in prepubertal girls: two-year data from the pediatric osteoporosis prevention (POP) study. *J Bone Miner Res*. 2006;21 (6):829–835.

41. Lindén C, Alwis G, Ahlborg H, et al. Exercise, bone mass and bone size in prepubertal boys: one-year data from the pediatric osteoporosis prevention study. *Scand J Med Sci Sports*. 2007;17(4):340–347.

42. Kato T, Yamashita T, Mizutani S, Honda A, Matumoto M, Umemura Y. Adolescent exercise associated with long-term superior measures of bone geometry: a cross-sectional DXA and MRI study. *Br J Sports Med*. 2009. Epub ahead of print.

43. Hoidrup S, Gronbaek M, Gottschau A, Lauritzen JB, Schroll M. Alcohol intake, beverage preference, and risk of hip fracture in men and women. *Am J Epidemiol*. 1999;149(11):993–1001.

44. Kanis JA, Johansson H, Johnell O, et al. Alcohol intake as a risk factor for fracture. *Osteoporos Int*. 2005; 16(7):737–742.

45. Lloyd T, Rollings NJ, Kieselhorst K, Eggli DF, Mauger E. Dietary caffeine intake is not correlated with adolescent bone gain. *J Am Coll Nutr*. 1998;17(5):454–457.

46. Packard PT, Recker RR. Caffeine does not affect the rate of gain in spine bone in young women. *Osteoporos Int*. 1996;6(2):149–152.

47. Harris SS, Dawson-Hughes B. Caffeine and bone loss in healthy postmenopausal women. *Am J Clin Nutr*. 1994;60(4):573–578.

48. Barrett-Connor E, Chang JC, Edelstein SL. Coffee-associated osteoporosis offset by daily milk consumption. The Rancho Bernardo Study. *JAMA*. 1994;271(4): 280–283.

49. Murray TM. Prevention and management of osteoporosis: consensus statements from the Scientific Advisory Board of the Osteoporosis Society of Canada. 4. Calcium nutrition and osteoporosis. *Can Med Assoc J*. 1996;155(7): 935–939.

50. Massey LK, Whiting SJ. Caffeine, urinary calcium, calcium metabolism and bone. *J Nutr*. 1993;123(9):1611–1614.

51. Greendale GA, Barrett-Connor E, Edelstein S, Ingles S, Haile R. Dietary sodium and bone mineral density: results of a 16-year follow-up study. *J Am Geriatr Soc*. 1994;42 (10):1050–1055.

52. Woo J, Kwok T, Leung J, Tang N. Dietary intake, blood pressure and osteoporosis. *J Hum Hypertens*. 2009;23(7):451–455.

53. Munger RG, Cerhan JR, Chiu BC. Prospective study of dietary protein intake and risk of hip fracture in postmenopausal women. *Am J Clin Nutr*. 1999;69(1):147–152.

54. Hu JF, Zhao XH, Jia JB, Parpia B, Campbell TC. Dietary calcium and bone density among middle aged and elderly women in China. *Am J Clin Nutr*. 1993;58:219–227.

55. Meyer HE, Tverdal A, Falch JA. Changes in body weight and incidence of hip fracture among middle aged Norwegians. *BMJ*. 1995;311(6997):91–92.

56. Keen RW. Burden of osteoporosis and fractures. *Curr Osteoporos Rep*. 2003;1(2):66–70.

57. Law MR, Wald NJ, Meade TW. Strategies for prevention of osteoporosis and hip fracture. *BMJ*. 1991;303:453–459.

58. Heinonen A, Kannus P, Sievanen H, et al. Randomised controlled trial of effect of high-impact exercise on selected risk factors for osteoporotic fractures. *Lancet*. 1996;348 (9038):1343–1347.

59. El Maghraoui A, Ghazi M, Gassim S, Mounach A, Ghozlani I, et al. Bone mineral density of the spine and femur in a group of healthy Moroccan men. *Bone*. 2009;44(5):965–969.

60. Palacios S. Advances in hormone replacement therapy: making the menopause manageable. *BMC Womens Health*. 2008;8:22.

61. Practice Committee of American Society for Reproductive Medicine. Estrogen and progestogen therapy in postmenopausal women. *Fertil Steril*. 2008;90(5 suppl):S88–S102.

62. Deady J. Clinical monograph: hormone replacement therapy. *J Manag Care Pharm*. 2004;10 (1):33–47.

63. Close P, Neuprez A, Reginster JY. Developments in the pharmacotherapeutic management of osteoporosis. *Expert Opin Pharmacother*. 2006;7 (12):1603–1615.

64. Napoli N, Thompson J, Civitelli R, Armamento-Villareal RC. Effects of dietary calcium compared with calcium supplements on estrogen metabolism and bone mineral density. *Am J Clin Nutr*. 2007;85(5): 1428–1433.

65. Bischoff-Ferrari HA, Rees JR, Grau MV, Barry E, Gui J, Baron JA. Effect of calcium supplementation on fracture risk: a double-blind randomized controlled trial. *Am J Clin Nutr*. 2008;87(6):1945–1951.

66. Going S, Lohman T, Houtkooper L, et al. Effects of exercise on bone mineral density in calcium-replete postmenopausal women with and without hormone replacement therapy. *Osteoporos Int*. 2003;14(8): 637–643.

67. Bendich A, Leader S, Muhuri P. Supplemental calcium for the prevention of hip fracture: potential health-economic benefits. *Clin Ther*. 1999;21(6):1058–1072.

68. Bischoff-Ferrari HA, Willett WC, Wong JB, et al. Prevention of nonvertebral fractures with oral vitamin D and dose dependency: a meta-analysis of randomized controlled trials. *Arch Intern Med*. 2009;169(6):551–561.

69. Zhu K, Devine A, Dick IM, Wilson SG, Prince RL. Effects of calcium and vitamin D supplementation on hip bone mineral density and calcium-related analytes in elderly ambulatory Australian women: a five-year randomized controlled trial. *J Clin Endocrinol Metab*. 2008;93(3): 743–749.

70. Cauley JA, Lacroix AZ, Wu L, et al. Serum 25-hydroxyvitamin D

concentrations and risk for hip fractures. *Ann Intern Med.* 2008;149(4):242–250.

71. Holick MF. Optimal vitamin D status for the prevention and treatment of osteoporosis. *Drugs Aging.* 2007;24(12):1017–1029.

72. Dawson-Hughes B. Serum 25-hydroxyvitamin D and functional outcomes in the elderly. *Am J Clin Nutr.* 2008;88(2):537S–540S.

73. Armas LA, Hollis BW, Heaney RP. Vitamin D2 is much less effective than vitamin D3 in humans. *J Clin Endocrinol Metab.* 2004;89 (11):5387–5391.

74. Holick MF, Biancuzzo RM, Chen TC, et al. Vitamin D2 is as effective as vitamin D3 in maintaining circulating concentrations of 25-hydroxyvitamin D. *J Clin Endocrinol Metab.* 2008;93(3): 677–681.

75. Iwamoto J, Takeda T, Ichimura S. Effect of combined administration of vitamin D3 and vitamin K2 on bone mineral density of the lumbar spine in postmenopausal women with osteoporosis. *J Orthop Sci.* 2000;5(6):546–551.

76. Knapen MH, Schurgers LJ, Vermeer C. Vitamin K2 supplementation improves hip bone geometry and bone strength indices in postmenopausal women. *Osteoporos Int.* 2007;18(7): 963–972.

77. Rapuri PB, Gallagher JC, Kinyamu HK, Ryschon KL. Caffeine intake increases the rate of bone loss in elderly women and interacts with vitamin D receptor genotypes. *Am J Clin Nutr.* 2001;74(5):694–700.

78. Ilich JZ, Brownbill RA, Tamborini L, Crncevic-Orlic Z. To drink or not to drink: how are alcohol, caffeine and past smoking related to bone mineral density in elderly women? *J Am Coll Nutr.* 2002;21(6):536–544.

79. Harrington M, Bennett T, Jakobsen J, et al. The effect of a high-protein, high-sodium diet on calcium and bone metabolism in postmenopausal women and its interaction with vitamin D receptor genotype. *Br J Nutr.* 2004;91(1): 41–51.

80. Rapuri PB, Gallagher JC, Haynatzka V. Protein intake: effects on bone mineral density and the rate of bone loss in elderly women. *Am J Clin Nutr.* 2003;77(6):1517–1525.

81. Vupadhyayula PM, Gallagher JC, Templin T, Logsdon SM, Smith LM. Effects of soy protein isolate on bone mineral density and physical performance indices in postmenopausal women – a 2-year randomized, double-blind, placebo-controlled trial. *Menopause.* 2009;16(2):320–328.

82. Ma DF, Qin LQ, Wang PY, Katoh R. Soy isoflavone intake inhibits bone resorption and stimulates bone formation in menopausal women: meta-analysis of randomized controlled trials. *Eur J Clin Nutr.* 2008;62(2):155–161.

83. Liu J, Ho SC, Su YX, Chen WQ, Zhang CX, Chen YM. Effect of long-term intervention of soy isoflavones on bone mineral density in women: a meta-analysis of randomized controlled trials. *Bone.* 2009;44(5):948–953.

84. Teucher B, Dainty JR, Spinks CA, et al. Sodium and bone health: impact of moderately high and low salt intakes on calcium metabolism in postmenopausal women. *J Bone Miner Res.* 2008;23(9):1477–1485.

85. Kannus P. Preventing osteoporosis, falls and fractures among elderly people. *Br Med J.* 1999;318:205.

86. Borer KT. Physical activity in the prevention and amelioration of osteoporosis in women: interaction of mechanical, hormonal and dietary factors. *Sports Med.* 2005;35 (9):779–830.

87. Ebrahim S, Thompson PW, Baskaran V, Evans K. Randomized placebo-controlled trial of brisk walking in the prevention of postmenopausal osteoporosis. *Age Ageing.* 1997;26(4):253–260.

88. Kuczyński M, Ostrowska B. Understanding falls in osteoporosis: the viscoelastic modeling perspective. *Gait Posture.* 2006;23 (1):51–58.

89. Pfeifer M, Begerow B, Minne HW, Suppan K, Fahrleitner-Pammer A, Dobnig H. Effects of a long-term vitamin D and calcium supplementation on falls and parameters of muscle function in community-dwelling older individuals. *Osteoporos Int.* 2009;20 (2):315–322.

90. Hourigan SR, Nitz JC, Brauer SG, O'Neill S, Wong J, Richardson CA. Positive effects of exercise on falls and fracture risk in osteopenic women. *Osteoporos Int.* 2008;19(7): 1077–1086.

91. Lord SR, Menz HB. Visual contribution to postural stability in older adults. *Gerontology.* 2000;46 (6):306–310.

92. Camacho PM, Lopez NA. Use of biochemical markers of bone turnover in the management of postmenopausal osteoporosis. *Clin Chem Lab Med.* 2008;46 (10):1345–1357.

Preventing cancer: red flags and risky choices

25

Cancer is the second most common cause of death in the US, exceeded only by heart disease.[1] About 2,437,180 new cancer cases were expected in the US in 2008; this included an anticipated 1 million cases of basal and squamous cell skin cancers.[1] In the US, men have an almost 1-in-2 lifetime risk of developing cancer; for women, the risk is a little more than 1 in 3.[1] More than 1 in 3 people in the UK will develop cancer during their lifetime.[2] Every 2 minutes someone is diagnosed with cancer in the UK, with around 285,000 new cases diagnosed each year.[2] In 2005 there were over 100,000 new cases of cancer diagnosed in Australia, a number projected to grow by over 3000 extra cases per year between 2006 and 2010.[3] About 77% of all cancers are diagnosed in persons aged 55 years and older.[1] In Australia in 2005 the risk of being diagnosed with cancer before age 75 was 1 in 3 and before age 85 was 1 in 2.[3] Around two-thirds of cancer deaths occur in people aged 65 and over.[2]

Breast, lung, bowel and prostate cancers account for over half of all new cancers each year in the UK.[2] In 2005 in Australia, cancer of the prostate, bowel, breast, lung and cutaneous melanoma made up 61% of all diagnoses.[3] Prostate cancer made up over 29% of all male cancers and breast cancer over 27% of all female cancers diagnosed in 2005.[3]

In the US and UK, cancer accounts for 1 in 4 deaths.[1,2] More than 1500 Americans die of cancer every day,[1] and every 4 minutes somebody dies of cancer in the UK.[2] Nonetheless, half of people diagnosed with cancer now survive for more than 5 years and the average 10-year cancer survival rate has doubled over the last 30 years.[2] The 5-year relative survival rate for all cancers is improving in the US and the National Institutes of Health estimated overall costs of cancer in 2007 to be $219.2 billion: $89.0 billion for direct medical costs (total of all health expenditures); $18.2 billion for indirect morbidity costs (cost of lost productivity due to illness); and $112.0 billion for indirect mortality costs (cost of lost productivity due to premature death).[1]

Carcinogenesis

Tumours result when the balance between cellular proliferation and death (apoptosis) is disrupted. All cancers involve the malfunction of genes controlling cell growth and division. Genetic malfunction may be inherited or result from DNA mutation. It is estimated that around 10% of cancers are inherited,[2] about half of which are strongly hereditary, in that an inherited genetic alteration confers a very high risk of developing one or more specific types of cancer.[1] Most cancers results from genetic mutation.

Carcinogenesis is postulated to be a two-stage process. Initiation involves DNA damage or mutation and is irreversible. Before the potential to develop cancer is realized, a promotion stage of accelerated cell proliferation is required. Initiators alter DNA, promotors modify cell proliferation. Promotion requires prolonged exposure and is reversible in the early stages. Promotors are only weakly carcinogenic to cells not previously exposed to initiators. There is a long delay between initiation, the primary causative event and overt disease. Carcinogenesis is a slow process involving either alteration of genetic material or genetic expression. The genetic structure of the cell may be changed either by irradiation or chemicals damaging DNA or by viruses inserting DNA or RNA into the genome. Papova, adeno and herpes viruses are oncogenic DNA viruses. Carcinogenesis leading to cell transformation due to a change in genetic expression may result from inactivation of tumour suppressor cells or from the activation of oncogenes.

The two mechanisms are stimulation of oncogenes and inhibition of tumour suppressor genes. Oncogenes cause hyperactivity; they encode for substances that stimulate growth. In cancer, the effect of the altered oncogene is dominant. The unaltered normal allele of that gene in a healthy cell is the proto-oncogene. Proto-oncogenes can be turned on by carcinogenic agents. Oncogenes can be inherited, e.g. familial breast cancer or familial polyposis coli. This represents a loss of function by mutation of a positive regulator. Anti-oncogenes inhibit tumour suppressor genes. In this instance, both alleles of the gene need to be inactivated to free the cell from growth inhibition. Inhibition of a gene causing inactivity results in malignant change. This represents a loss of function due to mutation by a negative regulator.

Carcinogenesis is a multistep process involving impaired differentiation and growth control. Cancer cells are characterized by their autonomy and their poor differentiation. Autonomous cells escape normal cellular control mechanisms and proliferate freely. Anaplastic cells fail to differentiate and specialize into recognizable organ tissue. Highly malignant cancers contain more anaplastic and less differentiated cells than do less relentless malignancies. Characteristics shared by malignant cells are:

- a local increase in cell numbers
- disruption of normal cellular arrangements
- variable cell size and shape
- increased nuclear size and density
- increased and abnormal mitotic activity
- increased metabolic demand.

Tumours are classified according to their tissue of origin, invasiveness and level of differentiation. Epithelial cancers are carcinomas, connective tissue cancers are sarcomas, lymphatic cancers are lymphomas, and blood cell cancers are leukaemias. Benign tumours are non-invasive, while malignant tumours are invasive. Carcinoma-in-situ is a pre-invasive epithelial tumour. Grade I tumours are well differentiated and therefore resemble their tissue of origin and maintain certain specialized function. In contrast, Grade IV tumours are very poorly differentiated and bear no resemblance to their tissue of origin.

Cancer progresses by invading tissues and establishing distal growth sites. Malignant tissue disrupts normal cell-to-cell communication. Dysplastic cells demonstrate localized disorganized growth and differentiation; anaplastic cells are dysplastic cells which in addition demonstrate progression and metastasis. Cancer cells invade normal tissue by a process called progression. This may be assisted by the tumour secreting plasminogen-activating factor, which activates plasminogen, producing plasmin. Plasmin degrades various proteins and assists tumour invasion by breaking down extracellular fluid. Cell surface glycoproteins and glycolipids are modified in tumour cells. Such changes may result in impaired cell-to-cell recognition, altered cell responsiveness to growth factors and modification of cell receptors, with respect to both density and configuration. Cancer cells metastasize or grow in a new environment as they lack the anchoring junctions which connect normal cells to their neighbours. Gap junctions, channels between adjacent cells important in cellular communication, are also disrupted. Prevention of cancer is best achieved before cellular growth has been disrupted. While it may be difficult to guard against initiators, it is highly feasible to limit exposure to a number of promoting agents. While it may not be practicable to prevent inheriting a gene that predisposes to a particular cancer, it is possible to identify those at risk and create a cellular environment that dissuades expression of a malignant phenotype. Major preventive effort to reduce cancer rates is consequently two-pronged. In the first instance, the aim is to create a cellular environment which does not favour tumour expression. The long lag time between initiation and promotion presents an opportunity to intervene, making cancer prevention a workable proposition. In the second instance, screening for early evidence of neoplasia creates the opportunity for timely intervention and a satisfactory clinical outcome. In the former, expression of a cancer genotype may be prevented; in the latter, progression of the disease may be halted.

Risky choices: orange flags

The most cost-effective approach to cancer control is primary prevention, and primary prevention is most effectively achieved by avoiding risky lifestyle choices. The American Cancer Society estimated that in 2008 30% of cancer deaths would be attributable to tobacco use with a further 33% or more being related to overweight or obesity, physical inactivity, and nutrition.[1] Diets low in fibre, fruit and vegetables and rich in red and processed meats, salt, saturated fats and alcohol are all risky choices. Exposure to occupational and environmental carcinogens contributes a further 6% to cancer prevalence.

It is estimated that almost 2 out of 3 cancer deaths in the US in 2008 could be prevented by health-promoting lifestyle choices. An estimated half of all cancer cases could be avoided if people made healthy lifestyle changes, such as stopping smoking, moderating alcohol intake, maintaining a healthy body weight and avoiding excessive sun exposure.[2] In the UK, more than a quarter of all deaths from cancer are linked to tobacco smoking and up to 12,000 cases of cancer could be avoided if everybody had a body mass index (BMI) of 25 or less.[2] Among postmenopausal women in the UK, 5% of all cancers (about 6000 annually) are attributable to being overweight or obese.[4] Even cancers attributable to infectious agents could be reduced by behavioural choices or vaccines. Behavioural change could avoid exposure to and the risk of developing cancer from hepatitis B virus (HBV), human papillomavirus (HPV) and human immunodeficiency virus (HIV).

Cancer prevention by avoiding risky choices requires apparently healthy people to commit to a lifetime of prudent choices. Risky choices can create an environment in which genes with the potential to permit and/or stimulate uncontrolled cellular proliferation can be expressed. Risky choices are orange flags for cancer prevention. They, along with a family history of cancer and increasing age, can designate particular individuals as 'high risk'.

Red flags

At least half of all new cancer cases in the US can be prevented or detected earlier by screening.[1] For individuals undergoing periodic health examinations, the American Cancer Society recommends a cancer-related check-up that encompasses health-related counselling and, depending on a person's age and gender, might include examination for cancers of the thyroid, oral cavity, skin, lymph nodes, testes, and ovaries, as well as for some non-malignant diseases.[1] They also strongly recommend routinely screening high-risk groups for biomarkers.

Detection of biomarkers suggesting early stages of cellular change creates the opportunity for early diagnosis and timely intervention. Screening followed by active intervention achieves a substantially better clinical outcome than treating clinically overt cancers. Histological and biochemical cell alterations characteristic of malignant transformation have been identified. Screening can detect pre-malignant changes in the cervix, colon, and rectum, allowing removal of aberrant tissue before it becomes malignant.[1] Screening also detects cancers of the breast, rectum, cervix, prostate, oral cavity, and skin at early stages. The 5-year relative survival rate for these cancers is about 85%, a reflection of real reductions in mortality and earlier diagnosis because of screening.[1]

Recognizing intermediate biomarkers of risk facilitates earlier diagnosis of the disease. Substances produced by cancer cells, collectively called tumour cell markers, are increasingly being used to screen individuals for cancer, diagnose specific types of cancer, and follow the clinical course of a cancer patient. Certain tumour cell markers that are emerging as useful diagnostic tags contain tumour-specific antigens that can be detected on routine immune surveillance. These are the same cell antigens targeted by a healthy immune system to eliminate detected tumour cells. Behavioural choices may influence the ability of the immune system to recognize cancer cells as non-self and destroy them. Just as the risk of acquiring cancer can be lessened, so too can the risk of dying of cancer.

Site-specific cancers

Cancer develops in response to damaged genes interacting with environmental factors. Cancer may occur sporadically or in families. In the latter case, cancer susceptibility may be inherited through acquiring a single dominant gene or through transmission of a number of strongly interacting genes. Persons are at greatest risk when they inherit a single dominant risky gene. In these cases, cancer presents at an earlier age. Cancer predisposition is characterized by vertical transmission, i.e. subsequent generations are susceptible to the site-specific cancer with offspring having a 50% chance of acquiring the defective gene. An autosomal dominant predisposition to one cancer may include a predisposition to other cancers. A family history provides valuable information in these instances. However, cancer is more often a sporadic occurrence. Although individuals may inherit a few aberrant genes, expression of a malignant phenotype depends on further genetic damage before carcinogenesis is initiated. Once initiated, development of clinically significant tumours depends on the cellular environment. The cellular environment is strongly influenced by lifestyle choices. Genes may predispose certain anatomical sites to carcinogenesis, but ultimately it is exposure to environmental variables that determines tumour progression.

Increasing BMI is associated with a significant increase in the risk of cancer. The absolute impact varies by site. For each 10-unit increase in BMI, the risk of endometrial cancer is increased 2.89-fold; that of adenocarcinoma of the oesophagus, 2.38×; kidney cancer, 1.53×; leukaemia, 1.50×; multiple myeloma, 1.31×, pancreatic cancer, 1.24×; non-Hodgkin lymphoma, 1.17×; ovarian cancer, 1.14×; breast cancer in postmenopausal women, 1.40×; colorectal cancer in premenopausal women, 1.61×; and all cancers combined, 1.12×.[4] Similar associations are found between BMI and risk of mortality from cancer.

While risk factors overlap, it is a unique combination of orange flags that determine the susceptibility to any one cancer. The outcome of the disease is determined by the aggressive nature of a malignancy, i.e. the rapidity of its growth and propensity to metastasize, the immune status of the patient, and the availability of early detection and successful intervention procedures.

Lung cancer

Fifteen percent (15%) of American men and 14% of women diagnosed with cancer in 2007 presented with cancer of the lung and bronchus.[1]* Yet, lung cancer is essentially a preventable disease. There is a clear dose–response relationship between smoking and lung cancer. Compared to lifelong non-smokers, male smokers are about 23 times and female smokers 13 times more likely to develop lung cancer.[1] Cigarette smoke byproducts are suspected to damage the multiple tumour suppressor 1 (*MTS1*) gene which acts on cell division. Smoking intensity, i.e. direct exposure, modifies risk with respect to years since quitting, age, method of inhalation, and type of cigarette.[5] Below 15 to 20 cigarettes a day, the excess odds ratio per pack-year increases with the number of cigarettes smoked. Risk appears greater when total exposure occurs over a shorter rather than a longer period.[6] Above 20 cigarettes per day, the converse is true, with risk being greater when total exposure is delivered over a longer period. Despite this paradox, the risk of lung cancer for a two-packets-a-day smoker is 20 times that of the non-smoker. Women are at risk after 10 pack-years compared to men who are at risk after 20 pack-years, i.e. smoking two packets a day over 20 years. For a fixed number of cigarettes smoked, the risk of lung cancer increases with age. Smoking increases the risk of at least 15 types of cancer, ranging from nasopharyngeal, pharyngeal and laryngeal cancers, through oral, oesophageal, stomach, pancreatic, cervical (uterine cervix), kidney and bladder cancers, to acute myeloid leukaemia.[1] Smoking is so potent a risk that it deserves the status of a red flag! **Handout 25.1** provides tips on how to reduce the risk of lung cancer. Handouts provided in Chapter 16 can be used to ascertain smoking behaviour and formulate a suitable quit strategy.

With the exception of lung cancer, cancer mortality rates have declined by 16% since 1950.[1] Although not the most common malignancy, cancer of the lung and bronchus is responsible for more cancer-related deaths annually in men (31%) and women (26%) than any other.[1] In the UK, more than 1 in 5 of all cancer deaths are from lung cancer.[2] Cigarette smoking is responsible for almost 9 in 10 lung cancer deaths.[2] The high mortality rate associated with lung cancer is partially attributable to it being diagnosed late. Non-invasive techniques such as chest X-ray and sputum cytology are of limited use. Low-dose spiral computed tomography scans and determination of molecular markers in sputum are promising; however, there is as yet no satisfactory early detection method.

As therapy is unsatisfactory, prevention of lung cancer remains the preferred approach to controlling this condition. Preventive efforts target smoking. Smokers who quit reduce their risk, albeit not to a never-smoker's level. At best, nutritional intervention based on a diet rich in green leafy vegetables offers a modicum of protection.[7] Never smoking and quitting are highly effective preventive measures; unfortunately, the tobacco industry continues to outspend tobacco control initiatives by a ratio of nearly 24 to 1.[8]

Colorectal cancer

Skin cancer aside, lung cancer is the second and colorectal cancer the third most common cancer in both sexes.[1]* Although risky lifestyle choices are an important consideration (see **Handout 25.2**), unlike lung cancer there is no single lifestyle choice that largely determines the likelihood of acquiring colorectal cancer. Obesity, physical inactivity, smoking, heavy alcohol consumption, a diet high in red or processed meat, and an inadequate intake of fruits and vegetables have all been implicated in the pathogenesis of this disease. A 12-year follow-up study identified a significant positive association between the Western dietary pattern and the risk of colon cancer.[9] The Western pattern is characterized by higher intakes of red and processed meats, high-fat dairy foods, refined grains, gravy and sauces, and high-fat and high-sugar desserts. A prudent pattern is characterized by higher intakes of fruits, vegetables, legumes, fish, poultry, and whole grains. Compared with the lowest intake, persons with the highest intake for total fruit, berries, fruit juice and green leafy vegetables had a 34%, 36%, 28%, and 26% reduced risk of colorectal adenomas, respectively.[10] Epidemiological evidence also suggests site-specific susceptibility to consumption patterns. Cancer of the distal colon is linked to fat and that of the rectum with alcohol consumption.[11] The risk of colon cancer is increased 1.24-fold in men with a higher BMI, that of rectal cancer 1.09-fold.[12] Genetic polymorphism explains these discrepancies. Variations in activity and inducibility of CYP2E1, in relation to alcohol or red meat intake, have been shown to contribute to the divergent susceptibility of colon and rectal cancer.[13]

Unlike lung cancer where primary prevention rests largely on one behavioural choice, prevention of colorectal cancer requires avoiding a number of risky dietary choices. Orange flags for colorectal cancer include:

- Alcohol. The risk of rectal cancer is moderately increased when intake exceeds 30 g a day. The hazard ratio for baseline alcohol intake is 1.07 for every 10 g per day increase.[14] Alcohol adversely affects folate metabolism and increases the risk of polyps. In the transition to carcinoma, bowel mucosa passes through a phase of adenomatous polyp formation.

- Fat. A case–control study found strongest positive associations between colon cancer risk and increased total fat intake. Significant positive associations were observed between proximal colon cancer risk in men and consumption of red meat and dairy products; and between distal colon cancer risk in women and total intake of meat and processed meat.[15] Another study found that although total and *trans*-monounsaturated fatty acids and palmitic, stearic and oleic acids were dose-dependently associated with colorectal cancer risk, these effects did not persist after further energy adjustment.[16] This suggests energy rather than these fats per se confer increased risk. Furthermore, significant dose-dependent reductions in risk were associated with increased consumption of omega-3 polyunsaturated fatty acids, an association which persisted after adjusting for energy both with respect to nutrient-energy and total fatty acid intake.[16] Meta-analyses of prospective cohort studies confirmed that consuming fish or omega-3 fatty acids tended to reduce colorectal cancer incidence.[17] Compared to those who have fish less than once a week, persons eating fish at least five times weekly reduced their risk of colorectal cancer by 40%.[18] Excess energy intake, regardless of the source, is a risky choice. When energy is derived from omega-3 fatty acids rather than saturated or *trans* fats, this risk is reduced.

- A low-fibre diet. Low-fibre diets favour constipation. Diets rich in insoluble fibre prevent constipation and are believed to protect against colon cancer by reducing mucosal exposure to carcinogens through a bulky stool diluting any carcinogens and shortening bowel transit time. A high fibre intake offers additional benefits by supporting multiplication of bacteria producing anticarcinogenic substances such as butyric acid. Butyric acid can modify nuclear architecture and, by changing the structure of chromatin, can induce apoptosis. In the case of the colon, butyric acid can overcome the resistance of cancer cells to normal programmed death.[19] A diet rich in fibre, although having no effect on rectal cancer, could cut the risk of developing colon cancer by about 40%.[20]

- Dairy products. In children, a high total dairy intake was associated with a near-tripling in the odds of colorectal cancer compared with low intake.[21] Evidence for a link between cancer risk and dairy consumption in adulthood is also increasing, and significant positive associations have been observed between proximal colon cancer risk in men and consumption of dairy products.[15] However, a significantly reduced risk of distal colon cancer was noted in women with increasing intake of dairy products.[15] Furthermore, a cohort study reported that the intake of dairy products was inversely associated with colorectal cancer risk, especially among non-users of supplemental calcium.[22] Total calcium intake and vitamin D intake were also inversely associated with colorectal cancer. Animal models have shown that intracellular calcium regulates proliferation of epithelial cells and dietary calcium inhibits hyperproliferation of colonic epithelial cells. A randomized, single-blind, controlled study found that the proliferative activity of colonic epithelial cells was decreased and markers of normal cellular differentiation restored by increasing the daily intake of calcium to 1200 mg via low-fat dairy food in subjects at risk for colonic neoplasia.[23] Whatever the final result, low-fat rather than full-cream dairy products are safer.
- A sedentary lifestyle. A sedentary lifestyle may predispose to constipation. Exercise reduces constipation. Increased leisure-time physical activity is associated with a modest reduction in colon, but not rectal, cancer risk.[24]

In addition to lifestyle choices influencing susceptibility to colorectal cancer, the increased incidence of this disease among family members suggests an inherited susceptibility in some instances. The risk of colorectal cancer increases from 4% in cases where there is no family history to 8% or 9% when one first-degree relative has either an adenomatous polyp or colorectal cancer and to 16% when that first-degree relative was diagnosed with colorectal cancer before the age of 45 years.[25] About 25%

of cases are thought to inherit genetic mutations. In less than 5% of cases, multiple family members present with familial adenomatous polyposis or hereditary non-polyposis colorectal cancer due to transmission of an autosomal dominant gene. Although 75% of colorectal cancer cases occur sporadically with no apparent evidence of an inherited disorder, genes play an important role in carcinogenesis. About 85% of colorectal cancers are due to events that result in chromosomal instability, while the remaining 15% are due to events that result in microsatellite instability or replication error.[25] Sixty-nine genes have been identified as relevant to the pathogenesis of colorectal cancer, with individual colorectal cancers containing an average of nine mutant genes per tumour. Mutation of DNA damage-repair genes may predispose colorectal epithelial cells to anaplasia; genes prone to replication errors can produce unstable tumours that progress rapidly from adenoma to carcinoma. The transformation of benign adenomatous polyps into colorectal cancers is well documented. More than 95% of colorectal cancers are carcinomas, and about 95% of these are adenocarcinomas. **Colorectal cancers usually grow slowly and may take 10–20 years to become malignant.** The protracted transition from normal mucosa through adenomatous polys to cancer offers opportunity for preventive interventions.

Both the incidence of and death rate from colorectal cancer has been decreasing over the last 2 decades. Rather than being attributable to prudent dietary choices, this improvement is largely due to improved screening.[1] The National Cancer Institute provides a colorectal cancer self-assessment tool which may be used prior to active screening.[26] The risk of colorectal cancer increases with age; more than 90% of cases are diagnosed in individuals aged 50 and older. Beginning at age 50, active screening for polyps and colorectal cancer is recommended.[27] The faecal occult blood test is useful because of its ease of administration. Annual occult blood testing is recommended for:

- everybody over the age of 50 years
- 40-year-olds who have a first-degree relative (parent, sibling, child) diagnosed with colorectal cancer at 50 years or older. Flexible sigmoidoscopy is recommended every 5 years
- 35-year-olds who either have a first-degree relative diagnosed with colorectal cancer before the age of 50 years or have two first-degree relatives with colorectal cancer. Colonoscopy should be performed every 3 to 5 years

- 25-year-olds who have three first-degree relatives with hereditary non-polyposis colorectal cancer. Colonoscopy should be performed at 2-yearly intervals
- 10-year-olds in a family with familial polyposis coli.

Persons with a history of breast, endometrial or ovarian cancer, previous bowel irradiation, or inflammatory bowel disease such as Crohn's disease or ulcerative colitis, are also at increased risk.

The usefulness of results derived from testing for occult blood depends on the underlying condition and the test used. Overall, in a standard at-risk population over the age of 40 years, 2–4% of tests will be positive. The false-negative rate for symptomatic cancer is about 30%, for large adenomatous polyps is about 20% and for small polyps is even greater.

Two types of occult blood tests are available. The traditional guaiac Hemoccult test is based upon the pseudoperoxidase activity of haem. The chemical guaiac test requires at least 10–20 mL/day of blood loss from the stomach or 1–2 mL/day of colonic blood loss before it is detectable. The guaiac test method detects between 40% and 80% of asymptomatic colorectal cancers and 30–40% of large adenomas. Up to 50% of cancers will be missed if the appropriate protocol is not followed. When dietary restrictions are followed, the Hemoccult test is highly specific. Between 98% and 99% of healthy subjects are negative. The newer Hemoccult SENSA variant works on a similar principle and is more sensitive and likely to detect 60–80% of colorectal cancers and 60% of large adenomas.

Immunochemical tests detect as little as 0.25–0.5 mL/day of colonic blood loss, while requiring over 100 mL of gastric blood loss before becoming positive. Immunochemical faecal occult blood tests are more sensitive than guaiac tests. They may detect up to 80–90% of bowel cancers and 60–75% of large adenomas.

The correct procedure for faecal occult blood testing requires that:

- reagents in the test kit have not exceeded their 'use by' date
- peroxidase-rich food not be ingested for 3 days before or during the test. Foods that may result in a false-positive result and must be excluded include: uncooked radishes, horseradish, raw broccoli, cauliflower, parsnips, bananas, cabbage, potatoes, cucumbers, mushrooms, artichokes, raw turnips, pineapples, melons and red meat

- certain medication be avoided. Vitamin C gives a false-negative result, while aspirin and other non-steroidal anti-inflammatory drugs (NSAIDs) may result in a false-positive result. Vitamin C must be avoided for 3 days and NSAIDs for 7 days prior to and during the test
- two smears are taken from each of three successive stools. The stool should be sampled from a normally passed bowel action and sampled from an area where blood may be present
- preliminary rehydration of slides with tap water is undertaken. This doubles slide sensitivity, decreasing the false-negative rate to 10% but increasing the false-positive rate
- any blue colour, no matter how transient, should be reported as positive. The test must be read in good light.

With specificity around 98%, any positive occult blood test serves as a red flag indicating the need for further investigation. Due to its low sensitivity (49%), persons at risk who have a negative annual faecal occult blood test or faecal immunochemical test also require further investigation. As fewer than 10% of colorectal cancers or adenomas develop within the potential reach of digital rectal examination, patients require more invasive investigations using a flexible sigmoidoscopy at 5-yearly intervals. The 60-cm flexible sigmoidoscopy identifies nearly all polyps and cancers greater than 1 cm in diameter. Up to 80% of polyps occur in the region of the bowel examined.[28] Colonoscopy every 10 years has also been suggested.[1] Indications for colonoscopy include:

- a positive occult blood test
- blood mixed with stool
- abdominal symptoms or a change in bowel habit
- a polyp, blood or mucosal changes on flexible sigmoidoscopy
- age over 40 years and a family history of colon cancer in a first-degree relative.

Persons with a personal or family history of colorectal cancer and/or polyps, or a personal history of chronic inflammatory bowel disease should be screened more frequently. It has been estimated that primary prevention through dietary modification may reduce the incidence of colorectal cancer by one-fifth, while secondary prevention by proctosigmoidoscopy may more than halve mortality. Double-contrast barium enema is another screening option available. Double-contrast barium enema allows examination of the entire bowel, but has low sensitivity for large polyps and cancers.[25]

Polyps or carcinomas are surgically removed. Patients are advised to screen their diets and minimize their intake of orange flags. They can also decrease their risk of polyp recurrence by taking aspirin and omega-3 fatty acid supplements. While the omega-6 arachidonic acid cascade has been linked to cancer formation and cell proliferation, an increased intake of omega-3 fatty acids may cut the risk of colorectal cancer in men not taking aspirin by 66%.[29] Epidemiological studies have consistently shown that chronic intake of NSAIDs, principally aspirin, can reduce the incidence of colorectal adenomas and carcinomas.[30] Aspirin and omega-3 fatty acids are thought to reduce the risk of colon cancer via altering prostaglandin metabolism in favour of less pro-inflammatory compounds. Overexpression of cyclooxygenase-2 in epithelial cells inhibits apoptosis and increases the invasiveness of tumour cells. Inhibitors of cyclooxygenases (Cox-1 and Cox-2) are chemopreventive and tumorigenesis is inhibited. Downregulation of Cox-1 and Cox-2 is a potentially important strategy for preventing cancer, as cyclooxygenases catalyse formation of prostaglandins, chemicals with multiple effects that favour tumour growth and development.[31] About half of inherited bowel cancers are due to germline mutations of mismatched repair genes and aspirin suppresses the accumulation of these mutations.

Randomized trials have shown that aspirin reduces the short-term risk of recurrent colorectal adenomas in patients with a history of adenomas or cancer.[32] In view of the slow growth rate of colorectal cancer, there is a latency period of about 10 years. Consumption of four to six aspirin tablets each week over 20 years was reported to reduce the risk of colorectal cancer by 50% in women.[33] As aspirin may prevent up to 15% of colorectal cancers,[34] persons with multiple risk factors for colorectal cancer may benefit from aspirin 300 mg (one tablet) daily. Use of 300 mg or more of aspirin a day for about 5 years appears to offer effective primary prevention of colorectal cancer.[32] At 300 mg, this aspirin dose is higher than the 80 mg/day required for cardiovascular protection. Folic acid may also have a preventive effect. A randomized, double-blind, placebo-controlled study suggested long-term high-dose supplementation with folic acid may inhibit recurrence of colorectal adenomas.[35]

Breast cancer

Breast cancer is the most commonly diagnosed cancer in women, making up 26% of new cancers detected annually in American women. Despite this, breast cancer is only responsible for 15% of cancer-related deaths.[1]* This is the converse of lung cancer. Although breast cancer lacks a single dominant risk factor as is the case with tobacco and lung cancer, early diagnosis and superior treatment outcomes make this a more manageable problem. Breast cancer bears many similarities to colorectal cancer insofar as between 5% and 10% of cases are inherited, multiple lifestyle choices are believed to influence pathogenesis, and population screening with early intervention provides a good clinical outcome in a substantial number of cases. According to estimates of lifetime risk, about 13.2% of women in the general population will develop breast cancer, compared with estimates of 36% to 85% of women with an altered breast cancer 1 (*BRCA1*) or *BRCA2* gene.[36] Women who have a first-degree relative (mother, sister, or daughter) with a history of breast cancer have about twice the risk of developing breast cancer compared to women who do not have a family history.[1]

The risk of breast cancer is increased three to seven times by the presence of altered *BRCA1* and *BRCA2* genes.[36]

The breast is a hormone-sensitive organ. Prolonged exposure to hormonal changes associated with the menstrual cycle is an important consideration when the personal risk of breast cancer is assessed. Woman at greatest risk are those who have an early menarche and late menopause and who are childless or had few children at an older age. Lifestyle choices also influence risk. Compared to teetotallers, consumption of 13.8 g of alcohol daily is associated with an increased risk for oestrogen receptor (ER+)/progesterone receptor (PR+) positive tumours.[37] Moderate alcohol consumption of 30 g a day is associated with a 32% increased risk for total breast cancer and a 43% increased risk for invasive breast cancer, compared to zero alcohol consumption.[38] A 10-g increase in daily intake of alcohol increases the odds ratio for breast cancer to 1.13[37] or increases the risk for ER+/PR+ tumours by 11%.[38] Alcohol-induced increases in circulating oestrogen or other hormones, reduction of folic acid levels, or a direct effect of alcohol or its metabolites on breast tissue are suspected to contribute to this increased risk.[1]

Regular consumption of even a few drinks per week has been associated with an increased risk of breast cancer in women.

Vigorous physical activity may decrease exposure of breast tissue to circulating oestrogen.[1] Compared with less active women, women who engage in regular strenuous physical activity at age 35 years have a 14% decreased risk of breast cancer.[39] Compared with inactive women, those who engage in the equivalent of 1.25 to 2.5 hours per week of brisk walking reduce their risk by 18%. Women with a BMI 24 or under benefit most. Exercise also protects against obesity and recent studies exploring intentional weight loss suggest that losing weight may reduce the risk of breast cancer.[1]

Increased adipose tissue may influence cancers of the reproductive system by altering the metabolic pathway of oestradiol, decreasing binding and facilitating oestrogen synthesis.[40] A study comparing the impact of four different diets on the risk of developing breast cancer concluded that BMI was likely responsible for the observed association.[41] Adherence to Western and prudent diet patterns were associated with an odds ratio for breast cancer of 1.32 and 1.42, respectively; a 'Native Mexican' diet of Mexican cheeses, soups, meat dishes, legumes and tomato-based sauces and a 'Mediterranean' diet rich in liquor, poultry, seafood, vegetables, salad greens and high-fat salad dressings were associated with an odds ratio for breast cancer of 0.68 and 0.76 respectively.[41] Compared to endogenous oestrogens, phytoestrogens have low potency. Nonetheless, in premenopausal women phytoestrogens tend to reduce stimulation of ER sites, while in postmenopausal women they tend to increase stimulation of these sites. Soy products are rich sources of isoflavones, well-known phytoestrogens. Compared to those consuming no more than 5 mg of isoflavones daily, those consuming 10 mg and 20 mg daily reduce their odds ratio of breast cancer to 0.88 and 0.71 respectively.[42] Approximately 10 mg of isoflavones can be obtained from a daily serve of tofu. Higher soy intake has been shown to be associated with a 33% reduced risk of breast cancer in postmenopausal women with a BMI above the median; in leaner postmenopausal women, the risk drops 17%.[43]

Equol is an isoflavonoid phytoestrogen produced from the soy isoflavone daidzein by gut microflora. Among women, dietary fibre or other components of a high-fibre diet may promote the growth and/or activity of bacterial populations responsible for equol production in the colon.[44] Compared to those with the lowest intake, a diet rich in fruit and cereal fibre confers a statistically significant reduced risk for overall and for ER+/PR+ cancer.[45] Benefit is most apparent in postmenopausal women who have used hormone replacement. Another study confirmed the protective effect of cereal fibre. Compared to those consuming 4 g or less, those consuming at least 13 g of cereal fibre daily appeared to reduce their risk of breast cancer by 41%.[46] Fruit and vegetables are also good sources of alpha-carotene, beta-carotene and lycopene, which have been shown to be inversely associated with the risk of ER+/PR+ invasive breast cancer,[47] and flavonols, flavones, flavan-3-ols and lignans, which are associated with a reduced risk of incident postmenopausal breast cancer.[48] Some flavonoids have been shown to bind to oestrogen receptors. There is little doubt that the risk of at least some cases of breast cancer is influenced by hormonal balance. The National Cancer Institute provides a breast cancer assessment tool which can be used for preliminary screening.[49]

Carbohydrate intake and glycaemic load have been associated with ER-negative breast cancer.[50] One study found a high glycaemic index to be associated with a 1.35-fold increased risk for breast cancer in overweight women and those in the highest category of waist circumference. An increased risk of breast cancer was also associated with a high glycaemic load and/or carbohydrate intake.[50] Another study reporting on a carbohydrate-rich diet, particularly one that imposed a high glycaemic load, confirmed an increase in the risk of breast cancer.[51] In addition to improving energy metabolism and weight control, physical activity may reduce circulating concentrations of insulin and related growth factors.[1] Exercise may reduce the risk of all types of breast cancer!

An association between dietary fat and breast cancer risk has long been suspected. While the result of high energy intake, i.e. increased BMI, has been linked, it is not only the energy provided by fat that seems pertinent. A significant inverse association has been observed between total omega-3 polyunsaturated fatty acids and the risk of breast cancer.[52] In fact, the inverse association with omega-3 fatty acids is most marked in women consuming the highest amounts of omega-6 PUFA.[53] Furthermore, the risk of breast cancer is inversely associated with intake of alpha-linolenic acid from fruits and vegetables and vegetable oils, but positively associated when alpha-linolenic acid is derived from processed foods and nut mixes.[53] There also appears to be a modest association between saturated fat intake and breast cancer risk.[54] Both pre- and post-menopausal women who consume the most red and processed meat have an increased risk of breast cancer;[55] on the other hand, two or more servings of dairy products daily appears to offer some protection.[56] Rather than saturated fat explaining the discrepancy between meat and dairy products, it appears likely that other constituents in dairy foods, such as calcium and vitamin D, may be protective.[57] Moreover, it appears that increased vitamin D, whether from sun exposure and/or diet, reduces the risk of breast cancer, irrespective of ER/PR status of the tumour.[58]

Primary prevention of breast cancer through prudent lifestyle choices is hampered by the lack of clear-cut modifiable lifestyle factors. The relatively low mortality rate of breast cancer, given its prevalence, is consequently largely attributable to early diagnosis through screening with subsequent successful treatment. Nonetheless, the U.S. Preventive Services Task Force (USPSTF) considers there to be insufficient evidence to recommend on routine clinical breast examination alone or on teaching women how to perform routine breast self-examination.[27] Even so, clinical breast examination detects about 60% of cancers detected by mammography, as well as some cancers not detected by mammography.[59] Conversely, the USPSTF does recommend screening mammography, with or without clinical breast examination, every 1 or 2 years for women aged 40 and older.[27] There is fair evidence that mammography screening every 12–33 months significantly reduces mortality from breast cancer; evidence is strongest for women aged 50–69 years of age.[27] The benefit:potential harm ratio for screening becomes more favourable as women age. In 2005, 66.5% of women aged 40 and older in the US reported getting a mammogram in the past 2 years.[7] Screening MRI is recommended for women with a 20% or greater lifetime risk of breast cancer.[1] This includes women with a strong family history of breast or ovarian cancer and women who were treated for Hodgkin disease.[1]

Despite the USPSTF's reticence, many believe that all women, but particularly those with risk factors, should perform breast self-examination. Women deemed at higher risk are those who: menstruated for more than 40 years; have a familial risk, i.e. have three or more close relatives on the same side of the family who have breast cancer; have a family member with breast cancer before the age of 45 and/or family members with ovarian cancer.

To be most effective, breast self-examination must be regularly performed. The median tumour size detected by either self- or clinician examination in one study was 2 cm.[59] Women untrained in breast self-examination can detect lumps of approximately 1.5 inches (3.8 cm) in size. Women who occasionally do breast self-examination are likely to detect a 1 inch (2.5 cm) mass, while those who regularly do breast self-examination are expected to be capable of detecting lumps of 0.5 inch (1.27 cm) in size. Mammography can detect lesions less than half this size. Nonetheless, breast self-examination does detect cancers that are smaller than those detected without screening. Furthermore, survival after a diagnosis of breast cancer tends to be longer among women who practise breast self-examination.[60] The optimal time for breast self-examination in a menstruating woman is a few days after the end of a menstrual period. Women should allow about 10 minutes each month for breast self-examination. **Handout 25.3** provides guidelines for breast self-examination.

Finding any abnormality on breast self-examination suggests the need for professional evaluation. In addition to professionals providing access to mammography, professional breast examination includes examination of the anterior, central, posterior and lateral axillary nodes as well as the supraclavicular and infraclavicular lymph nodes. Much of the breast drains into the anterior axillary nodes located along the lower border of pectoralis major.

In addition to routine breast self-examination, women at high risk should exercise regularly,[40] not smoke, avoid excess alcohol, and eat a diet low in fat and rich in fruits and vegetables.[41] Red and orange flags for breast cancer are listed in **Handout 25.4**.

Prostate cancer

The incidence of prostate cancer increased 1.7% over 15 years; it now affects 1 in 6 men in the US. One quarter of new male cases of cancer diagnosed annually are in the prostate, yet only 10% of men die from prostate cancer each year.[1]* Like breast cancer, there is a familial component but most cases are sporadic. Like breast cancer, lifestyle factors do play a role but which modifiable lifestyle factors and to what extent have yet to be determined. Like breast cancer, screening is available for prostate cancer but the cost:benefit ratio of routine screening is uncertain. In fact, the USPSTF feels there is insufficient evidence to recommend for or against routine screening for prostate cancer using prostate-specific antigen (PSA) testing or digital rectal examination (DRE).[27] The major reason for the discrepancy between the prevalence and mortality rates of prostate cancer is most likely associated with its slow growth. It has been suggested that more men die with prostate cancer than of the disease, as the estimated number of men with unrecognized prostate cancer exceeds the number with clinically detected disease. In fact, the increasing trend in the lifetime risk of prostate cancer may be attributable to longer life expectancy and better detection methods rather than any absolute increase in disease prevalence.[61]

Although the aetiology of prostate cancer remains obscure, certain non-modifiable risks are clearly defined. Age is a risk factor for prostate cancer: whereas 1 in 10,000 men under age 40 years will be diagnosed, the incidence rises to 1 in 38 in those aged 40 to 59, and more than doubles to 1 in 15 in the 60- to 69-year age group.[62] In fact, more than 65% of all prostate cancers are diagnosed in men over the age of 65. From 5% to 10% of prostate cancer cases are believed to be due primarily to high-risk inherited genetic factors for prostate cancer.[63] Men with a single first-degree relative – father, brother or son – with a history of prostate cancer are twice as likely to develop the disease, while those with two or more relatives are nearly four times as likely to be diagnosed.[62] Risk escalates if the affected family members were diagnosed at a young age, i.e. before 60 years of age.

The association between prostate cancer and modifiable lifestyle variables is obscure. Some dietary risk factors that possibly modulate prostate cancer risk are fat and/or meat consumption, dairy products/calcium/vitamin D and plant products/ phytoestrogen/vitamin E, lycopene, and selenium.[63] Fat has long been suspected of being associated with prostate cancer. Omega-3 fatty acids from fatty fish appear to lower the risk of developing advanced prostate cancer. In fact, eating the equivalent of three servings of fish per week may halve the risk of developing advanced prostate cancer.[62] Each additional daily intake of 0.5 g of marine fatty acid from food may decrease the risk of metastatic cancer by up to 24%.[64] On the other hand, studies suggest a high intake of alpha-linolenic acid, an omega-3 fatty acid found in green leafy vegetables, flaxseed and walnuts, is more likely to favour the development of prostate cancer and advanced prostate cancer.[62] While red meat does not appear to be associated with total or aggressive prostate cancer,

persons on a diet rich in dairy foods have a statistically significant reduced risk of aggressive prostate cancer.[65] Dairy foods protect current, but not former, smokers against aggressive cancer. Dairy foods are a major source of dietary calcium, yet a prospective study found that men with an intake of 2 g daily of calcium were at increased risk of prostate cancer.[66] Another study reported that blood levels of *trans* oleic acid (18:1n-9t), *trans* linoleic acid (18:2t), and total *trans*-fatty acids were positively associated with the risk of non-aggressive prostate tumours.[67] No association was found between blood levels of *trans*-fatty acids and risk of aggressive prostate tumours.

The relationship between plant products and prostate cancer is equally complex. Some researchers suggest lycopene or tomato-based regimens are ineffective for prostate cancer prevention;[68] others suggest four to five tomato-based meals per week may decrease the risk of prostate cancer by 25% and the risk of advanced prostate cancer by 60%.[69] Another group reported a statistically significant inverse association between higher plasma lycopene concentrations and prostate cancer risk.[70] They felt that tomato products may exhibit more potent protection against sporadic prostate cancer than against those with a stronger familial or hereditary component. Inverse associations between beta-carotene and prostate cancer risk were also detected among younger participants.[70] An increased intake of cruciferous vegetables, specifically cauliflower and broccoli, may reduce prostate cancer risk in a dose–response fashion.[71] Rat experiments showed a combination of broccoli and tomato reduced tumour weight more effectively than either vegetable alone.[72] Combining lycopene in tomatoes and glucosinolates in broccoli may enhance apoptosis, or programmed cell death, in cancer cells. Based on current results, researchers postulated that a 55-year-old man could improve his prostate health with daily consumption of 1.4 cups of raw broccoli and 2.5 cups of fresh tomato, or 1 cup of tomato sauce, or half a cup of tomato paste.[72] Eating whole foods is preferable, cooked tomatoes may be better than raw tomatoes, and chopping and heating may make the cancer-protective constituents of tomatoes and broccoli more bioavailable. Recently, a new prostate 'health food' has been identified. Pomegranate products and their polyphenols were shown to reduce tumour cell growth and induce apoptosis in both androgen-dependent and androgen-independent prostate cells.[73] Soy products are another dietary source influencing hormonal balance. Increased intake of soy isoflavones and their aglycones (genistein and daidzein) appears to significantly decrease the risk of prostate cancer.[74] The highest average isoflavone intake (89.9 mg/day) was associated with a 58% reduction in risk compared with the lowest average isoflavone intake (less than 30.5 mg/day).[74]

The relationship between physical activity and prostate cancer is complex. One study reported an inverse association between occupational but not leisure-time physical activity and prostate cancer risk.[75] In another study, vigorous physical activity failed to show a significant association with prostate cancer mortality.[76] As there is neither a satisfactory dietary nor exercise formula for prevention of prostate cancer, early detection of disease is a priority. However, the USPSTF has concluded that evidence is insufficient to determine whether the benefits of population screening outweigh the harm.[27]

Early detection relies upon the PSA test and/or DRE. The American Cancer Society recommends men 50 years and older be informed about the benefits and limitations of testing for early prostate cancer detection so they can make an informed decision. Men at high risk, including men of African descent and men with a first-degree relative diagnosed with prostate cancer at a young age, should begin screening at age 45.[1]

DRE requires the patient assume a side-lying position, hips and knees flexed with exposed buttocks close to the edge of the examining table. A gloved hand is used to part the buttocks and inspect the sacrococcygeal and perianal area. The patient is asked to strain, and as the anal sphincter relaxes, a lubricated gloved fingertip is inserted. The sphincter initially tightens, and when it again relaxes, the inserted finger is gently moved in the direction of the umbilicus. Anal sphincter tone, tenderness, induration or irregularities are noted. The posterior surface of the prostate is examined by rotating the hand clockwise with the finger deeply inserted. The patient will feel the urge to urinate. The examining finger is swept over the prostate to identify the lateral lobes and median sulcus. The size, shape and consistency of the prostate are noted. The normal prostate is rubbery and non-tender. Any tenderness and nodules are recorded. Malignancy should be suspected if a hard nodule or an irregular prostate is palpated. Failure to detect the median sulcus strengthens the likelihood of prostate cancer.

In men with a normal DRE, a PSA of 4–10 ng/mL carries a 25% probability and a PSA in excess of 10 ng/mL carries a 50% probability of cancer.[8] In patients with a PSA under 2.5 ng/mL, it is wise to screen every 12 months; with a PSA of 2.5–4.0 ng/mL, 6-monthly monitoring is recommended; and if the PSA is between 4 and 10 ng/mL, a free PSA should be ordered. Patients with a free PSA of 25% or more, or a total PSA in excess of 10 ng/mL, should have a biopsy and transrectal ultrasound. According to the 2005 NHIS, over 40% of American men aged 50 and older had had PSA tests within the past year.[8]

Handout 25.5 provides a self-screening tool for an increased risk of prostate cancer.

Cervical cancer

It was estimated there would be 11,070 new cervical cancers and 3870 cervical cancer deaths in the US in 2008.[77] However, an additional 1,250,000 women are diagnosed with precancerous cervical changes annually.[77] While Cancer Societies would prefer that all women over 40 years of age have an annual pelvic examination, cervical cancer is the only gynaecological malignancy for which screening is widely accepted and recommended. Early detection of cervical cellular changes followed by appropriate intervention prevents cervical cancer being listed amongst the top 10 cancers diagnosed in the US annually.[1] Effective secondary prevention and control of cervical cancer are attributable to the slow growth rate of the lesion and cytology screening, using the Papanicolaou (Pap) smear test. Cervical cancer develops through a continuum ranging from atypical squamous cells of undetermined significance, to low-grade cervical intraepithelial neoplasia (CIN1), to high-grade squamous intraepithelial lesions (CIN2 and CIN3), to invasive cancer. Lesions can regress, persist, or progress to an invasive malignancy. CIN1 lesions are more likely to regress spontaneously, while CIN2 and CIN3 are more likely to persist or progress. The average time for progression of CIN3 to invasive cancer is estimated to be 10 to 15 years.[77] Cervical cancer is a largely preventable condition. Progression to high-grade dysplasia or invasive cervical cancer cannot manifest without evidence of oncogenic human papillomavirus (HPV) infection.[78]

HPV infection is the initiating factor for cervical cancer. Cervical cancer is a sexually transmitted disease. It presents more frequently in women who initiate sexual activity at an early age and have multiple partners. Of the 30 or so types of HPV that infect the human genital tract, HPV types 16 and 18 are most often associated with invasive disease.[77] Promoting factors that increase the likelihood of cervical cancer include other infections, exposure to carcinogens in tobacco smoke, cervical trauma and hormonal stimuli. Other sexually transmitted factors such as herpes simplex virus 2 may play a co-causative role. Abstaining from sexual activity prevents HPV infection. Unprotected sex is the primary behavioural risk factor. Barrier protection, using a condom on all occasions, especially with spermicidal gels, offers substantial protection. Smoking is another orange flag. Among HPV-infected women, current and former smokers have approximately double or treble the incidence of CIN2, CIN3 or invasive cancer. Passive smoking increases risk to a lesser extent. High parity is a risk factor. The more full-term pregnancies reported, the greater the likelihood of cervical cancer among HPV-infected women. Oral contraceptive use is associated with increased risk. The longer the use, the greater the risk. Use of oral contraceptives for 10 years or longer appears to quadruple risk.

Secondary prevention of cervical cancer through screening is highly successful. Pap smears identify cellular dysplasia and provide an opportunity for intervention when cure is possible. In countries with ubiquitous Pap testing, the prevalence of cervical cancer has dropped 75%. This is directly attributed to screening alone.[78] Screening should begin approximately 3 years after a woman begins having vaginal intercourse, but no later than 21 years of age.[27] In 2005, 79.6% of American women aged 18 years and older reported having had a Pap test within the past 3 years.[8] Screening should be done every year with regular Pap tests or every 2 years using liquid-based tests in women between 18 and 30 years. Women aged 70 and older who have had three or more consecutive normal Pap tests in the last 10 years may choose to stop cervical cancer screening. Between the ages of 30 and 70, women who have had three normal test results in a row may get screened every second year.[77] Alternatively, women aged 30 years and over may be screened every 3 years if HPV DNA testing is combined with conventional Pap cytology.[79] HPV testing can identify high-grade cervical intraepithelial neoplasia earlier than Pap smears can, with acceptable rates of specificity. The USPSTF feels it may be premature to recommend for or against the routine use of HPV testing as a primary screening test for cervical cancer.[27] Prevention through vaccination against HPV is deemed to supplement rather than replace Pap screening.[77] Routine HPV vaccination is recommended for females aged 11–12 and those between 13 and 18 who missed or need to complete the vaccination series.[8] HPV vaccination is not currently recommended for women over 26 years of age or for men. Vaccination against HPV-16 and HPV-18 reduces incident infections and persistent infections by 91.6% and 100% respectively.[77] How long protection lasts is not known.

While prevention of cervical cancer rests firmly on the dual pillars of avoiding HPV infection and early detection of cervical epithelial cellular changes, diet should not be ignored. Compared to HPV-16-negative women with higher red cell folate, HPV-16-positive women with low red cell folate levels are significantly more likely to be diagnosed with CIN2 or more serious lesions.[80] Those with higher circulating concentrations of folate appear less likely to become positive for HPV and are more likely to become HPV-negative. Significant reduction in the risk of cervical cancer appears associated with diverse nutrients. Risk was significantly reduced with increased dietary fibre, vitamin C, vitamin E, vitamin A, alpha-carotene, beta-carotene, lutein, folate, and total fruit and vegetable intake.[81]

Like lung cancer, cervical cancer can be largely prevented by a single behavioural choice. However, unlike quitting, abstinence from sexual activity is currently not a viable option for survival of the human race. Vaccination and screening provide practical alternatives given the slow growth rate of cervical cancer. **Handout 25.6** provides a self-screening tool for an increased risk of cervical cancer.

Skin cancer

Although skin cancer is the most common form of cancer in the US*, the USPSTF considers there to be insufficient evidence to recommend on routine screening for skin cancer using total-body skin examination.[27]

Many of the more than 1 million skin cancers anticipated in 2008 in the US could have been prevented by protection from the sun's rays and avoiding indoor tanning.[1]

There are different types of skin cancer. The two most common types of skin cancer are highly curable. Basal and squamous cell carcinomas are so common and so treatable they are not tracked by central cancer registries.[82] Melanoma, the third most common skin cancer, is more dangerous, especially among young people. The estimated incidence in 2008 of melanoma in males was 34,950 and in females, 27,530, 5% and 4% respectively of all cancers diagnosed annually.[1]

Fair-skinned persons are 50 times more likely to be diagnosed and 22 times more likely to die of melanoma than are darker-skinned persons.[82] Up to 90% of melanomas are caused by exposure to ultraviolet (UV) light or sunlight.

Sun exposure is the most important orange flag for skin cancer. Exposure to sunlight hastens skin ageing and increases the risk of malignant change. Exposure of skin to both long-wavelength UVA (320–400 nm, tanning rays) and short-wavelength UVB (290–320 nm) stimulates melanin production, with increased pigment being produced within 24–48 hours and being dispersed over 5 to 10 days. Epidemiologic data suggest that most skin cancers can be prevented if children, adolescents, and adults are protected from UV radiation.[82]

The intensity, spectrum and duration of UV exposure all influence the risk of skin cancer. Ozone depletion, the level of UV light, latitude, altitude and weather conditions influence the emission of UV radiation reaching the earth's surface. UV exposure is greatest between 10:00 and 14:00 hours. Human skin is sensitive to UV radiation between a wavelength of 250 and 400 nm. Long-term repeated UVA exposure leads to photodamage and potentiates the effects of UVB on skin cancer formation. Epidemiological studies suggest that the action spectrum for skin cancers varies, with solar UVB being most important for squamous cell carcinoma, UVA being most important for melanoma, and both being important for basal cell carcinoma.[83] Lifetime sun exposure and sunburn increase the risk of squamous cell carcinoma, solar keratoses and, to a lesser degree, basal cell carcinoma.[84] By contrast, lifetime sun exposure appears associated with a lower risk of malignant melanoma. However, painful sunburns before the age of 20 years are associated with an increased risk of malignant melanoma and the development of its precursors, melanocytic naevi and atypical naevi.[84] Very high melanocytic naevi counts are associated with more than 4 hours daily of sun exposure and a history of sunburn. Persons with more than 200 naevi 2 mm or more in diameter

are at significant risk of malignant melanoma. Melanocytic naevus counts increase with age, fair skin colour and freckling.

The risk of sunburn and skin cancer decreases as natural skin pigmentation increases.[85] Skin type influences the risk associated with sun exposure.[82] Skin is categorized into six groupings, with Type I individuals being very fair skinned and always burning on sun exposure. Fair-skinned people, those with blue or green eyes and blond or red hair are at highest risk. Warning signs of being at risk are having a skin that burns, freckles, reddens easily, or becomes painful on limited sun exposure. Whereas Type I skin burns easily and never tans, Type II tans minimally and burns slightly less easily. Types III through to V are increasingly likely to tan rather than burn. Type VI persons are dark skinned and never burn but may still develop melanoma. Persons with certain types and/or a large number of moles are at increased risk, partially because early neoplastic changes may be missed.

The UV index provides a measure of UV overexposure. There is little risk at UV 0 but the risk increases as the index rises. UV intensity varies with latitude, being greatest where the ozone layer is thinnest. High altitude and reflection from snow and water also increase risk. An average of 3 hours at the beach can result in an estimated UV dose of 10.4 standard erythemal doses (SED). One SED is equivalent to an erythemally effective UV radiation exposure of 100 Joules per metre squared (J/m^2). A just-perceptible erythema is produced in unacclimatized skin by exposures of about 1.5 SED in Type I subjects, 2 SED in Type II subjects, and 3 SED in Type III subjects. Beachgoers may be exposed to five times the UVR dose required to result in erythema among unprotected fair-skinned populations.[86] Large epidemiological studies report that sun exposure on the beach or during water sports increases the risk of basal cell carcinoma, whereas skiers are at increased risk for squamous cell carcinoma.[87] Outdoor endurance sports increase the number of melanocytic naevi and solar lentigines. Sweating induced by heat or physical exercise significantly contributes to UV-related skin damage, increasing photosensitivity and augmenting the risk of sunburn.[87] Hydration of the horny layer is suspected to shift the UV absorption spectrum of the stratum corneum to shorter wavelengths and to decrease reflection and dispersion. Persons with a personal or family history of skin cancer are at increased risk.

Less common causes of skin cancer include ionizing radiation, environmental pollutants, chemical carcinogens and work-related exposures.[88] Viral infections such as HPV can cause squamous cell carcinomas. Exposure to artificial UV radiation (tanning beds and lamps), ageing, diet and smoking are attributable risks.[83] While increasing age provides an increased opportunity for sun exposure, the relationship with smoking and diet is more complex. Smoking appears to be a risk factor for non-melanoma skin cancers, but has been found inversely correlated with melanoma.[83] Meta-analysis suggests that vitamin D receptor polymorphisms may be important in the development of skin cancers; however, any association with vitamin D intake is less clear.[89] Unlike cigarette smoking, limited sun exposure is beneficial. Some 12 minutes in the midday sun or equivalent meets the daily requirement for vitamin D3, and vitamin D deficiency is so prevalent as to be viewed as a public health issue by some researchers.[90] Adult deficiency of vitamin D possibly precipitates or exacerbates osteopenia, osteoporosis, muscle weakness, fractures, autoimmune diseases, infectious diseases, cardiovascular diseases, type 1 diabetes and several types of cancer. Primary prevention of skin cancer is based on avoiding sun exposure, and inevitably impairs cutaneous vitamin D production.

Measures to reduce sun exposure and prevent these skin changes include:

- avoiding sunlight between 10:00 and 14:30 hours
- wearing protective clothing. This includes eye protection. Wraparound glasses or high impact resistant contact lenses that provide 100% UV filtration and high levels of blue light filtration are ideal[91]
- applying sunscreen with a solar protection factor (SPF) of at least 15. As 70–80% of ultraviolet rays penetrate the cloud layer, use of sunscreen is also required on overcast days. The amount of sunscreen applied also influences the protection afforded.

Of the 56% of American adults who practise at least one of the three sun-protective behaviours, 30% usually apply sunscreen, with 7% applying sunscreen with an SPF of 15 or higher; 18% report usually wearing some type of fully sun-protective clothing and 33% usually seek out shade.[82] Only 9% of high school students report routinely using a sunscreen with an SPF of 15 or higher and about 9% of teens aged 14–17 years use indoor tanning devices.[82]

In addition to primary prevention, the destructive effects of skin cancer can be avoided or limited by secondary prevention. Basal cell carcinoma is undoubtedly the most common malignant skin cancer and the most common of all human malignancies. UVB radiation is believed to play a dominant role in the pathogenesis of this cancer. UVB radiation damages DNA and its repair system, resulting in progressive genetic alterations and formation of neoplasm. UV-induced mutations in the TP53 tumour-suppressor gene have been found in about 50% of basal cell carcinoma cases.[92] This slow-growing malignancy is usually found in persons over the age of 35 years. A latency period of 20–50 years is typical between the time of UV damage and the clinical onset of basal cell carcinoma. Most cases are seen on the head and neck of chronically sun-exposed elderly people.

There are numerous variations in clinical presentation of basal cell carcinoma, including nodular, ulcerating, pigmented, sclerosing, superficial and fibroepithelioma variants.[93] Each varies in clinical presentation, histopathology and aggressive behaviour. Skin changes suggestive of basal cell carcinoma are a slow-growing, small, smooth-surfaced, well-defined pink/red nodule. Its pearly or translucent border is best seen by stretching the skin over the nodule. The nodule has overlying telangiectatic vessels and over time develops central ulceration and crusting, resulting in the typical 'rodent ulcer' with its rolled edge. Lesions most commonly occur around the orbit or at the side of the nose. Although rarely metastatic, the malignant nature of basal cell carcinoma is sometimes manifest as local tissue destruction, disfigurement, and even death if left untreated.

Solar keratoses are intraepidermal skin tumours that have the potential to progress to squamous cell carcinomas, second only to basal cell carcinoma as the most common type of skin cancer. Approximately 10% of solar keratoses will progress to squamous cell carcinomas in around 2 years.[94] This premalignant condition occurs on light-exposed areas and presents as erythematous dysplastic scaly lesions which sting if picked. These lesions come and go, often clearing in winter. The presentation of squamous cell carcinoma depends on the stage of the disease. The initial lesion is a progressive scaly erythematous patch on a sun-exposed area which undergoes cycles of macular and scaly erythematous lesions. The scaly lesions have a sandpaper texture on palpation and are often found in sun-damaged areas. In advanced cases, the lesion is either a hard enlarging flesh-coloured nodule or an ulcerated nodule with an everted edge and crusts. The tumour can metastasize.

Melanoma is a neoplasm of the pigmented cells of the skin and eye. Suspect lesions, particularly in an individual with a family history of dysplastic naevi, have a history of changing colour, shape or size. They are intermittently mildly itchy and bleed spontaneously or following minor trauma. Asymmetry, atypical network and blue-white structures are reproducible dermoscopic criteria with high sensitivity for the diagnosis of melanoma, even in the hands of non-experts.[95] Immediate further investigation is indicated for asymmetrical lesions of variable colour that are 5 mm or more in diameter with an irregular border.

Ocular malignant melanomas are most usually found in middle-aged individuals. The clinical presentation includes gradual painless loss of vision in an eye with an absent red reflex. Ophthalmoscopy reveals a pigmented tumour of the choroid visualized through the retina as a dark oval mass. Secondary retinal detachment may result from the malignant mass protruding into the vitreous. In sharp contrast to the other cutaneous malignancies, melanoma is one of the most aggressive forms of cancer. Survival depends largely on primary tumour thickness, ulceration and sentinel node status at the time of diagnosis. Once melanoma has metastasized to distant sites, the prognosis is fatal, with median survival times between 7 and 9 months.[96]

Handout 25.7 provides a self-screening tool for an increased risk of skin cancer. Danger signs vary depending on the type of skin cancer. See Figure 25.1.

A cancer-minimizing lifestyle

Lifestyle has a profound impact on cancer risk. Smoking alone accounts for at least 30% of all cancer deaths and an estimated 40% of the reduction in male cancer deaths between 1991 and 2003 can be attributed to smoking declines in the last half century.[8] Furthermore, about one-third of the cancer

deaths in the US each year are due to lifestyle factors such as nutrition and physical inactivity.[1] Overweight and obesity contribute 14–20% of all cancer-related deaths in that country.[1] Overweight and obesity are clearly associated with an increased risk for developing cancers of the breast, colon, endometrium, and kidney, and adenocarcinoma of the oesophagus.[1] Highly suggestive evidence suggests that obesity increases the risk for cancers of the pancreas, gallbladder, thyroid, ovary, and cervix, as well as for myeloma, Hodgkin lymphoma, and aggressive prostate cancer.[1] Maintaining a healthy weight throughout life by balancing energy intake and output is a proven recipe for good health.

Another proven recipe for good health is a plant-based diet. Not only does a diet rich in grains, pulses, vegetables and fruit favour weight loss,[97] it also is cancer protective. Amongst the protective constituents are vitamins, minerals, and natural cancer-protective phytonutrients including plant-based phenols, polyphenols, flavonoids, isoflavones, terpenes and glucosinolates.[98]

Limiting alcohol to 2 units or fewer each day further reduces cancer risk, particularly amongst smokers.[99] Alcohol causes cancers of the oral cavity, pharynx, oesophagus and liver, and a small increase in the risk for breast cancer. **Handout 25.8** provides some general guidelines for reducing the overall risk of cancer.

In perspective

Twenty years ago it was stated: 'The prevention of cancer will come from knowledge obtained from biomedical research, education of the public, and lifestyle changes made by individuals.'[100] The same remains true today.

Cancer is an important cause of death; primary prevention through prudent lifestyle choices and secondary prevention through screening are powerful tools for controlling this disease. Being cognizant of the orange and red flags for cancer risk can enable individuals to take preventative measures and reduce their personal risk of acquiring and dying from cancer. Researchers estimate 30–40% of all kinds of cancer could be prevented with a healthy lifestyle and dietary measures.[101]

---

*New case estimates made by the American Cancer Society exclude basal and squamous cell skin cancers and in situ carcinoma except urinary bladder.[1]

Examination of skin lesions includes:
- examination and magnification of any local lesions
- examination of the drainage area
- biopsy of the local lesion

Definitive diagnosis is made on biopsy.

Local lesions suggestive of malignancy vary depending on the underlying skin lesion.
Findings suggestive of malignant melanoma are:

- a change in: colour, shape or size
- a mild intermittent itch
- spontaneous bleeding or following minor trauma
- a family history of dysplastic naevi

Abrupt breakdown of pigment at the edge of the lesion and radial streaming beyond the border of the lesion (pseudopodia) are ominous signs.

Malignant melanoma should not be be confused with:

- seborrhoeic keratoses in the elderly. Seborrhoeic keratoses recur, are asymptomatic and may present as classical warty or brown slightly waxy lesions with discrete edges or be pale flesh-coloured, flat scaly lesions
- melanotic naevus in young people. Melanocytic naevi may be flat or raised and are evenly coloured with a sharp, well-demarcated edge. The colour does not fade in winter and varies from deep to light brown, or may even be flesh coloured.

The presence of a basal cell carcinoma is suggested by detecting a small nodule with:

- pink or red colour
- a well-defined edge
- a smooth surface
- a pearly or translucent border
- overlying telangiectatic vessels

Second and subsequent lesions are common especially in basal cell cancer.
Basal cell carcinoma may be confused with a chronic patch of eczema or psoriasis. On the trunk they are often scaly and erythematous rather than flat plaques. Check for basal cell carcinoma by stretching the skin to detect a pearly edge.

Findings suggestive of squamous cell carcinoma are:

- a change in a scaly erythematous patch in a sun-exposed area
- cycles of macular and scaly erythematous lesions
- a sandpaper texture on palpation

Lesions found on the scalp, retroauricular and nasolabial areas are often associated with a poorer prognosis.
Squamous cell carcinoma must be differentiated from solar keratosis, a premalignant condition with erythematous dysplastic scaly lesions that come and go, often clearing in winter. The lesions are found on light-exposed areas and sting if picked at. Check for squamous cell carcinoma by stretching the skin to detect an everted edge.

Figure 25.1 • Diagnosing skin cancer.

References

1. American Cancer Society. *Cancer Facts and Figures 2008*. http://www.cancer.org/docroot/stt/content/stt_1x_cancer_facts_and_figures_2008.asp; Accessed 12.02.09.

2. Cancer Research UK. http://info.cancerresearchuk.org/cancerstats/incidence/; Accessed 12.02.09.

3. AIHW. *Cancer Update December 2008*. http://www.aihw.gov.au/cancer/index.cfm; Accessed 12.02.09/.

4. Reeves GK, Pirie K, Beral V, et al. Cancer incidence and mortality in relation to body mass index in the Million Women Study: cohort study. *BMJ*. 2007;335(7630): 1134.

5. Lubin JH, Caporaso N, Wichmann HE, Schaffrath-Rosario A, Alavanja MC. Cigarette smoking and lung cancer: modeling effect modification of total exposure and intensity. *Epidemiology*. 2007;18(5):639–648.

6. Lubin JH, Alavanja MC, Caporaso N, et al. Cigarette smoking and cancer risk: modeling

total exposure and intensity. *Am J Epidemiol*. 2007;166(4):479–489.

7. Dosil-Díaz O, Ruano-Ravina A, Gestal-Otero JJ, Barros-Dios JM. Consumption of fruit and vegetables and risk of lung cancer: a case-control study in Galicia, Spain. *Nutrition*. 2008;24(5):407–413.

8. American Cancer Society. *Highlights, CPED 2008*. http://www.cancer.org/docroot/STT/content/STT_1x_Cancer_Prevention_Early_Detection_Facts__Figures_2008.asp; Accessed 14.02.09.

9. Fung T, Hu FB, Fuchs C, et al. Major dietary patterns and the risk of colorectal cancer in women. *Arch Intern Med*. 2003;163(3):309–314.

10. Wu H, Dai Q, Shrubsole MJ, et al. Fruit and vegetable intakes are associated with lower risk of colorectal adenomas. *J Nutr*. 2009;139(2):340–344.

11. Weisburger JH. Dietary fat and risk of chronic disease: mechanistic insights from experimental studies. *J Am Diet Assoc*. 1997;97(suppl): S16–S23.

12. Harriss DJ, Atkinson G, George K, et al. Lifestyle factors and colorectal cancer risk (1): systematic review and meta-analysis of associations with body mass index. *Colorectal Dis*. 2009;11(6):547–563.

13. Morita M, Le Marchand L, Kono S, et al. Genetic polymorphisms of CYP2E1 and risk of colorectal cancer: the Fukuoka Colorectal Cancer Study. *Cancer Epidemiol Biomarkers Prev*. 2009;18(1):235–241.

14. Thygesen LC, Wu K, Grønbaek M, Fuchs CS, Willett WC, Giovannucci E. Alcohol intake and colorectal cancer: a comparison of approaches for including repeated measures of alcohol consumption. *Epidemiology*. 2008;19(2):258–264.

15. Hu J, Morrison H, Mery L, DesMeules M, Macleod M. Canadian Cancer Registries Epidemiology Research Group. Diet and vitamin or mineral supplementation and risk of colon cancer by subsite in Canada. *Eur J Cancer Prev*. 2007;16(4):275–291.

16. Theodoratou E, McNeill G, Cetnarskyj R, et al. Dietary fatty acids and colorectal cancer: a case-control study. *Am J Epidemiol*. 2007;166(2):181–195.

17. Geelen A, Schouten JM, Kamphuis C, et al. Fish consumption, n-3 fatty acids, and colorectal cancer: a meta-analysis of prospective cohort studies. *Am J Epidemiol*. 2007;166(10):1116–1125.

18. Hall MN, Chavarro JE, Lee IM, Willett WC, Ma J. A 22-year prospective study of fish, n-3 fatty acid intake, and colorectal cancer risk in men. *Cancer Epidemiol Biomarkers Prev*. 2008;17(5):1136–1143.

19. Waldecker M, Kautenburger T, Daumann H, et al. Histone-deacetylase inhibition and butyrate formation: fecal slurry incubations with apple pectin and apple juice extracts. *Nutrition*. 2008;24(4):366–374.

20. Wakai K, Date C, Fukui M, et al. Dietary fiber and risk of colorectal cancer in the Japan collaborative cohort study. *Cancer Epidemiol Biomarkers Prev*. 2007;16(4):668–675.

21. van der Pols JC, Bain C, Gunnell D, Smith GD, Frobisher C, Martin RM. Childhood dairy intake and adult cancer risk: 65-y follow-up of the Boyd Orr cohort. *Am J Clin Nutr*. 2007;86(6):1722–1729.

22. Park SY, Murphy SP, Wilkens LR, Nomura AM, Henderson BE, Kolonel LN. Calcium and vitamin D intake and risk of colorectal cancer: the Multiethnic Cohort Study. *Am J Epidemiol*. 2007;165(7):784–793.

23. Holt PR, Atillasoy EO, Gilman J, et al. Modulation of abnormal colonic epithelial cell proliferation and differentiation by low-fat dairy foods: a randomized controlled trial. *JAMA*. 1998;280(12):1074–1079.

24. Harriss DJ, Atkinson G, Batterham A, et al. Lifestyle factors and colorectal cancer risk (2): a systematic review and meta-analysis of associations with leisure-time physical activity. *Colorectal Dis*. 2009;11(7):689–701.

25. National Cancer Institute. *Genetics of Colorectal Cancer*. http://www.cancer.gov/cancertopics/pdq/genetics/colorectal/healthprofessional; Accessed 16.02.09.

26. *Colorectal cancer assessment tool*. http://www.cancer.gov/colorectalcancerrisk/; Accessed 16.02.09.

27. U.S. Preventive Services Task Force Update, 2002 Release. *Guide to Clinical Preventive Services, 3rd Edition: Periodic Updates*. http://www.ahrq.gov/clinic/3rduspstf/preface.htm. Accessed 13.02.09.

28. Branch WT, Crouch M. Periodic health exams: what really matters? *Patient Care*. 1998;32:21–47.

29. Hall MN, Campos H, Li H, et al. Blood levels of long-chain polyunsaturated fatty acids, aspirin, and the risk of colorectal cancer. *Cancer Epidemiol Biomarkers Prev*. 2007;16(2):314–321.

30. Gwyn K, Sinicrope FA. Chemoprevention of colorectal cancer. *Am J Gastroenterol*. 2002;97(1):13–21.

31. Levy GN. Prostaglandin H synthases, nonsteroidal anti-inflammatory drugs, and colon cancer. *FASEB J*. 1997;11(4):234–247.

32. Flossmann E, Rothwell PM. British Doctors Aspirin Trial and the UK-TIA Aspirin Trial. Effect of aspirin on long-term risk of colorectal cancer: consistent evidence from randomised and observational studies. *Lancet*. 2007;369(9573):1603–1613.

33. Ruschoff J, Wallinger S, Dietmaier W, et al. Aspirin suppresses the mutator phenotype associated with hereditary nonpolyposis colorectal cancer by genetic selection. *Proc Natl Acad Sci USA*. 1998;95:11301–11306.

34. Vainio H, Morgan G, Kleihues P. An international evaluation of the cancer-preventive potential of nonsteroidal anti-inflammatory drugs. *Cancer Epidemiol Biomarkers Prev*. 1997;6(9):749–753.

35. Jaszewski R, Misra S, Tobi M, et al. Folic acid supplementation inhibits recurrence of colorectal adenomas: a randomized chemoprevention trial. *World J Gastroenterol*. 2008;14(28):4492–4498.

36. National Cancer Institute. *Genetic Testing for BRCA1 and BRCA2: It's Your Choice*. http://www.cancer.gov/cancertopics/factsheet/risk/brca; Accessed 16.02.09.

37. Deandrea S, Talamini R, Foschi R, et al. Alcohol and breast cancer risk defined by estrogen and progesterone receptor status: a case-control study. *Cancer Epidemiol Biomarkers Prev.* 2008;17(8):2025–2028.

38. Zhang SM, Lee IM, Manson JE, et al. Alcohol consumption and breast cancer risk in the Women's Health Study. *Am J Epidemiol.* 2007;165(6):667–676.

39. McTiernan A, Kooperberg C, White E, et al. Recreational physical activity and the risk of breast cancer in postmenopausal women: the Women's Health Initiative Cohort Study. *JAMA.* 2003;290 (10):1331–1336.

40. Shepard RJ, Shek PN. Association between physical activity and susceptibility to cancer. *Sports Med.* 1998;26:293–315.

41. Murtaugh MA, Sweeney C, Giuliano AR, et al. Diet patterns and breast cancer risk in Hispanic and non-Hispanic white women: the Four-Corners Breast Cancer Study. *Am J Clin Nutr.* 2008;87 (4):978–984.

42. Wu AH, Yu MC, Tseng CC, Pike MC. Epidemiology of soy exposures and breast cancer risk. *Br J Cancer.* 2008;98(1):9–14.

43. Wu AH, Koh WP, Wang R, Lee HP, Yu MC. Soy intake and breast cancer risk in Singapore Chinese Health Study. *Br J Cancer.* 2008;99 (1):196–200.

44. Lampe JW, Karr SC, Hutchins AM, Slavin JL. Urinary equol excretion with a soy challenge: influence of habitual diet. *Proc Soc Exp Biol Med.* 1998;217(3):335–339.

45. Suzuki R, Rylander-Rudqvist T, Ye W, Saji S, Adlercreutz H, Wolk A. Dietary fiber intake and risk of postmenopausal breast cancer defined by estrogen and progesterone receptor status—a prospective cohort study among Swedish women. *Int J Cancer.* 2008;122(2):403–412.

46. Cade JE, Burley VJ, Greenwood DC, et al. Dietary fibre and risk of breast cancer in the UK Women's Cohort Study. *Int J Epidemiol.* 2007;36(2):431–438.

47. Cui Y, Shikany JM, Liu S, Shagufta Y, Rohan TE. Selected antioxidants and risk of hormone receptor-defined invasive breast cancers among postmenopausal women in the Women's Health Initiative Observational Study. *Am J Clin Nutr.* 2008;87(4):1009–1018.

48. Fink BN, Steck SE, Wolff MS, et al. Dietary flavonoid intake and breast cancer risk among women on Long Island. *Am J Epidemiol.* 2007;165 (5):514–523.

49. National Cancer Institute. *Breast Cancer Risk Assessment Tool.* http://www.cancer.gov/bcrisktool/; Accessed 16.02.09.

50. Lajous M, Boutron-Ruault MC, Fabre A, et al. Carbohydrate intake, glycemic index, glycemic load, and risk of postmenopausal breast cancer in a prospective study of French women. *Am J Clin Nutr.* 2008;87(5):1384–1391.

51. Wen W, Shu XO, Li H, et al. Dietary carbohydrates, fiber, and breast cancer risk in Chinese women. *Am J Clin Nutr.* 2009;89 (1):283–289.

52. Sieri S, Krogh V, Ferrari P, et al. Dietary fat and breast cancer risk in the European Prospective Investigation into Cancer and Nutrition. *Am J Clin Nutr.* 2008;88 (5):1304–1312.

53. Thiebaut AC, Chajes V, Gerber M, et al. Dietary intakes of omega-6 and omega-3 polyunsaturated fatty acids and the risk of breast cancer. *Int J Cancer.* 2009;124(4):924–931.

54. Shannon J, King IB, Moshofsky R, et al. Erythrocyte fatty acids and breast cancer risk: a case-control study in Shanghai, China. *Am J Clin Nutr.* 2007;85(4):1090–1097.

55. Taylor EF, Burley VJ, Greenwood DC, Cade JE. Meat consumption and risk of breast cancer in the UK Women's Cohort Study. *Br J Cancer.* 2007;96 (7):1139–1146.

56. McCullough ML, Rodriguez C, Diver WR, Feigelson HS, Stevens VL. Dairy, calcium, and vitamin D intake and postmenopausal breast cancer risk in the Cancer Prevention Study II Nutrition Cohort. *Cancer Epidemiol Biomarkers Prev.* 2005;14 (12):2898–2904.

57. Lin J, Manson JE, Lee IM, Cook NR, Buring JE, Zhang SM. Intakes of calcium and vitamin D and breast cancer risk in women. *Arch Intern Med.* 2007;167 (10):1050–1059.

58. Blackmore KM, Lesosky M, Barnett H, et al. Vitamin D from dietary intake and sunlight exposure and the risk of hormone-receptor-defined breast cancer. *Am J Epidemiol.* 2008;168(8):915–924.

59. Güth U, Huang DJ, Huber M, et al. Tumor size and detection in breast cancer: self-examination and clinical breast examination are at their limit. *Cancer Detect Prev.* 2008;32 (3):224–228.

60. Weiss NS. Breast cancer mortality in relation to clinical breast examination and breast self-examination. *Breast J.* 2003; 9(suppl 2):S86–S89.

61. Merrill RM, Weed DL, Feuer EJ. The lifetime risk of developing prostate cancer in white and black men. *Cancer Epidemiol Biomarkers Prev.* 1997;6(10):763–768.

62. Prostate Cancer Foundation. http://www.prostatecancerfoundation.org/site/c.itIWK2OSG/b.70619/k.446E/Risk_Factors.htm; Accessed 16.02.09.

63. National Cancer Institute. *Genetic Testing for Prostate Cancer.* http://www.cancer.gov/cancertopics/pdq/genetics/prostate/healthprofessional; Accessed 16.02.09.

64. Augustsson K, Michaud DS, Rimm EB, Leitzmann MF, Stampfer MJ. A prospective study of intake of fish and marine fatty acids and prostate cancer. *Cancer Epidemiol Biomarkers Prev.* 2003;12(1):64–67.

65. Neuhouser ML, Barnett MJ, Kristal AR, et al. (n-6) PUFA increase and dairy foods decrease prostate cancer risk in heavy smokers. *J Nutr.* 2007;137 (7):1821–1827.

66. Mitrou PN, Albanes D, Weinstein SJ, et al. A prospective study of dietary calcium, dairy products and prostate cancer risk (Finland). *Int J Cancer.* 2007;120 (11):2466–2473.

67. Chavarro JE, Stampfer MJ, Campos H, et al. A prospective study of trans-fatty acid levels in blood and risk of prostate cancer. *Cancer Epidemiol Biomarkers Prev.* 2008;17(1):95–101.

68. Peters U, Leitzmann MF, Chatterjee N, Wang Y, Albanes D. Serum lycopene, other carotenoids, and prostate cancer risk: a nested

case-control study in the prostate, lung, colorectal, and ovarian cancer screening trial. *Cancer Epidemiol Biomarkers Prev.* 2007;16 (5):962–968.

69. Key TJ, Appleby PN, Allen NE, et al. Plasma carotenoids, retinol, and tocopherols and the risk of prostate cancer in the European Prospective Investigation into Cancer and Nutrition study. *Am J Clin Nutr.* 2007;86(3):672–681.

70. Wu K, Erdman Jr JW, Schwartz SJ, et al. Plasma and dietary carotenoids, and the risk of prostate cancer: a nested case-control study. *Cancer Epidemiol Biomarkers Prev.* 2004;13(2):260–269.

71. Kirsh VA, Peters U, Mayne ST, et al. Prospective study of fruit and vegetable intake and risk of prostate cancer. *J Natl Cancer Inst.* 2007;99 (15):1200–1209.

72. Canene-Adams K, Lindshield BL, Jeffery EH, Erdman JW. Combinations of tomato and broccoli enhance antitumor activity in Dunning R3327-H prostate adenocarcinomas. *Cancer Res.* 2007;67:836–843.

73. Young Hong M, Seeram NP, Heber D. Pomegranate polyphenols down-regulate expression of androgen-synthesizing genes in human prostate cancer cells overexpressing the androgen receptor. *J Nutr Biochem.* 2008;19(12):848–855.

74. Nagata Y, Sonoda T, Mori M, et al. Dietary isoflavones may protect against prostate cancer in Japanese men. *J Nutr.* 2007;137 (8):1974–1979.

75. Pierotti B, Altieri A, Talamini R, et al. Lifetime physical activity and prostate cancer risk. *Int J Cancer.* 2005;114(4):639–642.

76. Crespo CJ, Garcia-Palmieri MR, Smit E, et al. Physical activity and prostate cancer mortality in Puerto Rican men. *J Phys Act Health.* 2008;5(6):918–929.

77. National Cancer Institute. *Cervical Cancer Prevention.* http://www.cancer.gov/cancertopics/pdq/prevention/cervical/healthprofessional; Accessed 16.02.09.

78. Growdon WB, Del Carmen M. Human papillomavirus-related gynecologic neoplasms: screening and prevention. *Rev Obstet Gynecol.* 2008;1(4):154–161.

79. Lowy DR, Solomon D, Hildesheim A, Schiller JT, Schiffman M. Human papillomavirus infection and the primary and secondary prevention of cervical cancer. *Cancer.* 2008;113 (7 suppl):1980–1993.

80. Piyathilake CJ, Macaluso M, Brill I, Heimburger DC, Partridge EE. Lower red blood cell folate enhances the HPV-16-associated risk of cervical intraepithelial neoplasia. *Nutrition.* 2007;23 (3):203–210.

81. Ghosh C, Baker A, Moysich KB, et al. Dietary intakes of selected nutrients and food groups and risk of cervical cancer. *Nutr Cancer.* 2008;60(3):331–341.

82. CDC. *Skin Cancer.* http://www.cdc.gov/cancer/skin/; Accessed 18.02.09.

83. Grant WB. The effect of solar UVB doses and vitamin D production, skin cancer action spectra, and smoking in explaining links between skin cancers and solid tumours. *Eur J Cancer.* 2008;44(1):12–15.

84. Kennedy C, Bajdik CD, Willemze R, De Gruijl FR, Bouwes Bavinck JN. Leiden Skin Cancer Study. The influence of painful sunburns and lifetime sun exposure on the risk of actinic keratoses, seborrheic warts, melanocytic nevi, atypical nevi, and skin cancer. *J Invest Dermatol.* 2003;120 (6):1087–1093.

85. The Skin Cancer Foundation. http://www.skincancer.org/skin-types-and-at-risk-groups.html ; Accessed 19.02.09.

86. O'Riordan DL, Steffen AD, Lunde KB, Gies P. A day at the beach while on tropical vacation: sun protection practices in a high-risk setting for UV radiation exposure. *Arch Dermatol.* 2008;144 (11):1449–1455.

87. Moehrle M. Outdoor sports and skin cancer. *Clin Dermatol.* 2008;26 (1):12–15.

88. Saladi RN, Persaud AN. The causes of skin cancer: a comprehensive review. *Drugs Today (Barc).* 2005;41(1):37–53.

89. Gandini S, Raimondi S, Gnagnarella P, Doré JF, Maisonneuve P, Testori A. Vitamin D and skin cancer: a meta-analysis. *Eur J Cancer.* 2009;45 (4):634–641.

90. Hintzpeter B, Mensink GB, Thierfelder W, et al. Vitamin D status and health correlates among German adults. *Eur J Clin Nutr.* 2008;62(9):1079–1089.

91. Reichow AW, Citek K, Edlich RF. Ultraviolet and short wavelength visible light exposure: why ultraviolet protection alone is not adequate. *J Long Term Eff Med Implants.* 2006;16(4):315–325.

92. Situm M, Buljan M, Bulat V, Lugović Mihić L, Bolanca Z, Simić D. The role of UV radiation in the development of basal cell carcinoma. *Coll Antropol.* 2008;32 (suppl 2):167–170.

93. Buljan M, Bulat V, Situm M, Mihić LL, Stanić-Duktaj S. Variations in clinical presentation of basal cell carcinoma. *Acta Clin Croat.* 2008;47(1):25–30.

94. Fuchs A, Marmur E. The kinetics of skin cancer: progression of actinic keratosis to squamous cell carcinoma. *Dermatol Surg.* 2007; 33(9):1099–1101.

95. Soyer HP, Argenziano G, Zalaudek I, et al. Three-point checklist of dermoscopy. A new screening method for early detection of melanoma. *Dermatology.* 2004;208(1):27–31.

96. Rass K, Hassel JC. Chemotherapeutics, chemoresistance and the management of melanoma. *G Ital Dermatol Venereol.* 2009;144 (1):61–78.

97. Sartorelli DS, Franco LJ, Cardoso MA. High intake of fruits and vegetables predicts weight loss in Brazilian overweight adults. *Nutr Res.* 2008;28(4):233–238.

98. Uauy R, Solomons N. Diet, nutrition, and the life-course approach to cancer prevention. *J Nutr.* 2005;135:2934S–2945S.

99. Key TJ, Schatzkin A, Willett WC, Allen NE, Spencer EA, Travis RC. Diet, nutrition and the prevention of cancer. *Public Health Nutr.* 2004;7(1A):187–200.

100. Ames BN, Gold LS. Environmental pollution, pesticides, and the prevention of cancer: misconceptions. *FASEB J.* 1997;11(13):1041–1052.

101. Divisi D, Di Tommaso S, Salvemini S, Garramone M, Crisci R. Diet and cancer. *Acta Biomed Ateneo Parmense.* 2006; 77(2):118–123.

Index

ELSEVIER CD-ROM LICENCE AGREEMENT

PLEASE READ THE FOLLOWING AGREEMENT CAREFULLY BEFORE USING THIS PRODUCT. THIS PRODUCT IS LICENSED UNDER THE TERMS CONTAINED IN THIS LICENCE AGREEMENT ('Agreement'). BY USING THIS PRODUCT, YOU, AN INDIVIDUAL OR ENTITY INCLUDING EMPLOYEES, AGENTS AND REPRESENTATIVES ('You' or 'Your'), ACKNOWLEDGE THAT YOU HAVE READ THIS AGREEMENT, THAT YOU UNDERSTAND IT, AND THAT YOU AGREE TO BE BOUND BY THE TERMS AND CONDITIONS OF THIS AGREEMENT. ELSEVIER LIMITED ('Elsevier') EXPRESSLY DOES NOT AGREE TO LICENSE THIS PRODUCT TO YOU UNLESS YOU ASSENT TO THIS AGREEMENT. IF YOU DO NOT AGREE WITH ANY OF THE FOLLOWING TERMS, YOU MAY, WITHIN THIRTY (30) DAYS AFTER YOUR RECEIPT OF THIS PRODUCT RETURN THE UNUSED PRODUCT AND ALL ACCOMPANYING DOCUMENTATION TO ELSEVIER FOR A FULL REFUND.

DEFINITIONS As used in this Agreement, these terms shall have the following meanings:

'Proprietary Material' means the valuable and proprietary information content of this Product including without limitation all indexes and graphic materials and software used to access, index, search and retrieve the information content from this Product developed or licensed by Elsevier and/or its affiliates, suppliers and licensors.

'Product' means the copy of the Proprietary Material and any other material delivered on CD-ROM and any other human-readable or machine-readable materials enclosed with this Agreement, including without limitation documentation relating to the same.

OWNERSHIP This Product has been supplied by and is proprietary to Elsevier and/or its affiliates, suppliers and licensors. The copyright in the Product belongs to Elsevier and/or its affiliates, suppliers and licensors and is protected by the copyright, trademark, trade secret and other intellectual property laws of the United Kingdom and international treaty provisions, including without limitation the Universal Copyright Convention and the Berne Copyright Convention. You have no ownership rights in this Product. Except as expressly set forth herein, no part of this Product, including without limitation the Proprietary Material, may be modified, copied or distributed in hardcopy or machine-readable form without prior written consent from Elsevier. All rights not expressly granted to You herein are expressly reserved. Any other use of this Product by any person or entity is strictly prohibited and a violation of this Agreement.

SCOPE OF RIGHTS LICENSED (PERMITTED USES) Elsevier is granting to You a limited, non-exclusive, non-transferable licence to use this Product in accordance with the terms of this Agreement. You may use or provide access to this Product on a single computer or terminal physically located at Your premises and in a secure network or move this Product to and use it on another single computer or terminal at the same location for personal use only, but under no circumstances may You use or provide access to any part or parts of this Product on more than one computer or terminal simultaneously.

You shall not (a) copy, download, or otherwise reproduce the Product or any part(s) thereof in any medium, including, without limitation, online transmissions, local area networks, wide area networks, intranets, extranets and the Internet, or in any way, in whole or in part, except for printing out or downloading nonsubstantial portions of the text and images in the Product for Your own personal use; (b) alter, modify, or adapt the Product or any part(s) thereof, including but not limited to decompiling, disassembling, reverse engineering, or creating derivative works, without the prior written approval of Elsevier; (c) sell, license or otherwise distribute to third parties the Product or any part(s) thereof; or (d) alter, remove, obscure or obstruct the display of any copyright, trademark or other proprietary notice on or in the Product or on any printout or download of portions of the Proprietary Materials.

RESTRICTIONS ON TRANSFER This Licence is personal to You, and neither Your rights hereunder nor the tangible embodiments of this Product, including without limitation the Proprietary Material, may be sold, assigned, transferred or sublicensed to any other person, including without limitation by operation of law, without the prior written consent of Elsevier. Any purported sale, assignment, transfer or sublicense without the prior written consent of Elsevier will be void and will automatically terminate the Licence granted hereunder.

TERM This Agreement will remain in effect until terminated pursuant to the terms of this Agreement. You may terminate this Agreement at any time by removing from Your system and destroying the Product and any copies of the Proprietary Material. Unauthorized copying of the Product, including without limitation, the Proprietary Material and documentation, or otherwise failing to comply with the terms and conditions of this Agreement shall result in automatic termination of this licence and will make available to Elsevier legal remedies. Upon termination of this Agreement, the licence granted herein will terminate and You must immediately destroy the Product and all copies of the Product and of the Proprietary Material, together with any and all accompanying documentation. All provisions relating to proprietary rights shall survive termination of this Agreement.

LIMITED WARRANTY AND LIMITATION OF LIABILITY Elsevier warrants that the software embodied in this Product will perform in substantial compliance with the documentation supplied in this Product, unless the performance problems are the result of hardware failure or improper use. If You report a significant defect in performance in writing to Elsevier within ninety (90) calendar days of your having purchased the Product, and Elsevier is not able to correct same within sixty (60) days after its receipt of Your notification, You may return this Product, including all copies and documentation, to Elsevier and Elsevier will refund Your money. In order to apply for a refund on your purchased Product, please contact the return address on the invoice to obtain the refund request form ('Refund Request Form'), and either fax or mail your signed request and your proof of purchase to the address indicated on the Refund Request Form. Incomplete forms will not be processed. Defined terms in the Refund Request Form shall have the same meaning as in this Agreement.

YOU UNDERSTAND THAT, EXCEPT FOR THE LIMITED WARRANTY RECITED ABOVE, ELSEVIER, ITS AFFILIATES, LICENSORS, THIRD PARTY SUPPLIERS AND AGENTS (TOGETHER 'THE SUPPLIERS') MAKE NO REPRESENTATIONS OR WARRANTIES, WITH RESPECT TO THE PRODUCT, INCLUDING, WITHOUT LIMITATION THE PROPRIETARY MATERIAL. ALL OTHER REPRESENTATIONS, WARRANTIES, CONDITIONS OR OTHER TERMS, WHETHER EXPRESS OR IMPLIED BY STATUTE OR COMMON LAW, ARE HEREBY EXCLUDED TO THE FULLEST EXTENT PERMITTED BY LAW.

IN PARTICULAR BUT WITHOUT LIMITATION TO THE FOREGOING NONE OF THE SUPPLIERS MAKE ANY REPRESENTATIONS OR WARRANTIES (WHETHER EXPRESS OR IMPLIED) REGARDING THE PERFORMANCE OF YOUR PAD, NETWORK OR COMPUTER SYSTEM WHEN USED IN CONJUNCTION WITH THE PRODUCT, NOR THAT THE PRODUCT WILL MEET YOUR REQUIREMENTS OR THAT ITS OPERATION WILL BE UNINTERRUPTED OR ERROR-FREE.

EXCEPT IN RESPECT OF DEATH OR PERSONAL INJURY CAUSED BY THE SUPPLIERS' NEGLIGENCE AND TO THE FULLEST EXTENT PERMITTED BY LAW, IN NO EVENT (AND REGARDLESS OF WHETHER SUCH DAMAGES ARE FORESEEABLE AND OF WHETHER SUCH LIABILITY IS BASED IN TORT, CONTRACT OR OTHERWISE) WILL ANY OF THE SUPPLIERS BE LIABLE TO YOU FOR ANY DAMAGES (INCLUDING, WITHOUT LIMITATION, ANY LOST PROFITS, LOST SAVINGS OR OTHER SPECIAL, INDIRECT, INCIDENTAL OR CONSEQUENTIAL DAMAGES ARISING OUT OF OR RESULTING FROM: (I) YOUR USE OF, OR INABILITY TO USE, THE PRODUCT; (II) DATA LOSS OR CORRUPTION; AND/OR (III) ERRORS OR OMISSIONS IN THE PROPRIETARY MATERIAL.

IF THE FOREGOING LIMITATION IS HELD TO BE UNENFORCEABLE, OUR MAXIMUM LIABILITY TO YOU IN RESPECT THEREOF SHALL NOT EXCEED THE AMOUNT OF THE LICENCE FEE PAID BY YOU FOR THE PRODUCT. THE REMEDIES AVAILABLE TO YOU AGAINST ELSEVIER AND THE LICENSORS OF MATERIALS INCLUDED IN THE PRODUCT ARE EXCLUSIVE.

If the information provided in the Product contains medical or health sciences information, it is intended for professional use within the medical field. Information about medical treatment or drug dosages is intended strictly for professional use, and because of rapid advances in the medical sciences, independent verification of diagnosis and drug dosages should be made.

The provisions of this Agreement shall be severable, and in the event that any provision of this Agreement is found to be legally unenforceable, such unenforceability shall not prevent the enforcement or any other provision of this Agreement.

GOVERNING LAW This Agreement shall be governed by the laws of England and Wales. In any dispute arising out of this Agreement, you and Elsevier each consent to the exclusive personal jurisdiction and venue in the courts of England and Wales.